NURSING RESEARCH

Methods and Critical Appraisal for Evidence-Based Practice

7th Edition

NURSING RESEARCH

Methods and Critical Appraisal for Evidence-Based Practice

Geri LoBiondo-Wood, PhD, RN, FAAN

Director of Nursing Research and Evidence-Based Practice, Planning and Development
The University of Texas
MD Anderson Cancer Center
Houston, Texas

Adjunct Associate Professor
University of Texas Health Sciences Center
School of Nursing
Nursing Systems and Technology
Houston, Texas

Judith Haber, PhD, APRN, BC, FAAN

The Ursula Springer Leadership Professor in Nursing
Associate Dean for Graduate Programs
New York University
College of Nursing
New York, New York

MOSBY

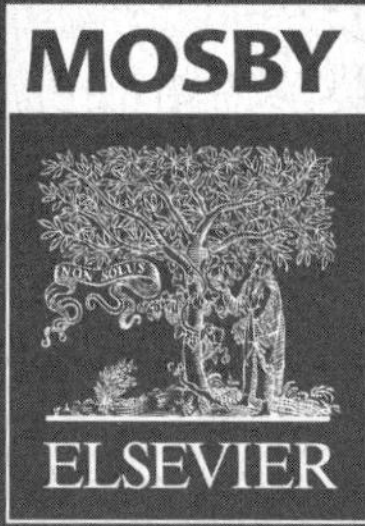

ELSEVIER

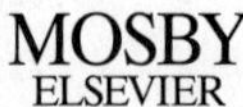

3251 Riverport Lane
St. Louis, Missouri 63043

NURSING RESEARCH: METHODS AND CRITICAL APPRAISAL FOR EVIDENCE-BASED PRACTICE, SEVENTH EDITION 978-0-323-05743-1

International Standard Book Number 978-0-323-05743-1

Managing Editor: Maureen Iannuzzi
Associate Developmental Editor: Mary Ann Zimmerman
Editorial Assistant: Julia Curcio
Publishing Services Manager: Jeffrey Patterson
Project Manager: Mary G. Stueck
Design Direction: Teresa McBryan

Printed in the United States of America

Last digit is the print number: 9 8 7 6 5 4 3 2

About the Authors

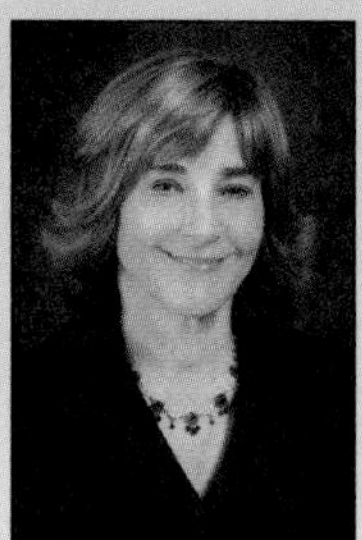

Geri LoBiondo-Wood, PhD, RN, FAAN, is the Director of Nursing Research and Evidence-Based Practice Planning and Development at the MD Anderson Cancer Center, Houston, Texas and an Adjunct Associate Professor at the University of Texas Health Sciences Center at Houston, School of Nursing (UTHSC-Houston). She received her Diploma in nursing at St. Mary's Hospital School of Nursing in Rochester, New York, her Bachelor's and Master's degrees from the University of Rochester, and her PhD in Nursing Theory and Research from New York University. At MD Anderson Cancer Center, Dr. LoBiondo-Wood developed and implemented the Evidence-Based Resource Unit Nurse (EB-RUN) Program, which is a hospital-wide program that involves all levels of nurses in the application of research evidence to practice. She also has implemented a mentorship program for nurses wishing to conduct research. Dr. LoBiondo-Wood also teaches research and evidence-based practice principles to undergraduate, graduate, doctoral, and doctor of nursing practice students at UTHSC-Houston School of Nursing. She has extensive experience guiding nurses and other health care professionals in the development and utilization of research in clinical practice. Dr. LoBiondo-Wood is currently a member of the Editorial Board of *Progress in Transplantation* and a reviewer for *Nursing Research* and *Nephrology Nursing Journal.* Her research and publications focus on chronic illness and the impact of solid organ transplantation on pediatric or adult recipients and their families throughout the transplant process. At MD Anderson her research focuses on symptom clusters in adult cancer patients.

Dr. LoBiondo-Wood has been active locally and nationally in many professional organizations, including the Southern Nursing Research Society, the Midwest Nursing Research Society, and the North American Transplant Coordinators Organization. She has received local and national awards for teaching and contributions to nursing. In 1997, she received the Distinguished Alumnus Award from New York University, Division of Nursing Alumni Association. In 2001 she was inducted as a Fellow of the American Academy of Nursing, and in 2007 to The University of Texas Academy of Health Science Education.

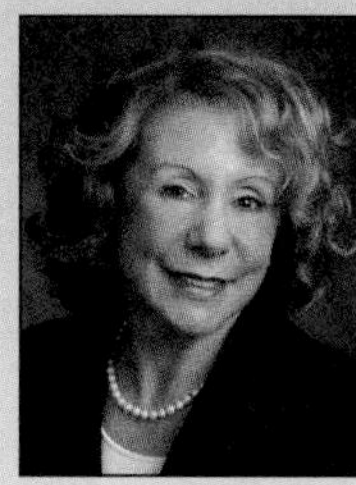

Judith Haber, PhD, APRN, BC, FAAN, is the Ursula Springer Leadership Professor in Nursing and Associate Dean for Graduate Programs in the College of Nursing at New York University. She received her undergraduate nursing education at Adelphi University in New York, and she holds a Master's degree in Adult Psychiatric–Mental Health Nursing and a PhD in Nursing Theory and Research from New York University. Dr. Haber is internationally recognized as a clinician and educator in psychiatric-mental health nursing. She has extensive clinical experience in psychiatric nursing, having been an advanced practice psychiatric nurse in private practice for over 30 years, specializing in treatment of families coping with the psychosocial sequelae of acute and chronic catastrophic illness. Dr. Haber is currently on the Editorial Board of the *Journal of the American Psychiatric Nurses Association (JAPNA).* Her areas of research involvement include tool development, particularly in the area of family functioning. She is internationally known for developing the Haber Level of Differentiation of Self Scale. Another program of research addresses physical and psychosocial adjustment to illness, focusing specifically on women with breast cancer and their partners. Based on this research, she and Dr. Carol Hoskins have written and produced an award-winning series of evidence-based psychoeducational videotapes, *Journey to Recovery: For Women with Breast Cancer and Their Partners,* which has been tested in a randomized clinical trial funded by the National Cancer Institute.

Dr. Haber has been active locally and nationally in many professional organizations, including the American Nurses Association, American Psychiatric Nurses Association, and the American Academy of Nursing. She has received numerous local, state, and national awards for public policy, clinical practice, and research, including the APNA Psychiatric Nurse of the Year Award in 1998 and 2005, the APNA Outstanding Research Award in 2005, and the 2007 NYU College of Nursing Distinguished Alumnus Award. In 1993, she was inducted as a Fellow of the American Academy of Nursing.

Contributors

Susan Adams, PhD, RN
Associate Director
Research Translation and Dissemination Core
Gerontological Nursing Interventions Research Center
College of Nursing
University of Iowa;
Director, National Nursing Practice Network
Iowa City, Iowa

Julie Barroso, PhD, ANP, APRN, BC, FAAN
Associate Professor and Specialty Director, Adult Nurse Practitioner Program
Research Development Coordinator, Office of Research Affairs
Duke University School of Nursing
Durham, North Carolina

Nancy Bergstrom, RN, PhD, FAAN
Theodore J. and Mary E. Trumble Professor of Aging Research
Director, Center on Aging
University of Texas Health Science Center
Houston, Texas

Carol Bova, PhD, RN, ANP
Associate Professor of Nursing and Medicine
Graduate School of Nursing
University of Massachusetts, Worcester
Worcester, Massachusetts

Stephanie Fulton, MSIS
Assistant Library Director
Research Medical Library
The University of Texas
MD Anderson Cancer Center
Houston, Texas

Susan Gennaro, RN, DSN, FAAN
Dean and Professor
Boston College
Chestnut Hill, Massachusetts

Carl A. Kirton, DNP, ANP-BC, ACRN
Vice President, Nursing and Nurse Practitioner
North General Hospital;
Adjunct Clinical Associate Professor
College of Nursing
New York University
New York, New York

Nancy E. Kline, PhD, RN, CPNP, FAAN
Director, Center for Evidence-Based Practice and Research
Department of Nursing
Memorial Sloan-Kettering Cancer Center
New York, New York

Barbara Krainovich-Miller, EdD, APRN, BC, ANEF, FAAN
Clinical Professor
College of Nursing
New York University
New York, New York

Marianne T. Marcus, EdD, RN, FAAN
John P. McGovern Professor in Addiction Nursing
Director
Center for Substance Abuse Education
Prevention and Research
Health Science Center School of Nursing
University of Texas–Houston
Houston, Texas

Helen J. Streubert, EdD, RN, CNE, ANEF
Vice President of Academic Affairs
Our Lady of the Lake University
San Antonio, Texas

Susan Sullivan-Bolyai, DNSc, CNS, RN
Associate Professor
Graduate School of Nursing and Department of Pediatrics
University of Massachusetts, Worcester
Worcester, Massachusetts

Kristen M. Swanson, RN, PhD, FAAN
Dean and Alumni Distinguished Professor
School of Nursing
University of North Carolina at Chapel Hill
Chapel Hill, North Carolina

Marita Titler, PhD, RN, FAAN
Professor of Nursing
Rhetaugh Dumas Endowed Chair
Associate Dean of Practice and Clinical Scholarship Development
University of Michigan School of Nursing
Ann Arbor, Michigan

Reviewers

Thomas L. Christenbery, PhD, RN
School of Nursing
Vanderbilt University
Nashville, Tennessee

Barbara Ferguson, RN, MSN, MHA, MBA
Queens University
Charlotte, North Carolina

Betsy Frank, RN, PhD, ANEF
College of Nursing
Indiana State University
Terre Haute, Indiana

Mary Tod Gray, PhD, RN
East Stroudsburg University
East Stroudsburg, Pennsylvania

JoAnne D. Joyner, PhD, PMHCNS-BC
University of the District of Columbia
Washington, DC

Sharon Kitchie, PhD, RN, ACNS-BC
Upstate Medical University
Syracuse, New York

Madelaine Lawrence, PhD, RN
Queens University
Charlotte, North Carolina

Joanne E. Layton, MS, RN, APN
University of Rochester School of Nursing
Rochester, New York

Ann Marie P. Mauro, PhD, RN, CNL
Seton Hall University
South Orange, New Jersey

Christina B. McSherry, RN, MA, PhD
William Paterson University
Wayne, New Jersey

Jacqueline M. O'Brien, MSN, RN, CIC
UPMC-St. Margaret
Pittsburgh, Pennsylvania

Sue Ellen Odom, RN, DSN
Clayton State University
Monow, Georgia

Teresa M. O'Neill, RNS, APRN, PhD
Our Lady of Holy Cross College
New Orleans, Louisiana

Sharon Souter, RN, PhD, CNE
University of Mary Hardin-Baylor
Belton, Texas

Shirley P. Toney, RN, PhD
Gardner-Webb University
Boiling Springs, North Carolina

Molly J. Walker, PhD, RN, CNS, CNE
Angelo State University
San Angelo, Texas

Fatma Youssef, DNSc, MPH, RN
Marymount University
Arlington, Virginia

To the Instructor

The foundation of the seventh edition of *Nursing Research: Methods and Critical Appraisal for Evidence-Based Practice* continues to be the belief that nursing research is integral to all levels of nursing education and practice. Over the past 22 years since the first edition of this textbook, we have seen the depth and breadth of nursing research grow, with more nurses conducting research and using research evidence to shape clinical practice, education, administration, and health policy.

The Institute of Medicine has challenged all health professionals to provide care based on the best available scientific evidence. This is an exciting challenge to meet. Nurses are using the best available evidence, combined with their clinical judgment and patient preferences to influence the nature and direction of health care delivery and document outcomes related to the quality and cost-effectiveness of patient care. As nurses continue to develop a unique body of nursing knowledge through research, decisions about clinical nursing practice will be increasingly evidence based.

As editors, we believe that all nurses need not only to understand the research process but also to know how to critically read, evaluate, and apply research findings in practice. We realize that understanding research, as a component of evidence-based practice, is a challenge for every student, but we believe that the challenge can be accomplished in a stimulating, lively, and learner-friendly manner.

Consistent with this perspective is a commitment to advancing implementation of the evidence-based practice paradigm. Understanding and applying nursing research must be an integral dimension of baccalaureate education, evident not only in the undergraduate nursing research course but also threaded throughout the curriculum. The research role of baccalaureate graduates calls for evidence-based practice competencies; central to this are critical appraisal skills—that is, nurses should be competent research consumers.

Preparing students for this role involves developing their critical thinking and reading skills, thereby enhancing their understanding of the research process, their appreciation of the role of the critiquer, and their ability to actually critically appraise research. An undergraduate course in nursing research should develop this basic level of competence, which is an essential requirement if students are to engage in evidence-informed clinical decision making and practice. This is in contrast to a graduate-level research course in which the emphasis is on carrying out research, as well as understanding and appraising it.

The primary audience for this textbook remains undergraduate students who are learning the steps of the research process, as well as how to develop clinical questions, critically appraise published research literature, and use research findings to inform evidence-based clinical practice. This book is also a valuable resource for students at the master's and doctoral levels who want a concise review of the basic steps of the research process, the critical appraisal process, as well as the principles and tools for evidence-based practice. This text is also a key resource for doctor of nursing practice (DNP) students who are preparing to be experts at leading evidence-based initiatives in clinical settings. Furthermore, it is an important resource for practicing nurses who strive to use research evidence as the basis for clinical decision making and development of evidence-based policies, protocols, and standards, rather than rely on tradition, authority, or trial and error. It is also an important resource for nurses who collaborate with nurse-scientists in the conduct of clinical research and evidence-based practice.

Building on the success of the sixth edition, we maintain our commitment to introduce evidence-based practice and research principles to baccalaureate students, thereby providing a cutting-edge, research consumer foundation for their clinical practice. *Nursing Research: Methods and Critical Appraisal for Evidence-Based Practice* prepares nursing students and practicing nurses to become knowledgeable nursing research consumers by doing the following:

- Addressing the evidence-based practice role of the nurse, thereby embedding evidence-based competence in the clinical practice of every baccalaureate graduate.
- Demystifying research, which is sometimes viewed as a complex process.
- Using an evidence-based approach to teaching the fundamentals of the research process.
- Teaching the critical appraisal process in a user-friendly, but logical and systematic, progression.
- Promoting a lively spirit of inquiry that develops critical thinking and critical reading skills, facilitating mastery of the critical appraisal process.
- Developing information literacy, searching, and evidence-based practice competencies that prepare students and nurses to effectively locate and evaluate the best available research evidence.
- Elevating the critical appraisal process and research consumership to a position of importance comparable to that of producing research. Before students become research producers, they must become knowledgeable research consumers.
- Emphasizing the role of evidence-based practice as the basis for informing clinical decision making and nursing interventions that support nursing practice, demonstrating quality and cost-effective outcomes of nursing care delivery.
- Presenting numerous examples of recently published research studies that illustrate and highlight each research concept in a manner that brings abstract ideas to life for students new to the research and critical appraisal process. These examples are a critical link for reinforcement of evidence-based concepts and the related research and critiquing process.
- Showcasing, in **Research Vignettes,** the work of renowned nurse researchers whose careers exemplify the links among research, education, and practice.
- Providing numerous pedagogical chapter features, including **Learning Outcomes, Key Terms, Key Points,** new **Critical Thinking Challenges, Helpful Hints, Evidence-Based Practice Tips,** revised **Critical Thinking Decision Paths,** as well as numerous tables, boxes, and figures. At the end of each chapter that presents a step of the research process we feature a revised section titled **Appraising the Evidence,** which reviews how each step of the research process should be evaluated from a consumer's perspective, and is accompanied by an updated **Critiquing Criteria** box.
- Offering an **Evolve site** with interactive Review Questions that provide chapter-by-chapter review in a format consistent with that of the NCLEX® Examination.
- Providing a **Study Guide** that promotes active learning and assimilation of nursing research content.
- Presenting a free **Evolve Resources for Instructors** that includes a test bank, instructor's manual, PowerPoint slides, audience response system questions, and an image collection. There also are Evolve resources for both the student and faculty that include **Critiquing Exercises** based on published studies with multiple-choice questions for additional practice in reviewing and appraising, quizzes, and a research article library for additional practice in reviewing and critiquing—as well as Content Updates. A Nursing Research Online course is also available to accompany this textbook.
- The seventh edition of *Nursing Research: Methods and Critical Appraisal for Evidence-Based Practice* is organized into four parts. Each part is preceded by an introductory section and opens with an exciting "Research Vignette" by a renowned nurse researcher.
- **Part I, Overview of Research and Evidence-Based Practice,** contains three chapters: Chapter 1, "Integrating the Processes of Research and Evidence-Based Practice," provides an excellent

overview of research and evidence-based practice processes that shape clinical practice. The chapter speaks directly to students and highlights critical thinking and critical reading concepts and strategies, thereby facilitating student understanding of the research process and its relationship to the critical appraisal process. The chapter introduces a model evidence hierarchy that is used throughout the text. The style and content of this chapter are designed to make subsequent chapters more user-friendly. The next two chapters address foundational components of the research process. Chapter 2, "Research Questions, Hypotheses, and Clinical Questions," focuses on how research questions, hypotheses, and evidence-based practice (EBP) questions are derived, operationalized, and critically appraised. Numerous clinical examples illustrating different types of research questions and hypotheses maximize student understanding. Students are also taught how to develop clinical questions that are used to guide evidence-based inquiry. Chapter 3, "Gathering and Appraising the Literature," showcases cutting-edge information literacy content, providing students and nurses with the tools necessary to effectively search, retrieve, manage, and evaluate research studies and their findings. This chapter also develops research consumer competencies that prepare students and nurses to critically read, understand, and appraise a study's literature review and framework.

- **Part II, Processes and Evidence Related to Qualitative Research,** contains three interrelated qualitative research chapters. Chapter 4, "Introduction to Qualitative Research," provides a framework for understanding qualitative research designs and literature as well as the significant contribution of qualitative research to evidence-based practice. Chapter 5, "Qualitative Approaches to Research," presents, illustrates, and showcases major qualitative methods using examples from the literature as exemplars. This chapter highlights the questions most appropriately answered using qualitative methods. Chapter 6, "Appraising Qualitative Research," synthesizes essential components of and criteria for critiquing qualitative research reports.
- **Part III, Processes and Evidence Related to Quantitative Research,** contains Chapters 7 to 16. This group of chapters delineates the essential steps of the quantitative research process, with published clinical research studies used to illustrate each step. Links between the steps and their relationship to the total research process are examined. These chapters make the case for linking an evidence-based approach with essential steps of the research process by teaching students how to critically appraise the strengths and weaknesses of each step of the research process and then weave them together in a synthesized critique of a research study. The steps of the quantitative research process, evidence-based concepts, and critical appraisal criteria are synthesized in Chapter 16.
- **Part IV, Application of Research and Evidence-Based Practice,** contains Chapters 17 and 18, which present a unique showcase of evidence-based practice models and tools to use in effectively solving patient problems. Chapter 17, "Developing an Evidence-Based Practice," provides a dynamic review of EBP models. These models can be applied, step by step, at the organizational or individual patient level, as frameworks for implementing and evaluating the outcomes of evidence-informed health care. Chapter 18, "Tools for Applying Evidence to Practice," is a vibrant, user-friendly, evidence-based toolkit with "real-life" exemplars that capture the totality of implementing high-quality evidence-informed nursing care. It "walks" students and practicing nurses through clinical scenarios and challenges them to consider the relevant EBP "tools" they would use to develop and answer the clinical questions that emerge from clinical situations. These chapters provide an inspirational conclusion to this text that we hope will motivate students and practicing nurses to advance their EBP knowledge base and clinical competence, thereby preparing to make an important contribution to improving health care delivery.

Stimulating critical thinking is a core value of this text. Innovative chapter features such as Critical Thinking Decision Paths, Evidence-Based Practice Tips,

Helpful Hints, and Critical Thinking Challenges enhance critical thinking and promote the development of evidence-based decision making skills. Consistent with previous editions, we promote critical thinking by including sections now called "Appraising the Evidence," which describe the critical appraisal process related to the focus of the chapter. Additionally, Critiquing Criteria are included in this section to stimulate a systematic and evaluative approach to reading and understanding qualitative and quantitative research literature and evaluating its strengths and weaknesses. Extensive Internet resources are provided on the accompanying Evolve site that can be used to develop evidence-based knowledge and skills.

The Evolve website that accompanies the seventh edition provides interactive learning activities that promote the development of critical thinking, critical reading, and information literacy skills designed to develop the competencies necessary to produce informed consumers of nursing research. Student resources include Critiquing Exercises, which consist of research articles and corresponding multiple-choice questions that review cross-chapter content to challenge students. Instructor resources are available at a passcode-protected website that gives faculty access to all instructor materials online, including the Instructor's Manual, Image Collection, Lecture Slides, and a Test Bank that allows faculty to create examinations using the ExamView test generator program.

The development and refinement of an evidence-based foundation for clinical nursing practice is an essential priority for the future of professional nursing practice. The seventh edition of *Nursing Research: Methods and Critical Appraisal for Evidence-Based Practice* will help students develop a basic level of competence in understanding the steps of the research process that will enable them to critically analyze research studies, judge their merit, and judiciously apply evidence in clinical practice. To the extent that this goal is accomplished, the next generation of nursing professionals will have a cadre of clinicians who inform their practice using theory and research evidence, combined with their clinical judgment, and specific to the health care needs of patients and their families in health and illness.

Geri LoBiondo-Wood
Geri.L.Wood@uth.tmc.edu
gwood@mdanderson.org

Judith Haber
jh33@nyu.edu

To the Student

We invite you to join us on an exciting nursing research adventure that begins as you turn the first page of the seventh edition of *Nursing Research: Methods and Critical Appraisal for Evidence-Based Practice.* The adventure is one of discovery! You will discover that the nursing research literature sparkles with pride, dedication, and excitement about the research dimension of professional nursing practice. Whether you are a student or a practicing nurse whose goal is to use research evidence as the foundation of your practice, you will discover that nursing research and a commitment to evidence-based practice positions our profession at the forefront of change. You will discover that evidence-based practice is integral to meeting the challenge of providing quality biopsychosocial health care in partnership with patients and their families/significant others, as well as with the communities in which they live. Finally, you will discover the richness in the "Who," "What," "Where," "When," "Why," and "How" of nursing research and evidence-based practice, developing a foundation of knowledge and skills that will equip you for clinical practice and making a significant contribution to quality patient outcomes!

We think you will enjoy reading this text. Your nursing research course will be short but filled with new and challenging learning experiences that will develop your evidence-based practice skills. The seventh edition of *Nursing Research: Methods and Critical Appraisal for Evidence-Based Practice* reflects cutting-edge trends for developing evidence-based nursing practice. The four-part organization and special features in this text are designed to help you develop your critical thinking, critical reading, information literacy, and evidence-based clinical decision making skills, while providing a user-friendly approach to learning that expands your competence to deal with these new and challenging experiences. The companion Study Guide, with its chapter-by-chapter activities, will serve as a self-paced learning tool to reinforce the content of the text. The accompanying Evolve website offers "summative" review material to help you tie the chapter material together and apply it to ten current research articles. You will also be able to access review questions to help you reinforce the concepts discussed throughout the book.

Remember that evidence-based practice skills are used in every clinical setting and can be applied to every patient population or clinical practice issue. Whether your clinical practice involves primary care or specialty care and provides inpatient or outpatient treatment in a hospital, clinic, or home, you will be challenged to apply your evidence-based practice skills and use nursing research as the foundation for your evidence-based practice. The seventh edition of *Nursing Research: Methods and Critical Appraisal for Evidence-Based Practice* will guide you through this exciting adventure, where you will discover your ability to play a vital role in contributing to the building of an evidence-based professional nursing practice.

Geri LoBiondo-Wood
gwood@mdanderson.org

Judith Haber
jh33@nyu.edu

Acknowledgments

No major undertaking is accomplished alone; there are those who contribute directly and those who contribute indirectly to the success of a project. We acknowledge with deep appreciation and our warmest thanks the help and support of the following people:

- Our students, particularly the nursing students at the University of Texas–Houston Health Science Center School of Nursing and the College of Nursing at New York University, whose interest, lively curiosity, and challenging questions sparked ideas for revisions in the seventh edition.
- Our chapter contributors, whose passion for research, expertise, cooperation, commitment, and punctuality made them a joy to have as colleagues.
- Our vignette contributors, whose willingness to share evidence of their research wisdom made a unique and inspirational contribution to this edition.
- Our colleagues, who have taken time out of their busy professional lives to offer feedback and constructive criticism that helped us prepare this seventh edition.
- Our editors, Maureen Iannuzzi, Mary Ann Zimmerman, Mary Stueck, and Julia Curcio, for their willingness to listen to yet another creative idea about teaching research in a meaningful way and for their timely help with manuscript preparation and production.
- Our families: Brian Wood, who now is pursuing his own graduate education, and over the years has sat in on classes, provided commentary, and patiently watched and waited as his mother rewrote each edition, as well as provided love, understanding, and support. Lenny, Andrew, and Abbe, Brett and Meredith Haber and Laurie, Bob, and Mikey, Benjy, and Noah Goldberg for their unending love, faith, understanding, and support throughout what is inevitably a consuming—but exciting—experience.

Geri LoBiondo-Wood

Judith Haber

Contents

PART I

OVERVIEW OF RESEARCH AND EVIDENCE-BASED PRACTICE

RESEARCH VIGNETTE

Braden Scale for Predicting Pressure Sore Risk

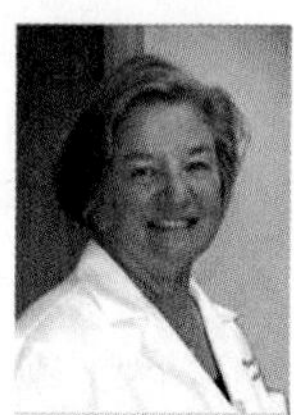

Nancy Bergstrom, PhD, RN, FAAN
Theodore J. and Mary E. Trumble Professor and Director for Aging Research
Director, Center on Aging
University of Texas–Houston Health Science Center
School of Nursing
Houston, Texas

I've always believed that "an ounce of prevention is worth a pound of cure." This philosophy is practical as it saves trouble/grief and expense. In my master's program in medical-surgical nursing at Loma Linda University, I focused on individuals with neurological problems (from multiple sclerosis to head trauma) and with recovery and rehabilitation concerns. Mostly, when working with individuals during acute care, I looked for ways to prevent complications that would prolong rehabilitation, such as pressure ulcers, contractures, footdrop, and more. I even worried about prevention of urinary retention following surgery, since catheterization was known to lead to bladder infections. My thesis involved using principles of neuromuscular facilitation to stimulate voiding postoperatively, and in 1969, this work resulted in my first publication. Little did I know that this early interest in prevention would become a lifelong focus.

While an assistant professor at Loma Linda University, I learned of a program (sponsored by the Western Interstate Commission for Higher Education) to stimulate faculty research. The program focused on bringing people together to collaborate on research. I found common ground with a group studying tube feeding, and our goal was to improve the safety and success of tube feeding. Two established investigators, Dr. Barbara Walike (later Hansen) and Dr. Geri Padilla, served as leaders, and Marcia Grant, Bob Hanson, Winnie Kubo, Hilda Luna Wong, and I began a great partnership that extended for more than 8 years. We may have been one of the first nursing consortium groups funded through the Department of Health, Education, and Welfare (DHEW) and, using a matrix design, one of the first to conduct both observational and experimental studies simultaneously. We enjoyed wonderful collegial relations while learning aspects such as the following: lactose in tube feeding diets caused diarrhea in individuals with relative lactose intolerance, teaching patients about procedures best prepared them for intubation, larger volumes of tube feeding could be tolerated when infused at slower rates, and more. At this time, I went to the University of Michigan for doctoral study, yet continued participating in the research. During my doctoral program, I wrote proposals related to nutrition and feeding problems of patients.

In my career, subtle shifts in direction have been driven by curiosity about a problem and new collegial opportunities. When I moved to Nebraska in the early 1980s, the University of Nebraska and Creighton University had a joint Robert Wood Johnson (RWJ) Teaching Nursing Home grant. With small seed funds from the RWJ project and funding from a University of Nebraska Foundation, I began studying nutrition in nursing home residents and this led to collaboration with Barbara Braden. Ultimately, we developed a tool that became known as the Braden Scale for Predicting Pressure Sore Risk.

During my doctoral program, I wrote proposals that built on nutritional variables (dietary intake, blood and serum levels, anthropometric measures, and so forth); later, combining these with a number of additional risk factors for pressure ulcers, Barbara Braden and I were funded by the Bureau of Health Professions (BHP), Department of Health and Human Services (DHHS), the only federal funding source for nursing research at that time. During these studies, we demonstrated that pressure ulcers could be predicted by the Braden Scale, that dietary intake of protein was a more important marker of pressure ulcer risk than serum albumin, and that blood pressure and body temperature were also important predictors of pressure ulcer risk. We also learned that older individuals who have higher levels of protein intake are less likely to develop pressure ulcers, those with moderate levels of intake may develop ulcers (but the ulcers healed during the study), and those with the lowest intake developed more ulcers and did not heal as quickly.

Our next study focused on the predictive validity of the Braden Scale for Predicting Pressure Sore Risk. This study was funded first by the National Center for Nursing Research (NCNR), which later became the National Institute for Nursing Research. I used the lessons learned about multisite consortium studies to prepare this proposal. We learned that the Braden Scale can be used with reliability and with good predictive validity in nursing homes, tertiary care settings, and Veterans Administration homes. After this study, we concluded that the critical cutoff point for assessing risk was a score of 18, and we knew that repeat assessments refined the score and increased the sensitivity and specificity. Finding that more than 800 individuals in three types of settings had similar scores let us know the tool was valid. However, we still had not tested whether the tool could be used to stimulate an accurate plan of care.

While this multisite study was in process, the Agency for Health Care Policy and Research (now the Agency for Healthcare Research and Quality) invited me to chair one of the first guideline development panels, the Panel for Pressure Sores. Once again, this was a unique opportunity to establish multidisciplinary collaboration and to focus on prevention. An elaborate process was established for reviewing the literature systematically, grading the resulting literature, and writing practice recommendations. The process was transformative in that investigators were taking time to systematically review the literature to determine which practices were supported and where more research was needed. The first guideline, "Predicting and Preventing Pressure Ulcers," was released in 1992, and the second, "Treatment of Pressure Ulcers," was released in 1994. These guidelines were discussed widely and efforts were made to change practice. Most guidelines written since this time follow the same conceptual outline.

Working with graduate students and small grants, most of my work at this point in my career focused on validating subscales of the Braden Scale or testing interventions. A significant personal event occurred during this period that ultimately challenged me to conduct a large intervention study. I received word that my mother had fallen and was hospitalized. I flew to Michigan, visited with my mother, and got her settled and positioned in her hospital bed for the night. When I returned in the morning, my mother was still in the same position. I have always been grateful that there wasn't a nurse around as, needless to say, I was frustrated that my own mother had not been turned and might develop a pressure ulcer. Furthermore, I was never aware of her being turned during the entire hospitalization.

Although I knew that studies of support surfaces showed that high-density, viscoelastic foam surfaces performed better than mattress overlays and the like, it was not until I saw the response of my mother's fragile skin on this surface that I was aware of the extent to which the newer surfaces could protect the skin of an older person. For a number of years, I worked with colleagues at the University of Texas Health Science Center in Houston to develop and pilot a randomized controlled trial (RCT) protocol to test alterations in turning intervals. Historically, because of the work of Kosiak, Hussain, and Linden, we turn patients every 2 hours. Norton and her colleagues, in observational studies, determined that people living in an "old folks home" who were turned every 2 or 3 hours had fewer pressure ulcers than those turned every 8 hours or once a day. Keep in mind that the mattresses of yesteryear were springs covered in heavy plastic that could be wiped with disinfectant. The surface was hard and caused a high degree of pressure in the interface between the mattress and the underlying bony prominences. The plastic coating on these old mattresses resulted in heat accumulation and caused sweating, which further compromised the skin.

We are currently conducting a multisite RCT to determine the optimal frequency of repositioning elderly nursing home residents who are at moderate or high risk (not mild or very high risk) according to the Braden Scale. Moderate-risk residents are randomly assigned to every 2, 3, or 4 hour turning, while high-risk subjects are randomly assigned to 2 or 3 hours. The subject's skin is extensively observed to ensure safety. This is one of the few studies to personalize the plan of care for residents based on the Braden Scale risk level and the subscale score. Whereas previous studies addressed subjects at every level of risk and treated them the same, this study represents a prototype to test the effectiveness of treatments according to a specific nursing assessment. We are hopeful that protecting skin while turning less often will promote better sleep and rest and improve quality of life. So, I'm at the same point as I started, believing that "an ounce of prevention (turning) is worth a pound of cure (treating ulcers)." Now we also believe that prevention improves quality of life.

We are pleased to report that the Braden Scale for Predicting Pressure Sore Risk is widely used in practice in the United States and throughout the world. It has been translated into many languages (e.g., Japanese, French, Italian, Portuguese, Croatian, Thai, Chinese, Korean, Icelandic, and more). Although the Braden Scale is copyrighted, free access can be obtained at www.bradenscale.com. Approximately 1,000 new clinical settings seek permission to use the Braden Scale for risk assessment each year. Many developers of electronic health records hold site licenses to include the Braden Scale, including two countries. We are looking forward to a time when nursing care is specifically tailored to the assessed risk and believe that health information technology will facilitate this integration.

1

Integrating the Processes of Research and Evidence-Based Practice

Geri LoBiondo-Wood and Judith Haber

KEY TERMS

clinical guidelines
consumer
critical appraisal
critical reading
critical thinking
evidence-based practice
evidence hierarchy
integrative review
meta-analysis
meta-synthesis
qualitative research
quantitative research
research
systematic review

LEARNING OUTCOMES

After reading this chapter, you should be able to do the following:

- State the significance of research to evidence-based nursing practice.
- Identify the role of the consumer of nursing research.
- Define evidence-based practice.
- Discuss evidence-based decision making.
- Explain the difference between quantitative and qualitative research.
- Explain the difference between types of systematic reviews: integrative review, meta-analysis, and meta-synthesis.
- Identify the importance of critical thinking and critical reading skills for critical appraisal of research studies.
- Discuss the format and style of research reports/articles.
- Discuss how to use a quantitative evidence hierarchy when critically appraising research studies.

STUDY RESOURCES

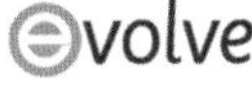

Go to Evolve at http://evolve.elsevier.com/LoBiondo/ for review questions, critiquing exercises, and additional research articles for practice in reviewing and critiquing.

We invite you to join us on an exciting nursing research adventure that begins as you read the first page of this chapter. The adventure is one of discovery! You will discover that the nursing research literature sparkles with pride, dedication, and excitement about this dimension of professional nursing practice. As you progress through your educational program you are taught how to ensure quality and safety in practice through acquiring knowledge of the various sciences and health care principles. Another critical component to clinical knowledge is research knowledge as it applies to practicing from an evidence base.

Whether you are a student or a practicing nurse whose goal is to use **research** as the foundation of your practice, you will discover that nursing research and **evidence-based practice** positions our profession at the cutting edge of change and improvement in patient outcomes. You will also discover that nursing research is integral with meeting the challenge of achieving the goal of providing quality biopsychosocial outcomes in partnership with clients, their families/significant others, and the communities in which they live. Finally, you will discover the cutting edge "Who," "What," "Where," "When," "Why," and "How" of nursing research and develop a foundation of evidence-based practice knowledge, and competencies that will equip you for twenty-first century clinical practice.

Your nursing research adventure will be filled with new and challenging learning experiences that develop your evidence-based practice skills. Your critical thinking, critical reading, and clinical decision-making skills will expand as you develop clinical questions, search the research literature, evaluate the research evidence found in the literature, and make clinical decisions about applying the "best available evidence" to your practice. For example, you will be encouraged to ask important clinical questions such as the following: What makes a telephone education intervention more effective with one group of patients with congestive heart failure but not another? What is the effect of computer learning modules on children's self-management of asthma? What research has been conducted in the area of identifying barriers to colon cancer screening in African-American men? What is the quality of studies conducted on therapeutic touch? What nursing-delivered smoking cessation interventions are most effective? This book will help you begin your adventure into evidence-based nursing practice by developing an appreciation of research as the foundation for evidence-based practice.

NURSING RESEARCH AND EVIDENCE-BASED PRACTICE

Professional nurses are constantly challenged to stay abreast of new information to provide the highest quality of patient care (Institute of Medicine Committee on Quality of Health Care in America, 2001). Nurses are challenged to expand their "comfort zone" by offering creative approaches to old and new health problems, as well as designing new and innovative programs that truly make a difference in the health status of our citizens. This challenge can best be met by integrating rapidly expanding research and evidence-based knowledge about biological, behavioral, and environmental influences on health into the care of patients and their families.

It is important to differentiate between research and evidence-based practice. **Research** is the systematic, rigorous, logical investigation that aims to answer questions about nursing phenomena. The conduct of research requires one to follow the steps of the scientific process, which are outlined later in this chapter and discussed in each chapter of this textbook. There are two types of research, quantitative and qualitative. The methods used by nurse researchers are the same methods used by other disciplines; the difference is that nurses study questions relevant to nursing practice. Nurse researchers also conduct research collaboratively with other disciplines. The conduct of research provides knowledge that is reliable and useful for practice. Studies are published in professional journals, read, and assessed for use in clinical practice. The methods and findings of studies provide evidence that is evaluated, and their applicability to practice is used to inform clinical decisions. Nursing research generates a specialized scientific knowledge base that empowers the nursing profession to anticipate and meet constantly shifting challenges and maintain our societal relevance.

Evidence-based practice is the collection, interpretation, and integration of valid research evidence, combined with clinical expertise, and an understanding of patient and family values and preferences to inform clinical decision making (Sackett, Straus, Richardson, et al., 2000). The evidence is research that has been completed and published. Research studies are gathered from the published literature and assessed so that decisions about application to clinical practice can be made, culminating in nursing practice that is evidence based. For example, to help you understand the importance of evidence-based practice, think about one of the latest reports from the Cochrane Collaboration by Rice and Stead (2008), which sought to determine which nursing interventions for smoking cessation provided the highest level of benefit (see Appendix E). They conducted a comprehensive search of the literature for studies on smoking cessation. Based on their search and synthesis of the literature, they put forth several conclusions regarding the benefits of smoking cessation advice that can be used by all nurses working with patients who are seeking to stop smoking.

When you first read about the research process and the evidence-based practice process, you will notice that both processes may seem similar. Each begins with a question. The difference is that in a research study the question is tested with a design appropriate to the question and specific methodology (sample, instruments, procedures, and data analysis) used to test the research question. In the evidence-based practice process, a question is used to search the literature for already completed studies that you will critically appraise in order to answer your clinical question.

It is proposed that all nurses share a commitment to the advancement of nursing science by conducting research and using research evidence in practice. Scientific investigation promotes accountability, which is one of the hallmarks of the nursing profession and a fundamental concept of the American Nurses Association (ANA) Code for Nurses (ANA, 2004). There is a consensus that the research role of the baccalaureate and master's graduate calls for the skills of **critical appraisal.** That is, the nurse must be a knowledgeable **consumer** of research, one who can **appraise** research evidence and use existing standards to determine the merit and readiness of research for use in clinical practice (AACN, 2008). Therefore to use research (evidence-based practice), one must not necessarily be able to conduct research but to understand and appraise the steps of the research process in order to read the research literature critically and use it to inform clinical decisions.

As you venture through this text, you will see the steps of the research process and evidence-based practice process as they unfold. The steps are systematic and orderly and relate to the development of evidence-based practice. Understanding the step-by-step process that researchers use will help you develop the assessment skills necessary to judge the soundness of research studies.

Throughout the chapters, research terminology pertinent to each step is identified and illustrated with many examples from the research literature. Five published research studies are found in the appendices and used as examples to illustrate significant points in each chapter. Judging not only the study's strength and quality but also a study's applicability to practice is key. Before you can judge a study it is important to understand the differences between and among studies. There are many different study designs that you will see as you read through this text and the appendices. There are standards not only for critiquing the soundness of each step of a study but also for judging the strength and quality of evidence provided by a study and determining its applicability to practice.

This chapter provides an overview of types of research studies, critical thinking, critical reading, and appraisal skills. It introduces the overall format of a research article and provides an overview of the subsequent chapters in the book. It also introduces the evidence-based practice process, an evidence hierarchy model, and other tools for helping you evaluate the strength and quality of evidence provided by a research study. These topics are designed to help you read research articles more effectively and with greater understanding, making this book more "user-friendly" as you learn about the research process so that you can make clinical decisions and practice from an evidence base and contribute to quality and cost-effective patient outcomes. The remainder of this book is devoted to helping you develop your evidence-based practice expertise.

TYPES OF RESEARCH: QUALITATIVE AND QUANTITATIVE

Research can be classified into two major categories: qualitative and quantitative. A researcher chooses between these categories based primarily on the question the researcher is asking. That is, a researcher may wish to test a cause-and-effect relationship or to assess if variables are related, or he or she may wish to discover and understand the meaning about an experience or process. A researcher would choose to conduct a **qualitative research** study if the question to be answered is about understanding the meaning of a human experience such a grief, hope, or loss. The meaning of an experience is based on the view that meaning varies and is subjective. The context of the experience also plays a role in qualitative research. That is, the experience of loss as a result of a miscarriage would be different than the experience from the loss of a parent.

Qualitative research is generally conducted in natural settings and uses data that are words or text rather than numeric to describe the experiences being studied. Qualitative studies are guided by research questions and data are collected from a small number of subjects, allowing an in-depth study of a phenomenon. For example, Landreneau and Ward-Smith (2007) explored in 12 subjects what patients on hemodialysis perceive about the types of renal replacement therapies (see Appendix D). Although qualitative research is systematic in its method, it uses a subjective approach. Data from qualitative studies help nurses to understand experiences or phenomena that affect patients; these data also assist in generating theories that lead clinicians to developing improved patient care and stimulates further research. Highlights of the general steps of qualitative studies and the journal format for a qualitative article are outlined in Table 1-1. Chapters 4 through 6 provide an in-depth view of qualitative research underpinnings, designs, and methods.

Whereas qualitative research looks for meaning, **quantitative research** encompasses the study of research questions and/or hypotheses that describe phenomena, test relationships, assess differences, and seek to explain cause-and-effect relationships between variables and test for intervention effectiveness. The numeric data in quantitative studies are summarized and analyzed using statistics. Quantitative research techniques are systematic, and the methodology is controlled. Appendices A, B, and C illustrate examples of different quantitative approaches

TABLE 1-1 Steps of the Research Process and Journal Format: Qualitative Research

Research Process Steps and/or Format Issues	Usual Location in Journal Heading or Subheading
Identifying the phenomenon	Abstract and/or in introduction
Research question study purpose	Abstract and/or in beginning or end of introduction
Literature review	Introduction and/or discussion
Design	Abstract and/or in introductory section or under method section entitled "Design" or stated in method section
Sample	Method section labeled "Sample" or "Subjects"
Legal-ethical issues	Data-collection or procedures section or in sample section
Data-collection procedure	Data-collection or procedures section
Data analysis	Methods section under subhead "Data Analysis" or "Data Analysis and Interpretation"
Results	Stated in separate heading: "Results" or "Findings"
Discussion and recommendation	Combined in separate section: "Discussion" or "Discussion and Implications"
References	At end of article

See Chapters 4, 5, and 6.

to answering research questions. Table 1-2 indicates where each step of the research process can usually be located in a quantitative research article and where it is discussed in this text. Chapters 2, 3, and 7 through 16 describe processes related to quantitative research.

The primary difference is that a qualitative study seeks to interpret meaning and phenomena whereas quantitative research seeks to test a hypothesis or answer research questions using statistical methods. Remember as you are reading research articles that a researcher may vary the steps slightly, depending on the nature of the research problem, but all of the steps should be addressed systematically.

Systematic Reviews

Other types of research articles that are appearing more frequently in the literature and that are important to understand for evidence-based practice are systematic reviews, **meta-analyses, integrative reviews** (sometimes called **narrative reviews**), and **meta-syntheses.** A **systematic review** is a summation and assessment of a group of quantitative studies that used similar designs based on a focused clinical question. If statistical techniques are used to summarize and assess the studies the systematic review is labeled as a meta-analysis. A **meta-analysis** summarizes a number of studies focused on a topic using a specific statistical methodology to synthesize the findings in order to draw conclusions about the area of focus. An **integrative review** is a focused review and synthesis of the literature on a specific area that follows specific steps of literature integration and synthesis without statistical analysis. At times in the literature the terms *systematic review* and *integrative review* are used interchangeably even though there is no statistical analysis. A **meta-synthesis** is a synthesis of a number of qualitative articles on a focused topic using specific qualitative methodology. The components of each of these will be discussed in greater detail in Chapters 5 and 9. These articles take a number of studies related to a clinical question and, using a specific set of criteria and method, evaluate those articles as a whole.

TABLE 1-2 Steps of the Research Process and Journal Format: Quantitative Research

Research Process Steps and/or Format Issue	Usual Location in Journal Heading or Subheading	Text Chapter
Research problem	Abstract and/or in introduction (not labeled) or in separately labeled heading: "Problem"	2
Purpose	Abstract and/or in introduction or at end of literature review or theoretical framework section, or labeled as separate heading: "Purpose"	2
Literature review	At end of heading "Introduction" but not labeled as such, or labeled as separate heading: "Literature Review," "Review of the Literature," or "Related Literature"; or not labeled or variables reviewed appear as headings or subheadings	3
Theoretical framework (TF) and/or conceptual framework (CF)	Combined with "Literature Review" or found in separate heading as TF or CF; or each concept or definition used in TF or CF may appear as separate heading or subheading	3
Hypothesis/research questions	Stated or implied near end of introductory section, which may be labeled or found in separate heading or subheading: "Hypothesis" or "Research Questions"; or reported for first time in "Results" section	3
Research design	Stated or implied in abstract or in introduction or under heading: "Methods" or "Methodology"	7, 8, and 9
Sample: type and size	"Size" may be stated in abstract, in methods section, or as separate subheading under methods section as "Sample," "Sample/Subjects," or "Participants"; "Type" may be implied or stated in any of previous headings described under size	10
Legal-ethical issues	Stated or implied in labeled headings: "Methods," "Procedures," "Sample," or "Subjects"	11
Instruments (measurement tools)	Found in headings labeled "Methods," "Instruments," or "Measures"	12
Validity and reliability	Specifically stated or implied in headings labeled "Methods," "Instruments," "Measures," or "Procedures"	13
Data-collection procedure	Stated in methods section under subheading "Procedure" or "Data Collection," or as separate heading: "Procedure"	12
Data analysis	Stated in methods section under subheading "Procedure" or "Data Analysis"	14
Results	Stated in separate heading: "Results"	14, 15
Discussion of findings and new findings	Combined with results or as separate heading: "Discussion"	15
Implications, limitations, and recommendations	Combined in discussion or presented as separate or combined major headings	15
References	At end of article	4
Communicating research results	Research articles, poster, and paper presentations	1, 17, 18

Clinical Guidelines

Clinical guidelines are another key reference for evidence-based practice. **Clinical guidelines** are systematically developed practice statements designed to assist clinicians about health care decisions for specific conditions or situations. Clinical guidelines are generally developed at the national level by governments or health care agencies and health care organizations. Two types of clinical guidelines will be discussed throughout this text: *consensus* or *expert-developed guidelines* and *evidence-based guidelines* that are developed based on research findings.

CRITICAL THINKING AND CRITICAL READING SKILLS

To develop an expertise in evidence-based practice you will need to be able to critically read all types of research literature. As you read a research article, you may be struck by the difference in style or format between a research article and a clinical article. The terms of a research article are new, and the focus of the content is different. You may also be thinking that the research article is hard to read or that it is too technical and boring. You may simultaneously wonder, "How will I possibly learn to appraise all the steps of a research study, the terminology, and the process of evidence-based practice? I'm only on Chapter 1. This is not so easy; research is as hard, as everyone says."

Try to reframe these thoughts with the "glass is half-full" approach. That is, tell yourself, "Yes, I can learn how to read and appraise research, and this chapter will provide the strategies for me to learn this skill." Remember that learning occurs with time and help. Reading research articles can be difficult and frustrating at first, but the best way to become a knowledgeable research consumer is to use critical thinking and reading skills when reading research articles. As a student, you are not expected to understand a research article or critique it perfectly the first time. Nor are you expected to develop these skills on your own. An essential objective of this book is to help you acquire critical thinking and reading skills so that you can use research in your practice. Remember that becoming a competent critical thinker and reader of research, similar to learning the steps of the research process, takes time and patience. Both skills will help you become a more effective evaluator of research studies.

Critical thinking is the examination of ideas, assumptions, principles, arguments, conclusions, beliefs, and actions (Paul & Elder, 2008). As applied to critically reading research, this means that you are engaged in the following:

- Systematic understanding of the research process
- Thinking that displays a mastery of the criteria for critiquing research and evidence-based practice
- The art of being able to make one's thinking better (i.e., clearer, more accurate, or more defensible) by clarifying what you understand and what you do not know

In other words, being a critical thinker means that you are consciously thinking about your thoughts and what you say, write, read, or do, as well as what others say, write, or do. While thinking about all of this, you are questioning the appropriateness of the content, applying standards or criteria, and seeing how information measure up.

Developing the ability to evaluate research critically requires not only critical thinking skills but also critical reading skills. **Critical reading** is defined as "an active, intellectually engaging process in which the reader participates in an inner dialogue with the writer" (Paul & Elder,

2008). A critical reader actively looks for **assumptions**, key concepts and ideas, reasons, justifications, supporting examples, implications and consequences, and any other structural features of the written text, to interpret and assess it accurately and fairly (Paul & Elder, 2008). Critical reading is a process that involves the following levels of understanding and allows you to critically assess a study's validity. Box 1-1 provides strategies for critical reading.

- *Preliminary:* familiarizing yourself with the content—skim the article
- *Comprehensive:* understanding the researcher's purpose or intent
- *Analysis:* understanding the parts of the study
- *Synthesis:* understanding the whole article and each step of the research process in a study

Critical thinking and critical reading skills are further developed by learning the research process. You will gradually be able to read an entire research article and reflect on it by identifying assumptions, identifying key concepts and methods, and determining whether the

BOX 1-1 Highlights of Critical Reading Process Strategies

Photocopy the article to be critiqued and make notations directly on the copy.

STRATEGIES FOR PRELIMINARY UNDERSTANDING

- Keep a research text and a dictionary by your side.
- Review the chapters in the text on various steps of the research process, critiquing criteria, key terms, etc.
- List key variables at the top of the photocopy.
- Highlight or underline on the photocopy new terms, unfamiliar terms, and significant sentences.
- Look up the definitions of new terms and write them on the photocopy.
- Review old and new terms before subsequent readings.
- Highlight or underline identified steps of the research process.

STRATEGIES FOR COMPREHENSIVE UNDERSTANDING

- Identify the main idea or theme of the article; state it in your own words in one or two sentences.
- Continue to clarify terms that may be unclear on subsequent readings.
- Before critiquing the article, make sure you understand the main points of each reported step of the research process that you identified.

STRATEGIES FOR ANALYSIS UNDERSTANDING

- Using the critiquing criteria, determine how well the study meets the criteria for each step of the process.
- Determine which level of evidence fits the study.
- Write cues, relationships of concepts, and questions on the photocopy.
- Ask fellow students to analyze the same study using the same criteria and then compare results.
- Consult faculty members about your evaluation of the study.

STRATEGIES FOR SYNTHESIS UNDERSTANDING

- Review your notes on the article and determine how each step discussed in the article compares with the critiquing criteria.
- Type a one-page summary in your own words of the reviewed study.
- Cite article references at the top according to American Psychological Association (APA) or another reference style.
- Briefly summarize each reported research step in your own words using the critiquing criteria.
- Briefly describe strengths and weaknesses in your own words.

conclusions are based on the study's findings. Once you have obtained this critical appraisal competency, you will be ready to synthesize the findings of multiple research studies to use in developing evidence-based practice. This will be a very exciting and rewarding process for you.

To read a research study critically will require several readings. A minimum of three or four readings is common. The first strategy is to keep your research textbook at your side as you read. As you read, use your research text for the following:

- Identify the steps of the research process and how the study was conducted
- Clarify unfamiliar concepts or terms
- Question assumptions and rationale
- Assess the study for validity

As you analyze and synthesize an article you are ready to begin the appraisal process that will help determine a study's worth. An illustration of how to use critical reading strategies is provided by the example in Box 1-2, which contains an excerpt from the abstract, introduction, literature review, theoretical framework literature, and methods and procedure section of a quantitative study (Meneses, McNees, Loerzel, et al., 2007) (see Appendix A). Note that in this particular article there is both a literature review and a theoretical framework section that clearly supports the objectives and purpose of the study. Also note that parts of the text of this section from the article were deleted to offer a number of examples within the text of this chapter.

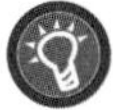

HELPFUL HINT

If you still have difficulty understanding a research study after using the strategies related to skimming and comprehensive reading, make another copy of your "marked-up" research article, include your specific questions or area of difficulty, and ask your professor to read it. Comprehensive understanding and synthesis are necessary to analyze a research article. Understanding the author's purpose and methods for the study reflects critical thinking and facilitates the evaluation of the study.

STRATEGIES FOR CRITIQUING RESEARCH STUDIES

The evaluation of a research article requires an appraisal or critique of the published study. The **critique** is the process of critical appraisal that objectively and critically evaluates a research report's content for scientific validity or merit and application to practice. It requires some knowledge of the subject matter and knowledge of how to critically read and use critiquing criteria. You will find

- Summarized examples of critiquing criteria for qualitative studies and an example of a qualitative critique in Chapter 6
- Summarized critiquing criteria and examples of a quantitative critique in Chapter 16
- An in-depth exploration of the criteria for evaluation required in quantitative research critiques in Chapters 7 through 15
- Criteria for qualitative research critiques presented in Chapters 4, 5, and 6
- General principles for qualitative and quantitative research in Chapters 1, 2, and 3

Critiquing criteria are the standards, appraisal guides, or questions used to judge (assess) an article. In analyzing a research report, the reader must evaluate each step of the research

BOX 1-2 Example of Critical Appraisal Reading Strategies

Introductory paragraphs, study's **purpose** and *aims*	Quality of life (QOL) during posttreatment breast cancer survivorship is a relatively new, emerging, and promising area of investigation. Numerous multidisciplinary studies conducted since the 1980s have documented QOL in several domains, including physical function, psychological distress, social and family concerns, and spiritual issues, among breast cancer survivors. Behavioral interventions to ameliorate QOL problems include a wide variety of methods such as psychoeducational support, individual and group counseling, expressive therapy, and cognitive behavioral therapy (Institute of Medicine & National Research Council, 2004). The preponderance of behavioral interventions has been delivered primarily during active cancer treatment. A small but growing number of multidisciplinary studies have reported interventions designed for the transition from cancer treatment to cancer survivorship. **The primary purpose of this article is to report the results of the effects of the Breast Cancer Education Intervention (BCEI) Study, a QOL survivorship intervention delivered using psychoeducational support and targeting women with early-stage breast cancer in the first year** of posttreatment survivorship. *The aims of this article are consistent with the study aims: (a) to describe the effect of the BCEI study on overall QOL, (b) to examine whether the intervention effects were retained over time, and (c) to describe the differential effects of the BCEI study on QOL in the domains of physical, psychological, social, and spiritual well-being.*
Literature review-concepts Quality of life and breast cancer	The literature on QOL and breast cancer is vast and synthesizing; it is outside the scope of this article. In general, however, multidisciplinary studies document the influence of breast cancer on overall QOL (Ashbury, Cameron, Mercer, Fitch, & Nielsen, 1998; Ashing-Giwa, Ganz, & Petersen, 1999).
Cancer survivorship intervention research	The number is small because most studies conducted during posttreatment survivorship did not have interventions and thus were excluded from the discussion. In addition, intervention studies in advanced breast cancer were excluded from the review.
Conceptual framework	QOL was the conceptual framework used to guide the identification and development of the BCEI study. QOL was defined as a multidimensional construct consisting of four domains: physical, psychological, social, and spiritual well-being (Dow et al., 1996; Ferrell, Dow, & Grant, 1995). Each domain contributes to an individual's perception of overall QOL. As individuals progress along the cancer continuum, QOL is considered dynamic. This study specifically focused on QOL in posttreatment survivorship, which is consistent with the NCI (2006) cancer survivorship research that concentrates on posttreatment concerns.
Methods Design	The BCEI study was a randomized trial with subjects assigned to the experimental group or the wait control group.
Specific aims and hypotheses	The specific aims and hypotheses of the study were to determine the effect of the BCEI study on overall QOL and on the individual QOL domains and to examine whether the effects of the intervention were durable over time.
Subject recruitment and accrual	Subjects were recruited from a regional cancer center and private oncology offices in the southeastern United States. Women at least 21 years of age, with histologically confirmed stage 0-II breast cancer and no evidence of local recurrence or metastatic disease, within 1 year of diagnosis, who had surgery at least 1 month before, who received radiation therapy or chemotherapy to recover from acute treatment side effects, and who were able to communicate in English were eligible to participate.
Procedure	Following study approval by the respective institutional review board of the university where the researchers were affiliated at the time of the study and the participating cancer centers, potential subjects were identified by the cancer center or private oncology office nursing staff using an eligibility checklist devised from consideration of the inclusion and exclusion criteria.
Intervention fidelity	Several strategies for treatment fidelity, including study design, interventionist's training, and intervention delivery and receipt, were incorporated into the BCEI study.

process and ask questions about whether each step of the process meets the criteria. For instance, the critiquing criteria in Chapter 3 ask if "the literature review identifies gaps and inconsistencies in the literature about a subject, concept, or problem" and if "all of the concepts and variables are included in the review." These two questions relate to critiquing the research question and the literature review components of the research process. Box 1-2 shows several places where the researchers in the study by Meneses and colleagues identified gaps in the literature, and how the study intended to fill these gaps by conducting a study for the stated objective and purpose (see Appendix A for the complete study). Remember that when you are doing a critique, you are pointing out strengths, as well as weaknesses. Developing critical reading skills will enable you to successfully complete a critique. The appraisal strategies that facilitate the understanding gained by reading for analysis are listed in Box 1-1. Standardized critical appraisal tools such as the Critical Appraisal Skills Programme—CASP Tools (www.phru.nhs.uk) also can be used by students and clinicians to systematically appraise the strength and quality of evidence provided in research articles (see Chapter 18).

Critiquing can be thought of as looking at a completed jigsaw puzzle. Does it form a comprehensive picture, or is there a piece out of place? What is the level of evidence provided by the study and its findings? What is the balance between the risks and benefits of the findings that contribute to clinical decisions? How can I apply the evidence to my patient, to my patient population, in my setting? In the case of reading several studies for synthesis, the interrelationship of the studies is assessed as is the overall strength and quality of evidence and its applicability to practice. Reading for synthesis is essential in critiquing research studies. Appraising a study helps for development of an evidence table (see Chapters 17 and 18 on writing an individual appraisal of a study; see also Chapters 6 and 16).

OVERCOMING BARRIERS: USEFUL CRITIQUING STRATEGIES

Throughout the text, you will find special features that will help refine the critical thinking and critical reading skills essential to developing your competence as a research consumer. A Critical Thinking Decision Path related to each step of the research process will sharpen your decision-making skills as you critique research articles. Look for Internet resources in chapters that will enhance your research consumer skills. Critical Thinking Challenges, which appear at the end of each chapter, are designed to reinforce your critical thinking and critical reading skills in relation to the steps of the research process. Helpful Hints, designed to reinforce your understanding and critical thinking, appear at various points throughout the chapters. Evidence-Based Practice Tips, which will help you apply evidence-based practice strategies in your clinical practice, are provided in each chapter.

When you complete your first appraisal, congratulate yourself; mastering these skills is not easy at the beginning, but we are confident that you can do it. Once you complete a research critique or two, you will be ready to discuss your critique with your fellow students and professor. Best of all, you can look forward to discussing the points of your appraisal because your critique will be based on objective data, not just personal opinion. As you continue to use and perfect critical analysis skills by critiquing studies, remember that these very skills are an expected clinical competency for delivering evidence-based nursing care.

EVIDENCE-BASED PRACTICE AND RESEARCH

Along with gaining comfort while reading and critiquing research studies, a final step must be undertaken. The final step of reading and appraising the research literature is deciding how, when, and if to apply a study or studies to your practice so that your practice is evidence based. **Evidence-based practice** allows you to systematically use the best available evidence with the integration of individual clinical expertise, as well as the patient's values and preferences, in making clinical decisions (Sackett et al., 2000). Evidence-based practice has processes and steps that are followed, as does the research process. These steps will be presented throughout the text. Chapter 17 provides an overview of evidence-based practice, and Chapter 18 conceptually introduces you to the steps and strategies associated with evidence-based practice.

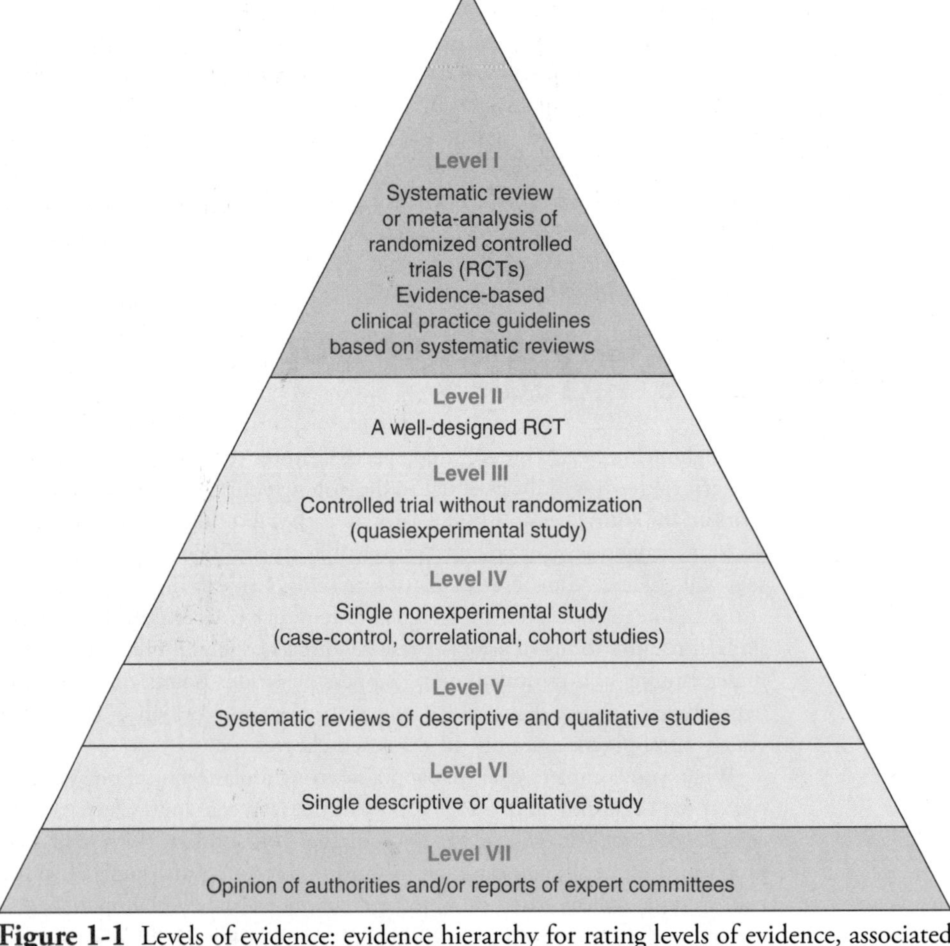

Figure 1-1 Levels of evidence: evidence hierarchy for rating levels of evidence, associated with a study's design. Evidence is assessed at a level according to its source.

When using evidence-based practice strategies, the first step is to be able to read a research article and understand how each section is linked to each step of the research process. The following section introduces you to the steps of the research process as presented in published articles. Once you read an article you decide which level of evidence a research article provides and how well the study was designed and executed. Figure 1-1 illustrates a model for determining the levels of evidence associated with the design of a study, ranging from systematic reviews of randomized clinical trials (RCTs) (see Chapters 8 and 9) to expert opinions. The rating system or evidence hierarchy model presented here is just one of many. Many hierarchies for assessing the relative worth of different types of research literature for both the qualitative and quantitative research literature are available. Early in the development of evidence-based practice, evidence hierarchies were thought to be very inflexible with systematic reviews or meta-analyses at the top and qualitative research at the bottom. When assessing a clinical question that measures cause and effect this may be true, but nursing and health care research is involved in a broader base of problem solving, and thus assessing the worth of a study within a broader context of applying evidence into practice requires a broader view.

The meaningfulness of an evidence rating system will become clearer to you as you read Chapters 7, 8, and 9) For example, the Meneses and colleagues (2007) study is Level II because of its experimental design whereas the Landreneau and Ward-Smith (2007) study is Level VI because of its qualitative design. The level in and of itself does not tell the full worth of a study but is another tool that helps you think about the strengths and weaknesses of a study and the nature of the evidence provided in the findings and conclusions. Chapters 6 and 16 will provide an understanding of how qualitative studies can be assessed for use in practice. You will use the evidence hierarchy presented in Figure 1-1 throughout the book as you develop your research consumer skills, so become familiar with its content.

This rating system represents an **evidence hierarchy** for judging the strength of a study's design, which is just one level of assessment that influences the confidence one has in the conclusions the researcher has drawn. Assessing the strength of scientific evidence or potential research bias provides a vehicle to guide nurses in evaluating research studies for their applicability in clinical decision making. In addition to identifying the level of evidence one needs to grade the strength of a body of evidence incorporating the three domains of: quality, quantity, and consistency (Agency for Healthcare Research and Quality, 2002):

- **Quality:** the extent to which a study's design, implementation, and analysis minimizes bias (see Chapters 4, 5, 7, 8, 9, 12, 13, and 14)
- **Quantity:** the number of studies that have evaluated the research question, including overall sample size across studies (see Chapters 5 and 10), as well as the strength of the findings from the data analyses (see Chapters 5 and 14)
- **Consistency:** the degree to which studies that have similar and different designs, but investigate the same research question, report similar findings (see Chapters 5, 8, 9, 13, 14, and 15)

Evidence-based practice has processes and steps that are followed, as does the research process. The steps of the evidence-based practice process are ask, gather, assess and appraise, act, and evaluate (Figure 1-2). Chapter 17 provides an overview of evidence-based practice, and Chapter 18 conceptually introduces you to the steps and strategies associated with evidence-based practice.

A number of studies are evaluated using specific criteria. These completed studies are evaluated in terms of their strength, quality, and consistency of evidence, which informs the nurse's

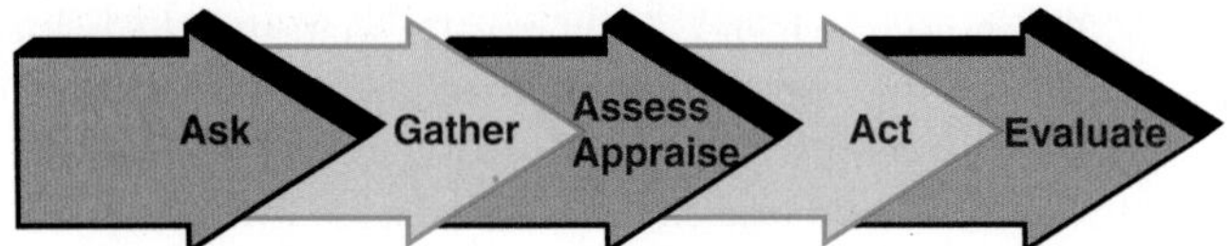

Figure 1-2 Evidence-based practice steps.

decision about whether the evidence supports a change in practice. Before one can proceed with an evidence-based project, it is necessary to understand the step of the research process found in research studies.

RESEARCH ARTICLES: FORMAT AND STYLE

Before you consider reading research articles, it is important to have a sense of their organization and format. Many journals publish research, either as the sole type of article in the journal or in addition to clinical or theoretical articles. Although many journals have some common features, they also have unique characteristics. All journals have guidelines for manuscript preparation and submission, which are published by each journal. A review of these guidelines will give you an idea of the format of articles that appear in specific journals.

It is important to remember that even though each step of the research process is discussed at length in this text, you may find only a short paragraph or a sentence in the research article that gives the details of the step in a specific study. Because of the journal's publishing guidelines, the published study that one reads in a journal is a shortened version of the complete work completed by the researcher(s). You will also find that some researchers devote more space in an article to the results, whereas others present a longer discussion of the methods and procedures. In recent years, most authors give more emphasis to the method, results, and discussion of implications than to details of assumptions, hypotheses, or definitions of terms. Decisions about the amount of material presented for each step of the research process are bound by the following:

- A journal's space limitations
- A journal's author guidelines
- The type or nature of the study
- An individual researcher's evaluation of what is the most important component of the study

The following discussion provides a brief overview of each step of the research process and how it might appear in an article. It is important to remember that a quantitative research article will differ from a qualitative research article. The components of qualitative research are discussed in Chapters 4 and 5 and summarized in Chapter 6.

Abstract

An **abstract** is a short, comprehensive synopsis or summary of a study at the beginning of an article. An abstract quickly focuses the reader on the main points of a study. A well-presented abstract is accurate, self-contained, concise, specific, nonevaluative, coherent, and readable.

Abstracts vary in length from 50 to 250 words. The length and format of an abstract are dictated by the journal's style. Both quantitative and qualitative research studies have abstracts that provide a succinct overview of the study. An example of an abstract can be found at the beginning of the study by Meneses and colleagues (2007) (see Appendix A). Their abstract follows an outline format that highlights the major steps of the study. It partially reads as follows:

> *Purpose/Objective:* "To examine the effectiveness of a psychoeducational intervention on quality of life (QOL) in breast cancer survivors in post-treatment survivorship..."

Within this example, the authors provide a view of the study variables. The remainder of the abstract provides a synopsis of the background of the study and the methods, results, and conclusions. The studies in Appendices A through D all have abstracts.

HELPFUL HINT

A journal abstract is usually a single paragraph that provides a general reference to the research purpose, research questions, and/or hypotheses and highlights the methodology and results, as well as the implications for practice or future research.

Introduction

Early in a research article, in a section that may or may not be labeled "Introduction," the researcher presents a background picture of the area researched and its significance to practice (see Chapter 2). When reading the study by Meneses and colleagues (2007), the reader can find the basis of the research question early in the report (see Appendix A):

> "Quality of life during post-treatment breast cancer survivorship is a relatively new, emerging and promising area of investigation....A small but growing number of multidisciplinary studies have reported interventions designed for the transition from cancer to cancer survivorship."

Another example can be found in the Landreneau and Ward-Smith (2007) study, as follows (see Appendix D):

> "The literature reveals a division as to either the study of dialysis therapy or the study of transplant therapy. The perceptions of the choice of renal replacement therapy for patients on hemodialysis remains unknown."

Definition of the Purpose

The purpose of the study is defined either at the end of the researcher's initial introduction or at the end of the "Literature Review" or "Conceptual Framework" section. The study's purpose may or may not be labeled as such (see Chapters 2 and 3), or it may be referred to as the study's aim or objective. The study by Landreneau and Ward-Smith (2007) has a sections entitled "Aim" (see Appendix D). The studies in Appendices A, B, C, and D state their purpose in the abstract and in the introductory paragraphs of the articles. The purpose of the Jones, Renger, and Kang (2007) study appears in the abstract and is repeated in the first sentence of the article (see Appendix B).

Literature Review and Theoretical Framework

Authors of studies and journal articles present the literature review and theoretical framework in different ways. Many research articles merge the "Literature Review" and the "Theoretical Framework." This section includes the main concepts investigated and may be called "Review of the Literature," "Literature Review," "Theoretical Framework," "Related Literature," "Background," or "Conceptual Framework"; or it may not be labeled at all (see Chapters 2 and 3). By reviewing Appendices A through D, the reader will find differences in the headings used. Meneses and colleagues (2007) have both a "Literature Review" and a "Conceptual Framework" section (see Appendix A); the studies in Appendices B and C use headings that reflect the theoretical concepts of the study but do not call it a literature review or a framework. All three studies have literature reviews and use a framework. One style is not better than another; all of the studies in the appendices contain all of the critical elements but present the elements differently.

Hypothesis/Research Question

A study's research questions or hypotheses can also be presented in different ways (see Chapter 2). Research reports in journals often do not have separate headings for reporting the "Hypotheses" or "Research Question." They are often embedded in the "Introduction" or "Background" section or not labeled at all (e.g., as in the studies in the appendices). If a study uses hypotheses, the researcher may report whether the hypotheses were or were not supported toward the end of the article in the "Results" or "Findings" section. Quantitative research studies have hypotheses or research questions. Qualitative research studies do not have hypotheses but have research questions and purposes. Meneses and colleagues (2007) (see Appendix A) and Jones, Renger, and Kang (2007) (see Appendix B) have hypotheses. The study by Horgas, Yoon, Nichols, and colleagues (2008) (see Appendix C) has research questions.

Research Design

The type of research design can be found in the abstract, within the purpose statement, or in the introduction to the "Procedures" or "Methods" section, or not stated at all (see Chapters 5, 8, and 9). For example, the studies in Appendices A, C, and D identify the design type in the abstract.

One of your first objectives is to determine whether the study is qualitative (see Chapters 4 and 5) or quantitative (see Chapters 7, 8, and 9) so that the appropriate criteria are used. Although the rigor of the critiquing criteria addressed do not substantially change, some of the terminology of the questions differs for qualitative and quantitative studies. For instance, in regard to Meneses and colleagues (see Appendix A), you might be asking if the hypotheses were generated from the theoretical framework or literature review and if the design chosen was appropriate and consistent with the study's questions and purpose (see Chapters 7, 8, and 9). With a qualitative study such as that by Landreneau and Ward-Smith (see Appendix D), however, you might be asking if the researchers conducted the study consistent with the principles of qualitative research and therefore focused on the identification of the themes of knowledge and choice (see Chapters 4 and 5).

Do not get discouraged if you cannot easily determine the design. More often than not, the specific design is not stated or, if an advanced design is used, the details are not spelled out. One of the best strategies is to review the chapters in this text that address designs (see

Chapters 5, 8, and 9) and to ask your professors for assistance. The following tips will help you determine whether the study you are reading employs a quantitative design:

- Hypotheses are stated or implied (see Chapter 2).
- The terms *control* and *treatment group* appear (see Chapter 8).
- The term *survey, correlational,* or *ex post facto* is used (see Chapter 9).
- The term *random* or *convenience* is mentioned in relation to the sample (see Chapter 10).
- Variables are measured by instruments or scales (see Chapter 12).
- Reliability and validity of instruments are discussed (see Chapter 13).
- Statistical analyses are used (see Chapter 14).

In contrast, generally qualitative studies do not usually focus on "numbers." Some qualitative studies may use standard quantitative terms (e.g., subjects) rather than qualitative terms (e.g., informants). Deciding on the type of qualitative design can be confusing; one of the best strategies is to review this text's chapters on qualitative design (see Chapters 4 and 5), as well as to critique qualitative studies (see Chapter 6). Begin trying to link the study's design with the level of evidence associated with that design as illustrated in Figure 1-1. This will give you a context for evaluating the strength and consistency of the findings and their applicability to practice. Reading Chapters 7, 8, and 9 will increase your understanding of how to link the levels of evidence with quantitative designs, and Chapters 4 and 5 will help you do the same with qualitative designs. Although many studies may not specify the particular design used, all studies inform the reader of the specific methodology used, which can help you decide the type of design used to guide the study.

HELPFUL HINT

Remember that not all research articles include headings related to each step or component of the research process, but that each step is presented at some point in the article.

Sampling

The population from which the sample was drawn is discussed in the section entitled "Methods" or "Methodology" under the subheadings of "Subjects" or "Sample" (see Chapter 10). For example, Meneses and associates (2007) discuss the sample under the title "Subject Recruitment and Accrual" (see Appendix A). However, Jones, Renger, and Kang (2007) present the sample selection criteria in a section labeled "Sample" (see Appendix B). Researchers should tell you both the population from which the sample was chosen and the number of subjects that participated in the study, as well as if they had subjects who dropped out of the study. The authors of all of the studies in the appendices discuss their samples in enough detail so that the reader is quite clear about who the subjects are and how they were selected.

Reliability and Validity

The discussion related to instruments used to measure the variables of a study is usually included in a "Methods" section under the subheading of "Instruments" or "Measures" (see Chapter 12). The researcher usually describes the particular measure (i.e., instrument or scale) used by discussing its reliability and validity (see Chapter 13). The studies in Appendices A through D discuss each of the measures used in their "Methods" section under the subheading "Measures" or "Instruments." The reliability and validity of each measure were presented.

In some cases, researchers do not report the reliability and validity of commonly used established instruments in an article and may refer you to other references. Ask assistance from your instructor if you are in doubt about the validity or reliability of a study's instruments.

Procedures and Data Collection Methods

The procedures used to collect data or the step-by-step way that the researcher(s) used the measures (instruments or scales) is generally given under the "Procedures" head (see Chapter 12). In each of the studies in Appendices A through D, the researchers indicate how they conducted the study in detail under the subheading "Procedure" or "Instruments and Procedures"; in the Meneses and colleagues (2007) study the term *intervention fidelity* (intervention and data collection consistency) was used as this was a randomized controlled study (see Chapter 8). Notice that the researchers in each study in Appendices A, B, and D also provided information that the studies were approved by an institutional review board (see Chapter 11), thereby ensuring that each meets ethical standards.

Data Analysis/Results

The data-analysis procedures (i.e., the statistical tests used and the results of descriptive and/or inferential tests applied in quantitative studies) are presented in the section labeled "Results" or "Findings" (see Chapters 14 and 15). Although qualitative studies do not use statistical tests, the procedures for analyzing the themes, concepts, and/or observational or print data are usually described in the "Method" or "Data Collection" section and reported in the "Results," "Findings," or "Data Analysis" section (see Appendix D and Chapters 5 and 6). Landreneau and Ward-Smith (2007) report the results of their qualitative analysis in the "Data Analysis and Findings" sections of the article (see Appendix D).

Meneses and colleagues (2007) has several sections, one entitled "Data Analysis," which describes how the data were analyzed, and four subsections under "Results," which describe the results of the hypotheses tested (see Appendix A).

Discussion

The last section of a research study is the "Discussion" section. As you will find when you read Chapter 15, in this section the researchers tie together all of the pieces of the study and give a picture of the study as a whole. The researchers go back to the literature reviewed and discuss how their study is similar to or different from other studies. Researchers may report the results and discussion in one section but usually report their results in separate "Results" and "Discussion" sections (see Appendices A, B, C, and D). One way is no better than the other. Journal and space limitations determine how these sections will be handled. Any new findings or unexpected findings are usually described in the "Discussion" section.

Recommendations and Implications

In some cases a researcher reports the implications, and limitations based on the findings, for practice and education and recommends future studies in a separate section labeled "Conclusions" (see Appendices B and D); in other cases this appears in several sections labeled with such titles as "Discussion" (see Appendix C), "Limitations," "Nursing Implications," "Implications for Research and Practice" (see Appendix A), and "Summary." Again, one way is not better than the other—only different.

References

All of the references cited in a research article are included at the end of the article. The main purpose of the reference list is to support the material presented by identifying the sources in a manner that allows for easy retrieval by the reader. Journals use various referencing styles to organize references.

Communicating Results

Communicating the results of a study can take the form of a research article, poster, or paper presentation (see Chapters 17 and 18). All are valid ways of providing nurses with the data and the ability to provide high-quality patient care based on research findings. Evidence-based nursing care plans and practice protocols, guidelines, or standards are outcome measures that effectively indicate communicated research.

As you develop critical thinking and reading skills by using the strategies presented in this chapter, you will become more familiar with the research and appraisal processes. Your ability to read and critique research articles will gradually improve. You will be well on your way to becoming a knowledgeable user of research from nursing and other scientific disciplines for application in nursing practice.

HELPFUL HINT

If you have to write a paper on a specific concept or topic that requires you to critique and synthesize the findings from several studies, you might find it useful to create an evidence table of the data (see Chapters 17 and 18). Include the following information: author, date, type of study, design, level of evidence, sample, data analysis, findings, and implications.

SYSTEMATIC REVIEWS: META-ANALYSES, INTEGRATIVE REVIEWS, AND META-SYNTHESES

Another variety of articles that are appearing more frequently in the literature and which are very important to understanding evidence-based practice are articles that are labeled as systematic reviews. Systematic reviews include meta-analyses, integrative reviews, and meta-syntheses. The components of each of these will be discussed in greater detail in Chapters 5, 9, and 18. These articles take a number of studies related to a clinical question and, using a specific set of criteria and method, evaluate those articles as a whole. The methods detailed here are not prescriptive but serve as a general outline of how you will find these articles formatted. Overall, though they vary somewhat in their approach, essentially these reviews are completed to better inform and develop evidence-based practice. The Cochrane Report in Appendix E is an example of a systematic review that is a meta-analysis.

The components of these types of articles are as follows:

- *Background:* The introduction will cover content related to the background of the clinical question, as well as clarify the specific question that the review will answer. The article's authors will clarify the definitions of the concepts in the question so the reader will know the definitions that were used in assessment.
- *Method:* The methods used for searching the literature will be detailed. The exact electronic databases, the years, and the key words used to conduct the search will be provided. In addition the article will detail the inclusion and exclusion criteria for the literature chosen to review and critique. If a number of articles were found and not used, the authors will detail why articles were excluded from the review.
- *Appraisal of the literature:* The articles that are included in the review will be discussed in the body of the article and an evidence table will be used to present a snapshot of the highlights of each article (see Chapters 17 and 18). The author will use the evidence table to discuss the articles, critique them for scientific validity, and discuss how well they answer the clinical question. If the review uses a meta-analysis format, a statistical summary of the data will be presented (see Chapter 18).
- *Conclusions/Summary:* The summary will pull together the strength, quality, and consistency of the data as it applies to practice. It make recommendations about which aspects of practice are supported by the data in the articles and which aspects need further research to be done to more fully answer the question posed in the review.

CLINICAL GUIDELINES

Clinical guidelines are systematically developed statements or recommendations that serve as a guide for practitioners. Guidelines have been developed to assist in bridging practice and research. Guidelines are developed by professional organizations, government agencies, institutions, or convened expert panels. Guidelines provide clinicians with an algorithm for clinical management, or decision making for specific diseases (e.g., colon cancer) or treatments (e.g., pain management). Not all guidelines are well developed and, like research, must be assessed before implementation (see Chapter 9). Clinical guidelines, though they are systematically developed and make explicit recommendations for practice, may be formatted differently. Guidelines should present scope and purpose of the practice, detail who the development group included, demonstrate scientific rigor, be clear in its presentation, demonstrate clinical applicability, and demonstrate editorial independence. The AGREE Tool-Appraisal of Guidelines Research and Evaluation (www.agreecollaboration.org) has developed an instrument for assessing the quality of clinical guidelines. The components and assessment of clinical guidelines will be presented in Chapter 18.

As you venture through this textbook you will be challenged to think not only about reading and understanding research studies but applying the findings to your practice. Nursing has a rich legacy of research that has grown in depth and breath. Producers of research and clinicians must engage in a joint effort to translate findings into practice that will make a difference in the care of patients and families.

CRITICAL THINKING CHALLENGES

- How might a nurse differentiate research from evidence-based practice to her colleagues?
- From your clinical practice, discuss several strategies nurses can undertake to promote evidence-based practice.
- What are some strategies you can use to develop a more comprehensive critique of an evidence-based practice article?
- A number of different components are usually identified in a research article. Discuss how these sections link with one another to ensure continuity.

KEY POINTS

- The best way to develop skill in critiquing research studies is to use critical thinking and reading skills while reading research articles.
- Critical thinking and critical reading skills will enable you to question the appropriateness of the content of a research article, apply standards or critiquing criteria to assess the study's scientific merit for use in practice, or consider alternative ways of handling the same topic.
- Critical reading involves active interpretation and objective assessment of an article, looking for key concepts, ideas, and justifications.
- Critical reading requires four stages of understanding: preliminary (skimming), comprehensive, analysis, and synthesis. Each stage includes strategies to increase your critical reading skills.
- Critiquing is the process of objectively and critically evaluating the strengths and weaknesses of a research article for scientific merit and application to practice, theory, or education; the need for more research on the topic/clinical problem is also addressed at this stage.
- Critiquing criteria are the measures, standards, evaluation guides, or questions used to judge the worth of a research study.
- Each article should be reviewed for the design's level of evidence as a means of judging the application to practice.
- Research articles have different formats and styles depending on journal manuscript requirements and whether they are quantitative or qualitative studies.
- Basic steps of the research process are presented in journal articles in various ways. Detailed examples of such variations can be found in chapters throughout this text.
- Evidence-based practice begins with the careful reading and understanding of each article contributing to the practice of nursing, clinical expertise and an understanding of patient values.
- A level of evidence model is a tool for evaluating the strength (quality, quantity, and consistency) of a research study and its findings.
- Nursing research provides the basis for expanding the unique body of scientific evidence that forms the foundation of evidence-based nursing practice. Research links education, theory, and practice.

- Nurses become knowledgeable consumers of research through educational processes and practical experience. As consumers of research, nurses must have a basic understanding of the research process and critical appraisal skills that provide a standard for evaluating the strengths and weaknesses of research evidence provided by the findings of research studies before applying them in clinical practice.

REFERENCES

Agency for Healthcare Research and Quality: *Systems to rate the strength of scientific evidence. File inventory, Evidence Report/Technology Assessment No. 47*, AHRQ Publication No. 02-E016, Rockville, MD, 2002, The Author.

American Association of Critical Care Nursing (AACN): 2008.

American Nurses Association: *Code for nurses with interpretive statements*, Washington, DC, 2004, The Association.

Horgas AL, Yoon SL, Nichols AL, et al: The relationship between pain and functional disability in black and white older adults, *Res Nurs Health* 31(4):341-354, 2008.

Institute of Medicine Committee on Quality of Health Care in America: *Crossing the quality chasm: a new health system for the 21st century*, Washington, DC, 2001, National Academy Press.

Jones EG, Renger R, Kang Y: Self-efficacy for health-related behaviors among deaf adults, *Res Nurs Health* 30:185-192, 2007.

Landreneau, KJ, Ward-Smith, P: Perceptions of adult patients on hemodialysis concerning choice among renal replacement therapies, *Nephrol Nurs* 34(5):513-519, 525, 2007.

Meneses DK, McNees P, Loerzel W, et al: Transition from treatment to survivorship: effects of a psychoeducational intervention on quality of life in breast cancer survivors, *Oncol Nurs Forum* 34:1007-1016, 2007.

Publication Manual of the American Psychological Association, ed. 5, Washington, DC, 2001, American Psychological Association.

Rice VH, Stead LF: Nursing interventions for smoking cessation, *Cochrane Collaboration Issue 1*, Hoboken, NJ, 2008, John Wiley & Sons.

Sackett DL, Straus S, Richardson S, et al: *Evidence-based medicine: how to practice and teach EBM*, ed. 2, London, 2000, Churchill Livingstone.

FOR FURTHER STUDY

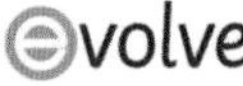

Go to Evolve at http://evolve.elsevier.com/LoBiondo/ for review questions, critiquing exercises, and additional research articles for practice in reviewing and critiquing.

2

Research Questions, Hypotheses, and Clinical Questions

Judith Haber

KEY TERMS

clinical question
complex hypothesis
dependent variable
directional hypothesis
hypothesis
independent variable
nondirectional hypothesis
population
purpose
research hypothesis
research question
statistical hypothesis
testability
theory
variable

LEARNING OUTCOMES

After reading this chapter, you should be able to do the following:

- Describe how the research question and hypothesis relate to the other components of the research process.
- Describe the process of identifying and refining a research question or hypothesis.
- Identify the criteria for determining the significance of a research question or hypothesis.
- Discuss the purpose of developing a clinical question.
- Discuss the appropriate use of the purpose, aim, or objective of a research study.
- Discuss how the purpose, research question, and hypothesis suggest the level of evidence to be obtained from the findings of a research study.
- Describe the advantages and disadvantages of directional and nondirectional hypotheses.
- Compare and contrast the use of statistical versus research hypotheses.
- Discuss the appropriate use of research questions versus hypotheses in a research study.
- Discuss the differences between a research question and a clinical question in relation to evidence-based practice.
- Identify the criteria used for critiquing a research question and hypothesis.
- Apply the critiquing criteria to the evaluation of a research question and hypothesis in a research report.

STUDY RESOURCES

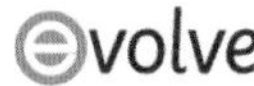

Go to Evolve at http://evolve.elsevier.com/LoBiondo/ for review questions, critiquing exercises, and additional research articles for practice in reviewing and critiquing.

As you read each chapter remember that each step of the research process will be defined and discussed as to how that particular step relates to evidence-based practice. All research studies begin with questions and hypotheses. The first step of the evidence-based practice process also asks a question, but it is a clinical question. The research questions and hypotheses in a research study discussed in the beginning of this chapter have different purposes than the clinical questions found in an evidence-based practice project. In a research study the research question and hypothesis lead to the development of a research study; the clinical question in an evidence-based practice project is the first step in the development of an evidence-based practice project.

At the beginning of this chapter you are going to learn about research questions and hypotheses from the perspective of the researcher, which, in the second part of this chapter, will help you to generate your own clinical questions that you will use to guide the development of evidence-based practice projects. From a clinician's perspective you have to understand the research question and hypothesis as it aligns with the rest of the study. As a practicing nurse, the clinical questions you will develop (see Chapters 17 and 18) represent the first step of the evidence-based practice process.

When nurses ask questions such as, "Why are things done this way?", "I wonder what would happen if … ?", "What characteristics are associated with … ?", or "What is the effect of … on patient outcomes?", they are often well on their way to developing a research question or hypothesis. Research questions are usually generated by situations that emerge from practice, leading nurses to wonder about the effectiveness of one intervention versus another for a specific patient population.

For an investigator conducting a study, the research question or hypothesis is a key preliminary step in the research process. The **research question** (sometimes called the problem statement) presents the idea that is to be examined in the study and is the foundation of the research study. The **hypothesis** attempts to answer the research question.

Hypotheses can be considered intelligent hunches, guesses, or predictions that help researchers seek a solution or answer a research question. Hypotheses are a vehicle for testing the validity of the theoretical framework assumptions and provide a bridge between **theory** (a set of interrelated concepts, definitions, and propositions) and the real world. In the scientific world, researchers derive hypotheses and research questions from theories and subject them to empirical testing. A theory's validity is not directly examined. Instead, it is through the hypotheses that the merit of a theory can be evaluated.

For a clinician making an evidence-informed decision about a patient care issue, a clinical question such as whether chlorhexidine or povidone-iodine is more effective in preventing central line catheter infections, would guide the nurse in searching for and retrieving the best available evidence that, combined with clinical expertise, and patient preferences, would provide an answer on which to base the most effective decision about patient care for this population.

You will often find research questions or hypotheses at the beginning of a research article. However, because of space constraints or stylistic considerations in such publications, they may be embedded in the purpose, aims, goals, or even in the results section of the research report. Nevertheless, it is equally important for both the consumer and the producer of research to understand the importance of research questions and hypotheses as the foundational elements of a research study. This chapter provides a working knowledge of quantitative research questions and hypotheses, as well as the standards for writing them and a set of criteria for evaluating them. It also highlights the importance of clinical questions and how to develop them.

DEVELOPING AND REFINING A RESEARCH QUESTION: STUDY PERSPECTIVE

A researcher spends a great deal of time refining a research idea into a testable research question. Unfortunately, the evaluator of a research study is not privy to this creative process because it occurs during the study's conceptualization. Although this section will not teach you how to formulate a research question, it is important to provide a glimpse of what the process of developing a research question may be like for a researcher.

Research questions or topics are not pulled from thin air. As shown in Table 2-1, research questions should indicate that practical experience, critical appraisal of the scientific literature, or interest in an untested theory was the basis for the generation of a research idea. The research question should reflect a refinement of the researcher's initial thinking. The evaluator of a research study should be able to discern that the researcher has done the following:

1. Defined a specific question area
2. Reviewed the relevant literature
3. Examined the question's potential significance to nursing
4. Pragmatically examined the feasibility of studying the research question

TABLE 2-1 How Practical Experience, Scientific Literature, and Untested Theory Influence the Development of a Research Idea

Area	Influence	Example
Practical experience	Clinical practice provides a wealth of experience from which research problems can be derived. The nurse may observe the occurrence of a particular event or pattern and become curious about why it occurs, as well as its relationship to other factors in the patient's environment.	Health professionals, including nurses, frequently advise patients to improve their health by stopping smoking. Nurse practitioners (NPs) working in a primary care practice starting a smoking cessation program want to find out if there are specific brief or intensive smoking cessation interventions led by nurses that are effective in increasing and maintaining the quit rate. Findings from a systematic review "*Nursing interventions for smoking cessation*" indicate that the effect of smoking cessation advice and/or counseling is most effective when interventions are provided by nurses whose main role is health promotion or smoking cessation. The challenge is to incorporate smoking behavior monitoring and cessation interventions as part of standard practice so that all patients are given the opportunity to be asked about their tobacco use and to be given advice and/or counseling to quit along with reinforcement and follow-up (Rice & Stead, 2008).

Continued

TABLE 2-1 How Practical Experience, Scientific Literature, and Untested Theory Influence the Development of a Research Idea—cont'd

Area	Influence	Example
Critical appraisal of the scientific literature	The critical appraisal of research studies that appear in journals may indirectly suggest a clinical problem area by stimulating the reader's thinking. The nurse may observe the outcome data from a single study or a group of related studies that provide the basis for developing a pilot study, quality improvement project, or clinical practice guideline to determine the effectiveness of this intervention in their own practice setting.	At a staff meeting, nurses, physicians, and other members of the interdisciplinary oncology team at a hospital specializing in treatment of cancer were discussing developing an algorithm to serve as an interdisciplinary protocol for the most effective interventions for treating adult cancer pain in specific treatment settings. Their search for and critical appraisal of existing clinical practice guidelines led to development of an interdisciplinary *Cancer Pain Practice Guideline,* based on National Cancer Institute (NCI) and National Cancer Consensus Network (NCCN) practice guidelines, for treatment of adult cancer pain in a variety of settings that were relevant to their patient population and clinical setting (MD Anderson Cancer Center, 2008).
Gaps in the literature	A research idea may also be suggested by a critical appraisal of the literature that identifies gaps in the literature and suggests areas for future study. Research ideas also can be generated by research reports that suggest the value of replicating a particular study to extend or refine the existing scientific knowledge base.	Rural adults have higher rates of chronic illness and physical limitations that might be prevented by increased physical activity, yet few studies have been focused on helping people increase their regular physical activity in rural environments. The study used a telephone-only motivational interviewing (MI) intervention that is different from other MI studies that included one or more in-person MI counseling sessions (Bennet, Lyons, Winter-Stone et al., 2008).
Interest in untested theory	Verification of an untested theory provides a relatively uncharted territory from which research problems can be derived. Inasmuch as theories themselves are not tested, a researcher may consider investigating a particular concept or set of concepts related to a particular nursing theory or a theory from another discipline. The researcher would pose questions such as the following: "If this theory is correct, what kind of behavior will I expect to observe in particular patients and under which conditions?" "If this theory is valid, what kind of supporting evidence will I find?"	Self-regulation theory (Johnson et al., 1997) proposes that individuals cope with illness according to their understanding of the experience. The theory emphasizes that patients need to have adequate information to gain knowledge and understanding of a specific health-related problem or risk (e.g., for breast cancer survivors, a health-related issue is lymphedema risk) and to make decisions and develop preventive or coping strategies (e.g., lymphedema risk reduction behaviors). Accordingly, patient education interventions that provide accurate information may be a critical component of lymphedema risk reduction. The use of self-regulation theory to test the effect of providing breast cancer survivors with lymphedema information on clinical outcomes has not been explored. Using Johnson's self-regulation theory to guide its development, the purpose of this study was to explore the effect of provision of lymphedema information on survivors' symptom experiences and practice of risk reduction behaviors (Fu et al., 2008).

Defining the Research Question

Brainstorming with teachers, advisors, or colleagues may provide valuable feedback that helps the researcher focus on a specific research question area. For example, suppose a researcher told a colleague that her area of interest was pain as a prevalent problem for older adults. The colleague may have said, "What is it about the topic that specifically interests you?" This conversation may have initiated a chain of thought that resulted in a decision to explore the relationship between pain and functional disability in older adults (Horgas et al., 2008) (see Appendix C). Figure 2-1 illustrates how a broad area of interest (pain as a prevalent problem for older adults) was narrowed to a specific research topic (persistent pain and its relationship to functional disability in older adults).

EVIDENCE-BASED PRACTICE TIP

A well-developed research question guides a focused search for scientific evidence about assessing, diagnosing, treating, or assisting patients with understanding of their prognosis related to a specific health problem.

Beginning the Literature Review

The literature review should reveal a relevant collection of individual studies and systematic reviews that have been critically examined. Concluding sections in such articles, that is, the recommendations and implications for practice, often identify remaining gaps in the literature, the need for replication, or the need for extension of the knowledge base about a particular research focus (see Chapter 3). In the previous example about persistent pain and functional disability in older adults, the researcher may have conducted a preliminary review of books and journals for theories and research studies on factors apparently critical to pain experience such as racial and/or ethnic differences in pain experience, pain treatment, and access to pain medications. These factors, termed *variables* in the language of research, should be potentially relevant, of interest, and measurable.

Possible relevant factors mentioned in the literature begin with an exploration of the relationship between self-reported pain intensity, acute versus chronic pain, pain management effectiveness, and functional disability. Other variables, called *demographic variables,* such as race, ethnicity, gender, age, income, education, and marital status, are also suggested as essential to consider. This information can then be used by the researcher to further define the research question and address a gap in the literature, as well as extend the knowledge base related to relationships among race (black or white), pain, and functional disability (physical and social functioning) in older adults. At this point the researcher could write the following tentative research question: "What are the relationships among race, pain, and disability in older adults?" Readers can envision the interrelatedness of the initial definition of the question area, the literature review, and the refined research question. Readers of research reports examine the end product of this process in the form of a research question and/or hypothesis, so it is important to have an appreciation of how the researcher gets to that point in constructing a study (Horgas et al., 2008) (see Appendix C).

HELPFUL HINT

Reading the literature review or theoretical framework section of a research article helps you trace the development of the implied research question and/or hypothesis.

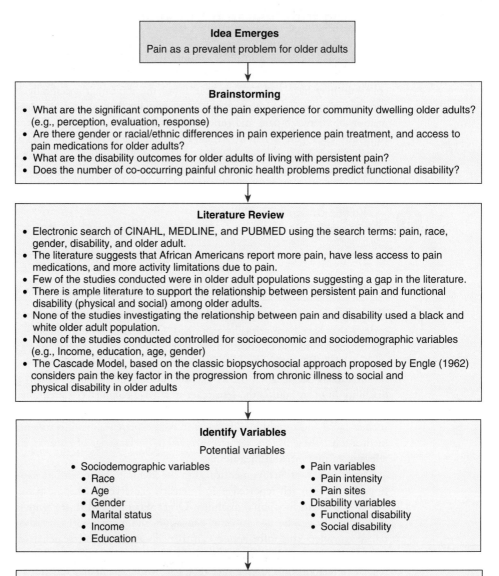

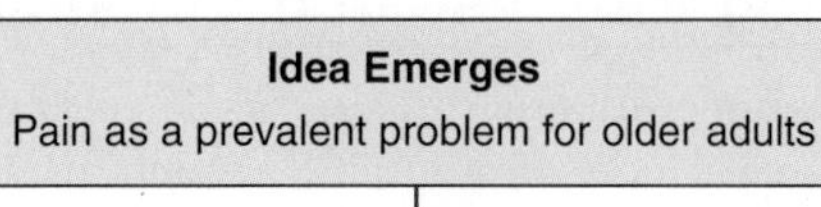

Brainstorming

- What are the significant components of the pain experience for community dwelling older adults? (e.g., perception, evaluation, response)
- Are there gender or racial/ethnic differences in pain experience pain treatment, and access to pain medications for older adults?
- What are the disability outcomes for older adults of living with persistent pain?
- Does the number of co-occurring painful chronic health problems predict functional disability?

Literature Review

- Electronic search of CINAHL, MEDLINE, and PUBMED using the search terms: pain, race, gender, disability, and older adult.
- The literature suggests that African Americans report more pain, have less access to pain medications, and more activity limitations due to pain.
- Few of the studies conducted were in older adult populations suggesting a gap in the literature.
- There is ample literature to support the relationship between persistent pain and functional disability (physical and social) among older adults.
- None of the studies investigating the relationship between pain and disability used a black and white older adult population.
- None of the studies conducted controlled for socioeconomic and sociodemographic variables (e.g., Income, education, age, gender)
- The Cascade Model, based on the classic biopsychosocial approach proposed by Engle (1962) considers pain the key factor in the progression from chronic illness to social and physical disability in older adults

Identify Variables

Potential variables

- Sociodemographic variables
  - Race
  - Age
  - Gender
  - Marital status
  - Income
  - Education
- Pain variables
  - Pain intensity
  - Pain sites
- Disability variables
  - Functional disability
  - Social disability

Research Question Formulated

What is the relationship among *race* (black/white), *pain* (pain sites and pain intensity), and *functional disability* (physical and social functional limitations) in older adults?

Figure 2-1 Development of a research question.

Examining Significance

When considering a research question, it is crucial that the researcher has examined the question's potential significance to nursing. The research question should have the potential to contribute to and extend the scientific body of nursing knowledge. Guidelines for selecting research questions should meet the following criteria.

- Patients, nurses, the medical community in general, and society will potentially benefit from the knowledge derived from the study.
- The results will be applicable for nursing practice, education, or administration.
- The results will be theoretically relevant.
- The findings will lend support to untested theoretical assumptions, extend or challenge an existing theory, fill a gap in the literature, or clarify a conflict in the literature.
- The findings will potentially provide evidence that supports developing, retaining, or revising nursing practices or policies.

If the research question has not met any of these criteria, it is wise to extensively revise the question or discard it. For example, in the previously cited research question, the significance of the question includes the following facts:

- Pain is a persistent problem in the daily lives of approximately 50% of community-dwelling older adults.
- Pain is due to the high prevalence of acute and chronic health problems in this population.
- Pain from acute and chronic conditions is a key indicator of physical and social functioning and quality of life.
- Data on racial and/or ethnic differences in pain experience indicate that African Americans report more pain, more untreated pain, and have less access to pain medications.
- Few of the studies conducted have been conducted in older adult populations.
- This study sought to fill a gap in the related literature by examining the relationships among race, pain, and functional disability in older adults.
- This study sought to extend the knowledge base about this phenomenon, thereby providing a foundation for the development and testing of interventions.

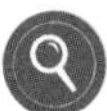

EVIDENCE-BASED PRACTICE TIP

Without a well-developed research question, the researcher may search for wrong, irrelevant, or unnecessary information. This will be a barrier to identifying the potential significance of the study.

Determining Feasibility

The feasibility of a research question must be pragmatically examined. Regardless of how significant or researchable a question may be, pragmatic considerations such as time; availability of subjects, facilities, equipment, and money; experience of the researcher; and any ethical considerations may cause the researcher to decide that the question is inappropriate because it lacks feasibility (see Chapters 4 and 7).

THE FULLY DEVELOPED RESEARCH QUESTION

When a researcher finalizes a research question, the following three characteristics should be evident:

- It clearly identifies the variables under consideration.
- It specifies the population being studied.
- It implies the possibility of empirical testing.

Because each of these elements is crucial to the formulation of a satisfactory research question, the criteria will be discussed in greater detail. These elements can often be found in the introduction of the published article; they are not always stated in an explicit manner.

HELPFUL HINT

Remember that research questions are used to guide all types of research studies, but are most often used in exploratory, descriptive, qualitative, or hypothesis-generating studies.

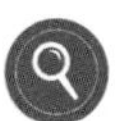

EVIDENCE-BASED PRACTICE TIP

The answers to questions generated by qualitative data reflect evidence that may provide the first insights about a phenomenon that has not been previously studied.

Variables

Researchers call the properties that they study variables. Such properties take on different values. Thus a **variable** is, as the name suggests, something that varies. Properties that differ from each other, such as age, weight, height, religion, and ethnicity, are examples of variables. Researchers attempt to understand how and why differences in one variable relate to differences in another variable. For example, a researcher may be concerned about the variable of pneumonia in postoperative patients on ventilators in critical care units. It is a variable because not all critically ill postoperative patients on ventilators have pneumonia. A researcher may also be interested in what other factors can be linked to ventilator-acquired pneumonia (VAP). There is clinical evidence to suggest that elevation of the head of the bed is also associated with VAP. You can see that these factors are also variables that need to be considered in relation to the development of VAP in postoperative patients.

When speaking of variables, the researcher is essentially asking, "Is **X** related to **Y**? What is the effect of **X** on **Y**? How are $\mathbf{X_1}$ and $\mathbf{X_2}$ related to **Y**?" The researcher is asking a question about the relationship between one or more independent variables and a dependent variable. (*Note:* In cases in which multiple independent or dependent variables are present, subscripts are used to indicate the number of variables under consideration.)

An **independent variable,** usually symbolized by **X,** is the variable that has the presumed effect on the dependent variable. In experimental research studies, the researcher manipulates the independent variable. For example, a nurse may study how different methods of administering pain medication affect the patient's perception of pain intensity. The researcher may manipulate the independent variable (i.e., the method of administering pain medication) by using nurse-controlled versus patient-controlled administration of analgesia (see Chapter 8). In nonexperimental research, the independent variable is not manipulated and is assumed to have occurred naturally before or during the study. For example, the researcher may be studying the relationship between gender and perception of pain intensity. The independent vari-

TABLE 2-2 Research Question Format

Type	Format	Example
QUANTITATIVE		
Correlational	Is there a relationship between **X** (independent variable) and **Y** (dependent variable) in the specified population?	Is there a relationship between pain and functional disability in black and white older adults? (Horgas et al., 2008)
Comparative	Is there a difference in **Y** (dependent variable) between people who have **X** characteristic (independent variable) and those who do not have **X** characteristic?	Do mothers who received a home-based nursing intervention for infant irritability report less parenting stress than mothers who did not receive the intervention? (Keefe et al., 2006)
Experimental	Is there a difference in **Y** (dependent variable) between Group A who received **X** (independent variable) and Group B who did not receive **X?**	What is the difference in physical, social, and emotional adjustment in women with breast cancer (and their partners) who have received phase-specific standardized education by video vs. phase-specific telephone counseling? (Budin et al., 2008)
QUALITATIVE		
Phenomenological	What is/was it like to have **X?**	What is the meaning of the health care provider (HCP) relationship for women with chronic illness and how they believe it affected their health? (Fox & Chesla, 2008)

able—gender—is not manipulated; it is just presumed to occur and is observed and measured as it naturally happens (see Chapter 9).

The **dependent variable,** represented by **Y,** is often referred to as the consequence or the presumed effect that varies with a change in the independent variable. The dependent variable is not manipulated. It is observed and assumed to vary with changes in the independent variable. Predictions are made from the independent variable to the dependent variable. It is the dependent variable that the researcher is interested in understanding, explaining, or predicting. For example, it might be assumed that the perception of pain intensity (i.e., the dependent variable) will vary in relation to a person's gender (i.e., the independent variable). In this case we are trying to explain the perception of pain intensity in relation to gender, that is, male or female. Although variability in the dependent variable is assumed to depend on changes in the independent variable, this does not imply that there is a causal relationship between **X** and **Y** or that changes in variable **X** cause variable **Y** to change.

Let us look at an example in which nurses' attitudes toward patients with hepatitis C were studied. The researcher discovered that older nurses had a more negative attitude about patients with hepatitis C than younger nurses. The researcher did not conclude that the nurses' negative attitudes toward patients with hepatitis C were because of their age, but at the same time it is apparent that there is a directional relationship between age and negative attitudes about patients with hepatitis C. That is, as the nurses' ages increase, their attitudes about patients with hepatitis C become more negative. This example highlights the fact that causal relationships are not necessarily implied by the independent and dependent variables; rather, only a relational statement with possible directionality is proposed. Table 2-2 presents a number of examples of research questions. Practice substituting other variables for the examples in Table 2-2. You will be surprised at the skill you develop in writing and critiquing research questions with greater ease.

Although one independent variable and one dependent variable are used in the examples just given, there is no restriction on the number of variables that can be included in a research question. Remember, however, that questions should not be unnecessarily complex or unwieldy, particularly in beginning research efforts. Research questions that include more than one independent or dependent variable may be broken down into subquestions that are more concise.

Finally, it should be noted that variables are not inherently independent or dependent. A variable that is classified as independent in one study may be considered dependent in another study. For example, a nurse may review an article about sexual behaviors that are predictive of risk for human immunodeficiency virus (HIV)/acquired immunodeficiency syndrome (AIDS). In this case, HIV/AIDS is the dependent variable. When another article about the relationship between HIV/AIDS and maternal parenting practices is considered, HIV/AIDS status is the independent variable. Whether a variable is independent or dependent is a function of the role it plays in a particular study.

Population

The **population** (a well-defined set that has certain properties) is either specified or implied in the research question. If the scope of the question has been narrowed to a specific focus and the variables have been clearly identified, the nature of the population will be evident to the reader of a research report. For example, a research question may ask, "What is the effect of a psychoeducational intervention on quality of life (QOL) in breast cancer survivors in posttreatment survivorship?" This question suggests that the population under consideration includes breast cancer survivors who have completed treatment for breast cancer (e.g., surgery, adjuvant therapy, reconstruction). It is also implied that some of the breast cancer survivors were involved in a psychoeducational intervention (consisting of face-to-face sessions and monthly follow-up sessions by telephone and in person) in contrast to other survivors (who received four monthly control telephone calls). The researcher or reader will have an initial idea of the composition of the study population from the outset (see Chapter 10).

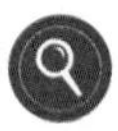

EVIDENCE-BASED PRACTICE TIP

Make sure that the population of interest and the setting have been clearly described so that if you were going to replicate the study, you would know exactly who the study population needed to be.

Testability

The research question must imply that it is **testable,** that is, measurable by either qualitative or quantitative methods. For example, the research question "Should postoperative patients control how much pain medication they receive?" is stated incorrectly for a variety of reasons. One reason is that it is not testable; it represents a value statement rather than a research question. A scientific research question must propose a relationship between an independent and a dependent variable and do this in such a way that it indicates that the variables of the relationship can somehow be measured. Many interesting and important clinical questions are not valid research questions because they are not amenable to testing.

The question "Should postoperative patients control how much pain medication they receive?" could be revised from a philosophical question to a research question that implies testability. Two examples of the revised research question might be the following.

TABLE 2-3 Components of the Research Question and Related Criteria

Variables	Population	Testability
Independent variable: Pain intensity Pain sites Race Health (number of limiting diagnoses) *Dependent variable:* Management effectiveness Functional status	Black and white older adults	Differential effect of pain intensity and number of painful sites on functional disability (physical and social functioning)

- Is there a relationship between patient-controlled analgesia (PCA) versus nurse-administered analgesia and perception of postoperative pain?
- What is the effect of PCA on pain ratings by postoperative patients?

These examples illustrate the relationship between the variables, identify the independent and dependent variables, and imply the testability of the research question.

Now that the elements of the formal research question have been presented in greater detail, this information can be integrated by formulating a formal research question about whether self-reported pain (pain sites and pain intensity) and disability (physical and social functional limitations) differ between black and white older adults. This research question was originally derived from a general area of interest—pain experiences of older adults of different racial groups. The topic was more specifically defined by delineating a particular research question, self-reported pain and outcomes (e.g., physical and social functional limitations). The question crystallized further after a preliminary literature review (Horgas et al., 2008). Table 2-3 identifies the components of this research question as they relate to and are congruent with the three research question criteria.

HELPFUL HINT

- Remember that research questions are often not explicitly stated. The reader has to infer the research question from the title of the report, the abstract, the introduction, or the purpose.
- Using your focused question, search the literature for the best available answer to your clinical question.

STUDY PURPOSE, AIMS, OR OBJECTIVES

Once the research question is developed and the literature review is critiqued in terms of the level, strength, and quality of evidence available for the particular research question, the purpose, aims, or objectives of the study become focused so that the researcher can decide whether a hypothesis should be tested or a research question answered.

The **purpose** of the study encompasses the aims or objectives the investigator hopes to achieve with the research, not the question to be answered. These three terms are synonymous with each other. For example, a nurse working with rehabilitation patients who have bladder dysfunction may be disturbed by the high incidence of urinary tract infections. The nurse may propose the following research question: "What is the optimum frequency of changing

BOX 2-1 Examples of Purpose Statements

- The purpose of this study was to evaluate the short and long-term effects of smoking cessation strategies tailored to the pregnant to attain and maintain abstinence (Albrecht et al., 2006).
- The aim of this study was to explore what patients on hemodialysis perceive concerning choice among three types of renal replacement therapies: transplantation, hemodialysis, and peritoneal dialysis (Landreneau & Ward-Smith, 2007).
- The primary purpose of this prospective randomized controlled trial of 56 cancer survivors was to test whether motivational interviewing (MI) would help long-term cancer survivors increase their participation in self-selected regular physical activities (Bennett et al., 2007).
- The objective of this study was to evaluate patient characteristics to predict selection and maintenance of a complementary therapy and the feasibility of a randomized clinical trial of complementary therapies (Wyatt, Sikorski, Siddiqi et al., 2007).
- The aims of this study were to determine whether a tailored, nurse-delivered adherence intervention program—Client Adherence Profiling and Intervention Tailoring (CAP-IT)—improved adherence to HIV medication compared to standard care (Holzemer et al., 2006).

urinary drainage bags in patients with bladder dysfunction to reduce the incidence of urinary tract infection?" If this nurse were to design a study, its purpose might be to determine the differential effect of a 1-week versus a 4-week urinary drainage bag change schedule on the incidence of urinary tract infections in patients with bladder dysfunction.

The purpose communicates more than just the nature of the question. Through the researcher's selection of verbs, the purpose statement suggests the manner in which the researcher planned to study the question and the level of evidence to be obtained through the study findings. Verbs such as *discover, explore,* or *describe* suggest an investigation of an infrequently researched topic that might appropriately be guided by research questions rather than hypotheses. In contrast, verb statements indicating that the purpose is to test the effectiveness of an intervention or compare two alternative nursing strategies suggest a study with a better-established knowledge base that is hypothesis testing in nature. You should remember that when the purpose of a study is to test the effectiveness of an intervention or compare the effectiveness of two or more interventions, the level of evidence is likely to have more strength and rigor than a study whose purpose is to explore or describe phenomena. Box 2-1 provides other examples of purpose, aims, and objectives.

EVIDENCE-BASED PRACTICE TIP

The purpose, aims, or objectives often provide the most information about the intent of the research question and hypotheses and suggest the level of evidence to be obtained from the findings of the study.

DEVELOPING THE RESEARCH HYPOTHESIS

Like the research question, hypotheses are often not stated explicitly in a research article. The evaluator will often find that hypotheses are embedded in the data analysis, results, or discussion section of the research report. Similarly, the population may not be explicitly stated but will have been identified in the background, significance, and literature review. It is then up to you to discern the nature of the hypotheses and population being tested. For example, in

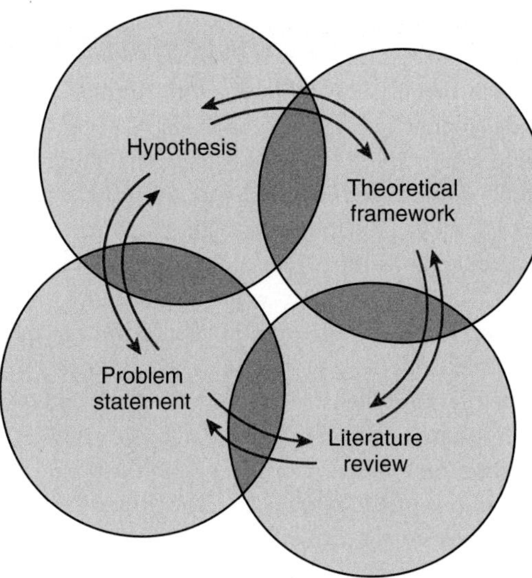

Figure 2-2 Interrelationships of research question, literature review, theoretical framework, and hypothesis.

the study by Meneses and colleagues (2007), the hypotheses are embedded in the Methods section of the article; you must interpret that the statement, "The overall hypotheses are to determine the effect of the breast cancer psychoeducational intervention (BCEI) on overall quality of life (QOL) and on the individual quality of life (QOL) and to examine whether the effects of the intervention were durable over time," represents the hypotheses that test the effect of the BCEI on QOL in female breast cancer survivors. In light of that stylistic reality, it is important for you to be acquainted with the components of hypotheses, how they are developed, and the standards for writing and evaluating them.

Hypotheses flow from the research question, literature review, and theoretical framework. Figure 2-2 illustrates this flow. A **hypothesis** is a statement about the relationship between two or more variables that suggests an answer to the research question. A hypothesis is a declarative statement that predicts an expected outcome. It explains or predicts the relationship or differences between two or more variables in terms of expected results or outcomes of a study. Hypotheses are formulated before the study is actually conducted because they provide direction for the collection, analysis, and interpretation of data.

HELPFUL HINT

When hypotheses are not explicitly stated by the author at the end of the Introduction section or just before the Methods section, they will be embedded or implied in the Results or Discussion section of a research article.

Characteristics

Nurses who are conducting research or critiquing published research studies must have a working knowledge about what constitutes a "good" hypothesis. Such knowledge will enable them to have a standard for evaluating their own work or the work of others. The following discussion about the characteristics of hypotheses presents criteria to be used when formulating or evaluating a hypothesis.

Relationship Statement

The first characteristic of a hypothesis is that it is a declarative statement that identifies the predicted relationship between two or more variables. This implies that there is a systematic relationship between an independent variable **(X)** and a dependent variable **(Y).** The direction of the predicted relationship is also specified in this statement. Phrases such as *greater than; less than; positively, negatively,* or *curvilinearly related;* and *difference in* connote the directionality that is proposed in the hypothesis. The following is an example of a directional hypothesis: "The rate of continuous smoking abstinence (dependent variable) at 6 months postpartum, based on self-report and biochemical validation, will be significantly higher in the treatment group (postpartum counseling intervention) than in the control group (independent variable)." The dependent and independent variables are explicitly identified, and the relational aspect of the prediction in the hypothesis is contained in the phrase *significantly higher than.*

The nature of the relationship, either causal or associative, is also implied by the hypothesis. A causal relationship is one in which the researcher can predict that the independent variable **(X)** causes a change in the dependent variable **(Y).** In research, it is rare that one is in a firm enough position to take a definitive stand about a cause-and-effect relationship. For example, a researcher might hypothesize that blood pressure telemonitoring plus usual care would lead to a greater reduction in blood pressure than usual care alone from baseline over a 12-month follow-up (Artinian et al., 2007). It would be difficult for a researcher to predict a strong cause-and-effect relationship, however, because of the multiple intervening variables (e.g., age, medication, and lifestyle changes) that might also influence the subject's health status.

Variables are more commonly related in noncausal ways; that is, the variables are systematically related but in an associative way. This means that the variables change in relation to each other. For example, there is strong evidence that asbestos exposure is related to lung cancer. It is tempting to state that there is a causal relationship between asbestos exposure and lung cancer. Do not overlook the fact, however, that not all of those who have been exposed to asbestos will have lung cancer and not all of those who have lung cancer have had asbestos exposure. Consequently, it would be scientifically unsound to take a position advocating the presence of a causal relationship between these two variables. Rather, one can say only that there is an associative relationship between the variables of asbestos exposure and lung cancer, a relationship in which there is a strong systematic association between the two phenomena.

Testability

The second characteristic of a hypothesis is its **testability.** This means that the variables of the study must lend themselves to observation, measurement, and analysis. The hypothesis is either supported or not supported after the data have been collected and analyzed. The predicted outcome proposed by the hypothesis will or will not be congruent with the actual outcome when the hypothesis is tested. Hypotheses advance scientific knowledge by confirming or refuting theories.

Hypotheses may fail to meet the criteria of testability because the researcher has not made a prediction about the anticipated outcome, the variables are not observable or measurable, or the hypothesis is couched in terms that are value-laden.

HELPFUL HINT

When a hypothesis is **complex** (i.e., it contains more than one independent or dependent variable), it is difficult for the findings to indicate unequivocally that the hypothesis is supported or not supported. In such cases, the reader must infer which relationships are significant in the predicted direction from the Findings or Discussion section.

Theory Base

A sound hypothesis is consistent with an existing body of theory and research findings. Whether a hypothesis is arrived at on the basis of a review of the literature or a clinical observation, it must be based on a sound scientific rationale. Readers should be able to identify the flow of ideas from the research idea to the literature review, to the theoretical framework, and through the research question(s) or hypotheses. For example, Jones and colleagues (2007) (Appendix B) investigated the effectiveness of the Deaf Heart Health Intervention (DHHI), which is an education program taught in sign language by a trained deaf lay heart-health teacher about modifiable cardiovascular disease (CVD) risk factors and principles of health behavior change. The study questioned whether DHHI increased self-efficacy for health behaviors related to risk for CVD among culturally deaf adults. Self-efficacy was a key construct used for the theoretical framework because it is a key factor in understanding and modifying health behaviors.

Wording the Hypothesis

As you read the scientific literature and become more familiar with it, you will observe that there are a variety of ways to word a hypothesis. Regardless of the specific format used to state the hypothesis, the statement should be worded in clear, simple, and concise terms. If this criterion is met, the reader will understand the following:

- The variables of the hypothesis
- The population being studied
- The predicted outcome of the hypothesis

Information about hypotheses may be further clarified in the Instruments, Sample, or Methods sections of a research report (see Chapters 10 and 12).

Statistical versus Research Hypotheses

Readers of research reports may observe that a hypothesis is further categorized as either a research or a statistical hypothesis. A **research hypothesis,** also known as a scientific hypothesis, consists of a statement about the expected relationship of the variables. A research hypothesis indicates what the outcome of the study is expected to be. A research hypothesis is also either directional or nondirectional. If the researcher obtains statistically significant findings for a research hypothesis, the hypothesis is supported. For example, in a study evaluating the effectiveness of a home-based nursing intervention in reducing parenting stress in three groups of families with irritable infants, the research hypothesis was that "Mothers who received the home-based nursing intervention (REST—reassurance, empathy, support, and time-out) for infant irritability will report less parenting stress than the mothers who did not receive the intervention" (Keefe et al., 2006). Because the findings for this hypothesis were

TABLE 2-4 Examples of How Hypotheses Are Worded

Variables*	Hypothesis	Type of Design; Level of Evidence Suggested
1. THERE ARE SIGNIFICANT DIFFERENCES IN SELF-REPORTED CANCER PAIN, SYMPTOMS ACCOMPANYING PAIN, AND FUNCTIONAL STATUS ACCORDING TO SELF-REPORTED ETHNIC IDENTITY.		
IV: Ethnic identity DV: Self-reported cancer pain DV: Symptoms accompanying pain DV: Functional status	Nondirectional, research	Nonexperimental; Level IV
2. INDIVIDUALS WHO PARTICIPATE IN USUAL CARE (UC) PLUS BLOOD PRESSURE (BP) TELEMONITORING (TM) WILL HAVE A GREATER REDUCTION IN BP FROM BASELINE TO 12-MONTH FOLLOW-UP THAN WOULD INDIVIDUALS WHO RECEIVE UC ONLY.		
IV: Telemonitoring (TM) IV: Usual care (UC) DV: Blood pressure	Directional, research	Experimental; Level II
3. THERE WILL BE A GREATER DECREASE IN STATE ANXIETY SCORES FOR PATIENTS RECEIVING STRUCTURED INFORMATIONAL VIDEOS BEFORE ABDOMINAL OR CHEST TUBE REMOVAL THAN FOR PATIENTS RECEIVING STANDARD INFORMATION.		
IV: Preprocedure structured videotape information IV: Standard information DV: State anxiety	Directional, research	Experimental; Level II
4. THE INCIDENCE AND DEGREE OF SEVERITY OF SUBJECT DISCOMFORT WILL BE LESS AFTER ADMINISTRATION OF MEDICATIONS BY THE Z-TRACK INTRAMUSCULAR INJECTION TECHNIQUE THAN AFTER ADMINISTRATION OF MEDICATIONS BY THE STANDARD INTRAMUSCULAR INJECTION TECHNIQUE.		
IV: Z-track intramuscular injection technique IV: Standard intramuscular injection technique DV: Subject discomfort	Directional, research	Experimental; Level II
5. NURSES WITH HIGH SOCIAL SUPPORT FROM CO-WORKERS HAVE LOW PERCEIVED JOB STRESS.		
IV: Social support DV: Perceived job stress	Directional, research	Nonexperimental; Level IV
6. THERE WILL BE NO DIFFERENCE IN ANESTHETIC COMPLICATION RATES BETWEEN HOSPITALS THAT RELY PRIMARILY ON CERTIFIED REGISTERED NURSE ANESTHETIST (CRNA) OBSTETRICAL ANESTHESIA VERSUS THOSE THAT RELY PRIMARILY ON ANESTHESIOLOGISTS.		
IV: Type of anesthesia provider (CRNA or MD) DV: Anesthesia complication rates	Nondirectional; null	Nonexperimental; Level IV
7. THERE WILL BE NO SIGNIFICANT DIFFERENCE IN THE DURATION OF PATENCY OF A 24-GAUGE INTRAVENOUS LOCK IN A NEONATAL PATIENT WHEN FLUSHED WITH 0.5 ml OF HEPARINIZED SALINE (2 U/ml), STANDARD PRACTICE, COMPARED WITH 0.5 ml OF 0.9% NORMAL SALINE.		
IV: Heparinized saline IV: Normal saline DV: Duration of patency of intravenous lock	Nondirectional; null	Experimental; Level II

*Abbreviations: *IV*, independent variable; *DV*, dependent variable.

TABLE 2-5 Examples of Statistical Hypotheses

Hypothesis	Variables*	Type of Hypothesis	Type of Design Suggested
Oxygen inhalation by nasal cannula of up to 6 L/min does not affect oral temperature measurement taken with an electronic thermometer.	IV: Oxygen inhalation by nasal cannula DV: Oral temperature	Statistical; null	Experimental
There will be no difference in the performance accuracy of adult nurse practitioners (ANPs) and family nurse practitioners (FNPs) in formulating accurate diagnoses and acceptable interventions for suspected cases of domestic violence.	IV: Nurse practitioner (ANP or FNP) category DV: Diagnosis and intervention performance accuracy	Statistical; null	Nonexperimental

*Abbreviations: *IV*, independent variable; *DV*, dependent variable.

not statistically significant, the hypothesis was not supported, thereby indicating that the REST intervention did not significantly reduce parenting stress for parents with irritable infants. The examples in Table 2-4 represent research hypotheses.

A **statistical hypothesis,** also known as a null hypothesis, states that there is no relationship between the independent and dependent variables. The examples in Table 2-5 illustrate statistical hypotheses. If, in the data analysis, a statistically significant relationship emerges between the variables at a specified level of significance, the null hypothesis is rejected. Rejection of the statistical hypothesis is equivalent to acceptance of the research hypothesis. For example, a study by Simonson and colleagues (2007) that sought to identify differences in the rates of anesthetic complications in hospitals whose obstetrical anesthesia is provided solely by certified registered nurse anesthetists (CRNAs) compared to hospitals with only anesthesiologists. The null hypothesis, that there would be no differences in anesthetic complication rates between the hospitals that rely primarily on CRNA obstetrical anesthesia versus those that rely primarily on anesthesiologists, was supported, thereby indicating that there were no differences in anesthesia-related complications according to the type of provider, nurse anesthetist or physician. Because the difference in outcomes was not greater than expected by chance, the null hypothesis was accepted (see Chapter 18).

Some researchers refer to the null hypothesis as a statistical contrivance that obscures a straightforward prediction of the outcome. Others state that it is more exact and conservative statistically, and that failure to reject the null hypothesis implies that there is insufficient evidence to support the idea of a real difference. You will note that when hypotheses are stated, research hypotheses are generally used more often than statistical hypotheses because they are more desirable to state the researcher's expectation. Readers then have a more precise idea of the proposed outcome. In any study that involves statistical analysis, the underlying null hypothesis is usually assumed without being explicitly stated.

Directional versus Nondirectional Hypotheses

Hypotheses can be formulated directionally or nondirectionally. A **directional hypothesis** is one that specifies the expected direction of the relationship between the independent and dependent variables. The reader of a directional hypothesis may observe not only the proposal of a relationship but also the nature or direction of that relationship. The following is an example of a directional hypothesis: "Culturally deaf adults who receive the DHHI would demonstrate greater self-efficacy for targeted health-related behaviors than deaf adults who do not receive the DHHI" (Jones et al., 2007) (see Appendix B). Examples of directional hypotheses can also be found in examples 2 through 7 in Table 2-4.

Whereas a **nondirectional hypothesis** indicates the existence of a relationship between the variables, it does not specify the anticipated direction of the relationship. For example, in a study to determine if proteins expressed in nipple aspirate fluid (NAF) serve to detect inflammatory or premalignant states, the following nondirectional hypothesis was used: "A relation exists between women's reproductive, nutritional, and body composition, and activity factors and the amount of C-reactive protein (CRP) in NAF" (Lithgow, Nyamathi, & Elashoff et al., 2006). Nurses who are learning to critique research studies should be aware that both the directional and the nondirectional forms of hypothesis statements are acceptable. They should also be aware that there are definite pros and cons pertaining to each one.

Proponents of the nondirectional hypothesis state that this format is more objective and impartial than the directional hypothesis. It is argued that the directional hypothesis is potentially biased, because the researcher, in stating an anticipated outcome, has demonstrated a commitment to a particular position.

On the other side of the coin, proponents of the directional hypothesis argue that researchers naturally have hunches, guesses, or expectations about the outcome of their research. It is the hunch, the curiosity, or the guess that initially leads them to speculate about the question. The literature review and the conceptual framework provide the theoretical foundation for deriving the hypothesis. For example, the theory (e.g., self-efficacy theory) will provide a critical rationale for proposing that relationships between variables will have particular outcomes. When there is no theory or related research to draw on for rationale or when findings in previous research studies are ambivalent, a nondirectional hypothesis may be appropriate. As you read research articles, you will note that directional hypotheses are much more commonly used than nondirectional hypotheses.

In summary, when you evaluate a hypothesis you should know that there are several advantages to directional hypotheses, making them appropriate for use in most studies. The advantages are as follows:

- Directional hypotheses indicate that a theory base has been used to derive the hypotheses and that the phenomena under investigation have been critically examined and interrelated. You should realize that nondirectional hypotheses may also be deduced from a theory base. Because of the exploratory nature of many studies using nondirectional hypotheses, however, the theory base may not be as developed.
- They provide you with a specific theoretical frame of reference, within which the study is being conducted.
- They suggest to that the researcher is not sitting on a theoretical fence, and as a result, the analyses of data can be accomplished in a statistically more sensitive way.

The important point for you to keep in mind about the directionality of the hypotheses is whether there is a sound rationale for the choice the researcher has proposed regarding directionality.

TABLE 2-6 Elements of a Clinical Question

Population	Intervention	Comparison Intervention	Outcome
People with advanced cancer	Pain diaries	No pain diaries	Increased pain control

RELATIONSHIP BETWEEN THE HYPOTHESIS, THE RESEARCH QUESTION, AND THE RESEARCH DESIGN

Regardless of whether the researcher uses a statistical or a research hypothesis, there is a suggested relationship between the hypothesis, the research design of the study, and the level of evidence provided by the results of the study. The type of design, experimental or nonexperimental (see Chapters 8 and 9), will influence the wording of the hypothesis. For example, when an experimental design is used, the research consumer would expect to see hypotheses that reflect relationship statements, such as the following:

- $\mathbf{X_1}$ is more effective than $\mathbf{X_2}$ on **Y.**
- The effect of $\mathbf{X_1}$ on **Y** is greater than that of $\mathbf{X_2}$ on **Y.**
- The incidence of **Y** will not differ in subjects receiving $\mathbf{X_1}$ and $\mathbf{X_2}$ treatments.
- The incidence of **Y** will be greater in subjects after $\mathbf{X_1}$ than after $\mathbf{X_2}$.

Such hypotheses indicate that an experimental treatment (i.e., independent variable **X**) will be used and that two groups of subjects, experimental and control groups, are being used to test whether the difference in the outcome (i.e., dependent variable **Y**) predicted by the hypothesis actually exists. Hypotheses reflecting experimental designs also test the effect of the experimental treatment (i.e., independent variable **X**) on the outcome (i.e., dependent variable **Y**). This would suggest that the strength of the evidence provided by the results would be Level II (experimental design) or Level III (quasi-experimental design).

In contrast, hypotheses related to nonexperimental designs reflect associative relationship statements, such as the following:

- **X** will be negatively related to **Y.**
- There will be a positive relationship between **X** and **Y.**

This would suggest that the strength of the evidence provided by the results of a study that examined hypotheses with associative relationship statements would be at Level IV (nonexperimental design).

Table 2-6 provides additional examples of this concept. The Critical Thinking Decision Path shown in the following diagram will help you determine the type of hypothesis presented in a study, as well as the study's readiness for a hypothesis-testing design.

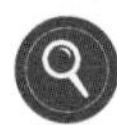

EVIDENCE-BASED PRACTICE TIP

Think about the relationship between the wording of the hypothesis, the type of research design suggested, and the level of evidence provided by the findings of a study using each kind of hypothesis. You may want to consider which type of hypothesis potentially will yield the strongest results applicable to practice.

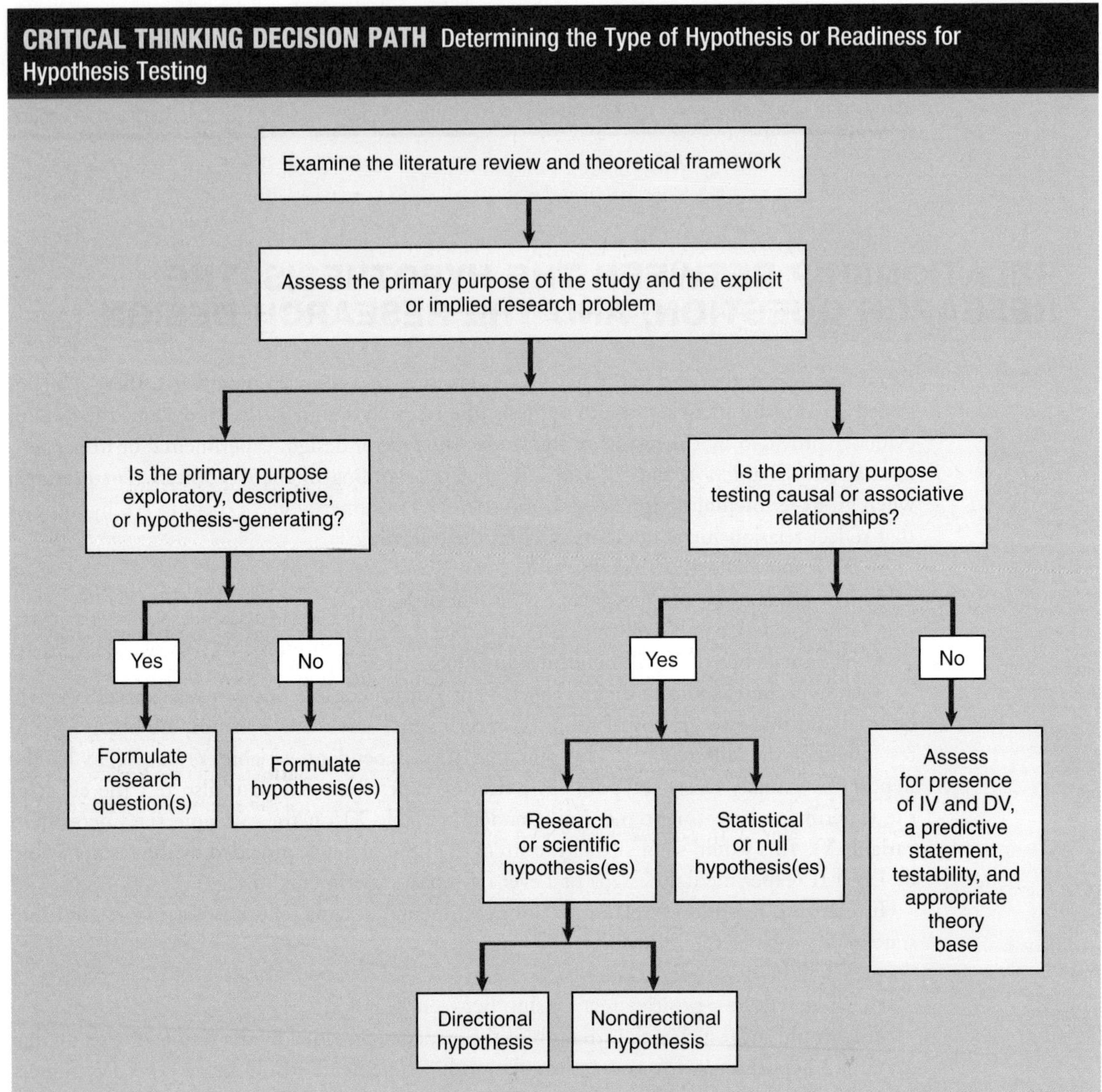
CRITICAL THINKING DECISION PATH Determining the Type of Hypothesis or Readiness for Hypothesis Testing
Examine the literature review and theoretical framework
Assess the primary purpose of the study and the explicit or implied research problem
Is the primary purpose exploratory, descriptive, or hypothesis-generating?
Is the primary purpose testing causal or associative relationships?
Yes
No
Yes
No
Formulate research question(s)
Formulate hypothesis(es)
Research or scientific hypothesis(es)
Statistical or null hypothesis(es)
Assess for presence of IV and DV, a predictive statement, testability, and appropriate theory base
Directional hypothesis
Nondirectional hypothesis

BOX 2-2 Components of a Clinical Question Using the PICO Format

Population: The individual patient or group of patients with a particular condition or health care problem (e.g., adolescents age 13 to 18 with type 1 insulin-dependent diabetes)

Intervention: The particular aspect of health care that is of interest to the nurse or the health team (e.g., a therapeutic [inhaler or nebulizer for treatment of asthma], a preventive [pneumonia vaccine], a diagnostic [measurement of blood pressure], or an organizational [implementation of a bar coding system to reduce medication errors] intervention)

Comparison intervention: Standard care or no intervention (e.g., antibiotic in comparison to ibuprofen for children with otitis media); a comparison of two treatment settings (e.g., rehabilitation center or home care)

Outcome: More effective outcome (e.g., improved glycemic control, decreased hospitalizations, decreased medication errors)

DEVELOPING AND REFINING A CLINICAL QUESTION: A CONSUMER'S PERSPECTIVE

Practicing nurses, as well as students, are challenged to keep their practice up-to-date by searching for, retrieving, and critiquing research articles that apply to practice issues that are encountered in their clinical setting (Cullum, 2000). Practitioners strive to use the current best evidence from research in making clinical and health care decisions. Although research consumers are not conducting research studies, their search for information from practice is also converted into focused, structured clinical questions that are the foundation of evidence-based practice. **Clinical questions** often arise from clinical situations for which there are no ready answers. You have probably had the experience of asking, *What is the most effective treatment for … ?* or *Why do we still do it this way?*

Using similar criteria related to framing a research question, focused clinical questions are used as a basis for searching the literature to identify supporting evidence from research. Clinical questions have four components:

- Population
- Intervention
- Comparison
- Outcome

The four components, known as PICO, a format that is effective in helping nurses develop searchable clinical questions. Box 2-2 presents each component of the clinical question.

The significance of the clinical question becomes obvious as the research evidence from the literature is critiqued. The research evidence is used side by side with clinical expertise and the patient's perspective to develop or revise nursing standards, protocols, and policies that are used to plan and implement patient care (Cullum, 2000; Sackett et al., 2000; Thompson et al., 2004). Issues or questions can arise from multiple clinical and managerial situations. Using the example of pain, albeit from a different perspective, a nurse working in a palliative care setting wondered whether completing pain diaries was a useful thing in the palliative care of patients with advanced cancer. She wondered whether time was being spent developing something that had previously been shown to be useless or even harmful. After all, it is conceivable that monitoring one's pain in a diary actually heightens one's awareness and experience

BOX 2-3 Examples of Clinical Questions

- What are the most effective decision aids to support oncology patients' participation in clinical decision making? (Stacey et al., 2008)
- In overweight or obese people with type 2 diabetes, does an intensive lifestyle intervention reduce weight and cardiovascular disease risk factors? (Pi-Sunyer et al., 2007)
- Are diet and/or exercise effective for weight reduction in postpartum women? (Amorim et al., 2007)
- In patients with multiple behavioral risk factors for cardiovascular disease, is sequential counseling (SQC) that targets one behavior at a time more effective than simultaneous counseling that targets multiple behaviors? (Hyman et al., 2007)
- In patients requiring mechanical ventilation for greater than 48 hours, is oral decontamination with chlorhexidene (CHX) or CHX plus colistin (COL) effective for reducing ventilator-associated pneumonia (VAP)? (Koeman et al., 2006)
- What is the effect of arch supports on balance, functional mobility, and back pain and lower extremity joint pain in older adults? (Mulford et al., 2008)
- Is there a significant difference in the effect of different body positions on blood pressure in healthy young adults? (Eser et al., 2007)
- In people with impaired glucose tolerance, do lifestyle or pharmacological interventions prevent or delay onset of type 2 diabetes? (Gillies et al., 2007)
- What are the experiences of middle-aged people living with chronic heart failure? (Nordgren et al., 2007)

of pain. To focus the nurse's search of the literature, she developed the following question: *Does the use of pain diaries in the palliative care of patients with cancer lead to improved pain control?* Sometimes it is helpful for nurses who develop clinical questions from a consumer perspective to consider three elements as they frame their focused question: (1) the situation, (2) the intervention, and (3) the outcome:

- The situation is the patient or problem being addressed. This can be a single patient or a group of patients with a particular health problem (palliative care of patients with cancer).
- The intervention is the dimension of health care interest and often asks whether a particular intervention is a useful treatment (pain diaries).
- The outcome addresses the effect of the treatment (intervention) for this patient or patient population in terms of quality and cost (decreased pain perception/low cost). It essentially answers whether the intervention makes a difference for the patient population.

The individual parts of the question are vital pieces of information to remember when it comes to searching for evidence in the literature. One of the easiest ways to do this is to use a table as illustrated in Table 2-6. Examples of clinical questions are highlighted in Box 2-3. Chapter 3 will provide examples of how to effectively search the literature to find answers to questions posed by researchers and research consumers.

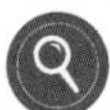

EVIDENCE-BASED PRACTICE TIP

You should be formulating clinical questions that arise from your clinical practice. Once you have developed a focused clinical question using the PICO format, you will search the literature for the best available evidence to answer your clinical question.

The Research Question and Hypothesis

The care that the researcher takes when developing the research question or hypothesis is often representative of the overall conceptualization and design of the study. In a quantitative research study, the remainder of a study revolves around answering the research question or testing the hypothesis. In a qualitative research study, the objective is to answer the research question. This may be a time-consuming, sometimes frustrating endeavor for the researcher, but in the final analysis the product, as evaluated by the consumer, is most often worth the struggle. Because this text focuses on the nurse as a critical consumer of research, the following sections will primarily pertain to the evaluation of research questions and hypotheses in published research reports.

CRITIQUING THE RESEARCH QUESTION

The following Critiquing Criteria box provides several criteria for evaluating the initial phase of the research process—the research question. Because the research question represents the basis for the study, it is usually introduced at the beginning of the research report to indicate the focus and direction of the study to the readers. You will then be in a position to evaluate whether the rest of the study logically flows from its foundation—the research question(s). The author will often begin by identifying the background and significance of the issue that led to crystallizing development of the unanswered question. The clinical and scientific background and/or significance will be summarized, and the purpose, aim, or objective of the study is identified. Finally, the research question and any related subquestions will be proposed before or after the literature review.

The purpose of the introductory summary of the theoretical and scientific background is to provide the reader with a glimpse of how the author critically thought about the research question's development. The introduction to the research question places the study within an appropriate theoretical framework and sets the stage for the unfolding of the study. This introductory section should also include the significance of the study (i.e., why the investigator is doing the study). For example, the significance may be to solve a problem encountered in the clinical area and thereby improve patient care, to resolve a conflict in the literature regarding a clinical issue, or to provide data supporting an innovative form of nursing intervention that is of equal or better quality and is also cost-effective. In a study by Holzemer and colleagues (2006) that tested a tailored nurse-delivered HIV/AIDS medication adherence intervention program compared with standard care, the significance of the research question was related to the known relationship between patient adherence and treatment outcomes across chronic health conditions and the ongoing challenge of improving patient adherence to HIV/AIDS therapeutic medication regimens and, thereby, improving patient outcomes.

Sometimes you will find that the research question is not clearly stated at the conclusion of this section. In some cases it is only hinted at, and you are challenged to identify the research question. In other cases the research question is embedded in the introductory text or purpose statement. To some extent, this depends on the style of the journal. Nevertheless, you, the evaluator, must remember that the main research question should be implied if it is not clearly identified in the introductory section—even if the subquestions are not stated or implied.

You will look for the presence of three key elements that are described and illustrated in an earlier section of this chapter. They are the following:

- Does the research question express a relationship between two or more variables, or at least between an independent and a dependent variable?
- Does the research question specify the nature of the population being studied?
- Does the research question imply the possibility of empiric testing?

You will use these three elements as criteria for judging the soundness of a stated research question. It is likely that if the question is unclear in terms of the variables, the population, and the implications for testability, then the remainder of the study is going to falter. For example, a research study contained introductory material on anxiety in general, anxiety as it relates to the perioperative period, and the potentially beneficial influence of nursing care in relation to anxiety reduction. The author concluded that the purpose of the study was to determine whether selected measures of patient anxiety could be shown to differ when different approaches to nursing care were used during the perioperative period. The author did not go on to state the research question. A restatement of the question might be as follows:

$$(Y_1)(X_1, X_2, X_3)$$

What is the difference in patient anxiety level in relation to different approaches to nursing care during the perioperative period?

If this process is clarified at the outset of a research study, all that follows in terms of the design can be logically developed. You will have a clear idea of what the report should convey and can knowledgeably evaluate the material that follows. When critically appraising clinical questions, think about the fact that they should be focused and specify the patient or problem being addressed, the intervention, and the outcome for a particular patient population. There should be evidence that the clinical question guided the literature search and suggests the design and level of evidence to be obtained from the study findings.

CRITIQUING THE HYPOTHESIS

As illustrated in the following Critiquing Criteria box, several criteria for critiquing the hypothesis should be used as a standard for evaluating the strengths and weaknesses of hypotheses in a research report.

1. When reading a research study, you may find the hypotheses clearly delineated in a separate hypothesis section of the research article (i.e., after the literature review or theoretical framework section[s]). In many cases the hypotheses are not explicitly stated and are only implied in the Results or Discussion section of the article. In cases such as that, you must infer the hypotheses from the purpose statement and the type of analysis used. You should not assume that if hypotheses do not appear at the beginning of the article, they do not exist in the particular study. Even when hypotheses are stated at the beginning of an article, they are reexamined in the Results or Discussion section as the findings are presented and discussed.
2. If a hypothesis or set of hypotheses are presented, the data analysis should directly answer the hypotheses. Its placement in the research report logically follows the literature review, and the theoretical framework, because the hypothesis should reflect the culmination and expression of this conceptual process. It should be consistent with both the literature review and the theoretical framework.

3. Although a hypothesis can legitimately be nondirectional, it is preferable, and more common, for the researcher to indicate the direction of the relationship between the variables in the hypothesis. You will find that when there are a lack of data available for the literature review (i.e., the researcher has chosen to study a relatively undefined area of interest), a nondirectional hypothesis may be appropriate. There simply may not be enough information available to make a sound judgment about the direction of the proposed relationship. All that could be proposed is that there will be a relationship between two variables. Essentially, you will want to determine the appropriateness of the researcher's choice regarding directionality of the hypothesis.
4. The notion of testability is central to the soundness of a hypothesis. One criterion related to testability is that the hypothesis should be stated in such a way that it can be clearly supported or not supported. Although the previous statement is very important to keep in mind, readers should also understand that ultimately theories or hypotheses are never proven beyond the shadow of a doubt through hypothesis testing. Researchers who claim that their data have "proven" the validity of their hypothesis should be regarded with grave reservation. You should realize that, at best, findings that support a hypothesis are considered tentative. If repeated replication of a study yields the same results, more confidence can be placed in the conclusions advanced by the researchers. An important thing to remember about testability is that although hypotheses are more likely to be accepted with increasing evidence, they are ultimately never proven.
5. Another point about testability to consider is that the hypothesis should be objectively stated and devoid of any value-laden words. Value-laden hypotheses are not empirically testable. Quantifiable words such as greater than; less than; decrease; increase; and positively, negatively, or related convey the idea of objectivity and testability. You should immediately be suspicious of hypotheses that are not stated objectively.
6. You should recognize that how the proposed relationship of the hypothesis is phrased suggests the type of research design that will be appropriate for the study, as well as the level of evidence to be derived from the findings. For example, if a hypothesis proposes that treatment $\mathbf{X}_1$ will have a greater effect on **Y** than treatment $\mathbf{X}_2$, an experimental (Level II evidence) or quasi-experimental design (Level III evidence) is suggested (see Chapter 8). If a hypothesis proposes that there will be a positive relationship between variables **X** and **Y,** a nonexperimental design (Level IV evidence) is suggested (see Chapter 9). A review of Table 2-4 provides you with additional examples of hypotheses, the type of research design, and the level of evidence that is suggested by each hypothesis. This factor has important implications for the remainder of the study in terms of the appropriateness of sample selection, data collection, data analysis, interpretation of findings, and—ultimately—the conclusions advanced by the researcher.
7. If the research report contains research questions rather than hypotheses, you will want to evaluate whether this is appropriate to the study. One criterion for making this decision, as presented earlier in this chapter, is whether the study is of an exploratory, a descriptive, or a qualitative nature. If it is, then it is appropriate to have research questions rather than hypotheses.

CRITIQUING CRITERIA: *Developing Research Questions and Hypotheses*

The Research Question

1. Was the research question introduced promptly?
2. Is the research question stated clearly and unambiguously?
3. Does the research question express a relationship between two or more variables or at least between an independent and a dependent variable, implying empirical testability?
4. How does the research question specify the nature of the population being studied?
5. How has the research question been substantiated with adequate experiential and scientific background material?
6. How has the research question been placed within the context of an appropriate theoretical framework?
7. How has the significance of the research question been identified?
8. Have pragmatic issues, such as feasibility, been addressed?
9. How have the purpose, aims, or goals of the study been identified?
10. Are research questions appropriately used (i.e., exploratory, descriptive, or qualitative study or in relation to ancillary data analyses)?

The Hypothesis

1. How does the hypothesis relate to the research problem?
2. Is the hypothesis concisely stated in a declarative form?
3. Are the independent and dependent variables identified in the statement of the hypothesis?
4. How are the variables measurable or potentially measurable?
5. Is each hypothesis specific to one relationship so that each hypothesis can be either supported or not supported?
6. Is the hypothesis stated in such a way that it is testable?
7. Is the hypothesis stated objectively, without value-laden words?
8. Is the direction of the relationship in each hypothesis clearly stated?
9. How is each hypothesis consistent with the literature review?
10. How is the theoretical rationale for the hypothesis made explicit?
11. Given the level of evidence suggested by the research question, hypothesis, and design, what is the potential applicability to practice?

The Clinical Question

1. Does the clinical question specify the patient population, intervention, comparison intervention, and outcome?

CRITICAL THINKING CHALLENGES

- Discuss how the wording of a research question or hypothesis suggests the type of research design and level of evidence that will be provided.
- Using the study about breast cancer survivors by Meneses et al. in Appendix A, diagram how the hypotheses flow from the theoretical framework and literature review.
- Using the Horgas study in Appendix C, describe how the significance of the research problem and purpose of the study are linked to the research questions.
- A nurse is caring for patients in a clinical situation that produces a clinical question having no ready answer. The nurse wants to develop and refine this clinical question using the PICO approach so that it becomes the basis for an evidence-based practice project. How can the nurse accomplish that objective?

KEY POINTS

- Formulation of the research question and stating the hypothesis are key preliminary steps in the research process.
- The research question is refined through a process that proceeds from the identification of a general idea of interest to the definition of a more specific and circumscribed topic.
- A preliminary literature review reveals related factors that appear critical to the research topic of interest and helps to further define the research question.
- The significance of the research question must be identified in terms of its potential contribution to patients, nurses, the medical community in general, and society. Applicability of the question for nursing practice, as well as its theoretical relevance, must be established. The findings should also have the potential for formulating or altering nursing practices or policies.
- The feasibility of a research question must be examined in light of pragmatic considerations (e.g., time); availability of subjects, money, facilities, and equipment; experience of the researcher; and ethical issues.
- The final research question consists of a statement about the relationship of two or more variables. It clearly identifies the relationship between the independent and dependent variables, specifies the nature of the population being studied, and implies the possibility of empirical testing.
- Focused clinical questions arise from clinical practice and guide the literature search for the best available evidence to answer the clinical question.
- A hypothesis attempts to answer the question posed by the research question. When testing the validity of the theoretical frameworks' assumptions, the hypothesis bridges the theoretical and real worlds.
- A hypothesis is a declarative statement about the relationship between two or more variables that predicts an expected outcome. Characteristics of a hypothesis include a relationship statement, implications regarding testability, and consistency with a defined theory base.
- Hypotheses can be formulated in a directional or a nondirectional manner. Hypotheses can be further categorized as either research or statistical hypotheses.
- Research questions may be used instead of hypotheses in exploratory, descriptive, or qualitative research studies. Research questions may also be formulated in addition to hypotheses to answer questions related to ancillary data.
- The purpose, research question, or hypothesis provides information about the intent of the research question and hypothesis and suggests the level of evidence to be obtained from the study findings.
- The critiquing criteria provide a set of guidelines for evaluating the strengths and weaknesses of the problem statement and hypotheses as they appear in a research report.
- The critiquer assesses the clarity of the research question, as well as the related subquestions, the specificity of the population, and the implications for testability.
- The interrelatedness of the research question, the literature review, the theoretical framework, and the hypotheses should be apparent.
- The appropriateness of the research design suggested by the research question is also evaluated.
- The purpose of the study (i.e., why the researcher is doing the study) should be differentiated from the research question.

- The reader evaluates the wording of the hypothesis in terms of the clarity of the relational statement, its implications for testability, and its congruence with a theory base. The appropriateness of the hypothesis in relation to the type of research design and level of evidence suggested by the design is also examined. In addition, the appropriate use of research questions is evaluated in relation to the type of study conducted.

REFERENCES

Albrecht SA, Caruthers D, Patrick T, et al: A randomized controlled trial of a smoking cessation intervention for pregnant adolescents, *Nurs Res* 55(6):402-410, 2006.

Amorim AR, Linne YM, Laurenco PMC: Diet or exercise or both, for weight reduction in women after childbirth, *Cochrane Database of Systematic Reviews* (3):CD005627, 2007.

Artinian NT, Flack JM, Nordstrom CK, et al: Effects of nurse-managed telemonitoring on blood pressure at 12 month follow-up among urban African Americans, *Nurs Res* 56(5):312-322, 2007.

Bennett JA, Lyons KA, Winters-Stone K, et al: Motivational interviewing to increase physical activity in long-term cancer survivors: a randomized clinical trial, *Nurs Res* 56(1):18-27, 2008.

Budin WC, Hoskins CN, Haber J, et al: Breast cancer: education, counseling, and adjustment among patients and partners: a randomized clinical trial, *Nurs Res* 57(3):199-213, 2008.

Cullum N: User's guides to the nursing literature: an introduction, *Evidence-Based Nurs* 3(2):71-72, 2000.

Eser I, Korshid L, Gunes UY, et al: The effect of different body positions on blood pressure, *J Clin Nurs* 16(1):137-140, 2007.

Fox S, Chesla C: Living with chronic illness: a phenomenological study of the health effects of the patient-provider relationship, *J Am Acad Nurse Pract* 20:109-117, 2008.

Fu MR, Axelrod D, Haber J: Breast cancer–related lymphedema, *J Nurs Scholarship* 40(40):341-348, 2008.

Gillies CL, Abrams KR, Lambert PC, et al: Pharmacological and lifestyle interventions to prevent or delay type 2 diabetes in people with impaired glucose tolerance: systematic review and meta-analysis, *BMJ* 334:299, 2007.

Holzemer WL, Bakken S, Portillo C, et al: Testing a nurse-tailored HIV medication adherence intervention, *Nurs Res* 55(3):189-197, 2006.

Horgas AL, Yoon SL, Nichols AL, et al: The relationship between pain and functional disability in black and white older adults, *Res Nurs Health* 31(4):341-354, 2008.

Hyman DJ, Pavlik VN, Taylor WC: Simultaneous vs sequential counseling for multiple behavior change, *Arch Intern Med* 167:1152-1158, 2007.

Jones EG, Renger R, Kang Y: Self-efficacy for health-related behaviors among deaf adults, *Res Nurs Health* 30:185-192, 2007.

Johnson JE, Fielder VK, Jones LS, et al: *Self-regulation theory: applying theory to your practice,* Pittsburgh, 1997, Oncology Nursing Press.

Keefe MR, Karlsen KA, Lobo ML, et al: Reducing parenting stress in families with irritable infants, *Nurs Res* 55(3):198-205, 2006.

Koeman M, van der Ven AJ, Hak E, et al: Oral decontamination with chlorhexidine reduces the incidence of ventilator-associated pneumonia, *Am J Respir Crit Care* 173:1348-1355, 2006.

Landreneau KJ, Ward-Smith P: Perceptions of adult patients on hemodialysis concerning choice among renal transplant therapies, *Nephrol Nurs J* 34(5):513-525, 2007.

Lithgow D, Nyamathi A, Elashoff D, et al: C-reactive protein in nipple aspirate fluid, *Nurs Res* 55(6):418-425, 2006.

MD Anderson Cancer Center: *Adult cancer pain interdisciplinary clinical practice guideline,* Houston, 2008, The Author.

Meneses KD, McNees P, Loerzei VW, et al: Transition from treatment to survivorship: effects of a psychoeducational intervention on quality of life in breast cancer survivors, *Oncol Nurs Forum* 34(5):1007-1016, 2007.

Mulford D, Taggart HM, Nivens A, et al: Arch support use for improving balance and reducing pain in older adults, *Appl Nurs Res* 21(3):153-158, 2008.

Nordgren L, Asp M, Fagerberg I: Living with moderate-severe chronic heart failure as a middle-aged person, *Qualitative Health Res* 17:4-13, 2007.

Pi-Sunyer X, Blackburn G, Brancati FL, et al: Reduction in weight and cardiovascular risk factors in overweight and obese people with type 2 diabetes: one year results of the Look AHEAD trial, *Diabetes Care* 30:1374-1383, 2007.

Rice VH, Stead LF: Nursing interventions for smoking cessation, *Cochrane Database of Systematic Reviews* (1):CD001188. DOI: 10.1002/14651858.CD001188.pub3, 2008.

Sackett D, et al: *Evidence-based medicine: how to practice and teach EBM,* London, 2000, Churchill Livingstone.

Simonson DC, Ahern MM, Hendryx MS: Anesthesia staffing and anesthetic complications during cesarean delivery: a retrospective analysis, *Nurs Res* 56(1):9-17, 2007.

Stacey D, Samant R, Bennett C: Decision making in oncology: a review of patient decision aids to support patient participation, *CA Cancer J Clin* 58(5):293-304, 2008.

Thompson C, Cullum N, McCaughan D, et al: Nurses, information use, and clinical decision making: the real world potential for evidence-based decisions in nursing, *Evidence-Based Nurs* 7(3):68-72, 2004.

Wyatt G, Sikorski A, Siddiqi A, et al: Feasibility of a reflexology and guided imagery intervention during chemotherapy: results of a quasi-experimental study, *Oncol Nurs Forum* 34(3):635-642, 2007.

FOR FURTHER STUDY

evolve

Go to Evolve at http://evolve.elsevier.com/LoBiondo/ for review questions, critiquing exercises, and additional research articles for practice in reviewing and critiquing.

3

Gathering and Appraising the Literature

Stephanie Fulton and Barbara Krainovich-Miller

KEY TERMS

Boolean operator
citation management software
concept
conceptual definition
conceptual framework
controlled vocabulary
literature review
online database
operational definition
primary source
print indexes
refereed, or peer-reviewed, journals
secondary source
theoretical framework
theory
Web browser

LEARNING OUTCOMES

After reading this chapter, you should be able to do the following:

- Discuss the relationship of the literature review to nursing theory, research, education, and practice.
- Discuss the purposes of the literature review from the perspective of the research investigator and the research consumer.
- Discuss the use of the literature review for quantitative designs and qualitative methods.
- Discuss the purpose of reviewing the literature in development of evidence-based practice.
- Differentiate between primary and secondary sources.
- Compare the advantages and disadvantages of the most commonly used online databases and print database sources for conducting a literature review.
- Identify the characteristics of an effective electronic search of the literature.
- Critically read, appraise, and synthesize primary and secondary sources used for the development of a literature review.
- Apply critiquing criteria to the evaluation of literature reviews in selected research studies.

STUDY RESOURCES

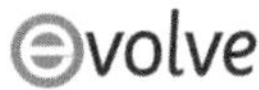

Go to Evolve at http://evolve.elsevier.com/LoBiondo/ for review questions, critiquing exercises, and additional research articles for practice in reviewing and critiquing.

You may wonder why an entire chapter of a research text is devoted to appraising and gathering the literature. The main reason is because searching for, retrieving, and critically appraising the literature is a key step in the research process for researchers and also for nurses involved in evidence-based practice. A more personal question you might ask is, "Will knowing more about how to critically appraise and gather the literature really help me as a student or later as a practicing nurse?" The answer is that it most certainly will! Your ability to locate and retrieve research studies, critically appraise them, and decide that you have the best available evidence to inform your clinical decision making is a skill essential to your current role as a student and your future role as a nurse who is a competent research consumer (American Association of Colleges of Nursing, 2008).

Your critical appraisal, also called a critique of the literature, is an organized systematic approach to evaluating a research study or group of research studies using a set of established critical appraisal criteria to objectively determine the strength, quality, and consistency of evidence provided by literature to determine its applicability to research, education, or practice. As a research consumer, you will become skilled at critically appraising research studies, combining the evidence with your clinical expertise and the patient population that you are caring for, to make an evidence-informed decision about the applicability of a particular nursing intervention for your patient or patient population in your practice setting.

The section of a published research report titled "Literature Review" generally appears near the beginning of the report. It provides an abbreviated version of the complete literature review conducted by a researcher and represents the building blocks of and foundation for the study. Therefore the **literature review,** a systematic and critical appraisal of the most important literature on a topic, is a key step in the research process that provides the basis of a research study.

The **conceptual framework** or **theoretical framework** of a research report is a structure of concepts and/or theories pulled together as a map for the study that provides rationale for the development of research questions or hypotheses. This section of a research report is often located as a titled subsection of the literature review and may be accompanied by a diagram illustrating the proposed relationships between and among the concepts. Alternatively, the conceptual/theoretical framework may not be separately identified and may be embedded in the literature review section of an article or simply not included. The links between theory, research, education, and practice are intricately connected; together they create the knowledge base for the nursing discipline as shown in Figure 3-1.

The purpose of this chapter is to introduce you to the literature review as it is used in research and evidence-based practice projects. It provides you with the systematic tools to

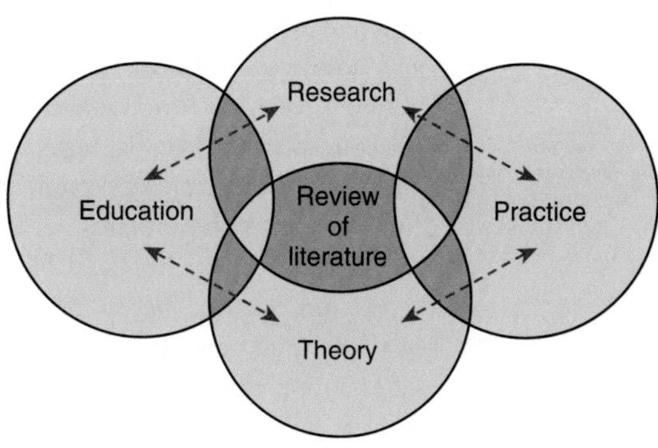

Figure 3-1 Relationship of the review of the literature to theory, research, education, and practice.

(1) consider how the theoretical or conceptual framework guides development of a research study; (2) critically appraise a research study or group of research studies; (3) locate, search for, and retrieve research studies, systematic reviews (see Chapters 1, 8, 9, and 18), documents, and statistical reports; and (4) differentiate between a research article and a conceptual article or book. This set of tools will help you develop your research consumer competencies and prepare your academic papers and evidence-based practice projects.

THE CONCEPTUAL OR THEORETICAL FRAMEWORK

The conceptual or theoretical framework of a research report is a structure of concepts and/or theories that provides the basis for development of research questions or hypotheses. A **concept** is an image or symbolic representation of an abstract idea. The researcher uses a concept, a set of concepts, or a particular theory or set of theories to build the theoretical foundation of the study. Concepts are the major components of theory and convey the abstract ideas within a theory. A **theory** is a set of interrelated concepts, definitions, and propositions that present a systematic view of phenomena for the purpose of explaining and making predictions about those phenomena. A **conceptual definition** includes the general meaning of a concept. An **operational definition** includes the method used to measure the concept; once the concept is linked to a measurement method or instrument, it is regarded as a variable.

For example, in the study by Meneses and colleagues (2007) investigating the effect of a psychoeducational telephone counseling intervention on the quality of life (QOL) for breast cancer survivors, QOL was the conceptual framework used to guide the identification and development of the study. QOL was conceptually defined as "a multidimensional construct consisting of four domains: physical, psychological, social, and spiritual well being. Each domain contributes to overall quality of life" and was operationally defined as the score on the Quality of Life–Breast Cancer Survivors measurement instrument, which is a rating scale to describe overall QOL, that is, problems or concerns within those four domains. There was a goodness of fit between the QOL conceptual framework and the conceptual and operational definitions that provided a strong theoretical foundation for this study. The content related to the conceptual framework is identified in a separately titled section of the article, and follows the presentation and critical appraisal of the QOL literature and cancer survivorship intervention literature related to breast cancer and QOL (see Appendix A).

As suggested in the introduction to this chapter, the theoretical or conceptual framework of a research study is often illustrated using a diagram. For example, see the study by Horgas and colleagues (2008), reprinted here in Appendix C, which investigates the relationship between pain and functional disability in black and white older adults. Figure 1 of this article is a conceptual model diagram that depicts the nature of the relationships between background and health characteristics, pain, and disability. Figure 2, in the same study, is the final structural model with statistical data explaining the quantitative strength of those conceptual relationships diagrammed in Figure 1.

As you can see, theory, practice, and research are interconnected: practice enables testing of theory and generates research questions; research contributes to theory building and provides supporting evidence for effective nursing interventions in clinical practice. Therefore what is learned through practice, theory, and research interweaves to create the knowledge fabric of the discipline of nursing, which then ends up being taught to you courses.

REVIEW OF THE LITERATURE

The Literature Review: The Researcher's Perspective

The overall purpose of the literature review in a research study is to present a strong knowledge base for the conduct of the research study. Specific objectives 1 through 7 listed in Box 3-1 reflect the purposes of a literature review for the conduct of quantitative research and most qualitative research. It is important to understand when reading a research article that the researcher's main goal when developing the literature review is to develop the knowledge foundation for a sound study and to generate research questions and hypotheses.

An extensive literature review is essential to all steps of the quantitative research process and to some qualitative methods. From this perspective the review is broad and systematic, as well as in-depth. It is a critical collection and evaluation of the important published literature in journals, monographs, books, and book chapters, as well as unpublished research print and computer-accessed materials (e.g., doctoral dissertations and masters' theses), audiovisual materials (e.g., audiotapes and videotapes), and sometimes personal communications (e.g., conference presentations and one-on-one interviews).

From a researcher's perspective the objectives in Box 3-1 direct the questions the researcher asks while reading the literature to determine a useful research question(s) or hypothesis(es) and how best to design a particular study.

The following brief overview about the use of the literature review in relation to the steps of the quantitative and qualitative research process will help you to understand the researcher's

BOX 3-1 Overall Purposes of a Literature Review

MAJOR GOAL

To develop a strong knowledge base to carry out a research study or an evidence-based practice project

OBJECTIVES

A review of the literature does the following:

1. Determines what is known and unknown about a subject, concept, or problem
2. Determines gaps, consistencies, and inconsistencies in the literature about a subject, concept, or problem
3. Discovers conceptual traditions used to examine problems
4. Generates useful research questions and hypotheses
5. Determines an appropriate research design, methodology, and analysis for answering the research question(s) or hypothesis(es) based on an assessment of the strengths and weaknesses of earlier works
6. Determines the need for replication of a study or refinement of a study
7. Synthesizes the strengths and weaknesses and findings of available studies on a topic/problem
8. Uncovers a new practice intervention(s), or gains supporting evidence for revising or maintaining current intervention(s), protocols, and policies
9. Promotes evidence-based revision and development of new practice protocols, policies, and projects/activities related to nursing practice
10. Generates clinical questions that guide development of evidence-based practice projects

focus. A critical review of relevant literature affects the steps of the quantitative research process as follows:

- *Theoretical or conceptual framework:* A literature review reveals conceptual traditions, concepts, and/or theories or conceptual models from nursing and other related disciplines that can be used to examine problems. This framework presents the context for studying the problem and can be viewed as a map for understanding the relationships between or among the variables in quantitative studies. The literature review provides rationale for the variables and explains concepts, definitions, and relationships between or among the independent and dependent variables used in the theoretical framework of the study.
- *Primary and secondary sources:* The literature review mainly should use **primary sources,** that is, articles and books by the original author. Sometimes it is appropriate to use **secondary sources,** which are published articles or books that are written by persons other than the individual who developed the theory or conducted the research study. The studies selected for the literature review should offer the strongest and most consistent level of evidence available on the topic (Table 3-1).
- *Research question and hypothesis:* The literature review helps to determine what is known and not known; to uncover gaps, consistencies, or inconsistencies; and/or to disclose unanswered questions in the literature about a subject, concept, theory, or problem that generate or allow for refinement of research questions and/or hypotheses.

TABLE 3-1 Primary and Secondary Sources

Primary: Essential	Secondary: Useful
Material written by the original person who conducted the study, developed the theory (model), or prepared the scholarly discussion on a concept, topic, or issue of interest (i.e., the original author). Primary sources can be published or unpublished. Research example: An investigator's report of his or her research study (e.g., articles in Appendixes A through D). Theoretical example: quality of life (QOL) is the theoretical framework used by Meneses et al. (2007) in their study investigating the effectiveness of a psychoeducational intervention on quality of life in breast cancer survivors. The QOL theoretical framework used in this study was developed by Dow et al. and Ferrell, Dow, and Grant and cited as such in the research report (see Appendix A). Other primary source examples include autobiographies, diaries, films, letters, artifacts, periodicals, and tapes. HINT: Critical evaluation of mainly primary sources is essential to a thorough and relevant review of the literature.	Material written by a person(s) other than the person who conducted the research study or developed a theory. This is someone other than the original who writes about or presents the author's original work. The material is usually in the form of a summary or critique (i.e., analysis and synthesis) of someone else's scholarly work or body of literature. Secondary sources can be published or unpublished. Secondary source examples are the following: response/commentary/critique articles of a research study, a theory/model, or a professional view of an issue; review of literature article published in a refereed scholarly journal; abstracts of a published work written by someone other than the original author; examples: a biography or a systematic review. HINT: Use secondary sources sparingly; however, secondary sources—especially of studies that include a research critique—are a valuable learning tool for a beginning research consumer.

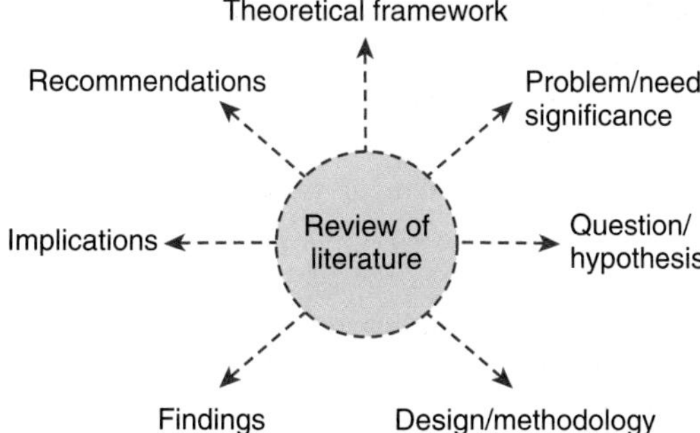

Figure 3-2 Relationship of the review of the literature to the steps of the quantitative research process.

- *Design and method:* The literature review exposes the strengths and weaknesses of previous studies in terms of designs and methods and helps the researcher choose an appropriate new, replicated, or refined design, including data-collection method, sampling strategy and size, valid and reliable measurement instruments, an effective data analysis method, and appropriate informed consent forms. Often, because of journal space limitations, researchers only include abbreviated information about this in their journal article.
- *Outcome of the analysis (i.e., findings, discussion, implications, and recommendations):* The literature review is used to help the researcher accurately interpret and discuss the results/findings of a study. In the discussion section of a research article, the researcher returns to the research studies and theoretical articles or books presented earlier in the article in the literature review and uses this conceptual and research literature to interpret and explain the study's findings (see Chapters 14 and 15). For example, in the discussion section of the article by Meneses and colleagues (2007), the authors comment that "study results add further evidence in the literature that demonstrates enhanced psychological and social adjustment with psychoeducational interventions." The literature review also helps to develop the implications of the findings for practice, education, and further research. For example, in the "Implications for Research and Practice" section of the same study, it is noted that the findings of this study contribute "to a clearer articulation and description of the actual components of the intervention to help future researchers clarify their respective descriptions of delivery methods." Figure 3-2 relates the literature review to all aspects of the quantitative research process.

The Literature Review: The Consumer Perspective

From the perspective of the research consumer, you review a number of studies to answer a clinical question or to solve a clinical problem. Therefore you will search the literature widely and gather multiple resources to answer your question using an evidence-based practice approach. The evidence-based practice process includes the following: (1) asking clinical questions; (2) identifying and gathering the evidence; (3) critically appraising and synthesizing the evidence or literature; (4) acting to change practice by using the best available evidence, coupled with your clinical expertise and patient preferences (values, setting, and resources);

and (5) evaluating the use of the research evidence found to assess applicability of the research findings to the practice change. In addition to objectives 1 through 7 in Box 3-1, objectives 7, 8, and 9 specifically reflect the purposes of a literature review for nurses involved in evidence-based practice projects.

As a student or practicing nurse you may be asked to generate a clinical question for an evidence-based practice project and search for, retrieve, review, and critically appraise the literature to identify the "best available evidence" that provides the answer to a clinical question and informs your clinical decision making. A clear and precise articulation of a question is critical to finding the best evidence. Evidence-based questions may sound like research questions, but they are questions used to search the existing literature for answers. The evidence-based practice process uses the PICO format to generate clinical questions. For example, students in an adult health course were asked to generate a clinical question related to health promotion for older women using the PICO format. The PICO format is as follows:

P Problem/patient population; specifically defined group
I Intervention; what intervention or event will be studied?
C Comparison of intervention; with what will the intervention be compared?
O Outcome; what is the effect of the intervention?

One group of students was interested in whether regular exercise prevented osteoporosis for postmenopausal women who had osteopenia. The PICO format for the clinical question that guided their search was as follows:

P Postmenopausal women with osteopenia
I Regular exercise program
C No regular exercise program
O Prevention of osteoporosis

Their assignment required that they do the following:

- Search the literature using electronic databases (e.g., Cumulative Index to Nursing and Allied Health Literature [CINAHL via EBSCO], MEDLINE, SCOPUS, and Cochrane Database of Systematic Reviews) for the background information that enabled them to identify the significance of osteopenia and osteoporosis as a woman's health problem
- Identify systematic reviews, practice guidelines, and individual research studies that provided the "best available evidence" related to the effectiveness of regular exercise programs on prevention of osteoporosis
- Critically appraise systematic reviews, practice guidelines, and research studies based on standardized critical appraisal criteria (e.g., CASP Tools) (see Chapter 18)
- Synthesize the overall strengths and weaknesses of the evidence provided by the literature
- Draw a conclusion about the strength, quality, and consistency of the evidence
- Make recommendations about applicability of the evidence to clinical nursing practice that guides development of a health promotion project about osteoporosis risk reduction for postmenopausal women with osteopenia

As a practicing nurse you will be called on to develop new and/or to revise or continue current evidence-based practice protocols, practice standards, or policies in your health care organization. This will require that you know how to retrieve and critically appraise research articles, systematic reviews, and practice guidelines to determine the degree of support or nonsupport found in the literature. A critical appraisal of the literature related to a specific clinical question uncovers data that contribute evidence to support current practice and clinical decision making, as well as for making changes in practice.

Research Conduct and Consumer of Research Purposes: Differences and Similarities

How does the literature review differ when it is used for research purposes versus consumer of research purposes? The literature review in a research study is used to develop a sound research proposal for a research study that will generate knowledge. From a broader perspective, the major focus of reviewing the literature as a consumer is to uncover multiple sources of evidence on a given topic that have been generated by researchers in their research studies that can potentially be used to improve clinical practice and patient outcomes.

From a student perspective, the ability to critically appraise the literature is essential to acquiring a skill set for successfully completing scholarly papers, presentations, debates, and evidence-based practice projects. Both types of literature reviews are similar in that both should be framed in the context of previous research and theoretical literature and pertinent to the objectives presented in Box 3-1.

HELPFUL HINT

Remember, the findings of one study on a topic do not usually provide sufficient evidence to support a change in practice; be cautious when a nurse colleague tells you to change your practice based on the results of one study.

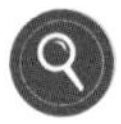

EVIDENCE-BASED PRACTICE TIP

For a research consumer, formulating a clinical question provides a focus that guides the literature review.

SEARCHING FOR EVIDENCE

In your student role, when you are preparing an academic paper you read the required course materials, as well as additional literature retrieved from the library. Students often state, "I know how to do research." Perhaps you have thought the same thing because you "researched" a topic for a paper in the library. In this situation, however, it would be more accurate for you to say that you have been "searching" the literature to uncover research and conceptual information to prepare an academic term paper on a certain topic. You will search for **primary sources,** which are articles, books, or other documents written by the person who conducted the study, developed the theory, or prepared the scholarly discussion on a concept, topic, problem, or issue of interest. You will also search for **secondary sources,** which are materials written by persons other than the individual(s) who conducted a research study or developed a particular theory. Table 3-1 provides more extensive definitions and examples of primary and secondary sources.

Although reviewing the literature for research purposes and research consumer activities requires the same critical thinking and reading skills, a literature review for a research proposal is usually much more extensive and comprehensive, and the critiquing process is more in-depth. From an academic standpoint, requirements for a literature review for a particular assignment differ depending on the level and type of course, as well as the specific objective of the assignment. These factors determine whether a student's literature search requires a limited, selective review or a major or extensive review. Regardless, discovering knowledge is the goal of any search; therefore a consumer of research must know how to search the litera-

TABLE 3-2 Steps and Strategies for Conducting a Literature Search

Steps of Literature Review	Strategy
Step I: Determine clinical question or research topic	Keep focused on the types of patients/clients you deal with in your work setting. You know what works and does not work in the delivery of nursing care. In your student role, keep focused on the assignment's objective; use the literature to support opinions or develop a concept under discussion.
Step II: Identify key variables/terms	Ask your reference librarian for help, and read the research guide books usually found near the computers that are used for student searches; include "research" as one of your variables.
Step III: Conduct computer search using at least two recognized online databases	Conduct the search yourself or with the help of your librarian; it is essential to use at least two health-related databases, such as CINAHL via EBSCO, MEDLINE, PsycINFO, or ERIC.
Step IV: Review abstracts online and weed out irrelevant articles	Scan through your search, read the abstracts provided, and mark only those that fit your topic; select "references," as well as "search history" and "full-text articles" if available, before printing, saving, or e-mailing your search.
Step V: Retrieve relevant sources	Organize by article type or study design and year and reread the abstracts to determine if the articles chosen are relevant and worth retrieving.
Step VI: Print articles, if unable to print directly from database, and/or order through interlibrary loan	Save yourself time and money; buy a library copying card ahead of time or bring plenty of change so that you avoid wasting time midway to secure change or bring a thumb drive to download PDF versions of your articles. Print the entire article (including the references), making sure that you can clearly read the name of the journal, year, volume number, and pages; this can save you an immense amount of time when you are word-processing your paper.
Step VII: Conduct preliminary reading and weed out irrelevant sources	Review critical reading strategies (see Chapter 1; e.g., read the abstract at the beginning of the articles; see the example in this chapter).
Step VIII: Critically read each source (summarize and critique each source)	Use the critical appraisal strategies from Chapter 1 (e.g., use a standardized critiquing tool), take time to word-process each summary and critical appraisal (no more than one page long), include the references in APA style at the top or bottom of each abstract, and staple the copied article to the back of the summary. Invest time in learning a citation management software tool. This will save you the hassle of formatting all of your citations.
Step IX: Synthesize critical summaries of each article	Decide how you will present your synthesis of overall strengths and weaknesses of the reviewed articles (e.g., chronologically or according to type: research or conceptual) and word-process the synthesized material and a reference list.

ture. Reference librarians are excellent people to ask about various sources of scholarly literature. If you are unfamiliar with the process of conducting a scholarly computer search, your reference librarian can help. Table 3-2 provides you with steps and strategies for conducting a literature search.

Prioritizing the Search for Evidence

In Chapter 1 an evidence hierarchy is presented for grading the strength and quality of evidence provided by individual studies or resources that are located during a search. In this chapter, an evidence-based model, called the "5S" pyramid, is used to help you identify the highest-level information resource to facilitate your search for the best evidence about the clinical question or problem that prompted your search (Haynes, 2007). This model, as illustrated in Figure 3-3, suggests that when searching the literature you consider prioritizing your search strategy so that you begin your search by looking for the highest-level information resource available. For example, individual original studies such as those found in MEDLINE or CINAHL (e.g., a randomized clinical trial) are at the lowest level of the information resource pyramid. Moving up the 5S pyramid to the next information resource level are systematic reviews (e.g., a Cochrane review), then evidence-based journal abstracts (e.g., the

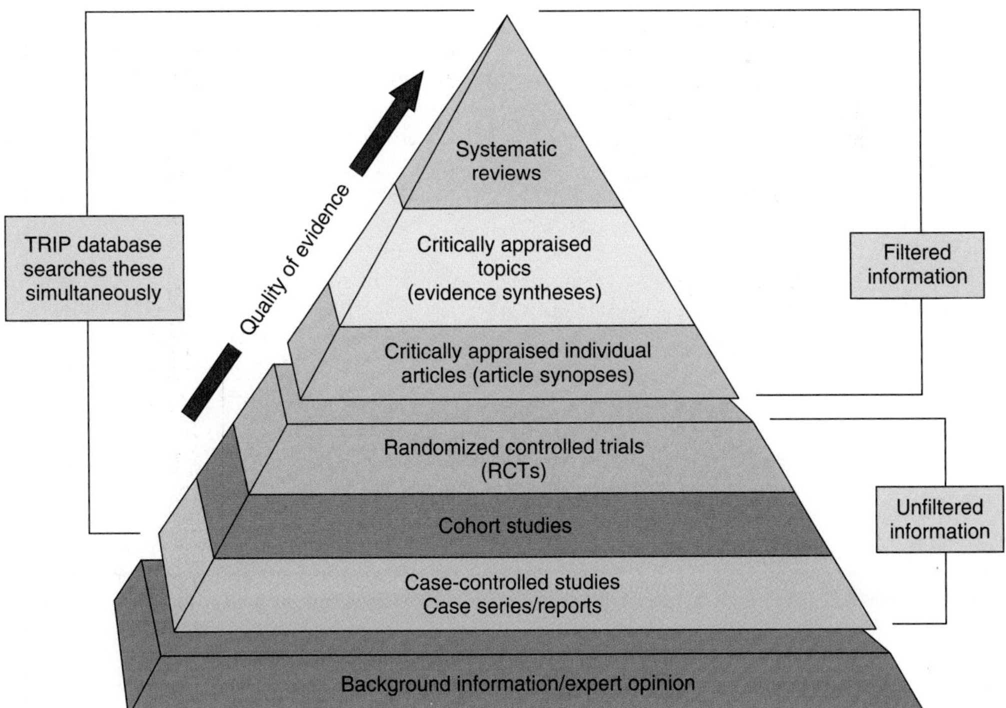

Figure 3-3 The 5S levels of organization of evidence from health care research.

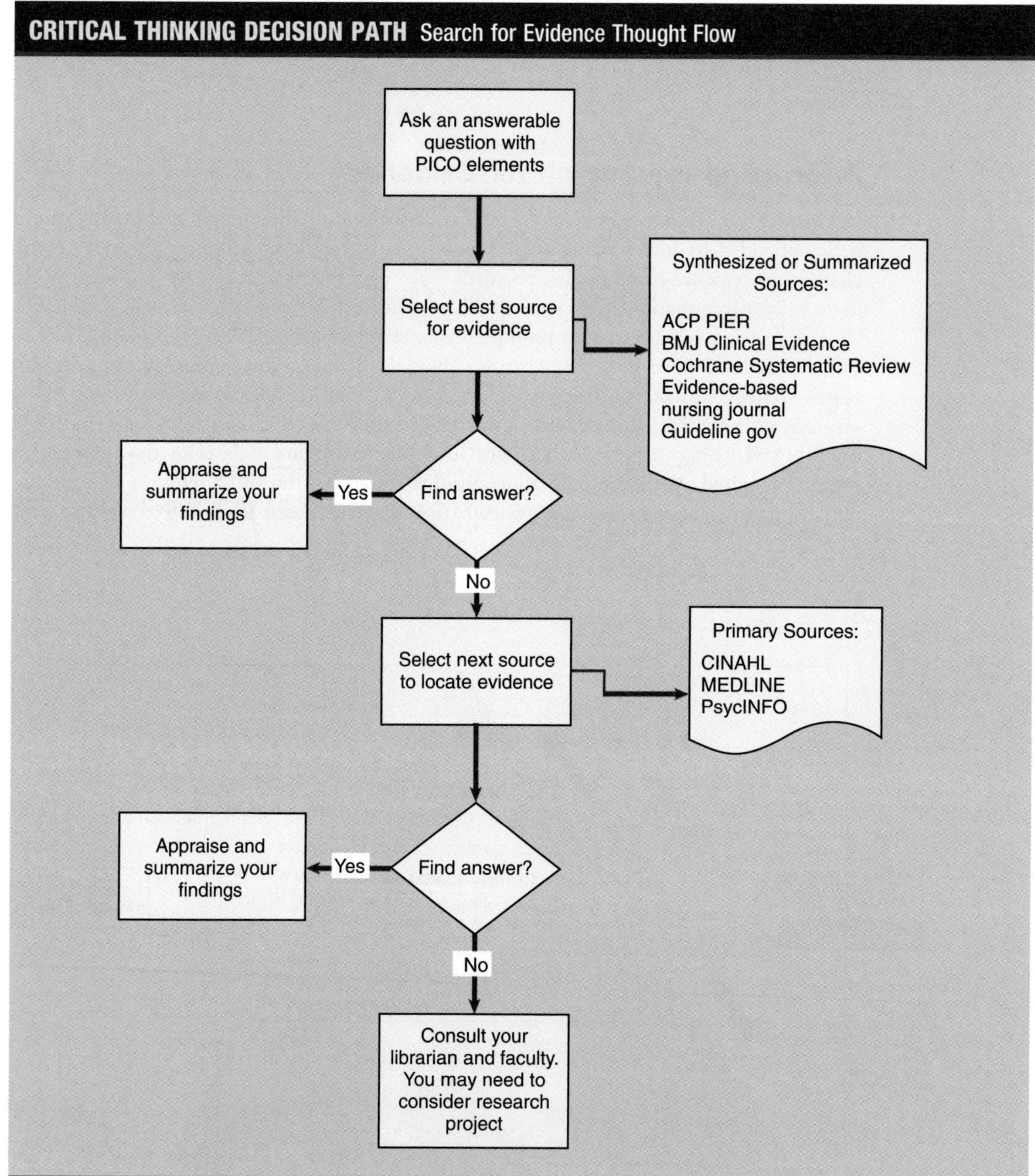

Adapted from Kendall, S. (2008). Evidence-based resources simplified. *Canadian Family Physician, 54*(2), p. 241-243.

one-page summary/commentary abstracts that appear in the journal *Evidence-Based Nursing*), or evidence-based textbooks.

The highest information resource level pertains to computerized decision support systems, a resource built into an electronic medical record that links your patient's distinctive needs with current evidence-based practice guidelines. The reality is that there are few such computerized systems at this time. But this does not mean that the information found within the other information resource levels are not useful or appropriate. The "5S" model is a tool that can help guide your search for the strongest and most relevant evidence. This model, although an important tool to guide your search for evidence-based information, does not replace the importance of critically reading each piece of evidence and assessing its quality and applicability for current practice.

HELPFUL HINT

- Make an appointment with your educational institution's reference librarian so you can take advantage of his or her expertise in accessing electronic databases.
- Take the time to set up your home/dorm computer for electronic library access.
- If the full text of an article is unavailable through your electronic search, read the abstract to determine if you want to order the article through interlibrary loan.

Performing an Online Database Search

Why Use an Online Database?

Perhaps you are still not convinced that online database searches are the best way to acquire information for a review of the literature. Maybe you have searched using Google or Yahoo and found relevant information. This is an understandable temptation, especially if your assignment only requires you to use five articles. Try to think about it once again from another perspective and ask yourself the following question: "Is this the most appropriate and efficient way to find out what is the latest and strongest research on a topic that affects patient care?" If you take the time to learn how to do a sound database search, you will have the essential competency needed for your career in nursing. The Critical Thinking Decision Path: Search for Evidence Thought Flow illustrates a path for locating evidence to support your research or clinical question.

TYPES OF RESOURCES

Print: Books, Journals, and Indexes

Most college/university libraries have an online card catalog to find print and online books, journals (titles only), videos and other media items, scripts, monographs, conference proceedings, masters' theses, dissertations, archival materials, and more.

Before the 1980s, a search was usually done by hand using **print indexes.** This was a tedious and time-consuming process. The print indexes are useful for finding sources that have not been entered into electronic (online) databases. Some of your professors might talk about the "Red Books" in referring to print version of what is now called CINAHL (Cumulative Index to Nursing and Allied Health Literature). The print index started in 1956 but is no longer produced. Print resources are still necessary if a search requires materials not entered into an electronic database before a certain year.

Print: Refereed Journals

A major portion of most literature reviews consists of journal articles. In contrast to books and textbooks, which take much longer to publish, journals are a ready source of the latest information on almost any subject. Therefore journals are the preferred mode of communicating the latest theory or results of a research study. As a beginning research consumer, you should use **refereed,** or **peer-reviewed, journals** as your first choice when looking for theoretical, clinical, or research articles. A refereed or peer-reviewed journal has a panel of internal and external reviewers who review submitted manuscripts for possible publication. The external reviewers are drawn from a pool of nurse scholars, and possibly scholars from other related disciplines, who are experts in various specialties. In most cases, the reviews are "blind"; that is, the manuscript to be reviewed does not include the name of the author(s). The reviewers use a set of scholarly criteria to judge whether a manuscript meets the publication standards of the journal. These criteria are similar to those used when you are critically appraising the strengths and weaknesses of a study (see Chapters 6 and 16). The credibility of a published theoretical or research article is strengthened by the peer-review process. Most refereed journals are available in print and accessible electronically through your library's online resources.

Internet: Online Bibliographic and Abstract Databases

Online databases are used to find journal sources (periodicals) of research and conceptual articles on a variety of topics (e.g., doctoral dissertations), as well as the publications of professional organizations and various governmental agencies. They contain bibliographic citation information such as the author, title, journal, and indexed terms for each record. Others also include the abstract. Box 3-2 lists examples of the more commonly used online databases.

Your college/university most likely enables you to access such databases from your residence whether on campus or not. The most relevant and frequently used source for nursing literature remains the Cumulative Index to Nursing and Allied Health Literature (CINAHL). Full text has been added to this database, so in many cases you will find the full article right at your fingertips. Another premier resource is MEDLINE, which is produced by the National Library of Medicine. MEDLINE focuses on the life sciences and dates back to the early 1950s.

Internet: Online Secondary or Summary Databases

Some databases contain more than just journal article information. These online resources contain either summaries or synopses of studies, overviews of diseases or conditions, or a summary of the latest evidence to support a particular treatment. American College of Physicians: The Physicians' Information and Education Resource (ACP PIER) is one such resource. You are able to enter a disease name and find out what treatment is supported by graded evidence (see Chapter 1). Another excellent resource is the Cochrane Library. This online resource consists of six databases, including the Cochrane Database of Systematic Reviews.

Using at least two electronic health-related databases such as CINAHL and MEDLINE (see Box 3-2) is recommended.

BOX 3-2 Online Databases

AMERICAN COLLEGE OF PHYSICIANS: THE PHYSICIANS' INFORMATION AND EDUCATION RESOURCE (ACP PIER)
- Produced by the American College of Physicians
- Designed to be a point-of-care evidence-based resource
- Covers over 300 disease modules
- Available online from ACP or through StatRef

CLINICAL EVIDENCE FROM THE *BRITISH MEDICAL JOURNAL (BMJ)*
- Produced by the *British Medical Journal*
- Systematic reviews that summarize the current state of knowledge or lack thereof on medical conditions
- Provide evidence reviews for more than 250 conditions
- Available online from BMJ and Ovid Technologies

CUMULATIVE INDEX TO NURSING AND ALLIED HEALTH LITERATURE (CINAHL)
- Initially called Cumulative Index to Nursing Literature
- Produced by CINAHL
- Print version known as the "Red Books"
- Electronic version available as part of the EBSCO online service
- Over 1,800 journals indexed for inclusion in database
- Citations in CINAHL are assigned index terms from a controlled vocabulary

THE COCHRANE LIBRARY
- Collection of databases that contain high-quality evidence
- Includes the Cochrane Database of Systematic Reviews
- Full Cochrane Library available from Wiley Interscience; other databases that make up the Cochrane Library available from other vendors, including Ovid
- Cochrane systematic reviews are indexed and searchable in both CINAHL and MEDLINE

EDUCATION RESOURCE INFORMATION CENTER (ERIC)
- Sponsored by the Institute of Education and the U.S. Department of Education
- Focuses on education research and information
- Currently indexes more than 600 journals and also includes references to books, conference papers, and technical reports
- Coverage begins in 1966
- ERIC is available from the ERIC Web site and by subscription from EBSCO, OCLC, and Ovid Technologies

MEDLINE (MEDICAL LITERATURE ANALYSIS AND RETRIEVAL SYSTEM ONLINE)
- Produced by the National Library of Medicine in the United States
- Premier bibliographic database for journal articles in life sciences
- Coverage begins in 1950 and approximately 5,200 worldwide journals are indexed
- Indexed with MeSH (Medical Subject Headings)
- MEDLINE is available for free via PubMed and by subscription from EBSCO, OCLC, and Ovid Technologies

PROQUEST DISSERTATIONS AND THESES
- Produced ProQuest
- Earliest records from 1637
- PDF downloads available for over 1 million dissertations
- Available from ProQuest

PSYCINFO
- Produced by the American Psychological Association (APA)
- An abstract database of the psychosocial literature beginning with citations dating back to 1800
- Covers more than 2,150 journals
- 98% are peer-reviewed journals
- Also includes book chapters and dissertations
- Indexed with the Thesaurus of Psychological Index Terms
- Available via APA PsycNET, EBSCO, Ovid Technologies, and ProQuest

Internet: Online Search Engines

You are probably familiar with accessing a **Web browser** (e.g., Internet Explorer, Mozilla FireFox, or Safari) to conduct searches for music or other entities and using search engines such as Google to find information or articles. However, "surfing" the Web is not a good use of your time for scholarly literature searches. Table 3-3 indicates sources of free online information. Review it carefully to determine if it is a good source of primary research studies. Note that it includes government Web sites such as www.hrsa.gov and www.nih.gov, which

TABLE 3-3 Selected Examples of Free Web Sites to Support Evidence-Based Practice

Web Site	Scope	Notes
Virginia Henderson International Nursing Library www.nursinglibrary.org	Access to the *Registry of Nursing Research* database, which contains nearly 30,000 abstracts of research studies and conference papers.	Service offered without charge; locate conference abstracts and research study abstracts. This library is supported by Sigma Theta Tau International, honor society of nursing.
National Guideline Clearinghouse www.guidelines.gov	Public resource for evidence-based clinical practice guidelines. There are over 1,900 guidelines, including non-U.S. publications.	Offers a useful online feature of side-by-side comparison of guidelines.
National Institute of Nursing Research www.nih.gov/ninr	Promotes science for nursing practice, funding for nursing and interdisciplinary research, and nurse scientist training programs; provides links to many nursing organizations and search sites; excellent site for graduate students.	Although able to link to CRISP (Computer Retrieval of Information on Scientific Projects) and PubMed (National Library of Medicine's search service), which accesses literature via MEDLINE and PreMEDLINE and other related material from online journals, this is a *limited* site for the beginning consumer of research for conducting scholarly review of nursing research literature because MEDLINE alone does not include all nursing literature; searching CINAHL and MEDLINE on your own would be your first choice; useful site for graduate students in addition to CINAHL and MEDLINE and a third database related to topic.
Turning Research into Practice (TRIP) www.tripdatabase.com	Content from a wide variety of free online resources, including synopses, guidelines, medical images, e-textbooks, and systematic reviews, is brought together under the TRIP search engine.	Check this tool out for a wide sampling of available evidence.
Agency for Health Research and Quality www.ahrq.gov	Over 160 evidence topic reports, 16 technical reports, as well as research reviews.	Free source of important government documents for both consumers and conductors of research; also searchable via PubMed.
Cochrane Collaboration www.cochrane.org	Provides free access to abstracts from the Cochrane Database of Systematic Reviews. Full text of reviews and access to the databases that are part of the Cochrane Library—Database of Abstracts of Reviews of Effectiveness, Cochrane Controlled Trials Register, Cochrane Methodology Register, Health Technology Assessment database (HTA), and NHS Economic Evaluation Database (NHS EED) are accessible via Wiley.	Abstracts of Cochrane Reviews are available without charge and can be browsed or searched; uses many databases in its reviews, including CINAHL via EBSCO and MEDLINE; some are primary sources (e.g., systematic reviews/meta-analyses); others (if commentaries of single studies) are a secondary source; important source for clinical evidence but limited as a provider of primary documents for literature reviews.

are sources of health information, and some clinical guidelines based on systematic reviews of the literature, but most Web sites are not a primary source of research studies. Less common and less used sources of scholarly material are audiotapes, videotapes, personal communications (e.g., letters or telephone or in-person interviews), unpublished doctoral dissertations, masters' theses, and conference proceedings.

Most searches using electronic databases include not only citation information but also the abstract of the article and options for obtaining the full text. When possible print the full text, which of course will include the abstract as well as the complete references. If the text is not available, choose the option *complete reference,* which will include the abstract. Reading the abstract (see Chapter 1) is critical to determining if you need to retrieve the article through another mechanism.

Use both CINAHL and MEDLINE electronic databases; it will facilitate all steps of critically reviewing the literature, especially the gaps.

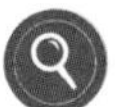

EVIDENCE-BASED PRACTICE TIP

Reading systematic reviews, if available, on your clinical question/topic will enhance your ability to implement evidence-based nursing practice because they generally offer the strongest and most consistent level of evidence.

How Far Back Must the Search Go?

Students often ask questions such as the following: "How many articles do I need?" "How much is enough?" "How far back in the literature do I need to go?" When conducting a search, you should use a rigorous focusing process or you may end up with hundreds or thousands of citations. Retrieving too many citations is usually a sign that there was something wrong with your search technique or you may have not sufficiently narrowed your clinical question.

Each online database offers an explanation of each feature; it is worth your time to click on each icon and explore the explanations offered because this will increase your confidence. Also keep in mind the types of articles you are retrieving. Many online resources allow you to limit your search by randomized controlled trials or systematic reviews. In CINAHL there is a limit for "Research" that will restrict the citations you retrieve to research articles. See Figure 3-4 as an example of using the "Research" limit to locate the Meneses article on breast cancer survivors (see Appendix A).

A general timeline for most academic or evidenced-based practice papers/projects is to go back in the literature at least 3 years, but preferably 5 years, although some research projects may warrant going back 10 or more years. Extensive literature reviews on particular topics or a concept clarification methodology study helps you to limit the length of your search.

As you scroll through and mark the citations you wish to include in your downloaded or printed search, make sure you include all relevant fields when you save or print. In addition to indicating which citations you want and choosing which fields to print or save, there is an opportunity to indicate if you want the "search history" included. It is always a good idea to include this information. It is especially helpful if your instructor suggests that some citations were missed, because then you can replicate your search and together figure out what variable(s) you missed so that you do not make the same error again. This is also your opportunity to indicate if you want to e-mail the search to yourself. If you are writing a paper and need to

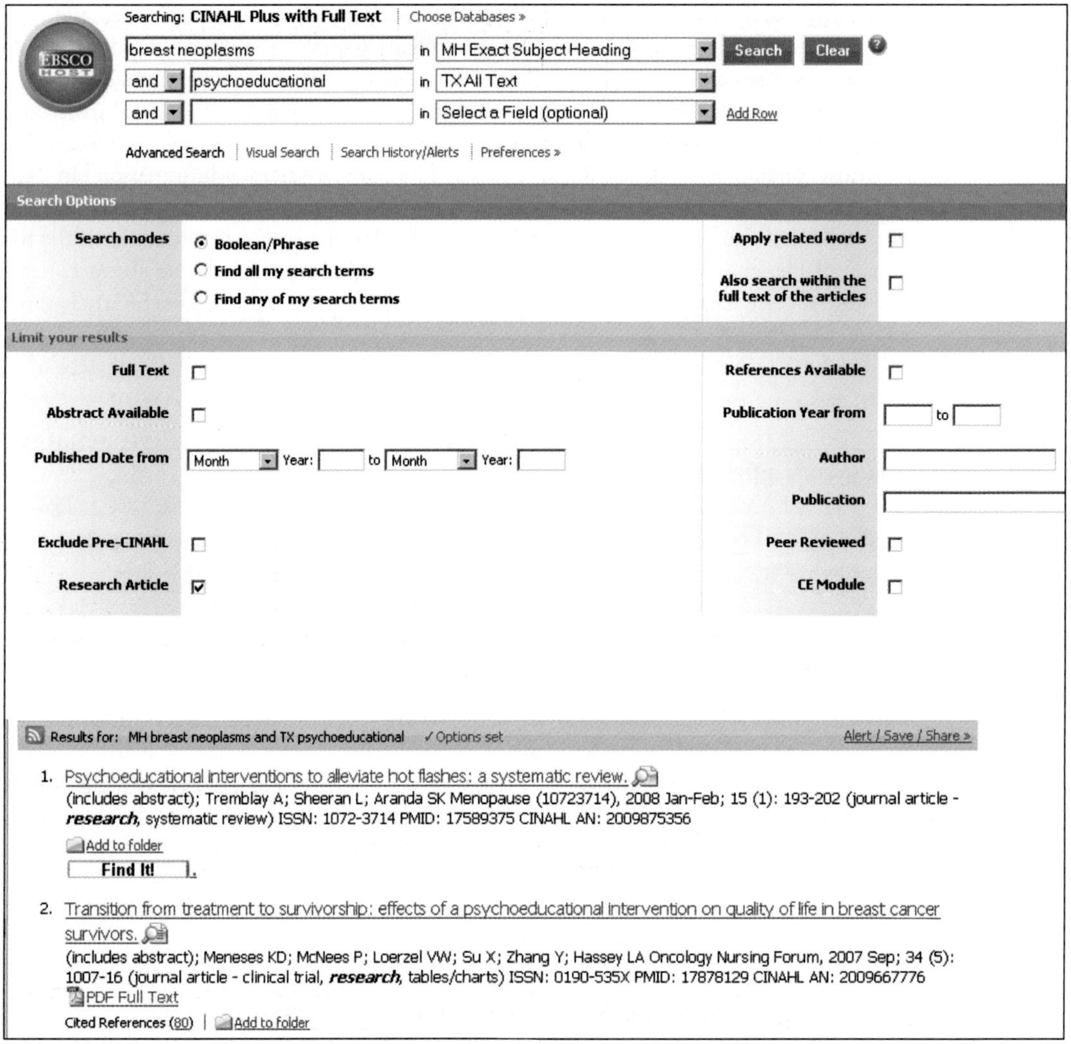

Searching: **CINAHL Plus with Full Text** | Choose Databases »

EBSCO HOST

breast neoplasms in MH Exact Subject Heading [Search] [Clear]
and psychoeducational in TX All Text
and in Select a Field (optional) Add Row

Advanced Search | Visual Search | Search History/Alerts | Preferences »

Search Options

Search modes	**Boolean/Phrase** **Find all my search terms** **Find any of my search terms**	**Apply related words** **Also search within the full text of the articles**	

Limit your results

Full Text	☐	**References Available**	☐
Abstract Available	☐	**Publication Year from**	to
Published Date from	Month Year: to Month Year:	**Author**	
		Publication	
Exclude Pre-CINAHL	☐	**Peer Reviewed**	☐
Research Article	☑	**CE Module**	☐

Results for: MH breast neoplasms and TX psychoeducational ✓Options set Alert / Save / Share »

1. Psychoeducational interventions to alleviate hot flashes: a systematic review.
(includes abstract); Tremblay A; Sheeran L; Aranda SK Menopause (10723714), 2008 Jan-Feb; 15 (1): 193-202 (journal article - ***research***, systematic review) ISSN: 1072-3714 PMID: 17589375 CINAHL AN: 2009875356
Add to folder
Find It!

2. Transition from treatment to survivorship: effects of a psychoeducational intervention on quality of life in breast cancer survivors.
(includes abstract); Meneses KD; McNees P; Loerzel VW; Su X; Zhang Y; Hassey LA Oncology Nursing Forum, 2007 Sep; 34 (5): 1007-16 (journal article - clinical trial, ***research***, tables/charts) ISSN: 0190-535X PMID: 17878129 CINAHL AN: 2009667776
PDF Full Text
Cited References (80) | Add to folder

Figure 3-4 Example of CINAHL Search Screen via EBSCO locating Meneses' survivorship article.

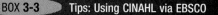

BOX 3-3 Tips: Using CINAHL via EBSCO

- Locate CINAHL from your library's home page. It may be located under databases, online resources, or nursing resources.
- In the Advanced Tab type in your key word or phrase (e.g., breast cancer, psychoeducational, quality of life). Do not use complete sentences. (Ask your librarian for the manual guide for each database or use feature in the database.)
- Before choosing "Search," make sure you mark "Research Articles," to ensure that you have retrieved only articles that are actually research. See the results in Figure 3-4.
- Note that in the Limit Your Results section you can limit by year, age-group, clinical queries, etc.
- Using the Boolean connector "and" between each of the above words you wish to use plus additional variables narrows your search. Using the Boolean "or" broadens your search.
- Note in Figure 3-4 that you can set up an RSS feed so that you are notified whenever new citations are added to the CINAHL database.
- Once the search results appear and you determine that they are manageable, you can decide whether to review them online, print, save, export, or e-mail them to yourself.

produce a bibliography you can export your citations to citation management software, which is a software program that formats and stores your citations so that they are available for electronic retrieval when they are needed to insert in a paper you are writing. Quite a few of these are available; some are free, such as Zotero, and others you or your institution must purchase, including EndNote and RefWorks.

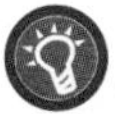

HELPFUL HINT

Ask your instructor for guidance if you are uncertain how far back you need to conduct your search. If you come across a systematic review on your specific clinical topic, scan it to see what years the review covers; then begin your search from the last year forward to the present.

What Do I Need to Know?

Each database usually has a specific search guide that provides information on the organization of the entries and the terminology used. The following suggestions and strategies as listed in Box 3-3 incorporate general search strategies, as well as those related to CINAHL and MEDLINE. Finding the right terms to "plug in" as keywords for a computer search is an important aspect of conducting a search. When possible, you want to match the words that you use to describe your question with the terms that indexers have assigned to the articles. In many online databases you can browse the controlled vocabulary terms and search. If you are still having difficulty, do not hesitate to ask your reference librarian.

Figure 3-4 is a screen shot of CINAHL in the EBSCO interface. As noted, you have the option of searching using the **controlled vocabulary** of CINAHL or a keyword search. If you wanted to locate the article "Transition from Treatment to Survivorship: Effects of a Psychoeducational Intervention on Quality of Life in Breast Cancer Survivors" (see Appendix A) you might take the approach of using both controlled vocabulary terms and keyword terms.

In this example, the two main concepts are your population of breast cancer survivors and the psychoeducational intervention. Breast cancer lends itself to a controlled term in the CINAHL subject headings, namely *breast neoplasms,* whereas *psychoeducational* is a unique term and is best searched in the text fields of the CINAHL database. Also note that these two concepts are connected with the **Boolean operator,** which defines the relationships between words or groups of words in your literature search. Examples of Boolean operators are words such as "AND," "OR," "NOT," and "NEAR." To restrict our retrieval to research, the "Research Article" limit has been applied.

Lawrence (2007) has a step-by-step presentation for conducting a search in CINAHL. She describes the controlled vocabulary, Boolean operators, and tips for narrowing your results in the EBSCO interface.

For further reading, a recent series in *Journal of Emergency Nursing* outlines the steps for embarking on an evidence-based search (Bernardo, 2008; Engberg & Schlenk, 2007; Klem & Northcutt, 2008), which covers the stages of evidence-based practice and basic search hints. This search was aimed at locating a known article to demonstrate some of the features of CINAHL. To broaden this search for other interventions that affect quality of life in breast cancer survivors you might change your terms entered to include *quality of life* and not focus on just *psychoeducational.* If the results from a broader search are to be saved for later use in a research paper for school, it is recommended that you export the bibliographic information to a citation manager, many of which have online interfaces so you can directly export from CINAHL, MEDLINE, and other databases. This software is designed to create bibliographies that conform to various styles such as the American Psychological Association (APA, 2008). If you have not used a package such as Zotero, EndNote, or RefWorks, consult your librarian.

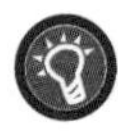

HELPFUL HINT

Look for useful tools within the search interfaces of online databases to make your searching more efficient. For example, when searching for a particular age-group, use the built-in limits of the database instead of relying on a keyword search. Other shortcuts include the Clinical Queries in CINAHL and MEDLINE that pull out therapy or diagnostic articles.

How Do I Complete the Search?

Now the truly important aspect of your searching begins: your critical reading of the retrieved materials. Critically reading scholarly material, especially research articles, requires several readings and the use of critiquing criteria (see Chapters 1, 6, and 16). Do not be discouraged if all of the retrieved articles are not as useful as you first thought; this happens to the most experienced reviewer of literature. If most of the articles are not useful, be prepared to do another search, but discuss the search terms you will use next time with your instructor and/or the reference librarian, and you may want to add a third database. In the previous example of a psychoeducational intervention for women who are breast cancer survivors, the third database of choice may be PsycINFO (see Box 3-2). Remind yourself how quickly you will be able to do it, now that you are experienced.

HELPFUL HINT

Read the abstract carefully (review the discussion on critical reading strategies in Chapter 2) to determine if it is a research article. It is also a good idea to review the references of your articles; if any seem relevant, you can retrieve them.

LITERATURE REVIEW FORMAT: WHAT TO EXPECT

Becoming familiar with the format of the literature review helps research consumers use critiquing criteria to evaluate the review. To decide which style you will use so that your review is presented in a logical and organized manner, you must consider the following:

- The research or clinical question/topic
- The number of retrieved sources reviewed
- The number and type of research versus conceptual materials

Some reviews are written according to the variables being studied and presented chronologically under each variable. Others present the material chronologically with subcategories or variables discussed within each time period. Still others present the variables and include subcategories related to the study's type or designs or related variables.

An example of a literature review, although brief, that is logically presented according to the variables under study was completed by Jones, Renger, and Kang (2007) (see Appendix B). The researchers stated that the purpose of their study was to "test the effectiveness of the Deaf Heart Health Intervention (DHHI) in increasing self-efficacy for health behaviors related to risk for cardiovascular disease (CVD) among culturally deaf adults." The authors did not have a titled "Literature" section in their report. Rather they had three titled sections, "Self-Efficacy for Health-Related Behaviors," "The Deaf Heart Health Intervention," and "Barriers to Accessing Health Information in Deaf Adults." All three sections contained literature related to the problem under study. For example, in the section on self-efficacy, the authors discussed that self-efficacy is a key construct in understanding and modifying behavior; they offer conceptual definitions, present earlier studies, critically appraise their strengths and weaknesses, and demonstrate how the study hypothesis was generated based on the relationships between and among those three conceptual areas. They concluded that "a clinical trial of the DHHI will be necessary to evaluate the theoretical correlations between self-efficacy and targeted behaviors, and the effectiveness of the DHHI in decreasing risk for CVD among culturally deaf adults."

In contrast to the styles of previous quantitative studies, the literature reviews of qualitative studies are usually handled in a different manner (see Chapters 4, 5, and 6). There is often little known about the topic under study. The literature may be conducted at the beginning of the study or after the data analysis is completed. The researchers always compare the literature review with their findings. In some cases, the reviewed literature is used during the analysis process as well.

EVIDENCE-BASED PRACTICE TIP

Sort the research articles you retrieve according to the levels of evidence model in Chapter 1. Remember that articles that are systematic reviews, especially meta-analyses, generally provide the strongest and most consistent evidence to include in a literature review.

HELPFUL HINT

When writing up your literature review you want to include enough information so that your professor or fellow students could re-create your search path and come up with the same results. This means including information regarding the databases searched, the date you searched, years of coverage, terms used, and any limits or restrictions that you used.

APPRAISING THE EVIDENCE:

Review of the Literature

Whether you were a researcher writing the literature review for the research study you were planning to conduct or a nurse writing a literature review for an evidence-based practice project, you would need to critically appraise individual research reports using appropriate criteria. If you are appraising an individual research study that is to be included in a literature review, it must be evaluated in terms of critical appraisal criteria that are related to each step of the research process (see the critical appraisal criteria at the end of Chapters 2, 3, 7 to 16 for quantitative studies and Chapters 4, 5, and 6 for qualitative studies) so that the strengths and weaknesses of each study can be identified. Standardized critical appraisal tools (e.g., CASP Tools and AGREE Guidelines) available for specific types of research designs (e.g., clinical trials, cohort studies, systematic reviews) can also be used to critically appraise an individual research study (see Chapters 1 and 18).

Critiquing the literature review of research or conceptual reports is a challenging task for seasoned consumers of research, so do not be surprised if you feel a little intimidated by the prospect of critiquing the published research. The important issue is to determine the overall value of the literature review, including both the research and theoretical materials. The purposes of a literature review (see Box 3-1) and the characteristics of a well-written literature review (Box 3-4) provide the framework for developing the evaluation criteria for a literature review.

The literature review should be presented in an organized manner. The theoretical and research literature can be presented chronologically from earliest studies to most recent; sometimes the theoretical literature that provided the foundation for the existing research will be presented first followed by the research studies that were derived from this theoretical base. Other times, the literature can be clustered by concept, grouped according to pro or con positions, or evidence that highlights differences in theoretical and/or research findings. The overall question to be answered is, "Does the review of the literature develop and present a knowledge base for a research study or an evidence-based practice project that builds on previ-

BOX 3-4 Characteristics of a Well-Written Review of the Literature

Each reviewed source of information reflects critical thinking and scholarly writing and is relevant to the study/topic/project, and the content satisfies the following criteria:

- Organizes the literature review using a systematic approach
- Summarizes each research or conceptual article succinctly and with appropriate references
- Uses established critical appraisal criteria for specific study designs to evaluate the study for strengths, weaknesses, or limitations, as well as for conflicts or gaps in information that relate directly or indirectly to the area of interest
- Provides evidence of a synthesis of the critiques that highlight the overall strengths and weaknesses of the studies reviewed
- Consists of mainly primary sources; there are a sufficient number of research sources
- Concludes with a synthesis of the reviewed material that reflects why the study or project should be implemented
- Identifies research questions and hypotheses or answers clinical questions

ous research, identifies a conflict or gap in the literature, and/or proposes to extend the current knowledge base?" (see Box 3-1).

However the literature review is organized, it should provide a strong knowledge base to carry out the research, educational, or clinical practice project. Questions related to the logical organization and presentation of the reviewed studies are somewhat more challenging for beginning research consumers. The more you read research studies, the more competent you become at differentiating a well-organized literature review from one that has no organizing framework.

Whenever possible, read both qualitative (meta-syntheses) and quantitative (meta-analyses) systematic reviews pertaining to a clinical question that provide Level I evidence (see Chapters 1, 9, and 18). Although systematic reviews are considered to be examples of secondary sources because they represent a body of completed research studies that have been critically appraised and synthesized by a team other than the original researchers, they often represent the best available evidence on a particular clinical issue. The systematic review on "Nursing Interventions for Smoking Cessation" (Rice & Stead, 2008) is an example of a quantitative systematic review that critically appraised and synthesized the evidence from research studies related to the effectiveness of smoking cessation interventions provided by registered nurses and advanced practice nurses (see Appendix E).

The Critiquing Criteria box summarizes general critiquing criteria for a review of the literature. Other sets of critiquing criteria may phrase these questions differently or more broadly. For instance, questions may be the following: "Does the literature search seem adequate?" "Does the report demonstrate scholarly writing?" These may seem to be difficult questions for you to answer; one place to begin, however, is by determining whether the source is a refereed

CRITIQUING CRITERIA: *Review of the Literature*

1. Are all of the relevant concepts and variables included in the review?
2. Does the search strategy include an appropriate and adequate number of databases and other resources to identify key published and unpublished research and theoretical sources?
3. Are both theoretical literature and research literature included?
4. Is there an appropriate theoretical/conceptual framework that guides the development of the research study?
5. Are primary sources mainly used?
6. What gaps or inconsistencies in knowledge does the literature review uncover?
7. Does the literature review build on earlier studies?
8. Does the summary of each reviewed study reflect the essential components of the study design (e.g., type and size of sample, reliability and validity of instruments, consistency of data-collection procedures, appropriate data analysis, identification of limitations)?
9. Does the critique of each reviewed study include strengths, weaknesses, or limitations of the design, conflicts, and gaps in information related to the area of interest?
10. Does the synthesis summary follow a logical sequence that presents the overall strengths and weaknesses of the reviewed studies and arrive at a logical conclusion?
11. Is the literature review presented in an organized format that flows logically (e.g., chronologically, clustered by concept or variables), enhancing the reader's ability to evaluate the need for the particular research study or evidence-based practice project?
12. Does the literature review follow the proposed purpose of the research study or evidence-based practice project?
13. Does the literature review generate research questions or hypotheses or answer a clinical question?

journal. It is reasonable to assume that a scholarly refereed journal publishes manuscripts that are adequately searched, use mainly primary sources, and are written in a scholarly manner. This does not mean, however, that every study reported in a refereed journal will meet all of the critiquing criteria for a literature review and other components of the study in an equal manner. Because of style differences and space constraints, each citation summarized is often very brief, or related citations may be summarized as a group and lack a critique. You still must answer the critiquing questions. Consultation with a faculty advisor may be necessary to develop skill in answering this question.

The key to a strong literature review is a careful search of the published and unpublished literature. Whether writing or critically appraising a literature review written for a published research study, it should reflect a synthesis or pulling together of the main points or value of all of the sources reviewed in relation to the study's research question or hypothesis (see Box 3-1). The relationship between and among these studies must be explained. The synthesis of a written review of the literature usually appears at the end of the review section before the research question or hypothesis reporting section. If not labeled as such, it is usually evident in the last paragraph of the introduction and/or the end of the review of the literature.

Searching the literature, like critiquing the literature, is an acquired skill. Practicing your search and critical appraisal skills on a regular basis will make a huge difference. Seeking guidance from faculty is essential to developing critical appraisal skills. Synthesizing the body of literature you have critiqued is even more challenging. Critiquing the literature will help you apply new knowledge from your critical appraisal to practice. This process is vital to the "survival and growth of the nursing profession and is essential to evidence-based practice" (Pravikoff & Donaldson, 2001).

HELPFUL HINT

- Use standardized critical appraisal criteria to evaluate your research articles.
- Make a table to represent the components of your study and fill in your evaluation to help you see the big picture of your analysis.
- Synthesize the results of your analysis to try and determine what was similar or different among and between these studies related to your topic/clinical question and then draw a conclusion.

CRITICAL THINKING CHALLENGES

- Using the PICO format, generate a clinical question related to health promotion for elementary school children.
- How does a research article's theoretical or conceptual framework interrelate concepts, theories, conceptual definitions, and operational definitions?
- A general guideline for a literature search is to use a timeline of 3 to 5 years. When would a nurse researcher need to search beyond this timeline?
- What is the relationship of the research article's literature review to the theoretical or conceptual framework?

KEY POINTS

- The review of the literature is defined as a broad, comprehensive, in-depth, systematic critique and synthesis of scholarly publications, unpublished scholarly print and online materials, audiovisual materials, and personal communications.
- The review of the literature is used for development of research studies, as well as other consumer of research activities such as development of evidence-based practice projects.
- The main objectives for the consumer of research in relation to conducting and writing a literature review are to acquire the ability to do the following: (1) conduct an appropriate electronic research and/or print research search on a topic; (2) efficiently retrieve a sufficient amount of materials for a literature review in relation to the topic and scope of project; (3) critically appraise (i.e., critique) research and theoretical material based on accepted critiquing criteria; (4) critically evaluate published reviews of the literature based on accepted standardized critiquing criteria; (5) synthesize the findings of the critique materials for relevance to the purpose of the selected scholarly project; and (6) determine applicability to practice.
- Primary research and theoretical resources are essential for literature reviews.
- Secondary sources, such as commentaries on research articles from peer-reviewed journals, are part of a learning strategy for developing critical critiquing skills.
- It is more efficient to use electronic rather than print databases for retrieving scholarly materials.
- Strategies for efficiently retrieving scholarly literature for nursing include consulting the reference librarian and using at least two online sources (e.g., CINAHL and MEDLINE).
- Literature reviews are usually organized according to variables, as well as chronologically.
- Critiquing and synthesizing a number of research articles, including systematic reviews, is essential to implementing evidence-based nursing practice.

REFERENCES

American Association of Colleges of Nursing: *The essentials of baccalaureate education for professional practice,* Washington, DC, 2008, The Author.

American College of Physicians: ACP PIER overview, 2008. Retrieved June 27, 2008, from http://pier.acponline.org/overview.html.

American Nurses Association: *Commission on nursing research: education for preparation in nursing research,* Kansas City, MO, 1989, The Association.

American Psychological Association: Databases—PsycINFO, 2008. Retrieved June 26, 2008, from www.apa.org/psycinfo/.

Bernardo LM: Finding the best evidence, part 1: understanding electronic databases, *J Emerg Nurs* 34(1):59-60, 2008.

Engberg S, Schlenk EA: Asking the right question, *J Emerg Nurs* 33(6):571-573, 2007.

Haynes B: Of studies, syntheses, synopses, summaries, and systems: the "5S" evolution of information services for evidence-based healthcare decisions, *Evidence-Based Nurs* 10(1):6-7, 2007.

Horgas AJ, Yoon SL, Nichols AL, et al: The relationship between pain and functional disability in black and white older adults, *Res Nurs Health* 31(4):341-354, 2008.

Jones EG, Renger R, Kang Y: Self-efficacy for health-related behaviors among deaf adults, *Res Nurs Health* 30:185-192, 2007.

Klem ML, Northcutt T: Finding the best evidence part 2: the basics of literature searches, *J Emerg Nurs* 34(2):151-153, 2008.

Lawrence JC: Techniques for searching the CINAHL database using the EBSCO interface, *AORN J* 85(4):779-780, 782-788, 790-791, 2007.

Meneses KD, McNees P, Loerzei VW, et al: Transition from treatment to survivorship: effects of a psychoeducational intervention on quality of life in breast cancer survivors, *Oncol Nurs Forum* 34(5):1007-1016, 2007.

National Library of Medicine: PubMed overview, 2008. Retrieved June 26, 2008, from www.ncbi.nlm.nih.gov/entrez/query/static/overview.html#Introduction.

Pravikoff D, Donaldson N: The online journal of clinical innovations, *Online J Issues Nurs* 5(1), 2001. Retrieved September 9, 2008 from: www.nursingworld.org/ojin/topic11/tpc11_6c.htm.

ProQuest: ProQuest dissertations and theses databases, 2008. Retrieved June 26, 2008, from www.il.proquest.com/products_pq/descriptions/pqdt.shtml.

Rice VH, Stead LF: Nursing interventions for smoking cessation, *Cochrane Database of Systematic Reviews* (1):CD001188. DOI: 10.1002/14651858.CD001188.pub3, 2008.

TRIP: Introduction and background—TRIP database, 2008. Retrieved June 27, 2008, from www.tripdatabase.com/AboutUs/Index.html.

Wiley Interface: Reference works, 2008. *The Cochrane Library 2008,* Issue 2. Retrieved June 26, 2008, from www3.interscience.wiley.com/cgi-bin/mrwhome/106568753/ProductDescriptions.html.

FOR FURTHER STUDY

evolve

Go to Evolve at http://evolve.elsevier.com/LoBiondo/ for review questions, critiquing exercises, and additional research articles for practice in reviewing and critiquing.

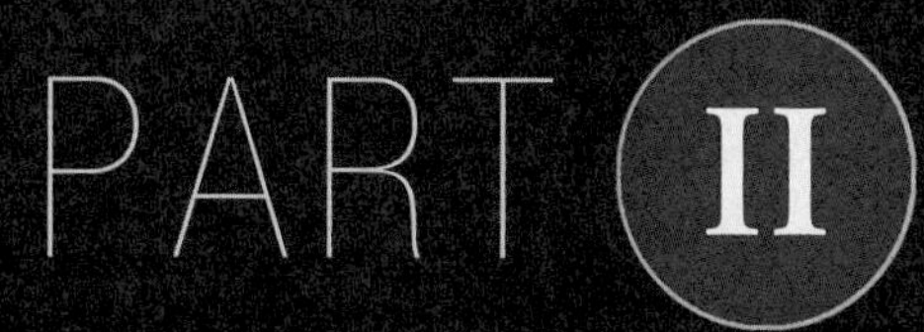

PROCESSES AND EVIDENCE RELATED TO QUALITATIVE RESEARCH

RESEARCH VIGNETTE

Program of Research on Miscarriage and Caring

Kristen M. Swanson, RN, PhD, FAAN
University of Washington, Seattle, Washington

The first few years of being a nurse I did things in twos: 2 years in practice, 2 years to get my masters in cardiac nursing, 2 years teaching medical-surgical nursing, and 2 years of course work toward my PhD in psychosocial nursing. Then I became a mother. Five weeks later I found myself sitting in a mothers' support group holding my infant son and listening to an obstetrician talking about spontaneous abortion. He lectured on the diagnosis, prognosis, treatment, and management of unexpected, unintended disruption of pregnancy before the point of expected fetal viability. When he finished, the women around me began to talk about what it had felt like to miscarry their babies. Two things happened that night: I looked down at my son and with a chill realized, "My God, I could have lost him!" Until that moment it had honestly never occurred to me. I was 29 years old and naively believed that if I worked hard enough, studied hard enough, or prayed hard enough, I could accomplish whatever I set my mind to. The reality of the fragility of life profoundly touched me. The second thing that happened that night was that I thought about the 1980 American Nurses Association (ANA) Social Policy statement that staked nursing's domain as the diagnosis and treatment of human responses to actual or potential health problems. That evening I became aware that while the obstetrician focused on the diagnosis and treatment of the actual or potential problems of spontaneously aborting, the women were living the human response to miscarriage of a beloved baby. Their very language was different. That night pretty much set my research program in motion.

As a doctoral student of Drs. Jean Watson and Jody Glittenberg, I had been fully exposed to the importance of context in making meaning of life events and the role of caring in supporting human healing. My philosophy of science and nursing theory courses exposed me to the limits of postpositivist empiricism when trying to understand human experiences. Yet, consistent with many nursing doctoral programs at that time (1980-1983), the research courses focused solely on quantitative methodologies. When it came time to do my dissertation, I found myself in quite a quandary. My question begged an interpretive approach, yet my skills in qualitative methods were lacking. Naively, I set out to do my own self-study. I drew inspiration about the importance of phenomenological interpretation of lived experiences from the writings of Giorgi (1970), figured out how to conduct open-ended interviews by reading about Spradley's ethnographic interviewing techniques (1979), and learned how to compare and contrast text data by reading Glaser and Strauss's classic text (1967) on grounded theory. My friend John Seidel showed me how to use a qualitative data management mainframe computer program he was developing. Hence I ended up weaving together a patchwork set of methods that facilitated my ability to analyze the rich stories shared by the 20 women who explained to me what it was like to miscarry and what caring meant in that context (Swanson-Kauffman, 1983). There were three outcomes of that dissertation study: (1)

the human experience of miscarriage model; (2) a model of caring in the context of miscarriage; and (3) reinforcement for John Seidel that set new directions for his fledgling computer program that went on to become "The Ethnograph" (available through www.qualisresearch.com/). In retrospect, I believe the methodology I used at that time might best be described as a descriptive phenomenology.

Subsequently, I completed two more phenomenological investigations of caring (see Swanson-Kauffman, 1986a, 1986b; and Swanson, 1990, 1991, 1993). I then combined these three studies and developed a middle-range theory of caring that I have subsequently tested through two randomized trials. The caring theory was also further validated through an in-depth review of 130 data-based publications on caring that I did during my sabbatical in 1996. Through that intensive review of the literature, I found approximately 60 studies that focused on caring as a way of practicing. In reviewing those studies, I found tremendous evidence of convergence across many different qualitative studies of nurse caring and was able to draw links between the discoveries of others and my own propositions about what constitutes caring. I never set out to be a nurse theorist. I really just wanted to understand how to care for women in a manner that helped them resolve their losses. Nonetheless, the caring theory I developed has taken on a life of its own, and there are now hospitals that use it as a practice model, schools that use it as a curriculum model, and other investigators who have explored and tested its relevance to their research populations of interest.

My dissertation led me to an exciting and rewarding program of research. It has included instrument development, model testing, descriptive studies, and randomized trials. In 1999 I published the results of an National Institute of Nursing Research (NINR)-funded Solomon four-group randomized trial of the longitudinal effects of treatment (caring-based counseling) and measurement (early vs. delayed) on women's healing during the first year after miscarriage (Swanson, 1999a, 1999b). That study was the first randomized trial to demonstrate treatment effectiveness in assisting women to resolve miscarriage. Briefly, there was evidence that compared with controls (no treatment beyond usual obstetrical care), women who received three 1-hour caring-based nurse counseling sessions in the first 3 months after miscarrying experienced less depression, anger, and overall disturbed moods during the first year after miscarriage.

Based on the findings from that first intervention study, I was invited by Evergreen Hospital and Medical Center in Kirkland, Washington, to set up a couples' miscarriage support group. My colleagues and I based the support group on the miscarriage model and trained group leaders to implement the caring theory. After helping to run several groups myself, I witnessed the healing power of working with couples versus women alone. Furthermore, in a secondary analysis of data from the first intervention study, we discovered that approximately one third of women claimed to be both interpersonally and sexually more distant from their mates 1 year after miscarriage (Swanson et al., 2003). Hence our recently completed study focused on couples. It was an NINR-funded randomized trial of three caring-based interventions against a control condition (no treatment). Our goal was to determine whether we could make a difference for women and their male mates during the first year after miscarriage. The main outcome variables included depression and grief. The interventions included the following: (1) nurse caring (three 1-hour nurse counseling sessions); (2) self-caring (three videotape and workbook modules mailed to couples for completion at home); and (3) combined caring (one nurse counseling session plus three videotape and workbook modules). After completion of outcome measures, the control group was mailed a complimentary set of the videotape and workbook modules. All interventions, based on the caring theory and miscarriage model, were delivered on the same time schedule. Outcome data were gathered 1, 3, 5, and 13 months after enrollment. There were many exciting and interesting components to this study. For the first time ever, I studied men's responses. Whereas there have been other investigators who have described men's responses to miscarriage, the size of our sample and the fact that it included couples in a randomized treatment protocol truly made this a unique study of how miscarriage takes its toll and how treatment can make a difference in how men and women heal after miscarriage. We have submitted our findings for publication and expect that results should be available in the not too distant future.

I love my work. Because my research is practice based, I still have hands-on experience in nursing. It is hard to believe that a research program born of curiosity has become a lifelong passion. I never cease to be amazed at how much there is to be learned about the ways in which men and women experience loss of pregnancy, and how grateful couples are that someone is studying their experience. I, in turn, am eternally grateful that couples have trusted us enough to allow us to witness their very personal transition through loss and healing.

REFERENCES

Giorgi A: *Psychology as a human science*, New York, 1970, Harper & Row.

Glaser BG, Strauss AL: *The discovery of grounded theory: strategies for qualitative research*, New York, 1967, Aldine.

Spradley JP: *The ethnographic interview*, New York, 1979, Holt, Rinehart, & Winston.

Swanson KM: Providing care in the NICU: sometimes an act of love, *Adv Nurs Sci* 13(1):60-73, 1990.

Swanson KM: Empirical development of a middle range theory of caring, *Nurs Res* 40(3):161-166, 1991.

Swanson KM: Nursing as informed caring for the well-being of others, *Image* 25(4):352-357, 1993.

Swanson KM: The effects of caring, measurement, and time on miscarriage impact and women's well-being in the first year subsequent to loss, *Nurs Res* 48(6):288-298, 1999a.

Swanson KM: Research-based practice with women who have had miscarriages, *Image* 31(4):339-345, 1999b.

Swanson KM, Karmali Z, Powell S, Pulvermahker F: Miscarriage effects on interpersonal and sexual relationships during the first year after loss: women's perceptions, *J Psychosomat Med* 65(5):902-910, 2003.

Swanson-Kauffman KM: *The unborn one: a profile of the human experience of miscarriage*, University of Colorado unpublished doctoral dissertation, 1983.

Swanson-Kauffman KM: A combined qualitative methodology for nursing research, *Adv Nurs Sci* 8(3):58-69, 1986a.

Swanson-Kauffman KM: Caring in the instance of unexpected early pregnancy loss, *Top Clin Nurs* 8(2):37-46, 1986b.

4

Introduction to Qualitative Research

Julie Barroso

KEY TERMS

context dependent
data saturation
exclusion criteria
"grand tour" question
inclusion criteria
naturalistic setting
paradigm
purposive sample
qualitative research

LEARNING OUTCOMES

After reading this chapter, you should be able to do the following:

- Describe the components of a qualitative research report.
- Differentiate between qualitative and quantitative research paradigms.
- Describe the beliefs generally held by qualitative researchers.
- Identify four ways qualitative findings can be used in evidence-based practice.

STUDY RESOURCES

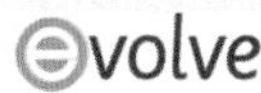

Go to Evolve at http://evolve.elsevier.com/LoBiondo/ for review questions, critiquing exercises, and additional research articles for practice in reviewing and critiquing.

Let's say that you are reading an article that reports findings that human immunodeficiency virus (HIV)–infected men are more adherent to their antiretroviral regimens than women. You wonder, why is that? Why would women be less adherent in taking their medications? Certainly, it is not solely because they are women. Or you are working on a postpartum unit and have just discharged a new mother who has debilitating rheumatoid arthritis. You wonder, what is the process by which disabled women decide to have children? How do they go about making that decision? These, like so many other questions we have as nurses, can be best answered through research conducted using qualitative methods. Qualitative research gives us the answers to those difficult "Why?" questions. Although it can be used at many different places in a program of research, you can most often find it answering questions we have when we understand very little about some phenomenon in nursing.

WHAT IS QUALITATIVE RESEARCH?

Qualitative research is a broad term that encompasses several different methodologies that share many similarities in the conduct of such research. It is a general term encompassing a varicty of philosophical underpinnings and research methods. According to Denzin and Lincoln (2005), "qualitative researchers study things in their natural settings, attempting to make sense of, or interpret, phenomena in terms of the meanings people bring to them." **Naturalistic settings** are ones that people live in every day. So, the researcher doing qualitative research goes wherever the participants are—in their homes, schools, communities, and sometimes in the hospital or an outpatient setting.

Qualitative studies most often help us to begin to formulate an understanding of a phenomenon. Although qualitative research has a long history in the social sciences, it is only within the past two decades that it has become more accepted in nursing research. For many years, doctoral nursing students were dissuaded from conducting qualitative studies; the push was for the traditional quantitative approach, which was viewed by many as being more credible to those in the "hard" sciences. So as nursing gained its foothold in academics, doctoral students were urged to conduct research using the quantitative **paradigm** or worldview, to help us gain legitimacy in academe. However, as academe and research evolved along two different but parallel channels, qualitative research found greater acceptance, and now we have a generation of nurse scholars who are trained in qualitative methods, and who encourage students to use the method that best answers their research questions, as opposed to using methods that might add a veneer of scientific legitimacy to its conduct but do not answer the research question at hand.

Qualitative research is discovery oriented; it is explanatory, descriptive in nature. It uses words, as opposed to numbers, to explain a phenomenon. Qualitative research lets us see the world through the eyes of another—the woman who struggles to take her antiretroviral medication, or the woman who has carefully thought through what it might be like to have a baby despite a debilitating illness. Qualitative researchers assume that we can only understand these things if we consider the context in which they take place, and this is why most qualitative research takes place in naturalistic settings.

Qualitative studies make the world of an individual visible to the rest of us. Qualitative research "encompasses modes of inquiry oriented toward how the social world is interpreted, understood, experienced, produced, or constituted" (Mason, 2002, p. 3). The Critical Thinking Decision Path illustrates a way of thinking about the different views of qualitative and

CRITICAL THINKING DECISION PATH Selecting a Research Process

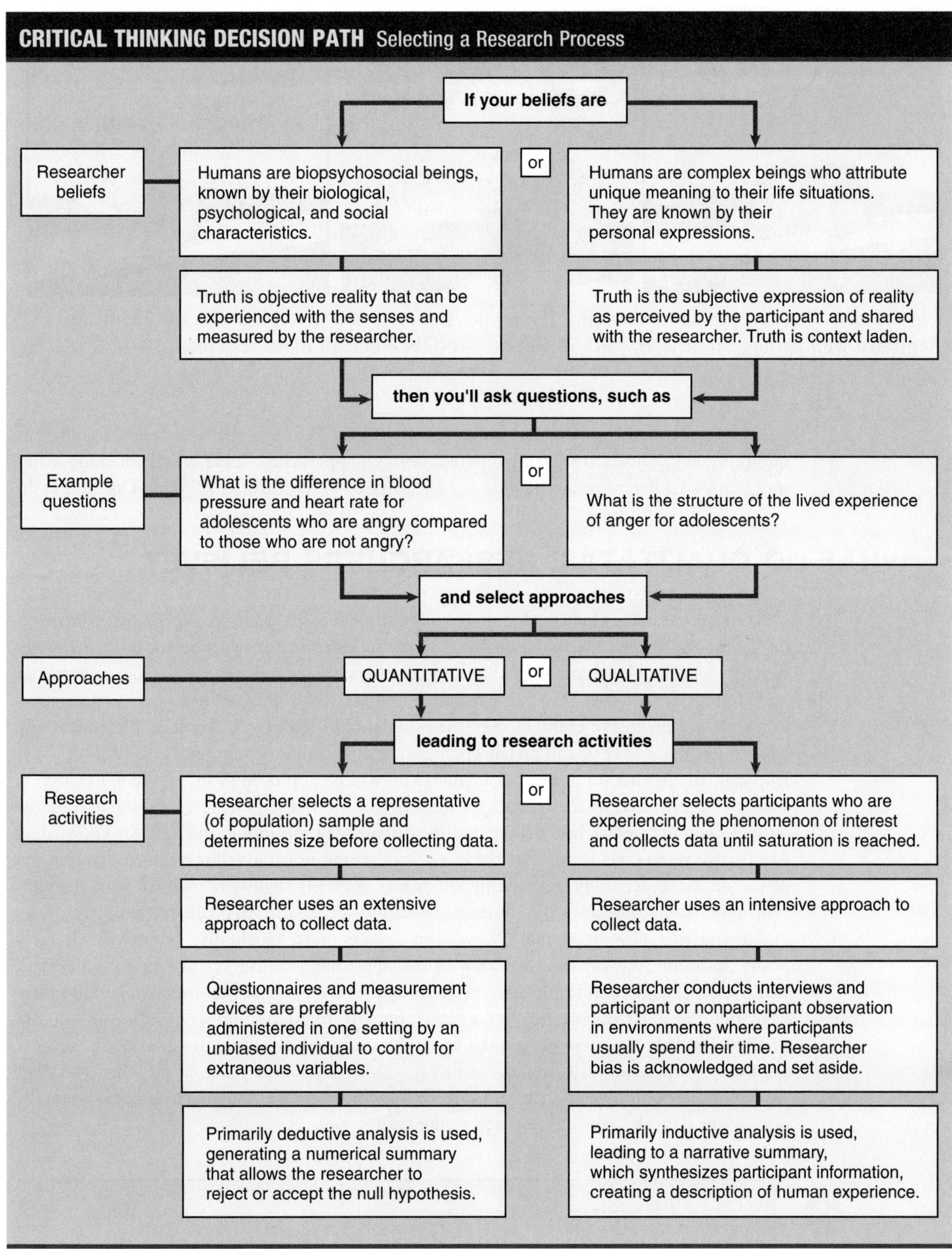
If your beliefs are
Researcher beliefs
Humans are biopsychosocial beings, known by their biological, psychological, and social characteristics.
or
Humans are complex beings who attribute unique meaning to their life situations. They are known by their personal expressions.
Truth is objective reality that can be experienced with the senses and measured by the researcher.
Truth is the subjective expression of reality as perceived by the participant and shared with the researcher. Truth is context laden.
then you'll ask questions, such as
Example questions
What is the difference in blood pressure and heart rate for adolescents who are angry compared to those who are not angry?
or
What is the structure of the lived experience of anger for adolescents?
and select approaches
Approaches
QUANTITATIVE
or
QUALITATIVE
leading to research activities
Research activities
Researcher selects a representative (of population) sample and determines size before collecting data.
or
Researcher selects participants who are experiencing the phenomenon of interest and collects data until saturation is reached.
Researcher uses an extensive approach to collect data.
Researcher uses an intensive approach to collect data.
Questionnaires and measurement devices are preferably administered in one setting by an unbiased individual to control for extraneous variables.
Researcher conducts interviews and participant or nonparticipant observation in environments where participants usually spend their time. Researcher bias is acknowledged and set aside.
Primarily deductive analysis is used, generating a numerical summary that allows the researcher to reject or accept the null hypothesis.
Primarily inductive analysis is used, leading to a narrative summary, which synthesizes participant information, creating a description of human experience.

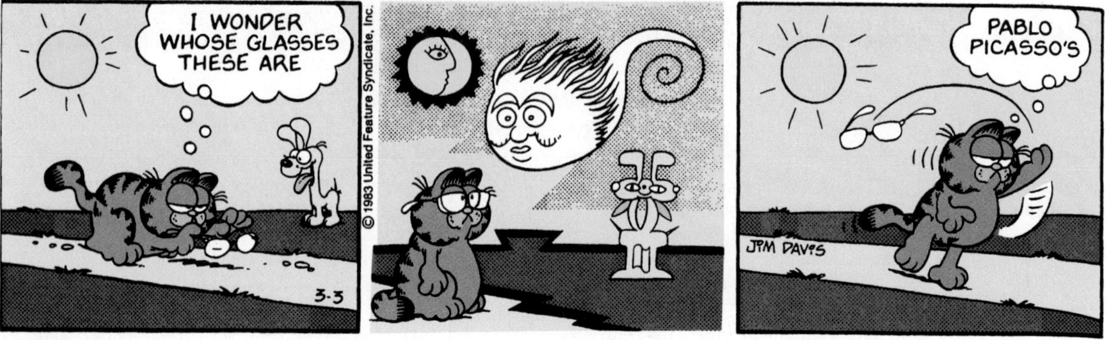
I WONDER WHOSE GLASSES THESE ARE
3-3
© 1983 United Feature Syndicate, Inc.
PABLO PICASSO'S
JIM DAVIS

Figure 4-1 Shifting perspectives: seeing the world as others see it. (GARFIELD, 1983 Paws, Inc. Reprinted with permission of UNIVERSAL PRESS SYNDICATE. All rights reserved.)

quantitative research processes. This decision algorithm illustrates that beliefs lead to different questions, which leads to selecting different research approaches. These beliefs and approaches lead to use of different research methods, as illustrated in the Critical Thinking Decision Path.

WHAT DO QUALITATIVE RESEARCHERS BELIEVE?

Qualitative researchers believe that there are multiple realities, that the experience of having a baby, though sharing some commonalities, is not the same for any two women, and is definitely different for a disabled mother. Qualitative researchers believe that reality is socially constructed and **context dependent.** That is, the meaning of an observation is defined by its circumstance or the environment. For example, even the experience of reading this book is different for any two students; one may be completely engrossed by the content, while another is reading but is worrying about whether or not her financial aid will be approved soon. Figure 4-1 is a great example of this; what we see depends on who we are and what experiences we bring to the situation. Qualitative researchers believe that the discovery of meaning is the basis for knowledge. Qualitative researchers know that there is a very strong imperative for them to describe the phenomenon under study well; ideally, the reader, if evenly slightly acquainted with the phenomenon, would have an "Aha!" moment in reading a well-written qualitative report.

So, you may now be saying, "Wow! This sounds great! Qualitative research is for me!" Many nurses do feel very comfortable with this approach, because we are educated in how to talk to people about the health issues concerning them; we are used to listening, and listening well. But the most important consideration for any research study is whether or not the methodology fits the question. It must fit, or the study will add little to our scientific knowledge base for practice. This is also the first question you should ask yourself when you read studies and are considering them as evidence on which to base your practice: does the methodology fit with the research question under study?

HELPFUL HINT

All research is based on a paradigm, but this is seldom specifically stated in a research report.

BOX 4-1 Steps in the Qualitative Research Process

Review of the literature	Data collection
Study design	Data analysis
Sample	Findings
Setting: recruitment and data collection	Conclusions

DOES THE METHODOLOGY FIT WITH THE RESEARCH QUESTION BEING ASKED?

As stated before, qualitative methods are often best for helping us to determine the nature of a phenomenon. Sometimes, authors will state that they are using qualitative methods because little is known about a phenomenon; that alone is not a good reason for conducting a study, though. Little may be known about a phenomenon because it does not matter! For us to ask people to participate in a study, to open themselves and their lives to us, we should be asking about things that will help us to make a difference in their lives, in how we provide nursing care. You should be able to articulate a valid reason for conducting a study, beyond "little is known about . . . ." In the examples at the start of this chapter, we need to know why HIV-infected women are less adherent to their medication regimens so we can work to change these barriers, and can anticipate these barriers when a woman is ready to start taking these pills. When we learn about the decision-making processes women use to decide whether or not to have a child when they are disabled, we can better answer the questions of the next woman who is going through this process. Next, let's discuss the parts of a qualitative research study. Box 4-1 outlines the steps of a qualitative study.

COMPONENTS OF A QUALITATIVE RESEARCH REPORT

Review of the Literature

The first step is one we have already discussed: being clear that a qualitative approach is the best way to answer the research question. Next, the author presents a review of the relevant literature. This may require creativity on the author's part, because there may not be any published research on the phenomenon in question. However, there are likely to be studies on similar subjects, or with the same patient population, or on a closely related concept. For example, the author may want to research how women who have a disabling illness make decisions about becoming pregnant. Although there may be no other studies in this particular area, there may be some on decision making in pregnancy when a woman does not have a disabling illness. These would be important to include in the review of the literature to show you as the reader that the author is familiar with the research on this process in a nondisabled woman. Or there may be literature on decision making in pregnancy when a woman has a different but not disabling illness, such as cancer or HIV infection. Reading all of this related literature will help you discern if the author really seems to know the field, and thus the kinds of questions they asked the subjects.

Let's say the author wanted to examine HIV-infected women's adherence to antiretroviral therapy. If there is no research on this direct topic, the author might examine research on adherence to therapy in other chronic illnesses, such as diabetes or hypertension. She or he might want to include studies that examine gender differences in medication adherence. Or the author might want to examine the literature on adherence in a stigmatizing illness, or to look at appointment adherence for women, to see what facilitates or acts as a barrier to attending health care appointments. The major point here is that even though there may be no literature on the author's exact subject, there should still be a review of the literature. In fact, it usually is more challenging to write the review of the literature for a qualitative study, because the authors must be creative and think of all of the other comparisons they need to make, whether it is on the study subject, relevant study concepts, or similar/dissimilar patient groups. At the conclusion of the review, you should feel clear about the most important points that you have learned, and should be able to articulate the problem to be studied and the purpose for studying it.

Study Design

In the next part of the report, the authors should explain the study design. In qualitative research, there may simply be a descriptive or naturalistic design, in which the researchers adhere to the general tenets of qualitative research, but do not commit to a particular methodology. However, there are different types of qualitative methods, which will be discussed in the next chapter. What is important, as you read from this point forward, is that the study design is congruent with the philosophical beliefs that qualitative researchers hold. In other words, you would not expect to see a random sample, or battery of questionnaires administered in a hospital outpatient clinic, or a multiple regression analysis. You may read about a pilot study in the opening of the design section; this is work the researchers did before undertaking the main study to make sure that the logistics of the proposed study were reasonable: Were they able to recruit participants? Did the questions they asked of them get the researchers the information they needed? Lack of a pilot study is not a deficit, however.

Sample

The next part of the report is the description of the sample and setting. There is critical information in this section that will allow you to see how qualitative research differs from quantitative research. In qualitative studies, the researchers are usually looking for a **purposive sample:** they are searching for a particular kind of person who can illuminate the phenomenon they want to study (see Chapter 10). Therefore, their recruitment materials must be very specific so that when people read their recruitment flyers, they know if they fit the criteria or not. So, if the researchers want to talk to HIV-infected women about adherence, they may distribute flyers looking for women who are adherent, and those who are not. Or they may want to talk to women who fit into only one of those categories. The researchers who are examining decision making in pregnancy among women with disabling conditions would clearly list the conditions they want to study. For example, they may describe wanting to talk to women with multiple sclerosis, or those with rheumatoid arthritis.

There may be other parameters—called **inclusion and exclusion criteria**—that the researchers impose as well, such as requiring that participants be over 18 years of age, or not using illicit drugs, or deciding about a first pregnancy (as opposed to subsequent pregnancies). It is critical that the authors make these criteria transparent to the reader, so the reader can make the judgment about the abilities of the participants to shed light on the phenomenon in question.

Often the researchers make decisions such as how to define a "long-term survivor" of a certain illness. In this case, they need to tell you, the reader, why and how they decided who would fit into this category. Is a long-term survivor someone who has had an illness for 5 years? For 10 years? What is the median survival time for people with this diagnosis? There should be sound scientific rationale for the decisions they make. Then, the researchers need to describe for you how they found these people. In the example of finding HIV-infected women who are having difficulties with adherence, they may report distributing flyers describing the study at acquired immunodeficiency syndrome (AIDS) service organizations, support groups for HIV-infected women, clinics, and other places where people with HIV may seek services. Again, this is one of the most critical parts of the qualitative research process, and one you should read with great care.

In qualitative research there is no set sample size as there is in a quantitative study (see Chapter 10). Qualitative researchers gather subjects until **data saturation** occurs. Data saturation is the point in a qualitative study when the information being shared with the researcher from subjects become repetitive; in other words, the ideas shared by the participants have been shared before by other subjects and no new ideas emerge.

Setting: Recruitment and Data Collection

The setting section may actually describe two settings: the settings in which recruitment of participants took place, and the settings in which data collection took place. We have already discussed the first; the settings in which data were collected are another critical area of difference between quantitative and qualitative studies. Data collection in a qualitative study is usually done in a naturalistic setting; we usually do not bring the participants into a clinic interview room to collect data. Often, the setting for data collection is the participant's home, and that can be an incredible window into other aspects of the participants' lives. To be in someone else's home is a great privilege, and helps the researcher to understand what that participant values. For example, one entire wall in my living room contains pictures of my daughter at all ages. Anyone who comes into my home would immediately understand the centrality of her to my life. Those who are ill may have everything they could need to get through a day clustered around a favorite chair: one would see an oxygen tank, glass of water, medications, telephone, *TV Guide,* Kleenex, and so on. This may be an indicator of someone for whom getting around is tremendously difficult. In any event, a good qualitative researcher will use this setting as additional data to help complete the complex, rich drawing that is being rendered in the study.

Data Collection

The next section, data collection, is another part of the process in which the two research paradigms differ tremendously. In a qualitative study, the data to be collected are usually words: the researcher may interview an individual, or may interview a group of people in what is called a focus group, or may observe an individual as she or he goes about a task such as sorting medications into a pill minder. But in each of these cases, the data collected are expressed in words. The researcher asks the participant about the phenomenon of interest, and then listens. However, they do not have to do this without some technical assistance! Most qualitative researchers use audio recorders so that they can be sure that they have captured what the participant says. This also takes some of the pressure off of researchers to try to write down every single word, and frees them up to listen fully. The recordings are usually transcribed verbatim, and then the researcher who conducted the interviews listens to the recordings for accuracy.

The data collection section should also contain details such as obtaining informed consent, and should describe in clear detail the steps from when a participant contacted the researcher to the end of the study visit. It is important to also know how long each interview or focus group lasted, and how much time overall the researcher spent "in the field" collecting data.

Another important component in this section is the description of when the researcher decided that there was a sufficient sample. In qualitative studies, researchers generally continue to recruit participants until they have reached **data saturation,** that is, nothing new is emerging from the interviews. As stated earlier, there usually is *not* a predetermined number of participants to be selected as there is in quantitative studies; rather, the researchers keep recruiting until they have the data they need. One important exception to this is if a researcher is very interested in getting different types of people in the study; for example, in the study of HIV-infected women and medication adherence, the researchers may want some women who were very adherent in the beginning but then became less so over time, or they may want women who were not adherent in the beginning but then became adherent, or they may want to interview women with children and those without children to determine the influence of being a mother on adherence. However, sample sizes tend to be fairly small (under 30 participants) because of the enormous amounts of written text that will need to be analyzed by the researcher.

Finally, you should read in this section about the kinds of questions the researchers asked the participants. These are different from the research question(s), which should be broad and encompassing and perhaps written in fairly esoteric language. The interview questions should be clear, be plain, and get at exactly what the researcher wants to know.

In qualitative studies, there may be a broad overview or **"grand tour" question,** such as "Tell me about taking your medications—the things that make it easier, and the things that make it harder," or "Tell me what you were thinking about when you decided to get pregnant." Along with this overview question, there are usually a series of prompts—additional questions—that were derived from the literature; these are areas that the researcher believes are important to cover, and that the participant will likely cover, but they are there to remind the researcher in case the material is not mentioned. For example, with regard to medication adherence, the researcher may have read in other studies that motherhood can influence adherence in two very different ways: children can become a reason to live, which would facilitate taking antiretroviral medication, and children can be all-demanding, leaving the mother with little to no time to take care of herself. So, a neutrally worded question about the influence of children would be a prompt if the participants do not mention it spontaneously.

The researcher may include a description of the sample in this section, or may wait and describe the sample in the findings section. In any event, besides the typical demographic data one sees collected in any study, a qualitative researcher should also report on key areas of difference in the sample—in a sample of HIV-infected women, there should be information about stage of illness, what kind/how many pills they must take, how many children they have, and so on. This information helps you, the reader, place the data into some context.

EVIDENCE-BASED PRACTICE TIP
Qualitative researchers use more flexible procedures than quantitative researchers. While collecting data for a project, they consider all of the experiences that may occur.

Data Analysis

Next is the description of data analysis. Here, the researcher tells you how he or she handled the raw data, which are usually transcripts of the recorded interviews in a qualitative study. Many qualitative researchers use computer-assisted data analysis programs to help with this task, which can seem overwhelming because of the sheer quantity of data to be dealt with. However, other researchers analyze the data themselves. In either situation, the goal is to find commonalities and differences in the interviews, and then to group these into broader, more abstract, overarching categories of meaning that capture much of the data. For example, in the case we have been using about decision making regarding pregnancy for disabled women, one woman might talk about discussing the need for assistance with her friends, and found that they were willing and able to help her with the baby. Another woman might talk about how she discussed the decision with her mother and sisters, and found them to be a ready source of aid. And yet a third woman may say that she talked about this with her church study group, and they told her that they could arrange to bring meals and help with housework during the pregnancy and afterward. On a more abstract level, these women are all talking about social support. So it is possible to find a term that is all-encompassing for these descriptions. In an ideal situation, the authors might even give you an example such as the one you just read, but the page limitations of most journals do not permit this level of detail.

Computer Management of Qualitative Data

At the completion of data collection, the qualitative researcher is faced with volumes of data requiring sorting, coding, and synthesizing. The researcher may use one of many computer programs available to assist with the task of data management. Meadows and Dodendorf (1999) categorize computer programs into three types:

- Code and retrieve, which assist in organizing and grouping data
- Theory builders, which move to a different level of data organization by connecting themes and categories
- Conceptual network builders, which incorporate graphics with theory-building capabilities

Unlike computer programs used with quantitative data, these programs do not actually analyze data. Data analysis and interpretation remain largely the task of the researcher. However, orderly organization and grouping of data make the job of analysis and interpretation much easier for the researcher.

Findings

Then, at last, we come to the results! First, the authors should tell you if they will be describing a process (such as in the decision-making example), or a list of things that are functioning in some way (such as a list of barriers and facilitators to taking medications for HIV-positive women), or a set of conditions that must be present for something to occur (what parents state they need to care for a ventilator-dependent child at home), or a description of what it is like to go through some health-related transition (what it is like to become the caretaker of a parent with dementia). This is by no means an all-inclusive list, but rather examples to help you know what you should be looking for.

After the description, the author presents the results, usually by breaking them down into units of meaning that help the data cohere and tell a story. It is very useful if the researchers tell you the logic for breaking down the units as they are: Are they telling you the themes from most prevalent to least prevalent? Are they describing a process in temporal terms? Are they starting with things that were most important to the subject, and then moving to less important?

After telling you how they are going to tell the story, they should proceed with a thorough description of the phenomenon, defining each of the themes for you, and fleshing out each of the themes with a thorough explanation of the role that it plays in the question under study. The authors should also provide quotations that support each of their themes. Ideally, they will stage the quote, giving you some information about the subject from whom it came: Was it a newly diagnosed HIV-infected woman of color, without children? Or was it a disabled woman who has chosen to become pregnant, but who has suffered two miscarriages? Staging of quotes allows you to put the information into some social context.

In a really good report of qualitative research, some of the quotes will give you an "Aha!" feeling—you will have a sense that the researcher has done an excellent job of getting to the core of the problem. Quotes are as critical to qualitative reports as numbers are to a quantitative study; you would not have a great deal of confidence in a quantitative report in which the author asks you to believe some finding without give you some statistical findings to back it up.

At the end of the report is the conclusion. Here, the researcher should summarize the results for you, and should compare his or her findings to the existing literature. How are these findings similar to and different from the existing literature? The author can also move into new extant findings or new conceptual conclusions here, because the findings may have led him or her into areas that were not anticipated at the beginning of the study. This is one of the great contributions of qualitative research: opening up new venues of discovery that were not heretofore anticipated. The researcher also makes suggestions regarding how to use the findings in practice, and further directions for future research.

The choice to conduct a qualitative research study is different from that of a quantitative research study (see Chapters 7, 8, and 9). The critical thinking decision path illustrates the beliefs and questions that lead a researcher to choose either a qualitative or a quantitative path.

HELPFUL HINT

Values are involved in all research. It is important, however, that they not influence the results of the research.

EVIDENCE-BASED PRACTICE

Because nursing is a practice discipline, the most important purpose of nursing research is to put research findings to use to improve the care of our patients. Qualitative methods are the best way to start to answer questions that have not been addressed or when a new perspective is needed in practice. The answers to questions provided by qualitative data reflect important evidence that may offer the first systematic insights about a phenomenon and the setting in which it occurs. Therefore broadening evidence models beyond a narrow hierarchical perspective is imperative.

Unfortunately, qualitative research studies do not fare well in the typical systematic reviews on which evidence-based practice recommendations are based. Randomized clinical trials and other types of intervention studies traditionally have been the major focus of evidence-based practice, as exemplified by the systematic reviews conducted by groups such as the Cochrane Collaboration. Typically, the selection of studies to be included in systematic reviews is guided by evidence hierarchies (see Chapter 1) that focus on the effectiveness of interventions according to their strength and consistency. Given that evidence models are hierarchical in nature, which perpetuates intervention studies, for example, randomized controlled studies (RCTs) (see Chapter 8) as the "gold standard" of research design, the value of qualitative studies and the evidence offered by their results have remained unclear. Qualitative studies historically have been ranked lower in a hierarchy of evidence, as a "weaker" form of research design.

Kearney (2001) developed a useful typology of levels and applications of qualitative research evidence (Table 4-1). She described five categories of qualitative findings that are distinguished from one another in their levels of complexity and discovery: those restricted by a priori (existing theory) frameworks, descriptive categories, shared pathway or meaning, depiction of experiential variation, and dense explanatory description. From these, Kearney proposed four modes of clinical application: (1) insight or empathy, (2) assessment of status or progress, (3) anticipatory guidance, and (4) coaching. She argued that the greater the complexity and discovery within qualitative findings, the stronger the potential for clinical application. The evidence that qualitative studies provide is used conceptually by the nurse: qualitative studies let nurses gain access to the experiences of patients, and help nurses expand their ability to understand, which should lead to more helpful approaches to care (Kearney, 2001). See Table 4-1 for explanation and examples.

Kearney argues that findings restricted by an existing set of ideas or a priori frameworks provide little or no evidence for practice; discovery is aborted when the analyst has obscured the findings with an existing theory. Descriptive categories can portray a high level of discovery when a phenomenon is vividly portrayed from a new perspective. For evidence-based nursing practice, these findings can serve as maps of previously uncharted territory in human experience. The third category, shared pathway or meaning, is more complex, in that these reports are a synthesis of a shared process or experience. There is an integration of concepts or themes that result in a logical, complex portrayal of the phenomenon. The researcher's ideas at this level reveal how discrete bits of data come together in a meaningful whole. For nursing practice, it allows us to reflect on the bigger picture and what it means for the human experience (Kearney, 2001).

The depiction of experiential variation is even more complex than shared pathways or meaning; it describes the main essence of an experience, but goes on to show how this experience varies, depending on the individual or context. For nursing practice, these

4-1 Kearney's Categories of Qualitative Findings, from Least to Most Complex

	Definition	Example
Restricted by a priori (existing theory) frameworks	Discovery aborted because researcher has obscured the findings with an existing theory	Use of the theory of "relatedness" to describe women's relationships, without substantiation in the data, and when there may be an alternative explanation to describe how women exist in relationship to others; the data seem to point to another explanation other than "relatedness"
Descriptive categories	Phenomenon is vividly portrayed from a new perspective; provides a map into previously uncharted territory in the human experience of health and illness	Children's descriptions of pain, including descriptors, attributed causes, and what constitutes good care during a painful episode
Shared pathway or meaning	Synthesis of a shared experience or process; integration of concepts that provides a complex picture of a phenomenon	Description of women's process of recovery from depression; each category was fully described, and the conditions for progression were laid out; able to see the origins of a phase in the previous phase
Depiction of experiential variation	Described the main essence of an experience, but also shows how the experience varies, depending on the individual or context	Description of how pregnant women recovering from cocaine addiction might or might not move forward to create a new life, depending on the amount of structure they imposed on their behavior and their desire to give up drugs and change their lives
Dense explanatory description	Rich, situated understanding of a multifaceted and varied human phenomenon in a unique situation; portray the full range and depth of complex influences; densely woven structure to findings	Unique cultural conditions and familial breakdown and hopelessness led young people to deliberately expose themselves to HIV infection in order to find meaning and purpose in life; describes loss of social structure and demands of adolescents caring for their diseased or drugged parents who were unable to function as adults

studies help us see a variety of viewpoints and realizations of a human experience, and the contextual sources of that variety. Conditional models that explain how different variables can produce different consequences broaden our thinking about a phenomenon. Finally, dense explanatory description is the highest level of complexity and discovery, and is a rich, situated understanding of a multifaceted and varied human phenomenon in a unique situation. These studies portray the full depth and range of complex influences that propel people to make decisions. Physical and social context are fully accounted for. There is a densely woven structure of findings in these studies that provide a rich fund of clinically and theoretically useful information for nursing practice, in which the layers of detail work together to increase understanding of human choices and responses in particular contexts (Kearney, 2001).

So how can we further use qualitative evidence in nursing? The simplest mode, according to Kearney, is to use the information to better understand the experiences of our patients, which in turn helps us to offer more sensitive support. Qualitative findings can also help us assess the patient's status or progress, through descriptions of trajectories of illness or through offering a different perspective on a health condition. They allow us to consider a range of possible responses from patients. We can then determine the fit of a category to a particular client, or try to locate them on an illness trajectory.

Anticipatory guidance includes sharing of qualitative findings directly with patients. Patients can learn about others with a similar condition, and can learn what to anticipate

TABLE 4-2 Kearney's Modes of Clinical Application for Qualitative Research

Mode of Clinical Application	Example
Insight or empathy: we can better understand our patients and offer more sensitive support	Nurse is better able to understand the behavio[illegible] patient, who is a woman recovering from depression
Assessment of status or progress: descriptions of trajectories of illness	Nurse is able to describe trajectory of recovery from depression, and can assess how her patient is moving through this trajectory
Anticipatory guidance: sharing of qualitative findings with the patient	Nurse is able to explain the phases of recovery from depression to her patient, and to reassure her that she is not alone, that others have made it through a similar experience
Coaching: advising patients of steps they can take to reduce distress or improve adjustment to an illness, according to the evidence in the study	Nurse describes the six stages of recovery from depression to her patient, and in ongoing contact, points out how the patient is moving through the stages, coaching her to recognize signs that she is improving and moving through the stages

ahead of them. This allows them to better obtain resources for what might lie ahead, or look for markers of improvement. Anticipatory guidance can also be tremendously comforting in that the sharing of research results can help patients realize they are not alone, that there are others who have been through a similar experience with an illness. Finally, Kearney argues that coaching is a way of using qualitative findings; in this instance, nurses can advise patients of steps they can take to reduce distress, improve symptoms, or monitor trajectories of illness (Kearney, 2001). See Table 4-2 for an overview of clinical applications of qualitative research. Sandelowski and Barroso (2003) have also suggested a typology of qualitative research. Most recently Grace and Powers (2009), building on the working of Kearney (2001) and Sandelowski and Barroso (2003), suggest a method of assessing qualitative studies for evidence-based practice not based on a hierarchical model but using a pyramid. The use of a pyramid removes the focus from a hierarchical design perspective to acknowledging the importance of the question, not the design.

EVIDENCE-BASED PRACTICE TIP

Qualitative research findings can be used in many ways, including improving ways clinicians communicate with patients and with each other.

Remember, the definition of evidence-based practice has three components: clinically relevant evidence, clinical expertise, and patient preferences. Qualitative research does not test interventions but does require the researcher to apply her or his clinical expertise to the choice of the research question and study design, as well as gaining a solid understanding of the patient's experience. Though qualitative research uses different methodologies and has different goals, it is important to explore how and when to use the evidence provided by findings of qualitative studies in practice. Remember too that when knowledge about a particular patient care situation is scarce, evidence obtained from data provided by qualitative studies may provide the best available evidence that informs a clinical question or decision about a patient population or patient care.

APPRAISING THE EVIDENCE

Foundation of Qualitative Research

A final example illustrates the differences in the methods discussed in this chapter and provides you with the beginning skills of how to critique qualitative research. The information in this chapter coupled with the information presented in Chapter 5 will provide the underpinnings of critical appraisal of qualitative research (see Critiquing Criteria box, Chapter 5). Consider the question of nursing students learning how to conduct research. The empirical analytical approach (quantitative research) might be used in an experiment to see if one teaching method led to better learning outcomes than another. The students' knowledge might be tested with a pretest, the teaching conducted, and then a posttest of knowledge given. Scores on these tests would be analyzed statistically to see if the different methods produced a difference in the results.

In contrast, a qualitative researcher may be interested in the process of learning research. The researcher might attend the class to see what occurs and then interview students to ask them to describe how their learning changed over time. They might be asked to describe the experience of becoming researchers or becoming more knowledgeable about research. The goal would be to describe the stages or process of this learning. Or a qualitative researcher might consider the class as a culture and could join to observe and interview students. Questions would be directed at the students' values, behaviors, and beliefs in learning research. The goal would be to understand and describe the group members' shared meanings. Either of these examples are ways of viewing a question with a qualitative perspective. The specific qualitative methodologies will be described in Chapter 5.

Many other research methods exist. Although it is important to be aware of the basis of the qualitative research methods used, it is most important that the method chosen is the one that will provide the best approach to answering the question being asked.

A helpful metaphor about the need to use a variety of research methods was used by Seymour Kety, a key figure in the development of biological research in psychiatry, who was the scientific director to the U.S. National Institute of Mental Health (NIMH) for many years. He invited readers to think about a civilization whose inhabitants, although very intelligent, had never seen a book (Kety, 1960). On discovering a library, they set up a scientific institute for studying books, which included anatomists, physical chemists, molecular biologists, behavioral scientists, and psychoanalysts. Each discipline discovered important facts, such as the structure of cellulose and the frequency of collections of letters of varying length. However, the meaning of a "book" continued to escape them. As he put it, "We do not always get closer to the truth as we slice and homogenize and isolate." He argued that a truer picture of a topic under study would emerge only from research by a variety of disciplines and techniques, each with its own virtues and particular limitations. Qualitative research methods could be added to understand how books are used by different groups and the meaning of books to the inhabitants.

This idea provides an important point for qualitative research. One research method does not rank higher than another. But rather a variety of methods based on different paradigms are essential for the development of a well informed and comprehensive approach to evidence-based nursing practice.

CRITICAL THINKING CHALLENGES

- Discuss how a researcher's values could influence the results of a study. Include an example in your answer.
- Can the metaphor "We do not always get closer to the truth as we slice and homogenize and isolate [it]" be applied to both qualitative and quantitative methods? Justify your answer.
- What is the value of qualitative research in evidence-based practice? Give an example.
- Using the model in Figure 4-2, discuss how you could apply the findings of a qualitative research study about coping with a miscarriage.

KEY POINTS

- All research is based on philosophical beliefs, a worldview, or a paradigm.
- Qualitative research encompasses different methodologies.
- Qualitative researchers believe that reality is socially constructed and is context dependent.
- Values should be kept as separate as possible from the conduct of research.
- Qualitative research like quantitative research follows a process but the components of the process vary.
- Qualitative research contributes to evidence-based practice.

REFERENCES

Denzin NK, Lincoln Y: Introduction: the discipline and practice of qualitative research. In Denzin NK, Lincoln Y, eds: *Handbook of qualitative research,* ed. 3, Thousand Oaks, CA, 2005, Sage.

Grace GT, Powers BA: Claiming our core: Appraising qualitative evidence for nursing questions about human response and meaning *Nurs Outlook*, 57:27-34, 2009.

Kearney MH: Levels and applications of qualitative research evidence, *Res Nurs Health* 24:145-153, 2001.

Kety S: A biologist examines mind and behavior, *Science*, 132(3443):1861-1870, 1960.

Mason J: *Qualitative researching,* ed. 2, Thousand Oaks, CA, 2002, Sage.

Meadows LM, Dodendorf DM: Data management and interpretation using computers to assist. In Crabtree B, Miller WL, eds: *Doing qualitative research,* ed. 2, Thousand Oaks, CA, 1999, Sage.

Sandelowski M, Barroso J: Classifying the findings in qualitative studies, *Qual Health Res*, 13, 905-923, 2003.

FOR FURTHER STUDY

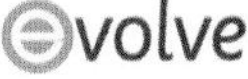

Go to Evolve at http://evolve.elsevier.com/LoBiondo/ for review questions, critiquing exercises, and additional research articles for practice in reviewing and critiquing.

5

Qualitative Approaches to Research

Julie Barroso

KEY TERMS

auditability
bracketing
case study method
community-based participatory research
constant comparative method
credibility
culture
data saturation
domains
emic view
ethnographic method
etic view
external criticism
fittingness
grounded theory method
historical research method
instrumental case study
internal criticism
intrinsic case study
key informants
lived experience
meta-synthesis
phenomenological method
primary sources
secondary sources
theoretical sampling
triangulation

LEARNING OUTCOMES

After reading this chapter, you should be able to do the following:

- Identify the processes of phenomenological, grounded theory, ethnographic, and case study methods.
- Recognize appropriate use of historical methods.
- Recognize appropriate use of community-based participatory research methods.
- Discuss significant issues that arise in conducting qualitative research in relation to such topics as ethics, criteria for judging scientific rigor, and combination of research methods.
- Apply critiquing criteria to evaluate a report of qualitative research.

STUDY RESOURCES

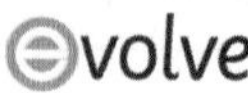

Go to Evolve at http://evolve.elsevier.com/LoBiondo/ for review questions, critiquing exercises, and additional research articles for practice in reviewing and critiquing.

Qualitative research combines the science and art of nursing to enhance the understanding of human health experience. This chapter focuses on four commonly used qualitative research methods: phenomenology, grounded theory, ethnography, and case study. Historical research as well as a newer methodology, community-based participatory research, is also presented. Each of these methods, although distinct from the others, shares characteristics that identify it as a method within the qualitative research approach.

In Chapter 1, how traditional hierarchies of research evidence categorize evidence from strongest to weakest, with an emphasis on support for the effectiveness of interventions, is presented. This perspective is very short-sighted, and does not take into account the ways that qualitative research can support practice, as discussed in the previous chapter. There is no doubt about the merit of qualitative studies; the problem is that no one has developed a satisfactory method for including them in the evidence hierarchies. In addition, qualitative studies can answer the critical "why?" questions that result from many evidence-based practice summaries; they may have figured out the answer to a research question, but they do not explain how it operates in the landscape of caring for people. You as a research consumer should know that qualitative methods are the best way to start to answer clinical and research questions about which little is known or when a new perspective is needed in practice. The very fact that qualitative research studies have increased exponentially in nursing and other social sciences speaks to the urgent need of clinicians to better understand the experience of illness. Thousands of reports of well-conducted qualitative studies exist on topics such as the following (Sandelowski, 2004; Sandelowski & Barroso, 2007):

- Personal and cultural constructions of disease, prevention, treatment, and risk
- Living with disease and managing the physical, psychological, and social effects of multiple diseases and their treatment
- Decision-making experiences with beginning and end-of-life, as well as assistive and life-extending, technological interventions
- Contextual factors favoring and mitigating against quality care, health promotion, prevention of disease, and reduction of health disparities

The answers provided by qualitative data reflect important evidence that provides valuable insights about a particular phenomenon, patient population, or clinical situation.

In this chapter, you are invited to look through the lens of human experience to learn about phenomenological, grounded theory, ethnographic, community-based participatory research, historical, and case study methods. You are encouraged to put yourself in the researcher's shoes as each method is introduced—to imagine how it would be to study an issue of interest from the perspective of each of these methods. No matter which method a researcher uses, there is a demand to embrace the wholeness of humans, focusing on the human experience in natural settings.

The researcher using these methods believes that each unique human being attributes meaning to his or her experience, and experience evolves from his or her social and historical context. So, one person's experience of pain is distinct from another's and can be known by the individual's subjective description of it. For example, the researcher interested in studying the lived experience of pain for the adolescent with rheumatoid arthritis will spend time in the adolescent's natural settings, such as the home and school, as discussed in Chapter 4. Efforts will be directed at uncovering the meaning of pain as it extends beyond the number of medications taken or a rating on a pain scale. Qualitative methods are grounded in the belief that objective data do not capture the whole of the human experience. Rather, the meaning of the adolescent's pain emerges within the context of personal history, current relationships, and future plans as the adolescent lives daily life in dynamic interaction with the environment.

The researcher using qualitative methods begins collecting bits of information and piecing them together, building a mosaic or a picture of the human experience being studied. As with a mosaic, when one steps away from the work, the whole picture emerges. This whole picture transcends the bits and pieces and cannot be known from any one bit or piece. In presenting study findings, the researcher strives to capture the human experience and present it so that others can understand it.

QUALITATIVE APPROACH AND NURSING SCIENCE

Qualitative research is particularly well suited to study the human experience of health, a central concern of nursing science. Because qualitative methods focus on the whole of human experience and the meaning ascribed by individuals living the experience, these methods extend understanding of health beyond traditional measures of isolated concepts to include the complexity of the human health experience as it is occurring in everyday living. The evidence provided by qualitative studies that consider the unique perspectives, concerns, preferences, and expectations each patient brings to a clinical encounter offers in-depth understanding of human experience and the contexts in which they occur. Qualitative research, in addition to providing unique perspectives, has the ability to guide nursing practice, contribute to instrument development (see Chapter 13), and develop nursing theory (Figure 5-1).

QUALITATIVE RESEARCH METHODS

Thus far an overview of the qualitative research approach has been presented (see Chapter 4), focusing on the importance of evidence offered by qualitative research for nursing science. An effort has been made to highlight how choice of a qualitative approach is reflective of one's worldview and research question. These topics provide a foundation for examining the qualitative methods discussed in this chapter. The Critical Thinking Decision Path introduces you to a process for recognizing differing qualitative methods by distinguishing areas of interest for each method and noting how the research question might be introduced for each distinct method. The phenomenological, grounded theory, ethnographic, case study, and community-based participatory research methods are described in detail for you.

Phenomenological Method

The **phenomenological method** is a process of learning and constructing the meaning of human experience through intensive dialogue with persons who are living the experience. The researcher's goal is to understand the meaning of the experience as it is lived by the participant. Meaning is pursued through a dialogic process, which extends beyond a simple interview and requires thoughtful presence on the part of the researcher. Each philosopher-guided (Husserl's eidetic phenomenology; Heidegger's interpretive phenomenology; Dutch hermeneutical phenomenology) base directs slight differences in research methods. Whatever the form of phenomenological research, you will find the researcher asking a question about the lived experience.

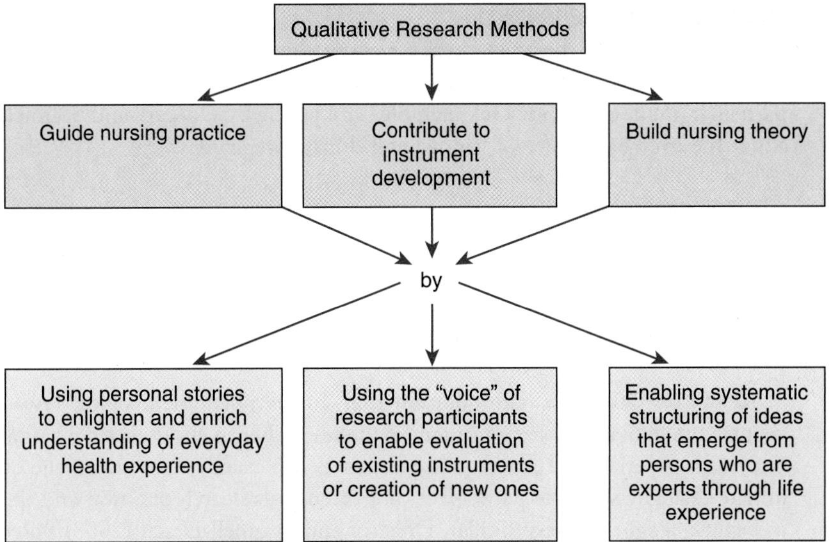

Figure 5-1 Qualitative approach and nursing science.

CRITICAL THINKING DECISION PATH Selecting a Qualitative Research Method

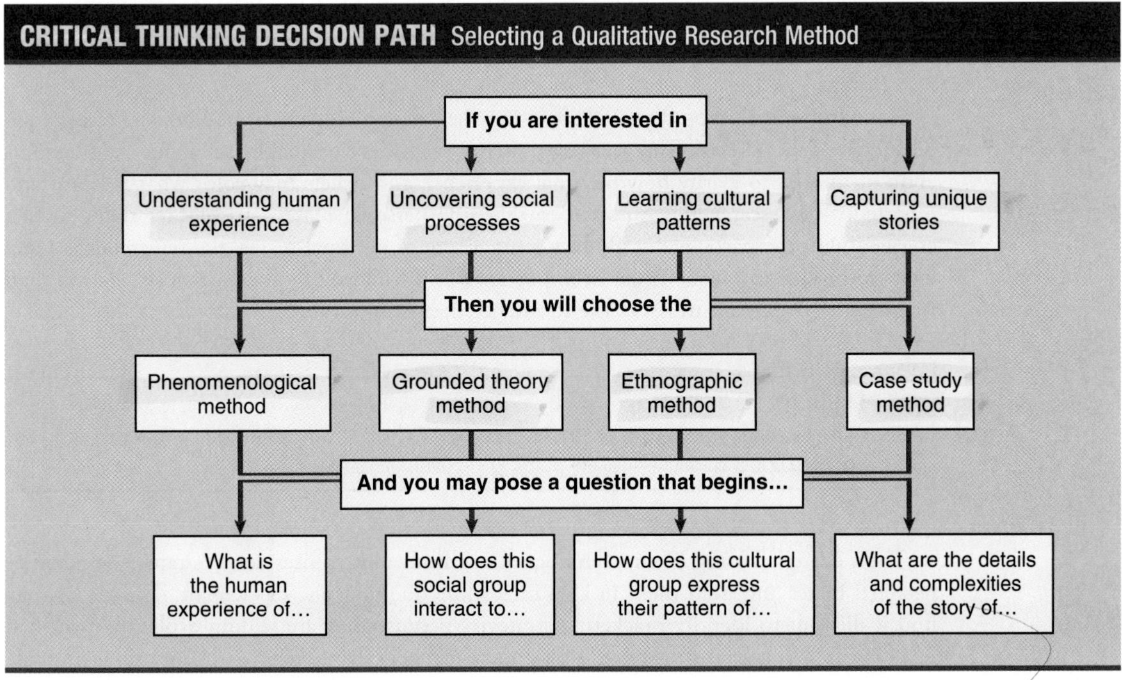

Identifying the Phenomenon

Because the focus of the phenomenological method is the **lived experience,** the researcher is likely to choose this method when studying some dimension of day-to-day existence for a particular group of people. Our example is an article by Doherty and Scannell-Desch (2008) about the lived experience of widowhood during pregnancy.

Structuring the Study

For the purpose of describing structuring, the following topics are addressed: the research question, the researcher's perspective, and sample selection. The issue of human subjects' protection has been suggested as a dimension of structuring (Parse et al., 1985); this issue is discussed generally with ethics in a subsequent section of the chapter.

Research Question. The question that guides phenomenological research always asks about some human experience. It guides the researcher to ask the participant about some past or present experience. The research question is not exactly the same as the question used to initiate dialogue with the participant, but often the research question and the question used to begin dialogue are very similar. Doherty and Scannell-Desch (2008) posed the following research question: What is the lived experience of widowhood during pregnancy? Four data-generating research questions guided the study and were asked of participants:

1. How would you describe your circumstance of becoming a widow?
2. What word, or words, or image comes to mind when you hear the word "widow"?
3. How would you describe your experience of becoming a widow while pregnant?
4. What else would you like to tell me about your experience?

Researcher's Perspective. When using the phenomenological method, the researcher's perspective is **bracketed.** That is, the researcher identifies personal biases about the phenomenon of interest to clarify how personal experience and beliefs may color what is heard and reported. The researcher is expected to set aside personal biases—to bracket them—when engaged with the participants. By becoming aware of personal biases, the researcher is more likely to be able to pursue issues of importance as introduced by the participant, rather than leading the participant to issues the researcher deems important.

HELPFUL HINT

Although the research question may not always be explicitly reported, it may be identified by evaluating the study's purpose or the question/statement posed to the participants.

The researcher using phenomenological methods always uses some strategy to identify personal biases and hold them in abeyance while querying the participant. The reader may find it difficult to identify bracketing strategies because they are seldom explicitly identified in a research manuscript. Sometimes, the researcher's worldview or assumptions provide insight into biases that have been considered and bracketed. There is nothing about bracketing in the Doherty and Scannell-Desch study; again, this is not unusual and does not detract from the quality of the report. Usually, you will find something about bracketing if there is something to report, but not if there are no bracketing issues.

Sample Selection. As you read a report of a phenomenological study you will find that the selected purposive sample either is living the experience the researcher is querying or has lived the experience in their past. Because phenomenologists believe that each individual's history is a dimension of the present, a past experience exists in the present moment. Even when a participant is describing an experience occurring in the present, remembered information is being gathered. The participants in the study by Doherty and Scannell-Desch were 10 widows; 7 of them lost their husbands in the terrorist attacks of September 11, 2001, and the other 3 were military widows. The mean length of time since becoming a widow was 4.25 years, and the mean age of participants at the time of their husbands' deaths was 29.5 years. Six were pregnant with their second child.

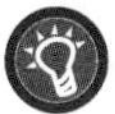

HELPFUL HINT

Qualitative studies often use purposive sampling (see Chapter 10).

Data Gathering

Written or oral data may be collected when using the phenomenological method. The researcher may pose the query in writing and ask for a written response or may schedule a time to interview the participant and tape-record the interaction. In either case, the researcher may return to ask for clarification of written or tape-recorded transcripts. To some extent, the particular data collection procedure is guided by the choice of a specific analysis technique. Different analysis techniques require different numbers of interviews. Data saturation usually guides decisions regarding how many interviews are enough. **Data saturation** is the situation of obtaining the full range of themes from the participants, so that in interviewing additional participants, no new data are emerging. In the example, Doherty and Scannell-Desch (2008) interviewed eight of the women in their homes, and two by telephone because of their geographic distance. The researchers state that the interviews took place over a 6-month period and continued until there was repetition of data without discovery of any new themes.

Data Analysis

Several techniques are available for data analysis when using the phenomenological method. For detailed information about specific techniques, the reader is referred to original sources (Colaizzi, 1978; Giorgi et al., 1975; Spiegelberg, 1976; van Kaam, 1969). Although the techniques are slightly different from each other, there is a general pattern of moving from the participant's description to the researcher's synthesis of all participants' descriptions. The steps generally include the following:

1. Thorough reading and sensitive reading of presence with the entire transcription of the participant's description
2. Identification of shifts in participant thought, resulting in division of the transcription into thought segments
3. Specification of significant phrases in each thought segment, using the participant's words
4. Distillation of each significant phrase to express the central meaning of the segment in the researcher's words
5. Grouping together of segments that contain similar central meanings for each participant

6. Preliminary synthesis of grouped segments for each participant with a focus on the essence of the phenomenon being studied
7. Final synthesis of the essences that have surfaced in all participants' descriptions, resulting in an exhaustive description of the lived experience

Doherty and Scannell-Desch (2008) used Colaizzi's method for analyzing data. Interviews were audiotaped and transcribed verbatim. The researchers listened to the audiotapes several times. After the tapes were transcribed verbatim, participants' descriptions were reviewed. Significant statements were extracted and categorized into related clusters. The researchers state that thematic content was validated by five study participants.

It is important to note here that giving verbatim transcripts to participants can have unanticipated consequences. It is not unusual for people to deny that they said something in a certain way, or that they said it at all. Even when the actual audiotape is played for them, they may have difficulty believing it. This is one of the more challenging aspects of any qualitative method: every time a story is told, it changes for the participant. The participant may sincerely feel that the story-as-recorded is not the story as it is now after being described.

Describing the Findings

When using the phenomenological method, the nurse researcher provides you with a path of information leading from the research question, through samples of participants' words and the researcher's interpretation, to the final synthesis that elaborates the lived experience as a narrative. When reading the report of a phenomenological study, the reader should find that detailed descriptive language is used to convey the complex meaning of the lived experience that offers the evidence for this qualitative method. Doherty and Scannell-Desch (2008) provide numerous quotes from participants to support their findings. They synthesized eight themes that described women's experience of widowhood during pregnancy:

1. *Denying versus dealing with reality:* He's not coming home
2. *Navigating pregnancy:* Flying solo while running on empty
3. *Planning for birth:* Gathering my team
4. *My safety net:* A band of sisters
5. *Unplanned journey:* A bittersweet homecoming
6. *Being there:* Network of family and friends
7. *Not being there:* Let down by others
8. *Re-creating home:* A new normal

These themes described the emotions, vulnerability, challenges, and issues experienced by these women. Direct participant quotes enable the reader to evaluate the connection between what the participant said and how the researcher labeled what was said.

EVIDENCE-BASED PRACTICE TIP

Phenomenological research is an important approach for accumulating evidence when studying a new topic about which little is known.

Grounded Theory Method

The **grounded theory method** is an inductive approach involving a systematic set of procedures to arrive at a theory about basic social processes. The emergent theory is based on observations and perceptions of the social scene and evolves during data collection and analysis as a product of the actual research process (Corbin & Strauss, 2008). The grounded theory method is used to construct theory where no theory exists or in situations where existing theory fails to provide evidence to explain a set of circumstances. According to Denzin (1998), grounded theory is the qualitative perspective most widely used by social scientists today, largely because it sets forth clearly defined steps for the researcher.

Developed originally as a sociologist's tool to investigate interactions in social settings (Glaser & Strauss, 1967), the grounded theory method is not bound to that discipline. Investigators from different disciplines may study the same phenomenon from varying perspectives (Corbin & Strauss, 2008; Denzin & Lincoln, 1998; Strauss & Corbin, 1994, 1997). As an example, in an area of study such as chronic illness, a nurse might be interested in coping patterns within families, a psychologist in personal adjustment, and a sociologist in group behavior in health care settings. Theory generated by each discipline will reflect the discipline and serve it in explaining the phenomenon of interest to the discipline (Liehr & Marcus, 2002). In grounded theory, usefulness stems from the transferability of theories from one study to another situation, making the key objective the development of more formal theories that are faithful to the cases from which they were derived (Sandelowski, 2004).

Identifying the Phenomenon

Researchers typically use the grounded theory method when they are interested in social processes from the perspective of human interactions, or patterns of action and interaction between and among various types of social units (Denzin & Lincoln, 1998). The basic social process is sometimes expressed as a ***gerund,*** indicating change across time as social reality is negotiated. Fenwick, Barclay, and Schmied (2008) described women's experiences of mothering in a neonatal intensive care nursery; their study will be used as an example of the grounded theory method.

Structuring the Study

Research Question. Research questions appropriate for the **grounded theory method** are those that address basic social processes that shape human behavior. In a grounded theory study, the research question can be a statement or a broad question that permits in-depth explanation of the phenomenon. For example, the reader will recognize Fenwick and colleagues' question implied in the study aim: to increase knowledge and understanding of how women begin their roles as mothers when their infant is in the neonatal intensive care nursery.

Researcher's Perspective. In a grounded theory study, the researcher brings some knowledge of the literature to the study, but you will notice that an exhaustive literature review may not be done. This allows theory to emerge directly from data and to reflect the contextual values that are integral to the social processes being studied. In this way, the theory product that emerges is "grounded in" the data.

Sample Selection. Sample selection involves choosing participants (purposive sample (see Chapter 10) who are experiencing the circumstance and selecting events and incidents related to the social process under investigation. Fenwick and colleagues (2008) recruited women whose infants were in special care nurseries.

Data Gathering

In the grounded theory method, you will find that data are collected through interviews and through skilled observations of individuals interacting in a social setting. Interviews are audiotaped and then transcribed, and observations are recorded as field notes. Open-ended questions are used initially to identify concepts for further focus. Fenwick and colleagues (2008) conducted two in-depth interviews with each of the 28 women, which resulted in over 300 hours of audiotape. They also took field notes and interviewed 20 nursery staff, 19 of whom were midwives. By collecting data from nursery staff as well as the mothers, the researchers were able to develop a more comprehensive grounded theory. Field notes allowed the researchers to have a fuller understanding of the physical surroundings in the special care nurseries and the impact they had on the women's abilities to mother their infants, which again contributed to the development of a more comprehensive grounded theory.

Data Analysis

A major feature of the grounded theory method is that data collection and analysis occur simultaneously. The process requires systematic, detailed record keeping using field notes and transcribed interview tapes. Hunches about emerging patterns in the data are noted in memos, and the researcher directs activities in the field by pursuing these hunches. This technique, called **theoretical sampling**, is used to select experiences that will help the researcher test ideas and gather complete information about developing concepts. The researcher begins by noting indicators or actual events, actions, or words in the data. Concepts, or abstractions, are developed from the indicators (Charmaz, 2000; Strauss, 1987).

The initial analytical process is called *open coding* (Strauss, 1987). Data are examined carefully line by line, broken down into discrete parts, and compared for similarities and differences (Corbin & Strauss, 2008). Data are compared with other data continuously as they are acquired during research. This is a process called the **constant comparative method**. Codes in the data are clustered to form categories. The categories are expanded and developed or they are collapsed into one another. Theory is constructed through this systematic process. As a result, data collection, analysis, and theory generation have a direct reciprocal relationship (Charmaz, 2000; Strauss & Corbin, 1990). Fenwick and colleagues (2008) describe how they drew together a number of previous publications that have described in detail the categories derived from the analysis that explain the actions, interactions, and reactions women engage in as they seek to "connect" with their infant.

HELPFUL HINT

In a report of research using the grounded theory method, you can expect to find a diagrammed model of a theory that synthesizes the researcher's findings in a systematic way.

Describing the Findings

Grounded theory studies are reported in sufficient detail to provide the reader with the steps in the process, the logic of the method, and the theory that has emerged. Reports of grounded theory studies use descriptive language and diagrams of the process as evidence to ensure that the theory reported in the findings remains connected to the data. Fenwick and colleagues (2008) described six major categories that, when combined, explained the intense emotional, cognitive, and worry "work" women undertook with both their infants and the nursery staff in an effort to learn how to mother in the nursery. Four explained how women worked to get to know and connect with their infants. The first three were labeled "just existing," "striving to be the baby's mother," and "trying to establish competence." The fourth, "learning and playing the game," overlays the first three and represents the reality of having to undertake these already difficult and unexpected activities of mothering in the nursery. Two categories—"becoming connected" and "struggling to mother"—were identified as the consequences of women's actions and interactions. A significant finding of the study was the impact of the interactions between nurses and mothers' mothering. The nurse-mother relationship had the potential to significantly affect how women perceived their connection to the infant and their confidence in caring for their infant, which occurred through a three-way interaction.

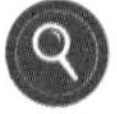

EVIDENCE-BASED PRACTICE TIP
When thinking about the evidence generated by the grounded theory method, consider whether the theory is useful in explaining, interpreting, or predicting the study phenomenon of interest.

Ethnographic Method

Derived from the Greek term *ethnos,* meaning people, race, or cultural group, the **ethnographic method** focuses on scientific description and interpretation of cultural or social groups and systems (Creswell, 1998). The reader should know that the goal of the ethnographer is to understand the natives' view of their world, or the emic view. The **emic** (insiders') **view** is contrasted to the **etic** (outsiders') **view** obtained when the researcher uses quantitative analyses of behavior. The ethnographic approach requires that the researcher enter the world of the study participants to watch what happens, listen to what is said, ask questions, and collect whatever data are available. The term *ethnography* is used to mean both the research technique and the product of that technique, the study itself (Creswell, 1998; Tedlock, 2000). Vidick and Lyman (1998) trace the history of ethnography, with roots in the disciplines of sociology and anthropology, as a method born out of the need to understand "other" and "self." Nurses use the method to study cultural variations in health and patient groups as subcultures within larger social contexts (Liehr & Marcus, 2002).

Identifying the Phenomenon

The phenomenon under investigation in an ethnographic study varies in scope from a long-term study of a very complex culture, such as that of the Aborigines (Mead, 1949), to a shorter-term study of a phenomenon within subunits of cultures. Kleinman (1992) notes the clinical utility of ethnography in describing the "local world" of groups of patients who are experiencing a particular phenomenon, such as suffering. The local worlds of patients have cultural, political, economical, institutional, and social-relational dimensions in much the same way as larger complex societies. To introduce you to ethnography, Clabo's (2008) study of pain assessment and the role of social context on two postoperative units will be highlighted.

Structuring the Study

Research Question. When reviewing the report of ethnographic research, notice that questions are asked about lifeways or particular patterns of behavior within the social context of a culture or subculture. **Culture** is viewed as the system of knowledge and linguistic expressions used by social groups that allows the researcher to interpret or make sense of the world (Aamodt, 1991). Ethnographic nursing studies address questions that concern how cultural knowledge, norms, values, and other contextual variables influence one's health experience. Clabo's (2008) research question is implied in her purpose statement: to examine nursing assessment of pain across two postoperative units. Remember that ethnographers have a broader definition of culture, where a particular social context is conceptualized as a culture. In this case, postoperative units are seen as a culture appropriate for ethnographic study.

Researcher's Perspective. When using the ethnographic method, the researcher's perspective is that of an interpreter entering an alien world and attempting to make sense of that world from the insider's point of view (Agar, 1986). Like phenomenologists and grounded theorists, ethnographers make their own beliefs explicit and *bracket,* or set aside, their personal biases as they seek to understand the worldview of others.

Sample Selection. The ethnographer selects a cultural group that is living the phenomenon under investigation. The researcher gathers information from general informants and from key informants. **Key informants** are individuals who have special knowledge, status, or communication skills and who are willing to teach the ethnographer about the phenomenon (Creswell, 1998). Clabo's (2008) research took place on two general surgical units that shared many common features. Each unit had a nurse manager and an assistant manager, ranged in size from 21 to 30 beds, and employed 27 to 30 registered nurses (RNs), with day shift staffing of 4 to 6 RNs providing care to similar mixed surgical populations.

HELPFUL HINT
Managing personal bias is an expectation of researchers using all of the methods discussed in this chapter.

Data Gathering

Ethnographic data gathering involves participant observation or immersion in the setting, interviews of informants, and interpretation by the researcher of cultural patterns (Crabtree & Miller, 1992). According to Boyle (1991), ethnographic research in nursing, as in other disciplines, involves "face-to-face interviewing, with data collection and analysis taking place in the natural setting." Thus fieldwork is a major focus of the method. Other techniques may include obtaining life histories and collecting material items reflective of the culture. Photographs and films of the informants in their world can be used as data sources. Spradley (1979) identified three categories of questions for ethnographic inquiry: descriptive, or broad, open-ended questions; structural, or in-depth, questions that expand and verify the unit of analysis; and contrast questions, or ones that further clarify and provide criteria for exclusion.

Ten of the 12 day-shift RNs on unit A and 10 of the 13 day-shift RNs on unit B agreed to be observed as they conducted pain assessments on individual clients and to be interviewed in relation to each assessment. The researcher observed each nurse in the conduct of between one and three assessments on different clients. The observations provided an overall sense of how any one nurse went about conducting a pain assessment, and the semistructured interviews captured more detail regarding the nurse's actual thinking, especially in regard to the approaches used to assess each client's pain. The interviews were conducted in a private space on the nursing unit, lasted from 10 to 30 minutes, and were audiotaped and transcribed verbatim. The next phase focused on expanding the understanding of the impact of nursing unit social context on the pain assessment practice of the individual nurse. A single focus group discussion, lasting 35 to 45 minutes, was held on each unit, facilitated by the researcher. Nurses were recruited through announcements posted on the units. These sessions were audiotaped and transcribed verbatim. The discussions followed a loosely scripted format. Initially, a rough sketch of the data was provided. Nurses were asked to describe the following: (1) the degree to which the picture presented represented their perception of pain assessment on the unit, (2) their perceptions regarding how this pattern of pain assessment was developed and maintained, and (3) their experiences (if any) with nurses whose pain assessment practice might differ from the predominant pattern on the unit.

Data Analysis

As with the grounded theory method, data are collected and analyzed simultaneously. Data analysis proceeds through several levels as the researcher looks for the meaning of cultural symbols in the informant's language. Analysis begins with a search for **domains** or symbolic categories that include smaller categories. Language is analyzed for semantic relationships, and structural questions are formulated to expand and verify data. Analysis proceeds through increasing levels of complexity until the data, grounded in the informant's reality and synthesized by the researcher, lead to hypothetical propositions about the cultural phenomenon under investigation. You are encouraged to consult Creswell (1998) for a detailed description of the ethnographic analysis process. Clabo (2008) describes a three-step data analysis plan for the second phase of her study. Initially, the conduct of each assessment was described and specific criteria used were identified. This was compared and contrasted across the number of clients assessed by any one nurse, followed by cross-nurse comparisons on any one unit and last between the two units. This approach resulted in a description of the pain assessment practice of any one nurse and the general pattern of pain assessment on each unit.

Describing the Findings

Ethnographic studies yield large quantities of data that reflect a wide array of evidence amassed as field notes of observations, interview transcriptions, and sometimes other artifacts such as photographs. Charmaz (2000) provided guidelines for ethnographic writing that are an excellent framework for you to use when you wish to critique descriptions of ethnographic studies. The five techniques recommended in Charmaz's guidelines are pulling the reader in, re-creating experiential mood, adding surprise, reconstructing ethnographic experience, and creating closure for the study. When critiquing, be aware that the report of findings usually provides examples from data, thorough descriptions of the analytical process, and statements of the hypothetical propositions and their relationship to the ethnographer's frame of reference. Evidence provided by complete ethnographies may be published as monographs. Clabo (2008) found that a predominant pattern of pain assessment existed on each unit. Nurses used assessment criteria from three spheres: the client's narrative, evident criteria, and a reference typology of assessment findings. Nurses used a single sphere as a primary filter through which data were processed. This filter was distinctive for each unit, and consistent with the unique pattern of nursing pain assessment on each unit. Clabo concluded that nurses' pain assessment practice is profoundly shaped by the social context of the unit on which practice occurs.

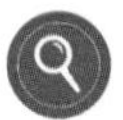

EVIDENCE-BASED PRACTICE TIP

Evidence generated by ethnographic studies will answer questions about how cultural knowledge, norms, values, and other contextual variables influence the health experience of a particular patient population in a specific setting.

Case Study

Case study research, which is rooted in sociology, is currently described slightly differently by Yin, Stake, Merriam, and Creswell, major thinkers who write about this method (Aita & McIlvain, 1999). For the purposes of introducing you to this research method, Stake's view is emphasized. The **case study method** is about studying the peculiarities and the commonalities of a specific case—familiar ground for practicing nurses. Stake (2000) notes that case study is not a methodological choice, but rather a choice of what to study. Case study can include quantitative and/or qualitative data, but it is defined by its focus on uncovering an individual case. Stake (2000) distinguishes intrinsic from instrumental case study. **Intrinsic case study** is undertaken to have a better understanding of the case—nothing more or nothing less. "The researcher at least temporarily subordinates other curiosities so that the stories of those 'living the case' will be teased out" (Stake, 2000). **Instrumental case study** is defined as research that is done when the researcher is pursuing insight into an issue or wants to challenge some generalization. Docherty and colleagues (2006) examined the daily symptom experience of a teenage girl undergoing treatment for cancer, in an attempt to ascertain patterns in daily experiences of pain, nausea, vomiting, retching, stress, sleep alterations, and anxiety.

Identifying the Phenomenon

Although some definitions of case study demand that the focus of research be contemporary, Stake's (1995, 2000) defining criterion of attention to the single case broadens the scope of phenomenon for study. By a single case, Stake is designating a focus on an individual, a family, a community, an organization—some complex phenomenon that demands close scrutiny for understanding. Docherty and colleagues (2006) wanted to explore symptom distress in children being treated for cancer, using critical case sampling, which involves choosing a case that has the highest potential to dramatically illustrate a phenomenon.

Structuring the Study

Research Question. The research question for a case study is one that provokes the curiosity of the researcher. Stake (2000) suggests that research questions be developed around issues that serve as a foundation to uncover complexity and pursue understanding. Although researchers pose questions to begin discussion, the initial questions are never all-inclusive. Rather, the researcher uses an iterative process of "growing questions" in the field. That is, as data are collected to address these questions, other questions will emerge to guide the researcher down another path in the process of untangling the complex story. Therefore research questions evolve over time and re-create themselves in case study research. In Docherty and colleagues' (2006) study, the first category of data collection involved self-report instruments. The second category entailed biobehavioral measures, including salivary cortisol levels and sleep actigraphy. The third category of data collection included narrative interviews. By using multiple ways of measuring symptoms, the researchers are better able to describe the phenomenon of interest, symptom distress of children.

Researcher's Perspective. When the researcher begins with questions developed around suspected issues of importance, the perspective of the researcher is reflected in the questions; this is sometimes referred to as an etic perspective. As the researcher begins engaging the phenomenon of interest, the story unfolds and leads the way, shifting from an etic (researcher) to an emic (story) perspective (Stake, 2000). The reader may recognize a shift from etic to emic perspective when stories spin off of the original questions posed by the researcher.

Sample Selection. This is one of the areas where scholars in the field present differing views, ranging from only choosing the most common cases to only choosing the most unusual cases (Aita & McIlvain, 1999). Stake (2000) advocates selecting cases that may offer the best opportunities for learning. For instance, if there are several heart transplant patients the researcher may study, practical factors will influence who offers the best opportunity for learning. Persons who live in the area and can be easily visited at home or in the medical center would be a better choice than someone living in another country. The researcher may want to choose someone who has an actively participating family, because most transplant patients exist in a family setting. No choice is perfect when selecting a case. There is much to learn about any one individual, situation, or organization when doing case study research, regardless of the contextual factors influencing the unit of analysis. As stated previously, Docherty and colleagues (2006) chose a case that they thought would best illuminate the phenomenon of symptom distress of children.

Data Gathering

Data are gathered using interview, observation, document review, and any other methods that accumulate evidence that enables understanding of the complexity of the case. The researcher will do what is needed to get a sense of the environment and the relationships that provide the context for the case. Stake (1995) advocates development of a data-gathering plan to guide the progress of the study from definition of the case through decisions regarding reporting. You may find little explicit information about data gathering in the report of research. As stated previously, Docherty and colleagues (2006) used multiple methods for collecting data, including a symptom diary. Docherty collected data from Abby, the subject, twice daily through six cycles (85 days) of chemotherapy. On four separate occasions during these data collection episodes, Docherty interviewed the patient for 60 to 90 minutes.

EVIDENCE-BASED PRACTICE TIP

Case studies are a way of providing in-depth evidence-based discussion of clinical topics that can be used to guide practice.

Data Analysis/Describing Findings

Data analysis is closely tied to data gathering and description of findings as the case study story is generated. "Qualitative case study is characterized by researchers spending extended time, on site, personally in contact with activities and operations of the case, reflecting, revising meanings of what is going on" (Stake, 2000). Reflecting and revising meanings are the work of the case study researcher, who has recorded data, searched for patterns, linked data from multiple sources, and arrived at preliminary thoughts regarding the meaning of collected data. This reflective dynamic evolution is the iterative process of creating the case study story that can be thought of as the evidence. The reader of a qualitative case study will have difficulty determining how data analysis was conducted because the research report generally does not list research activities. Findings are embedded in the following: (1) a chronological development of the case; (2) the researcher's story of coming to know the case; (3) the one-by-one description of case dimensions; and (4) vignettes that highlight case qualities (Stake, 1995). The primary focus of analysis in the Docherty and colleagues (2006) study was the appraisal of trend and cyclical patterns in the symptom data. Analysis consisted of four major components, including the search for trends, variation around the trends, deterministic cycles or patterns, and the analysis of random residual effects. A key finding was that the predictability evident in Abby's symptom patterns were in direct contrast to her perception that there was no predictability or pattern to her symptoms. Her perceived lack of control over her symptoms generated worry, anxiety, and depression and led Abby to question whether she could continue with the treatment. Abby represented a case of "fighting the treatment," as opposed to "fighting the cancer," and it is the difference between these responses that may explain children's overall ability to tolerate intensive chemotherapy.

Historical Research

The **historical research method** is a systematic approach for understanding the past through collection, organization, and critical appraisal of facts. One of the goals of the researcher using historical methodology is to shed light on the past so that it can guide the present and the future. Nursing's attention to historical methodology was initiated by Teresa E. Christy. Christy elaborated the method (1975) and the need (1981) for historical research long before most nurse scholars accepted it as a legitimate research method. More recently, Lusk (1997) summarized important information for the nurse interested in understanding historical research. She provided guidance for choosing a topic, acquiring data, addressing ethical issues, analyzing data, and reporting findings.

When appraising a study that used the historical method, expect to find the research question embedded in the phenomenon to be studied. The question is stated implicitly rather than explicitly. Data sources provide the sample for historical research. The more clearly a researcher delineates the historical event being studied, the more specifically data sources can be identified. Data may include written or video documents, interviews with persons who witnessed the event, photographs, and any other artifacts that shed light on the subject. Sometimes pivotal information cannot be retrieved and must be eliminated from the list of possible sources. To determine which data sources were used when reviewing a published study, the reader will look at the reference list. Sources of data may be primary or secondary. **Primary sources** are eyewitness accounts provided by varying sorts of communication appropriate to the time. **Secondary sources** provide a view of the phenomenon from another's perspective rather than a first-hand account.

Validity of documents is established by external criticism; reliability is established by internal criticism. **External criticism** judges the authenticity of the data source. The researcher seeks to ensure that the data source is what it seems to be. For instance, if the researcher is reviewing a handwritten letter of Florence Nightingale, some of the validity issues are the following:

- Are the ink, paper, and wax seal on the envelope representative of Nightingale's time?
- Is the wax seal one that Nightingale used in other authentic data sources?
- Is the writing truly Nightingale's?

Only if the data source passes the test of external criticism does the researcher begin internal criticism. **Internal criticism** concerns the reliability of information within the document (Christy, 1975). To judge reliability, the researcher must become familiar with the time in which the data emerged. A sense of the context and language of the time is essential to understanding a document. The meaning of a word in one era may not be equivalent to the meaning in another era. Knowing the language, customs, and habits of the historical period is critical for judging reliability. The researcher assumes that a primary source provides a more reliable account than a secondary source (Christy, 1975). The further a source moves from providing an eyewitness account, the more questionable is its reliability. The researcher using historical methods attempts to establish fact, probability, or possibility (Box 5-1). Adams (2007) was interested in research that suggests that backlashes to feminism may appear in the form of pro-family campaigns, so she conducted a socio-historical analysis of texts from a leading organized advocate of nineteenth-century pro-family reform that examined emergent rhetorical themes illustrative of a backlash to women's rights. She drew on critical feminist theory to suggest that these strategic rhetorical themes

BOX 5-1 Establishing Fact, Probability, and Possibility with the Historical Method

FACT
Two independent primary sources that agree with each other

Or

One independent primary source that receives critical evaluation and one independent secondary source that is in agreement and relieves critical evaluation and no substantive conflicting data

PROBABILITY
One primary source that receives critical evaluation and no substantive conflicting data

Or

Two primary sources that disagree about particular points

POSSIBILITY
One primary source that provides information but is not adequate to receive critical evaluation

Or

Only secondary or tertiary sources

Modified from Christy TE: The methodology of historical research: a brief introduction, *Image J Nurs Sch* 24(3):189-192, 1975.

were used to stimulate nineteenth-century women's ambivalence about family and independence. She also briefly engaged gender social movement's literature and research on current pro-family campaigns to point out similarities between the backlash rhetorical strategies of the historical and current movements. In accord with previous feminist scholarship, Adams' study is important in "making visible" the often hidden antifeminist bias in pro-family rhetoric.

HELPFUL HINT
When critiquing the historical method, do not expect to find a report of data analysis but simply a description of findings synthesized into a continuous narrative.

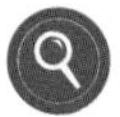

EVIDENCE-BASED PRACTICE TIP
The presentation of a historical study should be logical, consistent, and easy to follow.

Community-Based Participatory Research

Community-based participatory research (CBPR) is a method that systematically accesses the voice of a community to plan context-appropriate action. CBPR "provides an alternative to traditional research approaches that assume a phenomenon may be separated from its context for purposes of study.…CBPR recognizes the importance of involving members of a study population as active and equal participants, in all phases of the research project, if the research process is to be a means of facilitating change" (Holkup et al., 2004). Change or action is the intended "end-product" of CBPR, and *action research* is a term related to CBPR. Some scholars would consider CBPR a sort of action research and would group both action research and CBPR within the tradition of critical science (Fontana, 2004).

In his book entitled *Action Research,* Stringer (1999) distilled the research process into three phases: *look, think, act.* In the *look* phase Stringer (1999) talks about "building the picture" by getting to know stakeholders so that the problem is defined on their terms and the problem definition is reflective of the community context. The *think* phase addresses interpretation and analysis of what was learned in the *look* phase, where the researcher is charged with connecting the ideas of the stakeholders so that they provide evidence that is understandable to the community group (Stringer, 1999). Finally, in the *act* phase Stringer (1999) advocates for planning, implementing, and evaluating, based on information collected and interpreted in the other phases of research.

EVIDENCE-BASED PRACTICE TIP

Although qualitative in its approach to research, community-based participatory research leads to an action component in which a nursing intervention is implemented and evaluated for its effectiveness in a specific patient population.

Marcus and colleagues (2004) reported a study of CBPR to prevent substance use and human immunodeficiency virus (HIV)/acquired immunodeficiency syndrome (AIDS) in African-American adolescents. The research team used Stringer's phases of look, think, and act to frame their study within an African-American church community in the southwestern United States. In the *look* phase university research team members and church leaders formed a coalition, which met to consider the existing community situation and to evaluate the effectiveness of services already provided by the church to address substance use and HIV/AIDS in the adolescent congregation. Weekly meetings were convened to discuss evidence provided by relevant literature and apply the literature to the community situation. The coalition's *look* indicated that community youths could benefit from attention to substance use and HIV/AIDS prevention and the best course of action may be to begin with one community church, realizing that follow-up work could expand to the larger metropolitan community. In the *think* phase the coalition continued its work by analyzing and interpreting what was learned in the first phase of the research process. Analysis and interpretation were simultaneously connected with discussion of what could be done, and the collaborators initiated plans for Project BRIDGE to take African-American adolescents to a new level of understanding about everyday decisions that could seriously affect their health. Project BRIDGE integrated a faith component into structured programs supporting wise choices to reduce substance use and HIV/AIDS exposure. As plans for Project BRIDGE were formulated, the coalition was already moving into the *action* phase of research based on the strength of evidence generated in the previous phases. In the action phase Project BRIDGE was delivered to sixth-, seventh-, and eighth-graders within the structure of the community church environment. The church-university coalition members participated in all components of delivery and continued to meet to evaluate ongoing development, effectiveness, need for adjustment, and outcomes. Project BRIDGE is one example of CBPR that involved community members as equal participants in all phases of research to engage in context-appropriate action for affecting substance use and HIV/AIDS prevention in African-American youths.

TABLE 5-1 Characteristics of Qualitative Research Generating Ethical Concerns

Characteristics	Ethical Concerns
Naturalistic setting	Some researchers using methods that rely on participant observation may believe that consent is not always possible or necessary.
Emergent nature of design	Planning for questioning and observation emerges over the time of the study. Thus it is difficult to inform the participant precisely of all potential threats before he or she agrees to participate.
Researcher-participant interaction	Relationships developed between the researcher and participant may blur the focus of the interaction.
Researcher as instrument	The researcher is the study instrument, collecting data and interpreting the participant's reality.

ISSUES IN QUALITATIVE RESEARCH

Ethics

Inherent in all research is the demand for the protection of human subjects. This demand exists for both quantitative and qualitative research approaches. Human subjects' protection as applicable to the quantitative approach is discussed in Chapter 11. These basic tenets hold true for the qualitative approach. However, several characteristics of qualitative methodologies outlined in Table 5-1 generate unique concerns and necessitate an expanded view of protecting human subjects.

Naturalistic Setting

The central concern that arises when research is conducted in naturalistic settings focuses on the need to gain consent. The need to acquire informed consent is a basic researcher responsibility, but it is not always easy in naturalistic settings. For instance, when research methods include observing groups of people interacting over time, the complexity of gaining consent is apparent. These complexities generate controversy and debate among qualitative researchers. The balance between respect for human participants and efforts to collect meaningful data must be continuously negotiated. The reader should look for information that the researcher has addressed this issue of balance by recording attention to human participant protection.

Emergent Nature of Design

The emergent nature of the research design emphasizes the need for ongoing negotiation of consent with the participant. In the course of a study, situations change and what was agreeable at the beginning may become intrusive. Sometimes, as data collection proceeds and new information emerges, the study shifts direction in a way that is not acceptable to the participant. For instance, if the researcher were present in a family's home during a time when marital discord arose, the family may choose to renegotiate the consent. From another perspective,

Morse (1998) discusses the increasing involvement of participants in the research process, sometimes resulting in their request to have their name published in the findings or be included as a coauthor. If the participant originally signed a consent form and then chose an active identified role, Morse (1998) suggests that the participant then sign a "release for publication" form. The underlying nature of this discussion is that the emergent qualitative research process demands ongoing negotiating of researcher-participant relationships, including the consent relationship. The opportunity to renegotiate consent establishes a relationship of trust and respect characteristic of the ethical conduct of research.

Researcher-Participant Interaction

The nature of the researcher-participant interaction over time introduces the possibility that the research experience becomes a therapeutic one. It is a case of research becoming practice. There are basic differences between the intent of the nurse when conducting research or engaging in practice (Smith & Liehr, 2003). In practice, the nurse has caring-healing intentions. In research, the nurse intends to "get the picture" from the perspective of the participant. "Getting the picture" may be a therapeutic experience for the participant. Sometimes, talking to a caring listener about things that matter energizes healing, even though it was not intended. From an ethical perspective, the qualitative researcher is promising only to listen and to encourage the other's story. If this experience is therapeutic for the participant, it becomes an unplanned benefit of the research.

Researcher as Instrument

The responsibility to remain true to the data requires that the researcher acknowledge any personal bias, interpreting findings in a way that accurately reflects the participant's reality. This is a serious ethical obligation. To accomplish this, the researcher may return to the subjects at critical interpretive points and ask for clarification or validation.

Credibility, Auditability, and Fittingness

Quantitative studies are concerned with reliability and validity of instruments, as well as internal and external validity criteria, as measures of scientific rigor (see the Critical Thinking Decision Path), but these are not appropriate for qualitative work. The rigor of qualitative methodology is judged by unique criteria appropriate to the research approach. Credibility, auditability, and fittingness were scientific criteria proposed for qualitative research studies by Guba and Lincoln in 1981. Although these criteria were proposed decades ago, they still capture the rigorous spirit of qualitative inquiry and persist as reasonable criteria for appraisal. The meanings of **credibility, auditability,** and **fittingness** are briefly explained in Table 5-2.

Triangulation, Multimethods ... Or Is It Crystallization?

Triangulation is a term used in surveying and navigation. Triangulation has become a "buzzword" in qualitative research over the past several years and refers to the combination of several methods. There is discussion of theoretical triangulation (Kushner & Morrow, 2003), conceptual triangulation (Dabbs et al., 2004), and method triangulation, which is generally

TABLE 5-2 Criteria for Judging Scientific Rigor: Credibility, Auditability, Fittingness

Criteria	Criteria Characteristics
Credibility	Truth of findings as judged by participants and others within the discipline. For instance, you may find the researcher returning to the participants to share interpretation of findings and query accuracy from the perspective of the persons living the experience.
Auditabililty	Accountability as judged by the adequacy of information leading the reader from the research question and raw data through various steps of analysis to the interpretation of findings. For instance, you should be able to follow the reasoning of the researcher step-by-step through explicit examples of data, interpretations, and syntheses.
Fittingness	Faithfulness to everyday reality of the participants, described in enough detail so that others in the discipline can evaluate importance for their own practice, research, and theory development. For instance, you will know enough about the human experience being reported that you can decide whether it "rings true" and is useful for guiding your practice.

described as the collection of different kinds of data about a single complex phenomenon to bring clarity to the phenomenon that cannot be achieved with only one method. Triangulation provides an opportunity to more fully address the complex nature of the human experience. When referring to methods, **triangulation** can be defined as the expansion of research methods in a single study or multiple studies to enhance diversity, enrich understanding, and accomplish specific goals. It is important to know what triangulation is *not,* because it is frequently misused. It is not asking a woman for the name of her disabling illness, and then confirming that in a review of her medical record. Triangulation is using two pieces of information to find a third, unique finding. Richardson (2000) has suggested that the triangle be replaced by the crystal as a more appropriate metaphor for the multimethod approach. As you read nursing research, you will quickly discover that approaches and methods are being combined to contribute to theory building, guide practice, and facilitate instrument development. Table 5-3 synthesizes three manuscripts reporting multimethod analyses. The table notes the conceptual focus of the work, the study purposes, and whether the manuscript suggests implications for theory, practice, and instrument development.

From the perspective of crystallization, Swanson's work is most complete (see Table 5-3) because she has addressed implications for practice, instrument development, and theory building focused on the issue of caring for women who have had a miscarriage. Her research program has included an initial theory-building phase (studies 1 and 2), an instrument development phase (studies 3, 4, and 5), and a phase of testing a practice intervention (study 6). Swanson (1999) used the phenomenological method for studies 1 and 2 and quantitative methods for each of her other studies. In no study (see Table 5-3) does she use more than one method, but her use of multimethods during the course of research program development can be likened to examining different facets of one crystal—in this case, the experience of miscarriage. The crystallization process has contributed to theory building, nursing practice, and instrument development. Her practice contribution is highlighted by a case exemplar (Swanson, 1999), which synthesizes her years of work with women living through the life experience of miscarrying their baby. See Kristen Swanson's vignette on p. 82.

Both Hunter and Chandler (1999) and Liehr and colleagues (2000) reported pilot studies that include qualitative findings. Each study indicates plans for further investigation, based on the qualitative findings. Hunter and Chandler's study (1999) combined qualitative (phenomenological method, using focus groups, interview, and written stories) and quantitative

TABLE 5-3 Research Using Multimethod Approaches

				IMPLICATIONS		
Author/Date	**Conceptual Focus**	**Multimethod Approach**	**Study Purpose**	**Theory Building**	**Practice**	**Instrument Development**
Swanson (1999)	Miscarriage and caring	Six studies, each using one method	**Study 1:** Define common themes for women who had recently miscarried	Yes	Yes	
			Study 2: Describe the human experience of miscarriage and describe the meaning of caring	Yes	Yes	
			Study 3: Use descriptive data to create a survey instrument based on women's experience of miscarriage	Yes		Yes
			Study 4: Evaluate the relevance of the survey items to create miscarriage scale	Yes		Yes
			Study 5: Assess reliability and validity of the miscarriage scale	Yes		Yes
			Study 6: Test the effects of caring, measurement, and time on women's well-being in the first year after miscarriage	Yes	Yes	Yes
Hunter & Chandler (1999)	Adolescent resilience	One study using multimethods	Pilot study to explore the meaning of resilience for adolescents, and evaluate a resilience instrument	Yes	Yes	Yes
Liehr et al. (2000)	Adolescent hostility	One study using multimethods	Pilot study to test the reliability and validity of the adolescent version of the Cook-Medley Hostility scale with multiethnic sample			Yes

(Wagnild and Young's resiliency scale) methods to address their twofold study purpose (see Table 5-3). Data from the quantitative methods provided a different perspective than the one emerging from the qualitative methods—like differing facets of a crystal. The authors synthesize these differing perspectives in a model, entitled "Continuum of Resilience in Adolescents." They pose questions for further study related to (1) the health-promoting potential of resilience and (2) the likelihood of capturing adolescent resilience with a single paper-and-pencil measure.

The study reported by Liehr and associates (2000) (see Table 5-3) has a narrow focus. The purpose of the study was focused on instrument development. Within a quantitative context of reliability and validity testing, these researchers used a qualitative method (content analysis of adolescents' remembered descriptions of a time they experienced feeling angry) to evaluate the content validity of the adolescent version of the Cook-Medley Hostility Scale. The researchers note that the findings from this pilot study have led to changes in the scale for use in ongoing research.

These three manuscripts (see Table 5-3) present a range of approaches for combining methods in research studies, but the combining-methods picture is broader and growing. Although certain kinds of questions may be answered effectively by combining qualitative and quantitative methods in a single study, this does not necessarily make the findings and related evidence stronger. In fact, if a researcher inappropriately uses mixed methods, a study could be weaker and less credible. As a research consumer, you need to determine what led the researcher to choose a triangulated approach and whether this was an appropriate choice. You are encouraged to follow the ongoing debate about combining methods as nurse researchers strive to determine which research combinations promise enhanced understanding of human complexity and substantial contribution to nursing science.

EVIDENCE-BASED PRACTICE TIP

- Triangulation offers an opportunity for researchers to increase the strength and consistency of evidence provided by the use of both qualitative and quantitative research methods.
- The combination of stories with numbers (qualitative and quantitative research approaches) through use of triangulation may provide the most complete picture of the phenomenon being studied and therefore the best evidence for guiding practice.

Synthesizing Qualitative Evidence: Meta-Synthesis

The depth and breadth of qualitative research has grown over the years. It has become important to qualitative researchers to synthesize critical masses of qualitative findings. Qualitative **meta-synthesis** is a type of systematic review applied to qualitative research. Unlike quantitative research, which uses statistical approaches to aggregate or average data using meta-analysis (see Chapter 9), meta-synthesis integrates qualitative research findings on a topic and is based on comparative analysis and interpretative synthesis of qualitative research findings that seeks to retain the essence and unique contribution of each study (Sandelowski & Barroso, 2007).

Sandelowski and Barroso (2005) reported the results of a qualitative meta-synthesis and meta-summary that integrated the findings of qualitative studies of expectant parents who experienced a positive prenatal diagnosis. Using the methods of qualitative research synthesis (meta-analysis and meta-summary (see Sandelowski and Barroso, 2007), they analytically reviewed 17 qualitative studies retrieved from multiple databases. Based on the synthesis process detailed in the article, clinical implications and the need for further research in the area were identified.

Essentially, meta-synthesis provides a way for researchers to build up a critical mass of qualitative research evidence that is relevant to clinical practice. Sandelowski (2004) cautions that the use of qualitative meta-synthesis is laudable and necessary but requires researchers who use meta-synthesis methods to clearly understand qualitative methodologies, as well as the nuances of the various qualitative methods. It will be interesting for research consumers to follow the progress of researchers who seek to develop criteria for appraising a set of qualitative studies and using those criteria to guide the incorporation of these studies into systematic literature reviews.

APPRAISING THE EVIDENCE

Qualitative Research

Although general criteria for critiquing qualitative research are proposed in the following Critiquing Criteria box, each qualitative method has unique characteristics that influence what the research consumer may expect in the published research report, and journals often have page restrictions that penalize qualitative researchers, because it is difficult at times to fully explain all of the steps in Chapter 4 in a few pages. The criteria for critiquing are formatted to evaluate the selection of the phenomenon, the structure of the study, data gathering, data analysis, and description of the findings. Each question of the criteria focuses on factors discussed throughout the chapter. Appraising qualitative research is a useful activity for learning the nuances of this research approach. You are encouraged to identify a qualitative study of interest and apply the criteria for critiquing. Keep in mind that qualitative methods are the best way to start to answer clinical and/or research questions that previously have not been

CRITIQUING CRITERIA: *Qualitative Approaches*

Identifying the Phenomenon

1. Is the phenomenon focused on human experience within a natural setting?
2. Is the phenomenon relevant to nursing and/or health?

Structuring the Study

Research Question

3. Does the question specify a distinct process to be studied?
4. Does the question identify the context (participant group/place) of the process that will be studied?
5. Does the choice of a specific qualitative method fit with the research question?

Researcher's Perspective

6. Are the biases of the researcher reported?
7. Do the researchers provide a structure of ideas that reflect their beliefs?

Sample Selection

8. Is it clear that the selected sample is living the phenomenon of interest?

Data Gathering

9. Are data sources and methods for gathering data specified?
10. Is there evidence that participant consent is an integral part of the data-gathering process?

Data Analysis

11. Can the dimensions of data analysis be identified and logically followed?
12. Does the researcher paint a clear picture of the participant's reality?
13. Is there evidence that the researcher's interpretation captured the participant's meaning?
14. Have other professionals confirmed the researcher's interpretation?

Describing the Findings

15. Are examples provided to guide the reader from the raw data to the researcher's synthesis?
16. Does the researcher link the findings to existing theory or literature, or is a new theory generated?

addressed in research studies or that do not lend themselves to a quantitative approach. The answers provided by qualitative data reflect important evidence that may provide the first insights about a patient population or clinical phenomenon.

In summary, the term *qualitative research* is an overriding description of multiple methods with distinct origins and procedures. In spite of distinctions, each method shares a common nature that guides data collection from the perspective of the participants to create a story that synthesizes disparate pieces of data into a comprehensible whole that provides evidence and promises direction for building nursing knowledge.

CRITICAL THINKING CHALLENGES

- How can triangulation increase the effectiveness of qualitative research?
- How can a nurse researcher select a qualitative research method when he or she is attempting to accumulate evidence regarding a new topic about which little is known?
- How can the case study approach to research be applied to evidence-based practice?
- Describe characteristics of qualitative research that can generate ethical concerns.

KEY POINTS

- Qualitative research is the investigation of human experiences in naturalistic settings, pursuing meanings that inform theory, practice, instrument development, and further research.
- Qualitative research studies are guided by research questions.
- Data saturation occurs when the information being shared with the researcher becomes repetitive.
- Qualitative research methods include five basic elements: identifying the phenomenon, structuring the study, gathering the data, analyzing the data, and describing the findings.
- The phenomenological method is a process of learning and constructing the meaning of human experience through intensive dialogue with persons who are living the experience.
- The grounded theory method is an inductive approach that implements a systematic set of procedures to arrive at theory about basic social processes.
- The ethnographic method focuses on scientific descriptions of cultural groups.
- The case study method focuses on a selected phenomenon over a short or long time period to provide an in-depth description of its essential dimensions and processes.
- The historical research method is the systematic compilation of data and the critical presentation, appraisal, and interpretation of facts regarding people, events, and occurrences of the past.
- Community-based participatory research is a method that systematically accesses the voice of a community to plan context-appropriate action.
- Ethical issues in qualitative research involve issues related to the naturalistic setting, emergent nature of the design, researcher-participant interaction, and researcher as instrument.
- Credibility, auditability, and fittingness are criteria for judging the scientific rigor of a qualitative research study.
- *Triangulation* has shifted from a strategy for combining research methods to assess accuracy to expansion of research methods in a single study or multiple studies to enhance

diversity, enrich understanding, and accomplish specific goals. A better term may be *crystallization*.

- Multimethod approaches to research are controversial but promising.
- Qualitative research data can be managed through the use of computers, but the researcher must interpret the data.

REFERENCES

Aamodt AA: Ethnography and epistemology: generating nursing knowledge. In Morse JM, ed: *Qualitative nursing research: a contemporary dialogue*, Newbury Park, CA, 1991, Sage.

Adams M: Women's rights and wedding bells: 19th century pro-family rhetoric and (re)enforcement of the gender status quo, *J Fam Issues* 28:501-528, 2007.

Agar MH: *Speaking of ethnography*, Beverly Hills, CA, 1986, Sage.

Aita VA, McIlvain HE: An armchair adventure in case study research. In Crabtree B, Miller WL, eds: *Doing qualitative research*, ed 2, Thousand Oaks, CA, 1999, Sage.

Boyle JS: Field research: a collaborative model for practice and research. In Morse JM, ed: *Qualitative nursing research: a contemporary dialogue*, Newbury Park, CA, 1991, Sage.

Charmaz K: Grounded theory: objectivist and constructivist methods. In Denzin NK, Lincoln YS, eds: *Handbook of qualitative research*, ed 2, Thousand Oaks, CA, 2000, Sage.

Christy TE: The methodology of historical research: a brief introduction, *Image J Nurs Sch* 24(3):189-192, 1975.

Christy TE: The need for historical research in nursing, *Image J Nurs Sch* 4:227-228, 1981.

Clabo LML: An ethnography of pain assessment and the role of social context on two postoperative units, *J Adv Nurs* 61:531-539, 2008.

Colaizzi P: Psychological research as a phenomenologist views it. In Valle RS, King M, eds: *Existential phenomenological alternatives for psychology*, New York, 1978, Oxford University Press.

Corbin J, Strauss A: *Basics of qualitative research*, Los Angeles, 2008, Sage.

Crabtree BF, Miller WL: *Doing qualitative research*, Newbury Park, CA, 1992, Sage.

Creswell JW: *Qualitative inquiry and research design: choosing among five traditions*, Thousand Oaks, CA, 1998, Sage.

Dabbs ADV, Hoffman LA, Swigart V, et al: Using conceptual triangulation to develop an integrated model of the symptom experience of acute rejection after lung transplantation, *Adv Nurs Sci* 27(2):138-149, 2004.

Denzin NK: The art and politics of interpretation. In Denzin NK, Lincoln YS, eds: *Collecting and interpreting qualitative materials*, Thousand Oaks, CA, 1998, Sage.

Denzin NK, Lincoln YS: *The landscape of qualitative research*, Thousand Oaks, CA, 1998, Sage.

Docherty SL, Sandelowski M, Preisser JS: Three months in the symptom life of a teenage girl undergoing treatment for cancer, *Res Nurs Health* 29:294-310, 2006.

Doherty ME, Scannell-Desch E: The lived experience of widowhood during pregnancy, *J Midwife Womens Health* 53:103-109, 2008.

Fenwick J, Barclay L, Schmied V: Craving closeness: a grounded theory analysis of women's experiences of mothering in a special care nursery, *Women Birth* 21:71-85, 2008.

Fontana JS: A methodology for critical science in nursing, *Adv Nurs Sci* 27(2):93-101, 2004.

Giorgi A, Fischer CL, Murray EL, eds: *Duquesne studies in phenomenological psychology*, Pittsburgh, 1975, Duquesne University Press.

Glaser BG, Strauss AL: *The discovery of grounded theory: strategies for qualitative research*, Chicago, 1967, Aldine.

Guba E, Lincoln Y: *Effective evaluation*, San Francisco, 1981, Jossey-Bass.

Holkup PA, Tripp-Reimer T, Salois EM, Weinert C: Community-based participatory research: an approach to intervention research with a Native American community, *Adv Nurs Sci* 27(3):162-175, 2004.

Hunter AJ, Chandler GE: Adolescent resilience, *Image J Nurs Sch* 31(3):243-247, 1999.
Kleinman A: Local worlds of suffering: an interpersonal focus for ethnographies of illness experience, *Qual Health Res* 2(2):127-134, 1992.
Kushner KE, Morrow R: Grounded theory, feminist theory, critical theory: toward theoretical triangulation, *Adv Nurs Sci* 26(1):30-43, 2003.
Liehr P, Marcus MT: Qualitative approaches to research. In LoBiondo-Wood G, Haber J: *Nursing research: methods, critical appraisal, and utilization*, ed 5, St Louis, 2002, Mosby.
Liehr P, Meininger JC, Mueller WH, et al: Psychometric testing of the adolescent version of the Cook-Medley Hostility Scale, *Issues Compr Pediatr Nurs* 23(2):103-116, 2000.
Lusk B: Historical methodology for nursing research, *Image J Nurs Sch* 29(4):355-359, 1997.
Marcus MT, Walker T, Swint JM, et al: Community-based participatory research to prevent substance abuse and HIV/AIDS in African American adolescents, *J Interprofess Pract* 18(4):347-359, 2004.
Mead M: *Coming of age in Samoa*, New York, 1949, New American Library, Mentor Books.
Morse JM: The contracted relationship: ensuring protection of anonymity and confidentiality, *Qual Health Res* 8(3):301-303, 1998.
Parse RR, Coyne AB, Smith MJ: *Nursing research: qualitative and quantitative methods*, Bowie, MD, 1985, Brady.
Richardson L: Writing: a method of inquiry. In Denzin NK, Lincoln YS, eds: *Handbook of qualitative research*, ed 2, Thousand Oaks, CA, 2000, Sage.
Sandelowski M: Using qualitative research, *Qual Health Res* 14(10):1366-1386, 2004.
Sandelowski M, Barroso J: Creating metasummaries of qualitative findings, *Nurs Res* 52:226-233, 2003.
Sandelowski. M. Barroso J: The travesty of choosing after positive prenatal diagnosis. *J Obstet Gynecol Neonatal Nursing* 34(4):307-318, 2005.
Sandelowski M, Barroso J: *Handbook for synthesizing qualitative research*, Philadelphia, 2007, Springer.
Smith MJ, Liehr P: The theory of attentively embracing story. In Smith MJ, Liehr P, eds: *Middle range theory for nursing*, New York, 2003, Springer.
Spiegelberg H: *The phenomenological movement,* vols I and II, The Hague, 1976, Martinus Nijhoff.
Spradley JP: *The ethnographic interview*, New York, 1979, Holt, Rinehart, & Winston.
Stake RE: *The art of case study research*, Thousand Oaks, CA, 1995, Sage.
Stake RE: Case studies. In Denzin NK, Lincoln YS, eds: *Handbook of qualitative research*, ed 2, Thousand Oaks, CA, 2000, Sage.
Strauss AL: *Qualitative analysis for social scientists*, New York, 1987, Cambridge University Press.
Strauss A, Corbin J: *Basics of qualitative research: grounded theory procedures and techniques*, Newbury Park, CA, 1990, Sage.
Strauss A, Corbin J: Grounded theory methodology. In Denzin NK, Lincoln YS, eds: *Handbook of qualitative research*, Thousand Oaks, CA, 1994, Sage.
Strauss A, Corbin J, eds: *Grounded theory in practice*, Thousand Oaks, CA, 1997, Sage.
Stringer ET: *Action research*, ed 2, Thousand Oaks, CA, 1999, Sage.
Swanson KM: Research-based practice with women who have had miscarriages, *Image J Nurs Sch* 31(4):339-345, 1999.
Tedlock B: Ethnography and ethnographic representation. In Denzin NK, Lincoln YS, eds: *Handbook of qualitative research,* ed 2, Thousand Oaks, CA, 2000, Sage.
van Kaam A: *Existential foundations in psychology*, New York, 1969, Doubleday.
Vidick AJ, Lyman SM: Qualitative methods: their history in sociology and anthropology. In Denzin NK, Lincoln YS, eds: *The landscape of qualitative research: theories and issues*, Thousand Oaks, CA, 1998, Sage.

FOR FURTHER STUDY

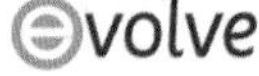

Go to Evolve at http://evolve.elsevier.com/LoBiondo/ for review questions, critiquing exercises, and additional research articles for practice in reviewing and critiquing.

6

Appraising Qualitative Research

Helen J. Streubert

KEY TERMS

auditability
credibility
emic view
fittingness
interpretive phenomenology
phenomena
saturation
theme
transferability
trustworthiness

LEARNING OUTCOMES

After reading this chapter, you should be able to do the following:

- Identify the influence of stylistic considerations on the presentation of a qualitative research report.
- Identify the criteria for critiquing a qualitative research report.
- Evaluate the strengths and weaknesses of a qualitative research report.
- Describe the applicability of the findings of a qualitative research report.
- Construct a critique of a qualitative research report.

STUDY RESOURCES

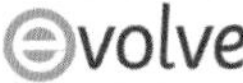

Go to Evolve at http://evolve.elsevier.com/LoBiondo/ for review questions, critiquing exercises, and additional research articles for practice in reviewing and critiquing.

Nurse scientists contribute significantly to the body of health care research. These contributions are evident in nursing, medical, health care, and business journals. Nurse researchers are partnering at an ever-increasing rate with other health care professionals to develop, implement, and evaluate a variety of evidence-based interventions to improve client outcomes. The methods used to develop evidence-based practice include quantitative, qualitative, and mixed research approaches. In addition to the increase in the number of research studies and publications, there is also a significant record of externally funded research by nurses adding to the credibility of the work. The willingness of private and publicly funded organizations to invest in nursing research attests to its quality and potential for affecting health care outcomes of individuals, families, groups, and communities. Quantitative, qualitative, and mixed research methods are all important to the ongoing development of a sound evidence-based practice; the focus of this chapter is on assessing the quality of qualitative research studies.

Qualitative and quantitative research methods come from strong traditions in the physical and social sciences. The two types of research are different in their purpose, approach, analysis, and conclusions. Therefore the use of each requires an understanding of the traditions on which the methods are based. The historical development of the methods identified as qualitative or quantitative can be discovered in this and other texts. This chapter aims to demonstrate a set of criteria that can be used to determine the quality of a qualitative research report. It is critical that nurses fully understand how to assess the value of qualitative research, particularly in light of the requirement that nursing practice be evidence based. According to Sackett and colleagues (2000), evidence-based practice requires that patient values, clinical expertise, and the best evidence from published research be used in combination.

As a framework for understanding the appraisal of qualitative research as a basis for evidence-based practice, a published research report, as well as critiquing criteria, will be presented. The criteria then will be used to demonstrate the process of appraising a qualitative research report.

STYLISTIC CONSIDERATIONS

Qualitative research differs from quantitative research in some very fundamental ways. Qualitative researchers represent a basic level of inquiry that seeks to discover and understand concepts, phenomena, or cultures. Jackson and colleagues (2007) state that the primary focus of qualitative research is to understand human beings' experiences in a humanistic and interpretive way (p. 21). In a qualitative study you should not expect to find hypotheses; theoretical frameworks; dependent and independent variables; large, random samples; complex statistical procedures; scaled instruments; or definitive conclusions about how to use the findings. Because the intent of the research is to describe, explain, or understand phenomena or cultures, the report is generally written in a narrative that is meant to convey the full meaning and richness of the phenomena or cultures being studied. This narrative includes subjective comments that are intended to provide the depth and richness of the phenomena under study.

The goal of a qualitative research report is to describe in as much detail as possible the "insider's" or emic view of the phenomenon being studied. The **emic view** is the view of the person experiencing the phenomenon reflective of his or her culture, values, beliefs, and experiences. What the qualitative researcher hopes to produce in the report is an understanding of what it is like to experience a particular phenomenon or be part of a specific culture.

One of the most effective ways to help the reader understand the emic view is to use quotes reflecting the phenomenon as experienced. For this reason the qualitative research report has a more conversational tone than a quantitative report. In addition, data are frequently reported using concepts or phrases that are called themes (see Chapter 5). A **theme** is a label. Themes represent a way of describing large quantities of data in a condensed format. To clearly demonstrate the application of a theme and how it helps the reader understand the emic view, the following is offered from a report published by Landreneau and Ward-Smith (2007). The authors' purpose is to "explore what patients on hemodialysis perceive concerning choice among three types of renal replacement therapies" (p. 513). The following quote is used by Landreneau and Ward-Smith to demonstrate the theme of *"choice."*

> *"I chose hemo because, I guess this is more, it's more sterile. I mean I'm more sterile, but if I was at home when you when you do the peritoneal you have to be real, well with this you have to be sterile too, but I don't know. This type was the best for me. You know, come in three days a week and let them do it. The other way it was at home, I guess, I think you can do it when you get home. Peritoneal you do it when you want to."*

The richness of the narrative provided in a qualitative research study cannot be shared in its entirety in a journal publication. Page limitations imposed by journals frequently limit research reports to 15 pages. Despite this limitation, it is the qualitative researcher's responsibility to illustrate the richness of the data and to convey to the audience the relationship between the themes identified and the quotes shared. This is essential in order to document the rigor of the research, which is called **trustworthiness** in a qualitative research study. It is important to point out that it is challenging to convey the depth and richness of the findings of a qualitative study in a published research report. A perusal of the nursing and health care literature will demonstrate a commitment by qualitative researchers and journal editors to publish qualitative research findings. Regardless of the page limit, Jackson and colleagues (2007) offer that it is the researcher's responsibility to ensure objectivity, ethical diligence, and rigor regardless of the method selected to conduct the study. Fully sharing the depth and richness of the data will also help practitioners to decide on the appropriateness of applying the findings to their practice.

There are some journals that by virtue of their readership are committed to publication of more lengthy reports. *Qualitative Health Research* is an example of a journal that provides the opportunity for longer research reports. Guidelines for publication of research reports are generally listed in each nursing journal or are available from the journal editor. It is important to note that criteria for publication of research reports are not based on a specific type of research method (i.e., quantitative or qualitative). The primary goal of journal editors is to provide their readers with high-quality, informative, timely, and interesting articles. To meet this goal, regardless of the type of research report, editors prefer to publish manuscripts that have scientific merit, present new knowledge, support the current state of the science, and engage their readership. The challenge for the qualitative researcher is to meet these editorial requirements within the page limit imposed by the journal of interest.

Nursing journals do not generally offer their reviewers specific guidelines for evaluating qualitative and quantitative research reports. The editors make every attempt to see that reviewers are knowledgeable in the method and subject matter of the study. This determination is often made, however, based on the reviewer's self-identified area of interest. It is important to know that research reports are often evaluated based on the ideas or philosophical viewpoints held by the reviewer. The reviewer may have strong feelings about particular types of qualitative or quantitative research methods. Therefore it is important to clearly state the qualitative approach used and, if appropriate, its philosophical base.

Fundamentally, principles for evaluating research are the same. Reviewers are concerned with the plausibility and trustworthiness of the researcher's account of the research and its potential and/or actual relevance to current or future theory and practice (Horsburgh, 2003, p. 308). The Critiquing Criteria: Qualitative Research box below provides general guidelines for reviewing qualitative research. For information on specific guidelines for appraisal of ethnography, grounded theory, historical, and action research, see Speziale and Carpenter (2007). If you are interested in additional information on the specifics of qualitative research design, see Chapters 4 and 5.

CRITIQUING CRITERIA: *Qualitative Research*

Statement of the Phenomenon of Interest

1. What is the phenomenon of interest and is it clearly stated for the reader?
2. What is the justification for using a qualitative method?
3. What are the philosophical underpinnings of the research method?

Purpose

1. What is the purpose of the study?
2. What is the projected significance of the work to nursing?

Method

1. Is the method used to collect data compatible with the purpose of the research?
2. Is the method adequate to address the phenomenon of interest?
3. If a particular approach is used to guide the inquiry, does the researcher complete the study according to the processes described?

Sampling

1. What type of sampling is used? Is it appropriate given the particular method?
2. Are the informants who were chosen appropriate to inform the research?

Continued

CRITIQUING CRITERIA: *Qualitative Research—cont'd*

Data Collection

1. Is data collection focused on human experience?
2. Does the researcher describe data collection strategies (i.e., interview, observation, field notes)?
3. Is protection of human participants addressed?
4. Is saturation of the data described?
5. What are the procedures for collecting data?

Data Analysis

1. What strategies are used to analyze the data?
2. Has the researcher remained true to the data?
3. Does the reader follow the steps described for data analysis?
4. Does the researcher address the credibility, auditability, and fittingness of the data?

Credibility

a. Do the participants recognize the experience as their own?
b. Has adequate time been allowed to fully understand the phenomenon?

Auditability

a. Can the reader follow the researcher's thinking?
b. Does the researcher document the research process?

Fittingness

a. Are the findings applicable outside of the study situation?
b. Are the results meaningful to individuals not involved in the research?
c. Is the strategy used for analysis compatible with the purpose of the study?

Findings

1. Are the findings presented within a context?
2. Is the reader able to apprehend the essence of the experience from the report of the findings?
3. Are the researcher's conceptualizations true to the data?
4. Does the researcher place the report in the context of what is already known about the phenomenon? Was the existing literature on the topic related to the findings?

Conclusions, Implications, and Recommendations

1. Do the conclusions, implications, and recommendations give the reader a context in which to use the findings?
2. How do the conclusions reflect the study findings?
3. What are the recommendations for future study? Do they reflect the findings?
4. How has the researcher made explicit the significance of the study to nursing theory, research, or practice?

APPLICATION OF QUALITATIVE RESEARCH FINDINGS IN PRACTICE

The purpose of qualitative research is to describe, understand, or explain phenomena or cultures. **Phenomena** are those things that are perceived by our senses. For example, pain and losing a loved one are considered phenomena. Unlike quantitative research, prediction and control of phenomena are not the aim of the qualitative inquiry. Therefore qualitative results are applied differently than more traditional quantitative research findings. Barbour and Barbour (2003, p. 185) state that

> *rather than seeking to import and impose templates and methods devised for another purpose, qualitative researchers and reviewers should look . . . for inspiration from their own modes of working and collaborating and seek to incorporate these, forging new and creative solutions to perennial problems, rather than hoping that these will simply disappear in the face of application of pre-existing sets of procedures.*

Further, Barbour and Barbour (2003) and Schepner-Hughes (1992) offer that qualitative research can provide the opportunity to give voice to those who have been disenfranchised and have no history. Therefore the application of qualitative findings will necessarily be context-bound (Russell & Gregory, 2003). This means that if a qualitative researcher studies, for example, the pain experience of individuals undergoing bone marrow biopsy, the application of these findings is confined to individuals who are similar to those in the study.

EVIDENCE-BASED PRACTICE TIP

Nurses using qualitative research findings should ask whether the evidence provided in the study enhances their understanding of particular patient care situations.

Qualitative research findings can be used to create solutions to practical problems (Glesne, 1999). Qualitative research also has the ability to contribute to the evidenced-based practice literature (Cesario et al., 2002; Gibson & Martin, 2003; Walsh & Downe, 2005). For instance, in the development of a phenomenological description of the health effects of the patient-provider relationship on individuals living with a chronic illness, Fox and Chesla (2008) share how important the patient-provider relationship is to improving the quality of life for patients living with chronic disease. As the authors carefully describe in their narrative the importance of patients feeling connected to their providers, current practitioners are invited to consider the value of such relationships in the care of their own patients.

It is important to view research findings within context, whether quantitative or qualitative. For instance, a quantitative study of survivorship in women breast cancer survivors (Meneses et al., 2007) should not be viewed as applicable to survivors of another "survivor" situation such as an epidemic. The findings must be used within context, or additional studies must be conducted to validate the applicability of the findings across situations and patient populations. This is true in qualitative research, as well. Nurses who wish to use the findings of qualitative research in their practice must validate them, through thorough examination and synthesis of the literature on the topic, through their own observations, or through interaction with groups similar to the study participants, to determine whether the findings accurately reflect the experience.

Morse and colleagues (2000) offer "qualitative outcome analysis (QOA) [as a] systematic means to confirm the applicability of clinical strategies developed from a single qualitative project, to extend the repertoire of clinical interventions, and evaluate clinical outcomes" (p. 125). Using this process, the researcher employs the findings of a qualitative study to develop interventions and then to test those selected. Qualitative outcome analysis allows the researcher/clinician to implement interventions based on the client's expressed experience of a particular clinical phenomenon. Morse and colleagues (2000) state, "QOA may be considered a form of participant action research" (p. 129). Application of knowledge discovered during qualitative data collection adds to our understanding of clinical phenomena by using interventions that are based on the client's experience. QOA is considered a form of evaluation research and as such has the potential to add to evidence-based practice literature either at Level V or at Level VI depending on how the study is designed.

Another use of qualitative research findings is to initiate examination of important concepts in nursing practice, education, or administration. For example, decision making as a concept has been studied using both qualitative and quantitative methods. It is considered a significant concept in nursing. Therefore studying its multiple dimensions is important. In a study by Hough (2008), the author examined ethical decision making by critical care nurses. The outcome of her research was the development of a new model of ethical decision making based on experiential learning. The study adds to the existing body of knowledge on ethical decision making and extends the current state of the science by examining a specific area of nursing practice and the experience of ethical decision making by critical care nurses. This type of study is at Level V or VI, which includes either systematic reviews or single studies that are descriptive or qualitative in their design (see Chapter 1).

EVIDENCE-BASED PRACTICE TIP

Qualitative research studies can be used to guide practice when they are applied within context. The question the nurse should ask is the following: "Does this study provide me with a direction for caring for a particular patient group?"

Finally, qualitative research can be used to discover evidence about phenomena of interest that can lead to instrument development. When qualitative methods are used to direct the development of structured measurement instruments, it is usually part of a larger empirical research project. Instrument development from qualitative research studies is useful to practicing nurses because it is grounded in the reality of human experience with a particular phenomenon and informs item development. A study completed by Richards (2008) illustrates the use of both qualitative and quantitative methods to develop, revise, and test a pain assessment instrument.

Critique of a Qualitative Research Study

The Research Study

The study "Living with Chronic Illness: A Phenomenological Study of the Health Effects of the Patient-Provider Relationship," by Sylvia Fox and Catherine Chesla, published in *Journal of the American Academy of Nurse Practitioners,* is critiqued. The article is presented in its entirety and followed by the critique on p. 146.

Living with Chronic Illness: A Phenomenological Study of the Health Effects of the Patient-Provider Relationship

Sylvia Fox, Catherine Chesla

Key Words

Interpretive phenomenology; chronic illness; health effects

Abstract

Purpose: To understand the patient–health care provider (HCP) relationship from the lived experience of women with chronic disease and determine how this relationship affects women's health.

Data Sources: Narrative accounts of 25 women's relationships with HCPs in repeated group and individual interviews were audio-taped and transcribed verbatim. Interpretive phenomenology was used to explore the data using three interconnected modes of paradigm cases, exemplars, and themes.

Conclusions: Women with chronic disease believed their health was significantly affected by their relationships with HCPs. The experienced a greater sense of well-being and security in connected relationships and had more confidence and motivation to manage their illness.

Implications for Practice: This research suggests that for women with chronic disease, relationships with HCPs that are connected, and characterized by partnerships, and personableness result in the women feeling better in many dimensions. The context of today's health care system often pushes the nurse practitioner (NP) to provide care more attuned to medical issues, leaving little time for the development of connected relationships. In spite of this pressure, NPs need to strive to develop relationships with patients that are intersubjective/connected.

BACKGROUND

The patient–health care provider (HCP) relationship has long been considered an important element in the delivery of health care. Cultural and social changes, such as patient rights,

Sylvia Fox, PhD, CNS, Psychiatric–Mental Health Clinical Specialist and Associate Professor of Nursing at Samuel Merritt College, Oakland, California; Catherine Chesla, DNSc, Professor, Department of Family Health Care Nursing at University of California, San Francisco, California. Correspondence to: Sylvia Fox, PhD, CNS; Nursing; Samuel Merritt College; 3100 Summit Street, Third Floor, Oakland, CA 94309. Tel: (510) 525-2838; Fax: (510) 594-7568; Email: s.fox@samuelmerritt.edu.

informed consent, and women's and gay rights, exert pressure on the system to be more responsive to patient concerns. Increased changes in health care delivery, especially with managed care, have resulted in doubt among patients of the once-sacrosanct authority of the HCP (McCloskey & Grace, 1997). Valuing women and women's experience, feminist scholars have given recognition to the nurturing and caring involved in the traditional practices of women and to their importance in relationships beyond the mother/child dyad, including health care relationships (McCloskey & Grace; Noddings, 1984; Tronto, 1994). However, there are multiple competing concerns in the health care arena. Positivist traditions and the search for positive outcomes have led to a press for evidence-based practice. Economic pressure and the commodification of health care have made it difficult for HCPs to develop personal caring relationships with patients (Benner, 2001; Lagana, 2000).

The literature reveals a persistent concern with qualities or characteristics of the patient-HCP relationship that influences the patient, the clinician, the relationship itself, and the outcomes of care (Crits-Christoph, 1998; Langford, Bowsher, Maloner, & Lillis, 1997; Norbeck & Anderson, 1988; Pieranunzi, 1997; Spiegel, Stroud, & Fyfe, 1998; Strupp, 1993; Yarcheski, Scoloveno, & Mahon, 1994). More specifically, several studies have examined relationships between patients and nurse practitioners (NPs) demonstrating the qualities of the relationship that are important in the delivery of care (Covington, 2005; Donohue, 2003; Lawson, 2002; Williams & Jones, 2006). Technical skill and biomedical competence are frequently believed to be the primary determinants of quality health care relationships and health outcomes. However, Balini (1957) pointed out almost a half century ago the importance of the provider's capacity to attend not only to the patient's symptoms but also to the patient's concerns and expectations.

Hall, Roter, and Katz (1988) conducted a meta-analysis to determine the relationship between physician communication and patient outcomes. They concluded that information giving, positive talk, partnership building, as well as the length of the visit are predictors of patient compliance and satisfaction with care. In another meta-analysis of literature that evaluated the effectiveness of three classes of interventions on patient compliance with health care regimens, 153 studies conducted between 1977 and 1994 were examined (Roter et al., 1998). Five classes of compliance were identified that were measured by direct and indirect measures. Interventions included educational, behavioral, and affective programs. All intervention types produced significant effects for all the compliance indicators. No single intervention strategy was more effective than another; programs with more than one intervention were most effective. Most importantly, patients with chronic diseases, such as diabetes or cancer, benefited highly from the interventions. The researchers concluded that building rapport with the patient can have a significant influence on patient compliance with treatment protocols.

In a review of 21 randomized clinical trials that studied physician communication and patient outcomes, several significant findings were reported (Stewart, 1996). Physician information giving, partnership building, and emotional support led to improvements in several categories of patient outcomes, including emotional health, symptom resolution, physical functioning, quality of life assessments, and physiological measures of disease management. These three overviews demonstrate that characteristics of the relationship between HCPs and patients and features that improve their communication do matter in health care.

The literature is unambiguous in noting the importance of NPs in the delivery of primary care with the positive health outcomes (Covington, 2005; Kinnersley, et al., 2000; Kleinman,

2004; Venning, Duric, Roland, Roberts, & Leese, 2000). Patients expect NPs to be caring and to engage them with mutuality (Alexander, 2004; Donohue, 2003; Heller & Solomon, 2005). Even though NPs perceive that they provide service that is caring (Green, 2004; Kleinman, 2004), current demands of health care systems that reduce appointment time and place an emphasis on medical care (Alexander; Williams & Jones, 2006) make it increasingly difficult to deliver care that lives up this ideal. As Lawson (2002) points out, particularly when patients who have chronic disease engage in behaviors detrimental to their health, NPs are less likely to involve them in negotiating plans for care.

In summary, there is a substantial body of empirical work that addresses how the encounter between the patient and the HCP affects patient health. In most of this research, an elemental or atomistic approach to the encounter has been taken. That is, the relationship and interaction have been broken down into its constituent parts, and researchers have attempted to identify elements that predict certain behaviors and responses and inhibit others. What has been learned is important. However, the elemental approach, by its very nature, blinds us to aspects of the relationship that may, in fact, be essential to understanding what makes it work, for example, the timing and pacing of the interaction, the feeling tone of the interaction, and the way in which the provider makes herself vulnerable to the risks that appear in the room when the patient is receiving a serious diagnosis or prognosis. The patients' perspectives and voices are also largely missing from this literature.

This research addressed the patient-HCP relationship and how it works from the patient's perspective. To date, no study has been found that attempted to understand the relationship from the patient's perspective. Additionally, little effort has been given to the process of patient-HCP relating. The dialogical process of qualitative research makes it possible for the lived experience to be transformed into a textual expression that is reflexive reliving of the experience. These animated descriptions based on human actions and lived experience demonstrate patients' meanings, concerns, and practices (Van Manen, 1990).

PURPOSE

The primary purpose of this research was to understand the patient-HCP relationship from the perspective of women with chronic disease. Our intent was to understand the meaning of the relationship for women and how they believed it affected their health. Specifically, we wanted to explore and articulate the full range of experiences women had with HCPs, including relationships they experienced as comforting and helpful as well as those they found oppressive and troublesome. Women's perceptions of how they believed their health was affected by the relationship were further explored.

CONCEPTUAL FRAMEWORK

Relational cultural theory is a theoretical approach that opens up ways of recognizing and talking about the experiences of patients in their relationships with HCPs. According to this model, the self is continuously developing in connection with others. "The movement of relating, of mutual initiative and responsiveness, is viewed as the ongoing central organizing dynamic of people's lives" (Jordan, 1997a, p. 343). According to this perspective, it is impossible to view oneself apart from or outside of relationships. The goal of development is not a separate, individuated self but rather the ability to participate in mutually empathic relationships, which foster the growth of all participants (Miller & Stiver, 1997). Relational confidence is the capacity to participate in a growing, moving, changing relationship. We seek to participate in connections that are meaningful and respectful. If successful, we have an increased sense of well-being, confidence, and vitality (Jordan, 1997b).

Relational cultural theory provided the framework and sensitizing concepts for our study of the health effects of the patient-provider relationship. Understanding the major concepts of the theory, empathy, mutuality, and empowerment provided the background against which the primary objective and the specific aims of the study were formulated.

SAMPLE

Study participants were women between the ages of 35-55 who had a diagnosis of a chronic disease, spoke and wrote English, had no major mental illness, and could consent for themselves. No time limit was established for the length of diagnosis and participation, but all women in the study had been chronically ill for a period of years. Twenty-five women participated in the study; all but three were Caucasian. Two of the women were in their 30s, 5 in their 40s, and 18 in their 50s. Three of the women had asthma, 1 breast cancer, 1 stroke, 1 hepatitis C, 1 IgA nephropathy, and the remaining 18 had diabetes. Two of the women with diabetes had a second chronic disease, one cancer, and the other multiple sclerosis. All but two of the women had some college education, and nine of them had graduate or professional education.

METHOD

The method for the study was interpretive phenomenology in the Heideggerian tradition, which holds that a person is self-interpreting and understands a situation directly according to the meaning it has for her (Levin, 1999). Accordingly, the researcher attempts to interpret what is always already understood, the taken for granted of everydayness. In this approach, it is believed that the nature of our everyday lived experience, the smooth functioning of everydayness, goes unnoticed or unarticulated and it is the work of interpretation to make explicit these aspects of human existence (Dreyfus, 1991).

In the process of interpreting, researchers must be attuned to everyday situations that they wish to articulate; this is influenced by the way the research is approached because it is believed that no objective stance is possible. Both researchers were mental health-psychiatric clinical specialists and had taught in university nursing programs extensively.

The University Committee on Human Research approved the study and written consents were obtained. All participants received $20.00 for each interview. Women were recruited through newspaper advertisement, flyers in private practitioner offices, a local health care center, support groups, and word of mouth. The interviews were conducted in private rooms at a local health center and hospital, in a private office, or in women's homes.

DATA COLLECTION

Narrative accounts of positive, neutral, and problematic experiences and relationships with HCPs were elicited in repeated group and individual interviews. Open-ended information probes were used to initiate the interviews, to follow up on something said, or to fill in gaps in the narratives. All the interviews were audio-taped and transcribed verbatim, and transcriptions were checked for accuracy against the tapes. All the participants were first interviewed in one of the five interview groups that met two times for 1.5 h. These were followed by 11 individual interviews each lasting 1.5 h. Women were selected to participate in individual interviews if their narratives were particularly vibrant or if they seemed to have insufficient opportunity in the group to complete their narratives. Women described experiences with a variety of HCPs, including NPs, physicians, physical therapists, occupational therapists, music therapists, and psychotherapists. Field notes of impressions were recorded after each interview.

DATA ANALYSIS

Analysis of the data involved multiple readings of the printed transcripts that began with the first group interview. The narratives of one respondent were contrasted to other respondent narratives. We examined both the whole and parts of the whole, returning repeatedly to the original text to uncover/discover meaning. We were looking for stories of both smooth functioning and also stories of breakdown, experiences that had not gone smoothly. Interpretive phenomenology includes the use of three interconnected modes of engaging the text: paradigm cases, exemplars, and themes. All three of these methods were used in this research. Paradigm cases and exemplars were identified. Paradigm cases are strong examples of particular ways of being, of concerns, or of practices (Benner, 1994). They illustrate dramatically the meaning of a person's lived experience. Exemplars are smaller units of analysis and reflect recurring themes. Finally, cross narrative comparisons were made to determine whether or not common meanings could be identified that showed up in more than one case. Thematic analysis works out the themes of the text. This occurred simultaneously with the reading, rereading, and discovery of paradigm cases and exemplars. As paradigm cases and exemplars were compared to one another, broader understanding or themes were derived. Going through the text slowly, again and again, it became a part of the interpretive findings.

FINDINGS

Relational Continuum-Connection

Narratives suggested that a link with the provider that opened up communication and closeness was essential to every encounter. Yet, women in the study experienced extreme variations in the qualities of connectedness so that two poles, connection and disconnection, became apparent. The quality of connection was especially clear in the paradigm cases of partnership and personableness.

Partnership

In partnered relationships, the women in the study trusted and believed in the HCP so that in times of difficulty, they were able to rely on the HCP's judgment. In this research, their terms "husband" and "coach" were used to describe the quality of relatedness some of the women experienced. They characterized a connected relationship as a "good" marriage and explained that they were better physically, emotionally, and spiritually as a result.

The case of Tillie was a paradigm for a connected relationship in which there was a partnership between her and the HCP. Tillie's story presented the give-and-take in the working relationship they established where they enjoyed genuine, honest communication.

Tillie (age 41) was first diagnosed with diabetes at age 13 when she was taken to an emergency room in a disoriented state and met her current HCP. She said, "He saved my life" because emergency room staff had assumed that she was under the influence of illicit drugs until he arrived and ordered blood sugar levels to be drawn. Their 28-year relationship developed connection over time. She said,

"It's a combination of husband, coach, and the other thing, partnership because Dr. L. is always involved with me. He would say, 'This isn't quite working. I think you should do this, this, and this.' I would say, 'I really don't think that will work' and I would explain why. And he would say, 'Okay.'"

In this example, Tillie described mutual respect. Both the HCP and the patient took responsibility, there was a give-and-take, and both were willing to listen to the other. They were able to be open and honest, say what they thought, and find a way to agree on the approach they would take. In another example, Tillie illustrated how this worked between her and her HCP.

"My doctor said, 'Well, you have this kind of, the dawn phenomenon. Get up at three and test your blood and let me know what it is.' And I said, 'You want me to call YOU at three?' He gives me the stern look, 'Don't you even think about it.' But when he tells me to something I don't want to do, I give him that uhhhhhh look and he goes, 'I know.' So he knows he's asking me to do something yucky. 'It won't be for long. I need this information.' And so, he understands like, it's a pain. But I understand it's going to help me. So, there's a give and take."

In this interchange the daily impact of managing was transparent. Neither wanted to have to be up at 3:00 a.m. and they teased about this. The HCP acknowledged that sometimes what he asked of her he understood to be burdensome. His empathic attunement was important to her. She knew that he was making decisions based on what was best for her, and this contributed to her ability to do as he asked.

The story of Tillie going on the insulin pump illustrated the closeness and intimacy of their connection. What happened to her mattered to him and she knew this. She believed that he shared in her experience and that what she did had an impact on him. This is the quality of "marriage" that Tillie and other women in the study talked about. She said,

"He would say, 'I really would like you to be on the insulin pump.' And say the reasons why. 'What about this?' And I said, 'No, I don't want to.' And he finally said, 'I'm really confused about you. Why are you resisting this?' And I said, 'You know that I faint when you give me a blood test. Don't like needles.' He said, 'Okay. I understand that.'"

There was between them a commitment to understand the concerns of the other and to negotiate the progress of treatment in a manner that was mindful of these concerns. Out of respect for Tillie's reluctance, the physician paced recommendations to her readiness. His willingness to wait and to puzzle with her about her reluctance to try the pump enabled her self-exploration. One can imagine that a more aggressive treatment approach may instead have invited from Tillie resistance, retrenchment, and postponement.

Instead, Tillie felt respected, particularly when her provider stopped bringing up the pump as an alternative.

"And then my cousin, who went on the pump a few months before I did, said, 'They have one of the MiniMed pumps.' And I called MiniMed immediately and said, 'Send the information on this thing.' And when I told my doctor, I said, 'Oh, by the way, I called MiniMed and let's talk about the pump.' And he almost fell over. And I said, 'Oh, I'm sorry. I should have warned you.'" From the narrative, it seems that the physician accepted Tillie's position on her diabetic management, and even though she did not want to do as he recommended, he continued to actively work with her to improve her health. His flexibility was key to how they worked together and, we might surmise, was key to her eventual willingness to take the leap.

"And when I told him, the smile that came across his face was like, I mean like a shock and a smile. He was *ecstatic!* He, I mean, I think if I had said that he had won the lottery he would have been less excited than when I said I want to do this. When I got the (blood glucose) results that he had been dreaming that I would have I said, 'Wow, that's pretty good.' And he said, 'No. That's *great!*' And it was sort of like, yeeaahhh. And it was exciting for both of us. it wasn't like it was just like my victory. It was, we both shared in that dream. sort of like getting the Gold Medal or something, it just was, it was a wonderful feeling."

From Tillie's perspective, the patience, encouragement, and support of the HCP were pivotal. His hope for better clinical management of her diabetes mattered to her as it paralleled her own hopes of better health. She believed that they were aligned in their desire for her to do better. When she succeeded, she believed that they shared in the success.

Having an HCP share the ups and downs of the chronic disease enabled Tillie not to feel alone. As she points out, she had several sources of help and support, but it was the support and caring of the HCP that mattered the most to her. He alone appreciated and understood the daily grind and threat of having a chronic disease. He had shared in moments of crisis and had helped her to survive them. His presence and help as she changed to the pump were essential to her. The results she was able to achieve, she believed, were the result of the efforts and hard work of both of them. These qualities of the relationship women in the study compared to a partnership or marriage were important in motivating Tillie and other women in the study.

The term *marriage* was an attempt by women in the study to capture the key qualities of their lived experience in which they shared with another person life and death struggles; emotional upheaval of fear, sadness, and joy; and finally the achievement of what had seemed impossible. The level of intimacy, while not what is usually considered when we think of a marriage, was significant enough for them to use the descriptive term as they described the relationship.

Personableness

Personableness was an important element that contributed to the strength and bonds of all relationships in this study. Women in the study expressed an ongoing need to be seen and recognized for whom they really were, and it was another qualitatively distinct aspect of connected relationships. Maintaining personableness was a dynamic process that enabled the women in the study to continuously represent their true experience within relationships as they arose. They did not feel a need to hold back, and they were able to discuss issues that were embarrassing or shameful. They felt comfortable asking questions, questioning advice, and disagreeing.

Meryl's narrative illustrates the quality of personableness. Meryl (age 55) was recovering from a cerebral vascular accident 6 years earlier. She had several HCPs who were part of her rehabilitation team whom she described as being "very real." In one narrative, she discussed her piano therapist, whom she described as relating to her in a manner that illustrates this notion of personableness.

"Well, she lives in a real cute bungalow. She has a great big music room that she added on. Two lovely grand pianos. And she has a nice sense of decorating. So she's always sitting in her chair. And I walk down through her garden, which is lovely . . . the piano lesson is a half an hour. But I can't play for a half an hour. So we kind of, I'll play my piece and then we'll talk about her ill mother or my ill mother. Or her kids. Or my kids. And then she'll say,

'Okay, let's try it again.' And it's always better the second time. And she'll occasionally put her hand on my shoulder because in my attempt to make my fingers work, my shoulder goes up. And she'll just gently put her hand on my shoulder. And she's a very touchy, feely kind of woman. And she has this loud laugh. It's a joyful laugh. And, she's just a wonderful person. So we talk about religion a lot. And we talk about rolfing. Because she likes rolfing and just whatever we're into. And when we're done, I feel like an equal and enjoy it and it's the one thing that I'm willing to do. Faithfully." In this narrative, we saw that the HCP opened up to Meryl in a very inclusive way, she invited her into her own environment, her personal world. She did this not only by giving the lessons in her own home, but also by giving personal information regarding her family, her beliefs, her values, and her unfolding experiences. She revealed herself personally. The positive influence on Meryl and her health was significant. In summing up her experiences, Meryl added,

"I think what I like in all of my health care providers is that they are willing to share, be open, to be authentic with me. I think about my psychotherapist. She occasionally brings up the issue of sexuality after the stroke. And without talking about her sex life, she shares what it's like to be a woman in her 50s and dealing with some of the same things. And with my piano teacher, she's also a professional, but she will say something real. She told me that she had had an affair when she was in her 30s and she had left her husband and left her children. I mean she seemed so strait-laced now. Can't imagine that she ever would have had that type of a life, but just the fact that she was willing to share that with me, to laugh about it you know, now, she's gone through it. She's still married. And then my occupational therapist, just to share her resentment toward her husband is an example of her being authentic with me. Think I crave that. I think we all crave that connection. I think this woman is sharing, all of these people are sharing a huge piece of their life. And how honored I feel that they're willing to do that even though I'm paying them. They wouldn't have to, you know. They wouldn't have to give of themselves, but they do."

Meryl expressed what others in the study have said: that connected relationships involved a degree of open, real communication from both the HCP and the patient, wherein they were able to experience each other as persons who had everyday struggles and concerns. In these relationships, the HCP was not the expert who was above question. On the contrary, when providers revealed their own struggles and real-life experiences, the patients felt more connected and often were moved by the stories. Self-disclosure, authentic relating, balanced the relationship in such a way that the women felt respected as persons rather than being treated as "patients" or passive recipients of care. The provider's willingness to disclose signaled that the women were valued as persons of substance and capability. Such signals strengthened their capacity to live with their illness and disclose weakness and difficulty.

RELATIONAL CONTINUUM-DISCONNECTION

Disconnection was apparent in several of the relationships women in the study experienced with their HCPs. In these relationships, HCPs were described by the women as being cold and distant, typically those in which the HCP maintained a professional/clinical manner. Disconnected relationships were characterized by what the women perceived to be disrespect, condescension, poor communication, and little information or teaching. In disconnected relationships, the women in the study experienced the HCP as being unapproachable and often defensive. At times, they believed they were put into a category of patient type, and the health care they received was based on that group rather than being individualized. They described their experience in these situations as being the result of a detached stance by the HCP whereby it was impossible for them to be known. Paradigm cases of power/control and clinical mismanagement helped to illustrate this pole of the relational continuum.

Power/Control

The use of power and control was seen in HCP behavior in which collaboration and support were either not present or inadequate. As a result the women who experienced this type of relationship experienced alienation, helplessness, hopelessness, oppression, paternalism, loss of a sense of control over their lives, and dependency (Gibson, 1991).

Jean's narrative was a paradigm of the negative consequences of encountering an HCP who related in terms of power and control. Jean (age 53) had type 2 diabetes. The relationship was problematic from the beginning, a "struggle" to use her description. The patient characterized the HCP as being very brusque, aggressive, and withholding of information and explanation. Jean described the HCP as being "grumpy, anesthetized, turned off, uncaring, an android." Jean asked to be assigned to another HCP but the constraints of the agency made that impossible. She told the story of an interaction she had with the HCP in which she asked why she had not been told that she needed to limit her protein intake to 40 g per day in order to prevent kidney disease. She said,

"And then that's when she said that 'Most people are type 2 diabetics, that most of them don't care about what they're eating or what they're doing or testing their blood. And most people are too stupid to know the information.'"

This was not the first time the HCP had made disrespectful remarks to Jean. It was a regular occurrence but its impact was immediate and significant. She was overwhelmed by the lack of caring demonstrated by the provider and found it inexcusable. Jean worried about the effect that not having her questions answered and not receiving adequate teaching might have on her health. In another example, she provided insight into the impact of not having the HCP respond to her needs and concerns regarding the management of her disease. The incident concerned her request of the HCP for an insulin pump.

"Well I was kind of caught between a rock and a hard place. I wanted the pump, and so I was told I had to do these certain things. I had to get my blood sugars between this level and I had to do this for a couple of months. So I did that for a couple of months. An then I was told that I didn't need the pump. I only wanted it for convenience because my blood sugars were in such great shape, what would I need the pump for? So it was kind of a power game. You know, because I kept pushing for it. You know, I kept asking when, when can I be eligible? When can I be eligible?"

When asked how this made her feel, she responded, "I did break down crying in front of her. You know, when I was told I was too good to have the pump. And she just said, 'We'll see you next visit.' And then left the room. That made me feel even worse. I cried all the way home."

In this narrative, the HCP acted with little regard for the patient and her concerns. She demonstrated a cold, detached manner as she used her power to control the situation. Her behavior and demeanor were disrespectful and cruel and diminished Jean and her concerns. Lacking empathy, her behavior was characteristic of the paternalism discussed by Henson (1997), in which care is similar to the style of strict fathers who intrusively impose values and choices. Jean felt helpless and hopeless and believed that the relationship with the HCP negatively affected her health.

At the time of the interview, Jean was considering whether or not to give up her health insurance altogether and manage her diabetes by herself. The quality of disconnection experienced by Jean was expressed by many women in the study. This relationship quality eliminated any possibility of collaboration between the women and their HCPs. The inappropriate use of power resulted in the women's sense of alienation, oppression, and a loss of control over their lives. They were less likely to ask questions, reveal important information, or to follow through with recommended treatment.

Clinical Mismanagement

The women in the study believed it was impossible to have a connected relationship with an HCP who did not manage their care competently. This was similar to research findings, which determined a link between clinical competence and interpersonal skills (Colliver, Swartz, Robbs, & Cohen, 1999). Women in the study entered HCP relationships assuming that the provider would be an excellent, knowledgeable clinician who stayed abreast of current practice standards.

Wanda described experiences with HCPs and the impact their mismanagement had on her health. Wanda (age 42) had numerous health problems, including obesity and hypertension. The interchange she described was with a new HCP to whom she had been assigned, the third in a short time, as a result of staffing changes. At the end of the first visit, the provider questioned why Wanda had an Accu-Check with her and then told her she was not a diabetic. Although she had not learned to use the Accu-Check and there had been no follow-up, Wanda had planned to ask for instructions during this visit with the new HCP. She explained that she did not know what to think. She wondered if the HCP had read her chart and worried about the consequences to her health and life if she was indeed diabetic. Wanda had a similar experience with a prior provider. She said,

"The other HCP wanted to meet with me and she said, 'Okay, your blood pressure is still a little high.' Then she said, 'How's your sugar?' And I go, 'My sugar?' And she's like, 'Yes.' She said, 'You're diabetic.' I go, 'Noooo.' She's like, 'Yeeessss.' She said, 'When you were diagnosed with the high blood pressure, didn't Carol tell you?' I said, 'No, she's only been treating me for the blood pressure.' So she said, 'No, you're diabetic. And you have to do this.' And she ordered the monitor. And they delivered it. So now, the new HCP, because of course both of the others are gone, she's saying, 'No, you're not.'

Wanda was not sure that she could believe anything that she was told or if any information that she was given was accurate. She had worried that the diagnosis of hypertension might not be accurate because of the way it was measured and now she was more certain that she probably did not have hypertension.

"See if it was the blood pressure, that's the one that I thought they really are off on because the cuff, because my arms are hellacious. They use the regular cuff; it doesn't give an accurate reading. I usually have to hold the cuff on because it wants to pop open and my arm feels like it's bruising. It's like bright red when they take it off. And she's wanting to up my medication, so I'm like, 'No.'"

Wanda believed that she was in a system where no one cared about her. She did not believe that she could trust anything she was told by any HCP. This narrative illustrates what can happen when a patient who needs clear direction, follow-up, and support finds herself in an environment in which error results in the misdiagnosis or miscommunication about diabetes and perhaps hypertension. The patient did not monitor her blood sugar levels and received no follow-up for the diagnosed diabetes. She did not know whether or not she was a diabetic. She had been on medication for hypertension but doubted that she was hypertensive. She had severe anemia as a result of continuous vaginal bleeding but had not agreed to recommended surgery. She was frightened for her health and her life. As a result of incompetent and/or incomplete teaching and advice, Wanda did not have information she needed to make important health decisions. At times in the interview, she sounded angry and helpless and seemed immobilized.

Mismanagement of chronic health care problems is a serious issue. Women in the study who had been misdiagnosed or had gone undiagnosed for significant periods of time found it difficult to trust, not just the initial provider but subsequent HCPs from whom they received care. In addition, there seemed to be a contagion factor. Feeling more vulnerable, they were wary of any information they were given. In relationships with HCPs who demonstrated that they were not trustworthy, women in the study found themselves in double jeopardy. Not only did they receive poor and at times dangerous health care management, information, and advice, but they also experienced the fear of being alone with their health concerns.

DISCUSSION

Articulated in the women's narratives are the contrasting poles of the relational continuum of connection and disconnection. Connected relationships, characterized as being genuine and honest, increase reciprocal respect and trust. This finding is supported by Finfgeld-Connett (2006), Dontje, Corser, Kreulen, and Teitelman (2004), Jordan (1997b), and Miller and Stiver (1997). Connected relationships set up the possibility for the HCP to believe in the patient and know that requests for care, attention, or time are based on the patient's legitimate needs and concerns (Benner, 2001). Significance increases as HCPs try to understand women's resistance to specific treatments and raises questions regarding current conceptions of patient compliance or adherence to planned care (Wuest, 1993).

Moreover, partnered relationships involve a level of intimacy in which women have a sense of equality, cooperation, negotiation, and shared decision making. In relational cultural theory, this is what Jordan (1997b) and Miller et al. (1999) refer to as mutuality, in that the patient and HCP are emotionally available to one another in a constantly changing process of receptivity and response.

Being connected in this way facilitates empathic attunement and compassion that is considerably different from technical, skilled empathy. In this study, women with chronic disease describe empathy that involves intersubjectivity described by Stolorow and Atwood (1992). It is also very similar to Halpern's (2001) description of emotional reasoning. These authors describe a process that is both affective and cognitive, in that identification allows for a perceptual grasp of the other's experience, which is assimilated and responded to in such deep attunement that traditional boundaries and a separate sense of self are altered. It is this intersubjective experience that makes possible the personal and professional growth of both the HCP and the patient (Kleinmen, 2004).

In addition, the personableness of the connection involves a degree of openness and exposure that enables both the HCP and the women to both reveal themselves and be seen and known for who they are. This is supported by Taylor's (1991) discussion of the ethos of authenticity in which we are all called upon to live our lives being true to ourselves and not in imitation or performance of prescribed roles (Farber et al., 2000; Halpern, 2001). In adopting a "clinical gaze," the HCP encounters the patient as essentially a collection of signs and symptoms (Benner, 2001; Toombs, 1993) rather than as a person.

IMPLICATIONS

This research suggests that for women with chronic disease, relationships that are connected, and that are characterized by partnership and personableness, result in the women being better off, as one of them said, "spiritually, mentally, and physically." These results support what Alexander (2004), Green (2004), and Kleinman (2004) express as being important for NPs in the delivery of primary care. The context of today's health care system often pushes the NP to provide care more attuned to medical issues, leaving little time for the development of connected relationships. In spite of this pressure, NPs need to strive to develop relationships with patients that are intersubjective/connected. As Kleinman points out, "Although NPs provide primary medical care, they define themselves as nurses who are, in the first instance, care-or-relationship-oriented, rather than disease-or-cure-oriented" (p. 268). This is particularly significant as we know that our patients expect care in which the NP is connected and present (Alexander; Donohue, 2003; Heller & Solomon, 2005).

NPs need to focus care that (a) is centered in the patient's life and illness experiences including specific cultural needs (Benner, 2001; Frank, 1995; Toombs, 1993), (b) is attuned to the patient's narrative of the illness/disease experience (Frank; Kleinman, 1988), (c) couples biomedical-clinical care with empathic attunement in which the NP is present authentically (Benner, 2001), and (d) uses emotional engagement and communication (Halpern, 2001). It is the relationship that helps to determine what experiences women will disclose to the NP. If the NP engages them with presence in connection, patients are more likely to disclose what matters to them.

CONCLUSION

Women with chronic disease believed their health was significantly affected by their relationships with HCPs. In connected relationships, the women experienced a sense of well-being in which they felt cared for and in which they were assured that they were not alone with their illness. Connectedness increased their sense of security and trust and reduced their levels of anxiety. Feeling more secure and trusting in the HCP enabled them to be themselves more completely in the relationship. They felt empowered, more confident in their ability to manage their illness, and were motivated to do the hard work their illness demanded both on a daily basis and during times of crisis. They were committed to the relationship with the HCP and engaged in self-exploration as a result.

Connected relationships also impacted the disease in more direct ways. The women reported that through connected relationships, they received more accurate diagnosis and treatments for their illness in a timely manner. They believed that the security and stability of the relationship enabled them to maintain continuity of care and increased their choices for care options and self-care activities. In general, the women described what they call better health care.

REFERENCES

Alexander, I.M. (2004). Characteristics of and problems with primary care interactions experienced by an ethnically diverse group of women. *Journal of the American Academy of Nurse Practitioners*, 16, 300-310.

Balini, M. (1957). *The doctor, his patient and the illness*. New York: International Universities.

Benner, P. (Ed.). (1994). *Interpretative phenomenology, embodiment, caring, and ethics in health and illness*. Thousand Oaks, CA: Sage.

Benner, P. (2001). The phenomenon of care. In S.K. Toombs (Ed.), *Handbook of phenomenology and medicine* (pp. 351-369). Boston: Kluwer Academic.

Colliver, J., Swartz, M., Robbs, R., & Cohen, D. (1999). Relationship between clinical competence and interpersonal and communication skills in standardized-patient assessment. *Academic Medicine*, 74, 271-274.

Covington, H. (2005). Caring presence, providing a safe space for patients. *Holistic Nursing Practice*, 19, 169-172.

Crits-Christoph, P. (1998). The interpersonal interior of psychotherapy. *Psychotherapy Research*, 8, 1-16.

Donohue, R.K. (2003). Nurse practitioner-client interaction as resource exchange in a women's health clinic: An exploratory study. *Journal of Clinical Nursing*, 12, 717-725.

Dontje, K., Corser, W., Kreulen, G., & Teitelman, A. (2004). A unique set of interactions: The MSU sustained partnership model of nurse practitioner primary care. *Journal of the American Academy of Nurse Practitioners*, 16, 63-69.

Dreyfus, H.L. (1991). *Being-in-the-world, a commentary on Heidegger's being and time.* Cambridge, MA: MIT Press.

Farber, N.J., Novak, D.H., Silverstein, J., Davis, E.B., Weiner, J., & Boyer, E.G. (2000). Physicians' experience with patients who transgress boundaries. *Journal of General Internal Medicine*, 15, 770-775.

Finfgeld-Connett, D. (2006). Meta-synthesis of presence in nursing. *Journal of Advanced Nursing*, 55, 708-714.

Frank, A.W. (1995). *The wounded storyteller, body, illness, and ethics.* Chicago: University of Chicago Press.

Gibson, C. (1991). A concept analysis of empowerment. *Journal of Advanced Nursing*, 16, 354-361.

Green, A. (2004). Caring behaviors as perceived by nurse practitioners. *Journal of the American Academy of Nurse Practitioners*, 16, 283-290.

Hall, J.A., Roter, D.L., & Katz, N.R. (1988). Meta-analysis of correlates of provider behavior in medical encounter. *Medical Care*, 26, 657-675.

Halpern, J. (2001). *From detached concern to empathy, humanizing medical practice.* Oxford, UK: Oxford University Press.

Heller, K.S., & Solomon, M.Z. (2005). Continuity of care and caring: What matters to parents of children with life-threatening conditions. *Journal of Pediatric Nursing*, 20, 335-346.

Henson, R. (1997). Analysis of the concept of mutuality. *Image: Journal of Nursing Scholarship*, 29, 77-81.

Jordan, J.V. (1997a). Relational development through mutual empathy. In A.C. Bohart & L.S. Greenberg (Eds.), *Empathy reconsidered, new directions in psychotherapy* (pp. 343-351). Woodbridge, VA: American Psychological Association.

Jordan, J.V. (Ed.). (1997b). *Women's growth in diversity.* New York: Guilford Press.

Kinnersley, P., Anderson, F., Parry, K., Clement, J., Archard, L., Turton, P., et al. (2000). Randomized controlled trial of nurse practitioner versus general practitioner care for patients requesting 'same day' consultations in primary care. *British Medical Journal*, 320, 1043-1048.

Kleinman, A. (1988). *The illness narratives, suffering, healing, and the human condition.* New York: Basic Books.

Kleinman, S. (2004). What is the nature of nurse practitioners' lived experiences interacting with patients? *Journal of the American Academy of Nurse Practitioners*, 16, 263-269.

Lagana, K. (2000). The "right" to a caring relationship: The law and ethic of care. *Journal of Perinatal and Neonatal Nursing*, 14(2), 12-33.

Langford, C.P., Bowsher, J., Maloner, J.P., & Lillis, P.P. (1997). Social support: A conceptual analysis. *Journal of Advanced Nursing*, 25, 95-100.

Lawson, M.T. (2002). Nurse practitioner and physician communication styles. *Applied Nursing Research*, 16, 60-66.

Levin, D.M. (1999). *The philosopher's gaze, modernity in the shadows of enlightenment.* Berkeley, CA: University of California Press.

McCloskey, J.C., & Grace, H.K. (Eds.). (1997). *Current issues in nursing.* St. Louis, MO: Mosby.

Miller, J.B., Jordan, J., Stiver, I., Walker, M., Stirrey, J., & Eldridge, N.S. (1999). *Therapists' authenticity. Work in progress, no. 82.* Wellesley, MA: Stone Center Working Paper Series.

Miller, J.B., & Stiver, I. P. (1997). *The healing connection: How women form relationships in therapy and in life.* Boston: Beacon Press.

Noddings, N. (1984). *Caring: A feminine approach to ethics and moral education.* Berkeley, CA: University of California Press.

Norbeck, J., & Anderson, N. (1988). Psychosocial predictors of pregnancy outcomes in low-income black, hispanic, and white women. *Nursing Research,* 38, 204-209.

Pieranunzi, V.R. (1997). The lived experience of power and powerlessness in psychiatric nursing: A Heideggerian hermeneutical analysis. *Archives of Psychiatric Nursing,* 11, 155-162.

Roter, D.I., Hall, J.A., Merisca, R., Nordstrom, B., Cretin, D., & Svarstad, B. (1998). Effectiveness of interventions to improve patient compliance, a meta-analysis. *Medical Care,* 36, 1138-1161.

Spiegel, D., Stroud, P., & Fyfe, A. (1998). Complementary medicine. *Western Journal of Medicine,* 168, 241-247.

Stewart, M.A. (1996). Effective physician-patient communication and health outcomes: A review. *Canadian Medical Association Journal,* 152, 1423-1433.

Stolorow, R.D., & Atwood, G.E. (1992). *Contexts of being: The intersubjective foundation of psychological life.* Hillsdale, NJ: Analytic Press.

Strupp, H.H. (1993). The Vanderbilt psychotherapy studies: Synopsis. *Journal of Consulting and Clinical Psychology,* 61, 431-433.

Taylor, C. (1991). *The ethics of authenticity.* Cambridge, MA: Harvard University Press.

Toombs, S. (1993). *The meaning of illness: A phenomenological account of the different perspectives of physician and patient.* Dordrecht, the Netherlands: Kluwer Academic.

Tronto, J.C. (1994). *Moral boundaries: A political argument for an ethic of care.* New York: Routledge.

Van Manen, M. (1990). *Researching lived experience, human science for an action sensitive pedagogy.* London: State University of New York Press.

Venning, P., Durie, A., Roland, C., Roberts, C., & Leese, B. (2000). Randomized controlled trial comparing cost-effectiveness of general practitioners and nurse practitioners in primary care. *British Medical Journal,* 320, 1048-1053.

Williams, A., & Jones, M. (2006). Patients' assessments of consulting a nurse practitioner: The time factor. *Journal of Advanced Nursing,* 53, 188-195.

Wuest, J. (1993). Removing the shackles: A feminist critique of noncompliance. *Nursing Outlook,* 41, 217-224.

Yarcheski, A., Scoloveno, M., & Mahon, N. (1994). Social support and well-being in adolescents: The mediating role of hopefulness. *Nursing Research,* 43, 288-292.

The Critique

The research report "Living with Chronic Illness: A Phenomenological Study of the Health Effects of the Patient-Provider Relationship" (Fox & Chesla, 2008) is critically examined for its rigor as a phenomenological study, its contribution to nursing, and its usefulness in practice. The criteria identified in the Critiquing Criteria box on pp. 129-130 are used to guide the critique. Comments will be offered to illustrate for the reader specific questions that might be asked of **interpretive phenomenology,** which is the understanding of the subject's meaning of an experience. Asking questions regarding the rigor of the study helps to determine its usefulness and applicability to practice.

STATEMENT OF THE PHENOMENON OF INTEREST

Fox and Chesla (2008) clearly state the phenomenon of interest. The researchers are interested in studying the "patient-health care provider (HCP) from the lived experience of women with chronic disease and to determine how this relationship affects women's health" (p. 109). To justify the need for the study, the authors offer a substantive evaluation of the current research from the perspective of physicians, as well as nurse practitioners (NPs). In addition to building a solid case for the study, the researchers tell the reader that the reason they are proposing to use interpretive phenomenology is because to date, no studies are available that focus on understanding the relationship from the patient's perspective (p. 110). They go on to share with the reader that the philosophical underpinnings of their study are based on the Heideggerian tradition. This gives the reader a clear context for understanding the focus and direction of the research. A number of interpretations of phenomenology are available; clearly stating the type—interpretive—and the tradition—Heideggerian—sets the stage for understanding the interpretation of the findings.

PURPOSE

The purpose of the research according to the authors is to "understand the patient-HCP relationship from the perspective of women with chronic disease" (p. 110). Fox and Chesla further state that their intent was to "understand the meaning of the relationship from women and how they believed it affected their health" (p. 110). A contrast of how these relationships unfolded was equally important to the researchers—they wanted to understand the comforting and helpful relationships, as well as the oppressive and troublesome ones.

There are those critics of phenomenology who would suggest that researchers who initiate a study with preconceived ides about what they expect to find alter the outcome of the study. However, Rapport and Wainwright (2006) share that two of the distinguishing differences between descriptive and interpretive phenomenology are "the degree to which it is possible to suspend preknowledge and presuppositions" and "the degree to which it is possible to know the world prior to conscious knowing" (p. 229). This means that interpretive phenomenologists accept that you cannot approach a study without having assumptions about the research and that it is important to recognize those assumptions, but there is no need to do anything about them. Recognizing this critical difference, the researchers in the study are being true to the interpretive tradition by not attending to suspension of their presuppositions.

METHOD

The method identified is interpretive phenomenology. Research "informed by interpretive phenomenology seeks to reveal and convey deep insight and understanding of the concealed meanings of everyday life experiences" (deWitt & Ploeg, 2006, pp. 216–217). Fox and Chesla (2008), in stating the purpose of their study, discuss the importance of exploring the patient-HCP relationship on a level not previously described. Since their focus is on understanding the phenomenon, use of interpretive phenomenology is appropriate.

SAMPLING

The sampling method used for this study is not clearly described. The researchers share that individuals with chronic diseases were interviewed. Their ages, educational levels, and races are offered, as are their chronic disease diagnoses. Because the researchers are interested in studying individuals with chronic illness, the participants are appropriate to inform the study.

In qualitative research, the most common type of sampling is purposive or purposeful sampling. According to Speziale and Carpenter (2007), "individuals are selected to participate in qualitative research based on their first-hand experience with a culture, social process, or phenomenon of interest" (p. 29). This ability to describe an experience from one's own perspective is what makes selection purposive.

EVIDENCE-BASED PRACTICE TIP

Qualitative studies are helpful in answering research questions about a concept or phenomenon that is not well understood or adequately covered in the literature.

Based on the assumption that the women in the study are in a patient-provider relationship and have a chronic disease, their selection as informants is appropriate. The reader would be better informed if the authors had more fully described how they determined which patients would be interviewed and why. Additionally, there is no reference to the length of the relationship with the providers mentioned in the study. The reader is left to conjecture about this. The researchers do state that the women were able to describe a variety of relationships with health care providers, including nurse practitioners, physicians, physical therapists, occupational therapists, music therapists, and psychotherapists. To fully use the findings in an evidence-based practice environment, it is critical to fully understand the sample so that practitioners can fully determine the applicability of the findings to their practice.

DATA COLLECTION

Fox and Chesla (2008) report that before data collection began, permission to conduct the study was obtained from the institutional review board. All participants were paid a stipend for the interview. Recruitment occurred through newspaper advertisement, through flyers in providers' offices, in a local health center, through support groups, and through word of mouth. The actual interviews were conducted in private areas of participants' homes, at the local health center, and in the hospital. These are appropriate methods for participant recruitment.

The researchers offer that they solicited narrative accounts of positive, negative, and neutral encounters with health care providers. It is not unusual in phenomenological research to encourage participants to share varying perspectives on their experience. The danger, however, is in giving participants the idea that they should have had all three types of experiences. It is important for the researcher to stay as neutral as possible when evoking descriptions of experiences from participants.

In addition to describing the prompts for the data collection, the researchers share that all interviews were audiotaped and transcribed verbatim. The transcripts were checked against the recordings to ensure accuracy. This is a common technique in qualitative research and ensures that the narratives of the subjects are recorded accurately.

The researchers started collecting data by using a group interview technique. Each group met for approximately one and one half hours at two different times. The women whose narratives were the most "vibrant" were invited to participate in a personal interview. It is unclear why the researchers chose to begin with group interviews or why they were followed up with individual interviews. The reader can assume that the later interviews were conducted in an effort to more fully probe the individual women's experiences. Without this being reported, however, the reader has no validation of this.

It is also unclear why Fox and Chesla chose to interview women exclusively. Although it can be surmised that the focus on women was related to having a clearer understanding of one group's experience, this is not stated.

Finally, there is no discussion of why 25 women were interviewed. Usually data are collected in phenomenological studies until no new data are revealed. This end point is called data **saturation.** The researchers do share that data analysis ended when the same theme showed up repeatedly. This statement speaks to the reason why data analysis was concluded but not why 25 women participated in the study.

DATA ANALYSIS

According to the researchers, "analysis of data involved multiple readings of the printed transcripts" (Fox & Chesla, 2008, p. 111). This began with the first group interview. The researchers compared narratives from each of the participants to those of other participants. The purpose of this process, according to the researchers, was to illustrate extremes in the relationships. Interpretive phenomenologists frequently speak of the need to observe paradigm cases, exemplars, and themes in the narratives of participants. The researchers state that they found all three of these in the data. There is clear description of the activities that were used in the data analysis.

Generally speaking, the measure of rigor in qualitative research is trustworthiness. Trustworthiness includes the concepts of **credibility, auditability,** and **fittingness/transferability.** In some sources, confirmability is offered as the fourth criterion for trustworthiness. Trustworthiness is seen as the relative equivalent of validity and reliability in quantitative research. These terms are defined in Chapter 5.

In this report, there is no mention of how credibility was obtained. It may be assumed that by virtue of the amount of time spent with the informants and by the iterative process of contrasting data, credibility of the findings was achieved. However, without attention to discussing this detail, the reader is making suppositions about the trustworthiness of these data.

Auditability (also called the audit trail) is the second assessment of rigor. The question to ask is as follows: Did the researcher present enough information for me to see how the raw data lead to the interpretation? In this case, the conclusion is that there is insufficient evidence to determine whether the raw data lead to the conclusions. There is one theme: relational continuum-disconnect that does not include any participant comments. Without these, the reader must accept the researchers' conclusions as fact without the benefit of an illustration of how the data lead to the theme identified.

Fittingness or transferability of the data is based on asking the following question: Is there enough detail here for me to evaluate the relevance and importance of these data for my own practice or for use in research or theory development? The themes as provided do provide insight into the experience of the provider-patient relationship for chronically ill women. It is up to the practitioner to determine the utility of the findings given his or her knowledge of similar populations.

EMPIRICAL GROUNDINGS OF THE STUDY: FINDINGS

In this section of the critique, the reader must ask whether the conceptualizations offered are true to the data. Do the researchers use the informant's words to guide the development of concepts/themes?

EVIDENCE-BASED PRACTICE TIP

Qualitative research may generate basic knowledge, hypotheses, and theories to be used in the design of other types of qualitative or quantitative studies. On the other hand, it is not necessarily a preliminary step to some other type of research. It is a complete and valuable end product in itself.

In most sections of the research report, the investigators offer subjective comments from the informants that help the reader understand the lived experience of women suffering from chronic disease who are engaged in HCP-patient relationships. For all but one of the themes identified, narrative comments are provided by the study participants. These annotations bring to life the lived experiences of women who participated. It is clear that the researchers have tried to stay close to the data by using the informants' words to illustrate the themes. The analyses offered in each of the theme sections of the report reflect careful attention to interpretation of meaning. This is very characteristic of interpretive phenomenology and helps you gain insights into the experience, adding to the ability to assess the usefulness of the findings.

In the discussion section of the report, the researchers share the relationship of their findings to those of other researchers. This is important. Contrasting what is discovered in a current phenomenological study with that which is already known places the study in context. The findings of this study are important to practice because as a Level V or VI research study, it informs practice in an area that was formally unknown or limitedly known.

CONCLUSIONS, IMPLICATIONS, AND RECOMMENDATIONS

The implications of this study are based on helping the reader understand that women with chronic disease need to feel like they are in partnership with their providers. This relationship should be of a strong, personable nature. With this information exposed, the researchers discuss the need for nurse practitioners to provide care that (a) is based on the life and illness experiences of the patient, taking into account his or her cultural needs; (b) is cognizant of the patient's narrative of the illness experience; (c) is based in biomedical/clinical care but remains authentic to the patients' needs; and (d) uses communication and engagement to enhance the quality of the relationship (p. 116). These focused points are necessary if this research is to provide clear direction for evidence-based care.

The conclusions available in this report reiterate the discussion and implication portion of the study. The major points made are that the relationship between the provider and the patient significantly affected the health outcomes of the participants in this study. Informants who believed that they have strong relationships with their providers felt empowered and confident in their ability to manage their disease. They also believed that they were provided with better factual information about their disease state. This is significant for the providers. If nurse practitioners are to provide care to individuals with chronic disease, it is important to develop the type of connected relationship described by the study participants. Patients suffering from chronic diseases will have long-term relationships with their providers, which, according to this study, will be enhanced and more likely to result in positive outcomes if *connected* relationships are developed.

The findings of the study are valuable. They provide important information about the provider-patient relationship. Unfortunately, the researchers do not provide the reader with direction for building on this study. It is always important to demonstrate the value of the research to future study development. By providing this information, the scientist is establishing the building blocks for a body of evidence on the topic.

The significance of this study is discussed within the context of the application of the findings to practice. Clearly, the researchers are most interested in influencing the HCP-patient relationship. Discussing the significance of the study to theory development and future research adds to the reader's understanding of the findings. The investigators did focus on the direct application of the findings to clinical practice. This is important. However, focusing only on practice and not how the findings contribute to building the body of nursing knowledge on this topic could be viewed as limiting.

The research report by Fox and Chesla (2008) provides evidence that adds to the body of nursing knowledge and provides direction on some of the important elements of the provider-patient relationship. The narratives provided give the reader a good understanding of how female patients with chronic illness perceive their professional relationships with their providers. This information is invaluable to practitioners.

REFERENCES

deWitt L, Ploeg J: Critical appraisal of rigour in interpretive phenomenological nursing research, *J Adv Nurs* 55(2):215-229, 2006.

Fox S, Chesla C: Living with chronic illness: a phenomenological study of the health effects of the patient-provider relationship, *J Am Acad Nurs Pract* 20:109-117, 2008.

Rapport F, Wainwright P: Phenomenology as a paradigm of movement, *Nurs Inquiry* 13(3):228-236, 2006.

Speziale HJS, Carpenter DR: *Qualitative research in nursing: advancing the humanistic imperative*, ed 4, Philadelphia, 2007, Lippincott.

CRITICAL THINKING CHALLENGES

- Discuss the similarities and differences between the stylistic considerations of reporting a qualitative study as opposed to a quantitative study in a professional journal.
- Discuss how one would go about incorporating qualitative research in evidence-based practice. Give an example.

REFERENCES

Barbour RS, Barbour M: Evaluating and synthesizing qualitative research: the need to develop a distinctive approach, *J Eval Clin Pract* 9(2):179-186, 2003.

Cesario S, Morin K, Santa-Donato A: Evaluating the level of evidence of qualitative research, *J Obstet Gynecol Neonat Nurs* 31(6):708-714, 2002.

Fox S, Chesla C: Living with chronic illness: a phenomenological study of the health effects of the patient-provider relationship, *J Am Acad Nurs Pract* 20:109-117, 2008.

Gibson BE, Martin DK: Qualitative research and evidence-based physiotherapy practice, *Physiotherapy* 89(6):350-358, 2003.

Glesne C: *Becoming qualitative researchers: an introduction*, ed 2, New York, 1999, Longman.

Horsburgh D: Evaluation of qualitative research, *J Clin Nurs* 12:307-312, 2003.

Hough MC: Learning, decisions and transformations in critical care nursing practice, *Nurs Ethics* 15(3):322-331, 2008.

Jackson RL, Drummond DK, Camara S: What is qualitative research? *Qual Rep Comm* 8(1):21-28, 2007.

Landreneau KJ, Ward-Smith P: Perceptions of adult patients on hemodialysis concerning choice among renal replacement therapies, *Nephrol Nurs J* 34(5):513-525, 2007.

Meneses KD, McNees P, Loerzel VW, et al: Transition from treatment to survivorship: effects of a psychoeducational intervention on quality of life in breast cancer survivors, *Oncol Nurs Forum* 34(5):1007-1016, 2007.

Morse JM, Penrod J, Hupcey JE: Qualitative outcome analysis: evaluating nursing interventions for complex clinical phenomena, *J Nurs Sch* 32(2):125-130, 2000.

Richards KM: RAP project: an instrument development study to determine common attributes for pain assessment among men and women who represent multiple pain-related diagnoses, *Pain Manage Nurs* 9(10):33-43, 2008.

Russell CK, Gregory DM: Evaluation of qualitative research studies, *Evidence-Based Nurs* 6(2):36-40, 2003.

Sackett DL, Strauss D, Richardson W, et al: *Evidence based medicine: how to practice and teach EBM*, Edinburgh, 2000, Churchill Livingstone.

Schepner-Hughes N: *Death without weeping: the violence of everyday life in Brazil*, Berkeley, CA, 1992, University of California Press.

Speziale HJS, Carpenter DR: *Qualitative research in nursing: advancing the humanistic imperative*, ed 4, Philadelphia, 2007, Lippincott.

Walsh D, Downe S: Meta-synthesis method of qualitative research: a literature review, *J Adv Nurs* 50(2):204-211, 2005.

FOR FURTHER STUDY

evolve

Go to Evolve at http://evolve.elsevier.com/LoBiondo/ for Web links, content updates, and additional research articles for practice in reviewing and critiquing.

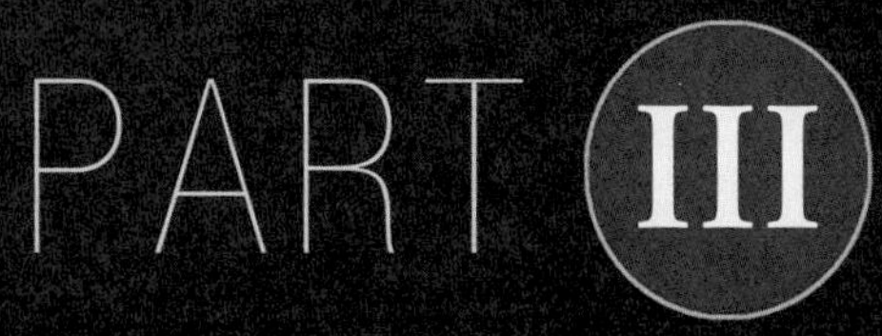

PROCESSES AND EVIDENCE RELATED TO QUANTITATIVE RESEARCH

RESEARCH VIGNETTE

Making Practice Perfect

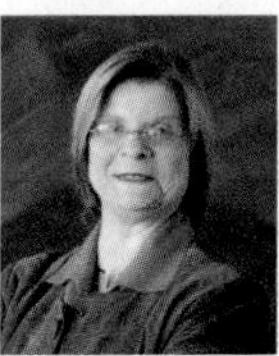

Susan Gennaro, RN, DSN, FAAN
Boston College, Chestnut Hill, MA

I started my research career as a neonatal nurse who was constantly frustrated because I had no way of determining which parents needed nursing care. Often what determined what parental support I could provide was how much time I had available. If I had lots of babies under my care, I could have a family that clearly was stressed but I might not be able to do much to provide support. If I had time I was always interested in providing parental support, but sometimes the support wasn't needed. Often families weren't available when the unit was calm, or sometimes I had a lighter patient load but the families who were in the nursery didn't need nursing care. I knew there had to be a better way to prioritize care than based on time available, so my first research question was to try to identify predictors of parental adaptation to a preterm baby.

This first question has led me to many others and has enabled me to do the following: identify teaching needs for families of preterm infants, suggest interventions to ease the transition when a preterm infant enters a family, and extend knowledge of the physiological responses to having a preterm infant as opposed to a term infant. Ultimately that first question has led to a research trajectory that has focused on the antecedents and consequences of stress in families with preterm infants. It's been a long and satisfying journey that has had many interesting side trips, and it's one of those side trips I'd like to share.

Early in my research career I was the Chair of the Research Committee for the Association of Women's Health, Obstetric and Neonatal Nurses (AWHONN, although in 1991 the organization was still called the Nurses' Association of the American College of Obstetricians and Gynecologists [NAACOG]). The previous chair, Karen Haller, had helped to identify that the committee was only addressing two out of its three goals. The research committee was supposed to facilitate the conduct, dissemination, and utilization of nursing research. We knew that the organization was helping the conduct of nursing research through our small grants program and the dissemination of nursing research in our journal (*Journal of Obstetric, Gynecologic, and Neonatal Nursing* [JOGNN]), but we weren't helping in the utilization of nursing research. As the incoming research chair I was challenged to help the Association facilitate the transfer of research into practice.

This seemed like an important thing to do as an organization, but this was 1991 and evidence-based nursing was in its infancy. The 1991 research committee decided that the first two tasks at hand were to understand what knowledge we had in perinatal nursing that could be immediately used in practice and then to determine how best to change practice through research.

To answer the first question (research ready to be used in practice), we had a research consultation and asked leaders in perinatal nursing research to identify areas of research that were practice ready. This might seem unnecessary, but this was before there were easily accessed

Web sites that evaluated nursing research, before the Cochrane Collaboration was readily available over the Internet, before there were journals and columns in journals to help translate research into practice. So we obtained information in a very old-fashioned way: by asking the experts.

To answer the second question about how best to change practice through research, I spoke with leaders in the American Association of Critical Care Nurses about the "Thunder Project," whose goal was to facilitate practice-based research by providing protocols to study the effect on patency of arterial pressure monitoring lines if heparinized or nonheparinized flushes were used (American Association of Critical-Care Nurses Thunder Project Task Force, 1995). Today I would have been able to tap into an ever-increasing body of research on how knowledge is translated into practice. I would have been able to access models of knowledge dissemination and I would have been able to learn about knowledge stakeholders, barriers to change, early adapters to practice change, and so on. However, our efforts occurred before knowledge about practice changes was so abundant and at a time when we didn't know that what we were trying to do was to develop evidence-based practice projects. We were still talking about "research utilization" (Gennaro, 1994), and we didn't realize that using research is only one step in the process of ensuring that practice is evidence based.

I remember being relieved to find out through our research consultation that there was a lot of research that was ready for practice but wasn't being used. We examined this research base and determined where there was knowledge from which practice guidelines could be written. We discussed thermoregulation, nonnutritive sucking, neonatal pain management, second-stage labor management, urinary incontinence, and many other topics. The 1992 project was the transition of the preterm infant to an open crib (Medoff-Cooper, 1995). I, as the Chair of the Research Committee, worked with two well-known neonatal researchers, Paula Meier and Barbara Medoff-Cooper, and with the research committee and site coordinators from around the country. We spent 2 days developing a guideline for transferring babies from isolettes to open cribs based on the extant research on neonatal thermoregulation. At that time weight and gestational age were the most common parameters being used to trigger transfer of a baby from an isolette to an open crib. We developed research-based guidelines in which babies who were medically stable could start the weaning process while in the isolette by being dressed (including a two-ply stocking cap on their head) and with careful monitoring. Slowly, the heat in the isolette was turned down as the infant was able to maintain his or her temperature without an additional heat source. When an infant demonstrated 4 hours of thermal stability, he or she was transferred to an open crib and monitoring continued.

We could have just disseminated this protocol after it was developed, but there were gaps in our knowledge base, and we weren't sure that what worked at sea level would work in the mountains, and so on. Much of the knowledge had been developed in England, and we weren't sure that what worked in English nurseries would work in America. We knew that babies are an extremely vulnerable population, and we wanted to make sure that what worked in research would work in practice. Finally, we were interested in learning about barriers to translating research into practice and so having communication with the site coordinators helped us to identify facilitators in the process of using research findings in practice.

This neonatal thermoregulation project was very successful and resulted in practice change. In fact, we had a difficult time continuing the project because the sites were so eager to adapt practice changes. One thing we learned from it was that having enthusiastic support from parents was a key reason why the project was successful. Parents couldn't wait to be able to have their babies in open cribs and so provided much positive reinforcement for practice change. Our first successful research utilization project rapidly led to a second project on second-stage labor management. At this point I no longer chaired the Research Committee but I worked informally as a consultant with the coordinator on this project, Linda Mayberry.

As practice changes, new research is often needed. An outgrowth of the second-stage labor management project was a question about whether upright positioning in second-stage labor worked as well with women who had epidurals as it did in women who were unmedicated (as were most of the women in the original studies). Across the country, epidural rates were rising and site coordinators questioned whether the research findings were applicable for women who had epidural analgesia. Dr. Mayberry and I were able to answer some of these questions with new research (Gilder, Mayberry, Gennaro et al., 2002; Mayberry, Strange, Supplee et al., 2003). So I learned another key lesson from being involved in evidence-based practice projects: there needs to be a feedback loop with new areas of knowledge continually being developed and continuing to inform practice.

Finally, I learned the importance of disseminating research-based guidelines so that others could benefit from our work. AWHONN as an organization has been involved in continuing to engage in evidence-based practice projects and to ensure that these projects then become part of the National Guideline Clearinghouse (www.guideline.gov).

AWHONN has clearly been a leader in improving the use of evidence in perinatal and women's health nursing. I am very proud to have been a part of this process and in helping to develop mechanisms that could be institutionalized in making nursing practice more perfect, that is, evidence based.

REFERENCES

American Association of Critical-Care Nurses Thunder Project Task Force: Nurses' perceptions of involvement in Thunder Project, *Clin Nurse Spec* 9:88-91, 1995.

Gennaro S: Research utilization: an overview, *J Obstet Gynecol Neonatal Nurs* 23:313-321, 1994.

Gilder K, Mayberry LJ, Gennaro S, et al: Maternal positioning in labor with epidural analgesia. Results from a multi-site survey, *AWHONN Lifelines* 6(1):40-45, 2002.

Mayberry LJ, Strange LB, Supplee PD, et al: Use of upright positioning with epidural analgesia: findings from an observational study, *MCN Am J Matern Child Nurs* 28(3):152-159, 2003.

Medoff-Cooper B: Transition of the preterm infant to an open crib, *J Obstet Gynecol Neonatal Nurs* 23:329-335, 1995.

7

Introduction to Quantitative Research

Geri LoBiondo-Wood

KEY TERMS

bias
constancy
control
control group
dependent variable
experimental group
external validity
extraneous or mediating variable
generalizability
history
homogeneity
independent variable
instrumentation
internal validity
intervening variable
intervention fidelity
maturation
measurement effects
mortality
pilot study
randomization
reactivity
selection
selection bias
testing

LEARNING OUTCOMES

After reading this chapter, you should be able to do the following:

- Define *research design.*
- Identify the purpose of research design.
- Define *control* as it affects research design and the outcomes of a study.
- Compare and contrast the elements that affect control.
- Begin to evaluate what degree of control should be exercised in a research study.
- Define *internal validity.*
- Identify the threats to internal validity.
- Define *external validity.*
- Identify the conditions that affect external validity.
- Identify the links between study design and evidence-based practice.
- Evaluate research design using critiquing questions.

STUDY RESOURCES

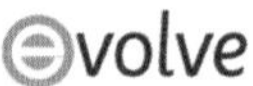

Go to Evolve at http://evolve.elsevier.com/LoBiondo/ for review questions, critiquing exercises, and additional research articles for practice in reviewing and critiquing.

The word *design* implies the organization of elements into a masterful work of art. In the world of art and fashion, design conjures up images of processes and techniques that are used to express a total concept. When an individual creates, process and form are employed. The form, process, and degree of adherence to structure depend on the aims of the creator. The same can be said of the research process. The research process does not need to be a sterile procedure, but one where the researcher develops a masterful work within the limits of a research question or hypothesis and the related theoretical basis. The framework that the researcher creates is the **design.** When reading a study, you should be able to recognize that the research question, purpose, literature review, theoretical framework, and hypothesis all interrelate with, complement, and assist in the operationalization of the design (Figure 7-1). The degree to which there is a fit between these design elements and the steps of the research process after the choice of a design strengthens the study and also your confidence in the evidence provided by the findings and their potential applicability to practice.

Nursing is concerned with a variety of structures that require varying degrees of process and form, such as the provision of quality and safe patient care, responses of patients to illness, and factors that affect caregivers. When patient care is administered, the nursing process is used. Previous chapters stress the importance of a clear research question or hypothesis, literature review, conceptual framework, and subject matter knowledge. How a researcher structures, implements, or designs a study affects the results of a research project and ultimately its application for evidence-based practice.

For you to understand the implications and the utility of a study for evidence-based practice, the central issues in the design of a research study must be understood. This chapter provides an overview of the meaning, purpose, and issues related to quantitative research design, and Chapters 8 and 9 present specific types of quantitative designs.

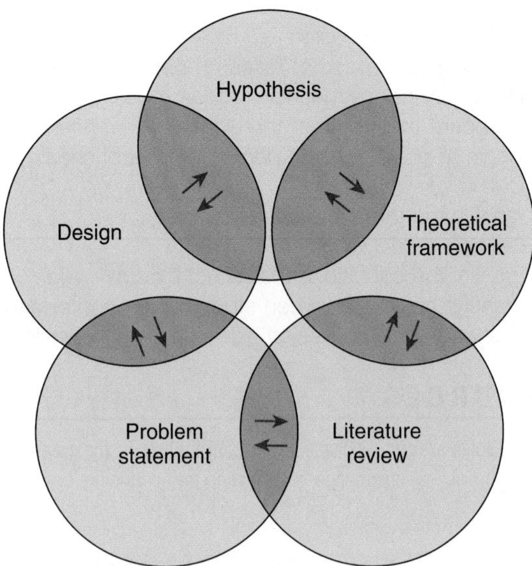

Figure 7-1 Interrelationships of design, research question, literature review, theoretical framework, and hypothesis.

PURPOSE OF RESEARCH DESIGN

The research design in quantitative research has multiple overlapping and yet unique purposes. The design

- Provides the plan or blueprint
- Is the vehicle for testing research questions and hypotheses
- Involves structure and strategy

These three design concepts guide a researcher in writing the hypotheses or research questions, conducting the study, and analyzing and evaluating the data. The overall purpose of the research design is twofold: to aid in the systematic solution of research questions or hypotheses and to maintain **control.** All research attempts to answer questions. The design coupled with the methods and analysis is the mechanism for finding solutions to research questions or hypotheses. *Control* is defined as the measures that the researcher uses to hold the conditions of the study uniform and avoid possible impingement of bias on the dependent variable or outcome variable. Control measures help to avoid **bias** or threats to the internal validity of the study.

A research example that demonstrates how the design can aid in the solution of a research question and maintain control is the study by Meneses and colleagues (2007; see Appendix A), whose aim was to evaluate the effect of a psychoeducational intervention on quality of life in breast cancer survivors. Subjects who fit the study's inclusion criteria were randomly assigned to either the experimental or wait control group. The two interventions were clearly defined. The authors also discuss how they maintained **intervention fidelity** or constancy of interventionists, data-collector training supervision, and follow-up throughout the study. By establishing the specific sample criteria and subject eligibility (inclusion criteria; see Chapter 10) and by clearly describing, designing, and distinguishing the experimental intervention, the researchers demonstrated that they had a well-developed plan and structure and were able to consistently maintain the study's conditions. A variety of considerations, including the type of design chosen, affect the successful completion of the study. These considerations include the following:

- Objectivity in conceptualizing the research question or hypothesis
- Accuracy
- Feasibility
- Control and intervention fidelity
- Validity—internal
- Validity—external

There are statistical principles behind the many forms of control, but it is more important that you have a clear conceptual understanding. The forms of control are important not only to assess the quality of the study but also application to a practice that is evidence based.

The type of design used in a study also affects its application to practice. The next two chapters present a number of experimental, quasi-experimental, and nonexperimental designs. As you will recall from Chapter 1, the type of design used in a study is linked to the level of evidence and, in turn, how a study's findings contribute to evidence-based practice. As you critically appraise the design, you must also take into account other aspects of a study's design. These aspects are reviewed in this chapter. How they are applied depends on the type of design (see Chapters 8 and 9).

OBJECTIVITY IN THE RESEARCH QUESTION CONCEPTUALIZATION

Objectivity in the conceptualization of the research question is derived from a review of the literature and development of a theoretical framework (see Figure 7-1). Using the literature, the researcher assesses the depth and breadth of available knowledge on the question. The literature review and theoretical framework should demonstrate that the researcher reviewed the literature critically and objectively (see Chapter 3), because this affects the type of design chosen. For example, a research question about the length of a breast-feeding teaching program in relation to adherence to breast-feeding may suggest either a correlational or an experimental design (see Chapters 8 and 9), whereas a question related to fatigue levels and amount of sleep at different points in cancer treatment may suggest a survey or correlational study (see Chapter 9). Therefore the literature review should reflect the following:

- When the question was studied
- What aspects of the question were studied
- Where it was investigated and with what populations
- By whom it was investigated
- The gaps or inconsistencies in the literature

HELPFUL HINT

A literature review that incorporates all aspects of the question allows you to judge the objectivity of the research question and therefore whether the design chosen matches the question.

ACCURACY

Accuracy in determining the appropriate design is also accomplished through the theoretical framework and review of the literature (see Chapter 3). Accuracy means that all aspects of a study systematically and logically follow from the research question or hypothesis. A beginning researcher may answer a question involving a few variables that will not require the use of sophisticated designs. The simplicity of a research project does not render it useless or of less value for practice. Although the scope of the project is limited or focused, the researchers should demonstrate how they maintained accuracy. You should feel that the researcher chose a design that was consistent with the question and offered the maximum amount of control. The issues of control are discussed later in this chapter.

Also, many research questions have not yet been researched. Therefore a preliminary or pilot study is also a wise approach. The key is the accuracy, validity, and objectivity used by the researcher in attempting to answer the question. Accordingly, when reading research you should read various types of studies and assess how and if the criteria for each step of the research process were followed. Many nursing journals publish not only sophisticated clinical research projects but also smaller clinical studies that can be applied to practice.

Howie-Esquivel and Dracup (2008) conducted a **pilot study** that investigated whether oxygen saturation (SaO_2) and distance walked during the 6-minute walk test, as well as other demographic variables, could predict early hospitalization risk in heart failure patients. This pilot study was done to test the influence of gender and heart failure indices on rehospitalization risk, the feasibility of the intervention for use in a larger follow-up study, to assist with sample size estimation for the larger follow-up study, and to help decide what would be an adequate number of research assistants to employ for a larger study. To understand the feasibility issues of a larger intervention study, the researchers decided first to conduct a pilot study to assess the feasibility and the intervention's usefulness. The researchers learned a great deal from this pilot study. Pilot studies such as this one are invaluable for maintaining accuracy and provide important information for future inquiry that is feasible and well grounded.

FEASIBILITY

When critiquing the research design one also needs to be aware of the pragmatic consideration of feasibility. Sometimes the reality of feasibility does not truly sink in until one does research. It is important to consider feasibility when reviewing a study, including availability of the subjects, timing of the research, time required for the subjects to participate, costs, and analysis of the data (Table 7-1). As indicated, a major objective of the Howie-Esquivel and Dracup (2008) pilot study was to test the feasibility of implementing the intervention.

TABLE 7-1 Pragmatic Considerations in Determining the Feasibility of a Research Question

Factor	Pragmatic Considerations
Time	The research question must be one that can be studied within a realistic period of time. All researchers have deadlines for completion of a project. The scope of the research question must be circumscribed enough to provide ample time for the completion of the entire project. Research studies generally take longer to complete than anticipated.
Subject availability	The researcher must determine whether a sufficient number of eligible subjects will be available and willing to participate in the study. If one has a captive audience (e.g., students in a classroom), it may be relatively easy to enlist their cooperation. If a study involves the subjects' independent time and effort, they may be unwilling to participate when there is no apparent reward for doing so. Potential subjects may have fears about harm or confidentiality and be suspicious of the research process. Subjects with unusual characteristics are often difficult to locate. People are generally fairly cooperative about participating, but a researcher should consider enlisting a larger subject pool than actually needed to prepare for subject unavailability. At times, when reading a research report the researcher may note how the inclusion criteria were liberalized or the number of subjects was altered, probably as a result of some unforeseen pragmatic consideration.
Facility and equipment availability	All research projects require some kind of equipment. The equipment may be questionnaires, telephones, stationery, stamps, technical equipment, or some other apparatus. Most research projects require the availability of some kind of facility. The facility may be a hospital site for data collection or laboratory space or computer programs for data analysis.
Money	Many research projects require some expenditure of money. Before embarking on a study the researcher probably itemized the expenses and projected the total cost of the project. This provides a clear picture of the budgetary needs for items such as books, stationery, postage, printing, technical equipment, telephone and computer charges, and salaries. These expenses can range from about $200 for a small-scale student project to hundreds of thousands of dollars for a large-scale federally funded project.
Researcher experience	The selection of the research problem should be based on the nurse's experience and interest. It is much easier to develop a research study related to a topic that is either theoretically or experientially familiar. Selecting a research question that is of interest to the researcher is essential for maintaining enthusiasm when the project has its inevitable ups and downs.
Ethics	Research questions that place unethical demands on subjects may not be feasible for study. Researchers must take ethical considerations seriously. The consideration of ethics may affect the choice of the design and methodology.

Before conducting a large experimental study, or a randomized controlled trial, it is helpful to first conduct a pilot study with a small number of subjects to determine the feasibility of subject recruitment, the intervention, the data-collection protocol, the likelihood that subjects will complete the study, the reliability and validity of measurement tools, and the costs of the study. These pragmatic considerations are not presented as a step in the research process as are the theoretical framework or methods, but they do affect every step of the process and, as such, should be considered when assessing a study. The student researcher may or may not have monies or accessible services. When critiquing a study, note the credentials of the author and whether the investigation was part of a student project or part of a fully funded grant project. If the project was a student project, the scope of the project may be more limited than that of a doctorally prepared, experienced researcher or clinician with funding. Finally, the pragmatic issues raised affect the scope and breadth of an investigation and the strength of evidence generated, and therefore its generalizability.

CONTROL AND INTERVENTION FIDELITY

A researcher attempts to use a design to maximize the degree of **control** or uniformity over the tested variables. **Intervention fidelity** is another key concept when considering a study's design. The word *fidelity* means trustworthiness or faithfulness. In a study, intervention fidelity means that the researcher actively standardized the intervention, and planned how to administer intervention to each subject in the same manner under the same conditions. Control and intervention fidelity involves holding the data procedures or conditions of the study constant and establishing specific sampling criteria. Control and intervention fidelity for administration of an intervention and ***data*** collection is described by Meneses and colleagues (2007; see Appendix A):

- The same instruments were used with all subjects and the instruments had established reliability and validity (see Chapters 12 and 13).
- The data-collection methods were standardized for each subject (intervention fidelity; see later discussion).
- The research associates who assisted with data collection were trained and assessed for standardization of procedures and supervised throughout the study to ensure that data were collected as instructed (intervention fidelity and interrater reliability; see Chapter 13).
- Women were invited to participate if they were at least 21 years of age, with histologically confirmed stage 0 to II breast cancer and no local recurrence or metastatic disease (establishing sampling inclusion and exclusion criteria; see Chapter 10).
- Baseline demographic variables were compared to determine whether any significant baseline differences existed between groups, but none were found (assessing for intervening or extraneous variables; see Chapter 8).

The Meneses and colleagues (2007) study reflects constancy of data collection in the sections that describe the intervention, procedure, and intervention treatment fidelity. An efficient design can maximize results, decrease bias, and control preexisting conditions that may affect outcomes. To accomplish these tasks, the research design and methods should demonstrate the researcher's efforts at control. This study illustrates how the investigators planned the design to apply controls. Control is important in all designs. When various research designs are critiqued, the issue of control is always raised but with varying levels of flexibility. The issues discussed here will become clearer as you review the various types of designs discussed in later chapters (see Chapters 8 and 9). Control is accomplished by ruling out extraneous or mediating variables that compete with the independent variables as an explanation for a study's outcome. An **intervening, extraneous, or mediating variable** is one that interferes with the operations of the variables being studied. An example would be the type of breast cancer treatment women experienced (Meneses et al., 2007). Also Horgas and colleagues (2008) noted that they had overlooked asking subjects if they had taken pain medication. In this example taking pain medication would be an intervening variable. Means of controlling extraneous variables include the following:

- Use of a homogeneous sample
- Use of consistent data-collection procedures
- Training and supervision of data collectors and interventionists
- Manipulation of the independent variable
- Randomization

The following example illustrates and defines these concepts:

An investigator might be interested in how a new stop-smoking program (independent variable) affects smoking behavior (dependent variable). The independent variable is assumed to affect the outcome or ***dependent variable.*** *An investigator needs to be relatively sure that the decrease in smoking is truly related to the stop-smoking program rather than to some other variable, such as motivation. The design of the research study alone does not inherently provide control. However, an appropriately designed study with the necessary controls can increase an investigator's ability to answer a research question. These examples illustrate how appropriate control strengthens a research study and offers you as a reader the following: (1) more confidence in the evidence provided by the findings, (2) a perspective about the degree to which the findings are generalizable, and (3) an assessment of readiness for use in practice.*

EVIDENCE-BASED PRACTICE TIP

As you read studies it is important to assess if the study includes a tested intervention and whether the report contains a clear description of the intervention and how it was controlled. If the details are not clear, it should make you think that the intervention may have been administered differently among the subjects, therefore affecting the interpretation of the results.

Homogeneous Sampling

In a stop-smoking study, extraneous variables may affect the dependent variable. The characteristics of a study's subjects are common extraneous variables. Age, gender, length of time smoked, amount smoked, and even smoking rules may affect the outcome in the stop-smoking example. These variables may therefore affect the outcome, even though they are extraneous or outside of the study's design. As a control for these and other similar problems, the researcher's subjects should demonstrate **homogeneity** or similarity with respect to the extraneous variables relevant to the particular study (see Chapter 10). Extraneous variables are not fixed but must be reviewed and decided on, based on the study's purpose and theoretical base. By using a sample of homogeneous subjects, based on inclusion and exclusion criteria, the researcher has used a straightforward step of control.

For example, in the study by Jones and colleagues (2007; see Appendix B), the researchers ensured homogeneity of the sample based on age and demographics. This control step limits the **generalizability** or application of the outcomes to other populations when analyzing and discussing the outcomes (see Chapter 15). As you start reading more studies you will often see the researchers limit the generalizability of the findings to like samples. Results can then be generalized only to a similar population of individuals. You may say that this is limiting. This is not necessarily so because no treatment or program can be applicable to all populations, nor is it feasible to examine a large number of different populations in one study. Thus as you appraise the research findings of studies, you must take the differences in populations into consideration.

HELPFUL HINT

When reviewing studies, remember that it is better to have a "clean" study that can be used to make generalizations about a specific population than a "messy" one that can generalize little or nothing.

If the researcher feels that one of the extraneous variables is important, it may be included in the design. In the smoking example, if individuals are working in an area where smoking is not allowed and this is considered to be important, the researcher could build it into the design and set up a control for it. This can be done by comparing two different work areas: one where smoking is allowed and one where it is not. The important idea to keep in mind is that before the data are collected, the researcher should have identified, planned for, or controlled the important extraneous variables.

Constancy in Data Collection

Another basic, yet critical, component of control is constancy in data-collection procedures. **Constancy** refers to the notion that the data-collection procedures should reflect to the consumer a cookbook-like recipe of how the researcher controlled the conditions of the study. This means that environmental conditions, timing of data collection, data-collection instruments, and data-collection procedures used to collect the data are the same for each subject (see Chapter 12). Constancy in data collection is also referred to as **intervention fidelity** (Santacroce et al., 2004; Whitmer et al., 2005).

The Meneses article (Appendix A; see intervention fidelity section of article) is an example of a well-controlled study. The investigators solicited volunteers who met the inclusion and exclusion criteria and tested a standardized intervention. To control conditions, subjects were randomized to a treatment or control group by the biostatistician. A review of this study shows that data were collected from each subject in the same manner and under the same conditions by trained data collectors. This type of control aided the investigators' ability to draw conclusions, discuss limitations, and cite the need for further research in this area. For the consumer it demonstrates a clear, consistent, and specific means of data collection. When interventions are implemented, researchers will often describe the training of and supervision of interventionists and/or data collectors that took place to ensure constancy.

Manipulation of Independent Variable

A third means of control is manipulation of the **independent variable.** This refers to the administration of a program, treatment, or intervention to only one group within the study and not to the other subjects in the study. The first group is known as the **experimental group** or **intervention,** and the other group is known as the **control group.** In a control group the variables under study are held at a constant or comparison level. For example, Meneses and colleagues (2007; see Appendix A) manipulated the provision of a psychoeducational support intervention for breast cancer survivors using an experimental design, whereas Jones and colleagues (2007; see Appendix B), using a quasi-experimental design, tested the effectiveness of a heart intervention for deaf individuals by recruiting deaf subjects from two different Arizona communities, Tucson and Phoenix.

Experimental and quasi-experimental designs use manipulation. These designs are used to test whether a treatment or intervention affects patient outcomes. Nonexperimental designs do not manipulate the independent variable. Lack of variable manipulation does not decrease the usefulness of a nonexperimental design, but the use of a control group in an experimental or quasi-experimental design is related to the level of the research question or hypothesis. For example, Horgas and colleagues (2008; see Appendix C) used a nonexperimental study to examine the relationship between pain and functional disability in older black and white adults. This study did not manipulate the pain experience (that would be unethical) but studied the relationship between race (black and white), pain, and functional disability, both physical and social limitations, in this group of older adults.

HELPFUL HINT

Be aware that the lack of manipulation of the independent variable does not mean a weaker study. The level of the question, the amount of theoretical development, and the research that has preceded the project all affect the researcher's choice of the design. If the question is amenable to a design that manipulates the independent variable, it increases the power of a researcher to draw conclusions; that is, if all of the considerations of control are equally addressed.

Randomization

Researchers may also choose other forms of control, such as randomization. **Randomization** is used when the required number of subjects from the population is obtained in such a manner that each subject in a population has an equal chance of being selected. Randomization eliminates bias, aids in the attainment of a representative sample, and can be used in various designs (see Chapters 10 and 12). Meneses and colleagues (2007; see Appendix A) randomized subjects to an intervention or control group.

Randomization can also be done with paper-and-pencil types of instruments. By randomly ordering items on the instruments, the investigator can assess if there is a difference in responses that can be related to the order of the items. This may be especially important in longitudinal studies where bias from giving the same instrument to the same subjects on a number of occasions can be a problem (see Chapter 9).

QUANTITATIVE CONTROL AND FLEXIBILITY

The same level of control or elimination of bias cannot be exercised equally in all types of designs. When a researcher wants to explore an area in which little or no literature and/or research on the concept exists, the researcher will probably use a qualitative study (see Chapters 4 through 6). In this type of study the researcher is interested in describing or categorizing a phenomenon in a group of individuals. Beginning in 1986, Swanson began developing the theory of caring, first in her work with women who had experienced a miscarriage. Over the years Swanson has used both qualitative and different quantitative designs to develop the middle range theory of caring (see Kristen Swanson's Research Vignette on p. 82). Swanson's beginning qualitative exploratory research with the subsequent testing of interventions using quantitative designs and the subsequent publications of these works is an excellent example of moving theory along a research continuum that ranged from a qualitative to a quantitative program of research to readiness for application of evidence to practice. In critiquing Swanson's various studies the issues of control would be viewed differently based on the design of each study.

If it is determined from a review of a study that the researcher intended to conduct a correlational study, or a study that looks at the relationship between or among the variables, the issue of control takes on a different importance (see Chapter 9). Control must be exercised as strictly as possible. At this intermediate level of design, it should be clear to you that the researcher considered all of the extraneous variables that may affect the outcomes.

All aspects of control are strictly applied to studies that use an experimental design (see Chapter 8). You should be able to locate in the research report how the researcher met the following criteria (i.e., the conditions of the research were constant throughout the study, random assignment of subjects was used, and intervention and control groups were used). The Meneses and colleagues (2007) study, which was previously discussed, is an example in which aspects of control were addressed. Because of the control exercised in the study, the reviewer can see that all issues related to control were considered and the extraneous variables were addressed.

EVIDENCE-BASED PRACTICE TIP

Remember that establishing evidence for practice is determined by assessing the validity of each step of the study, assessing if the evidence assists in planning patient care, and assessing if patients respond to the evidence-based care.

INTERNAL AND EXTERNAL VALIDITY

When reading research, you must be convinced that the results of a study are valid, based on precision, and faithful to what the researcher wanted to measure. For a study to form the basis of further research, practice, and theory development, it must be credible and dependable and needs to reflect how the researcher avoided bias. **Bias** can occur at any step of the research process. Bias can be a result of what questions are asked (see Chapter 2), what hypotheses are tested (see Chapter 2), how data are collected or observations made (see Chapter 12), number of subjects and how subjects are recruited and included (see Chapter 10), how groups are conceptualized in an intervention study (see Chapter 8), and how data are reported and analyzed (see Chapter 14). When bias occurs it is not that the researcher was careless or intended to cause bias, but as studies evolve and are carried out, problems can occur that need to be considered before studies are used to change practice. There are two important criteria for evaluating bias, credibility, and dependability of the results: internal validity and external validity. An understanding of the threats to internal validity and external validity is necessary for reading research and considering whether it is applicable to practice. Threats to validity are listed in Box 7-1, and discussion follows.

Internal Validity

Internal validity asks whether the independent variable really made the difference or the change in the dependent variable. To establish internal validity the researcher rules out other factors or threats as rival explanations of the relationship between the variables. There are a number of threats to internal validity, and these are considered by researchers in planning a

BOX 7-1 Threats to Validity

INTERNAL VALIDITY	EXTERNAL VALIDITY
• History	• Selection effects
• Maturation	• Reactive effects
• Testing	• Measurement effects
• Instrumentation	
• Mortality	
• Selection bias	

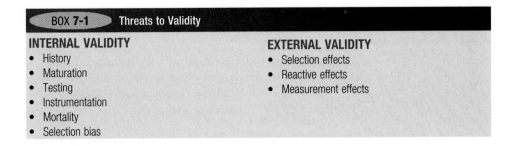

study and by clinicians such as you before implementing the results in practice (Campbell & Stanley, 1966). You should note that the threats to internal validity are most clearly applicable to experimental designs, but attention to factors that can compromise outcomes for all designs, and thereby the overall strength and quality of evidence of a study's findings, should be considered to some degree in all quantitative designs. If these threats are not considered as potential sources of bias, they could negate the results of the research study. How these threats may affect specific designs are addressed in Chapters 8 and 9. Threats to internal validity include history, maturation, testing, instrumentation, mortality, and selection bias. Table 7-2 provides examples of the threats to internal validity. Generally, researchers will note the threats to validity that they encountered in the discussion and or limitations section of a research article.

History

In addition to the independent variable, another specific event that may have an effect on the dependent variable may occur either inside or outside the experimental setting; this is referred to as **history**. For example, in a study of the effects of a breast-feeding teaching program on the length of time of breast-feeding, an event such as government-sponsored advertisements on the importance of breast-feeding featured on television and in newspapers may be a threat of history.

Another example may be that of an investigator testing the effects of a testicular self-examination teaching program on the incidence of testicular self-examination. Concurrently, a famous movie star or news correspondent is diagnosed as having testicular cancer. The occurrence of this diagnosis in a public figure engenders a great deal of media and press attention. In the course of the media attention, medical experts are interviewed widely and the importance of testicular self-examination is supported. If the researcher finds that testicular self-examination behavior is improved, the researcher may not be able to conclude that the change in behavior is the result of the teaching program because it may be the result of the diagnosis given to the known figure and the resultant media coverage. An example of history from a published study can be found in the study by Bull and colleagues (2000) (see Table 7-2).

Maturation

Maturation refers to the developmental, biological, or psychological processes that operate within an individual as a function of time and are external to the events of the investigation. For example, suppose one wishes to evaluate the effect of a specific teaching method on baccalaureate students' achievements on a skills test. The investigator would record the students' abilities before and after the teaching method. Between the pretest and posttest, the students have grown older and wiser. The growth or change is unrelated to the investigation and

TABLE 7-2 Examples of Internal Validity Threats

Threat	Example
History	Bull and colleagues (2000) tested a teaching intervention in one hospital and compared outcomes to those of another hospital in which usual care was given. During the final months of data collection, the control hospital implemented a congestive heart failure critical pathway; as a result, data from the control hospital (cohort) was not included in the analysis.
Maturation	Koniak-Griffin and colleagues (2003) evaluated the 2-year postbirth infant health and maternal outcomes of an early intervention program by public health nurses and noted that the lack of change in some of the variables and changes in other variables may have been due to the general maturation changes experienced by new mothers rather than the intervention.
Testing	Bennett and colleagues (2007) conducted a study to evaluate the effect of a motivational intervention on increasing physical activity in long-term cancer survivors. Several established instruments were used to measure the variables. The measure of physical activity was gained through self-report, which the researchers noted to be a possible limitation. The repeated self-measurements may have primed the patients' responses and influenced the results.
Instrumentation	Chang and colleagues (2008) conducted a study to test the effectiveness of an intervention on self-care among nursing home elder persons in Taiwan. The researchers noted that several of the instruments used in the study were developed in the United States and were translated into Chinese. "Although the translated instruments were validated by a panel of experts, it is possible that the meaning of the construct in the instrument may be different from culture to culture. Therefore, cultural adequacy of these translated instruments may be another limitation of the study" (p. 197).
	Newlin and colleagues (2008) conducted a study to examine the relations of religion and spirituality to glycemic control. In addition to established instruments they used a diabetes medication index that had not been established as a valid or reliable measure.
Mortality	Budin and colleagues (2008), in a randomized trial of a phase-specific evidence-based psychoeducational and telephone counseling intervention study for breast cancer patients and their partners, noted the attrition (mortality) rate in their study. The study had four different intervention groups. Each group experienced subject attrition. The researchers noted that they had planned for this potential and oversampled to end the study with 40 subjects per group, which they did.
Selection bias	Meneses and colleagues (2007) controlled for selection bias by establishing inclusion and exclusion criteria for participation. Once the potential subject's interest was established, the research nurse contacted her for written consent and completion of baseline measure. After completion of this phase of the study, the biostatistician randomly assigned subjects to the treatment arm or the wait control group.
	Thompson and colleagues (2008), in a study that explored the effect of generic and specialist experience on ability to detect the need for nursing action in acute care and the impact of time pressure on nurses' decision-making performance, noted that the "non-random nature of the majority of the sample also raises selection bias in the results" (p. 309).

may explain the differences between the two testing periods rather than the experimental treatment.

Maturation could also occur in a study focused on investigating the relationship between two methods of teaching about children's knowledge of self-care measures. Posttests of student learning must be conducted in a relatively short time period after the teaching sessions are completed. A relatively short interval allows the investigator to conclude that the results were the result of the design of the study and not maturation in a population of children who are learning new skills rapidly. It is important to remember that maturation is more than change resulting from an age-related developmental process but could be related to physical changes as well (see Table 7-2).

Testing

Taking the same test repeatedly could influence subjects' responses the next time a measure is completed. For example, the effect of taking a pretest on the subject's posttest score is known as **testing.** The effect of taking a pretest may sensitize an individual and improve the score of the posttest. Individuals generally score higher when they take a test a second time, regardless of the treatment. The differences between posttest and pretest scores may not be a result of the independent variable but rather of the experience gained through the testing. Table 7-2 provides an example.

Instrumentation

Instrumentation threats are changes in the measurement of the variables or observational techniques that may account for changes in the obtained measurement. For example, a researcher may wish to study various types of thermometers (e.g., tympanic, digital, electronic, chemical indicator, plastic strip, and mercury) to compare the accuracy of using the mercury thermometer to other temperature-taking methods. To prevent instrumentation threat, a researcher must check the calibration of the thermometers according to the manufacturer's specifications before and after data collection.

Another example that fits into this area is related to techniques of observation or data collection. If a researcher has several raters collecting observational data, all must be trained in a similar manner so that they collect data using a standardized approach, thereby ensuring interrater reliability (see Chapter 13) and treatment fidelity. Lack of treatment fidelity weakens the strength of the findings.

If data collectors are not similarly trained, or even if they are similarly trained but unable to conduct the study as planned, a lack of consistency may occur in their ratings, and therefore a threat to internal validity will occur. For examples, see Table 7-2. At times, even though the researcher takes steps to prevent problems of instrumentation, this threat may still occur. When an appraiser finds such a threat, it must be evaluated within the total context of the study.

Mortality

Mortality is the loss of study subjects from the first data-collection point (pretest) to the second data-collection point (posttest). If the subjects who remain in the study are not similar to those who dropped out, the results could be affected. The loss of subjects may be from the sample as a whole, or in a study that has both an experimental and a control group, there may be differential loss of subjects. Differential loss of subjects means that more of the subjects in one group dropped out than the other group. In a study of the ways a media campaign affects the incidence of breast-feeding, if most dropouts were non–breast-feeding women, the perception given could be that exposure to the media campaign increased the number of breast-feeding women, whereas it was the effect of experimental mortality that led to the observed results. See Table 7-2 for an example of mortality.

Selection Bias

If the precautions are not used to gain a representative sample, **selection bias** could result from the way the subjects were chosen. Selection effects are a problem in studies in which the individuals themselves decide whether to participate in a study. Suppose an investigator wishes to assess if a new stop-smoking program contributes to smoking cessation. If the new program is offered to all, chances are only individuals who are more motivated to learn about how to stop smoking will take part in the program. Assessment of the effectiveness of the program is problematic, because the investigator cannot be sure if the new program encouraged smoking-cessation behaviors or if only highly motivated individuals joined the program. To avoid selection bias, the researcher could randomly assign subjects to either the new teaching method group or a control group that receives a different type of instruction. Table 7-2 provides another example of selection bias.

HELPFUL HINT

The list of internal validity threats is not exhaustive. More than one threat can be found in a study, depending on the type of study design. Finding a threat to internal validity in a study does not invalidate the results and is usually acknowledged by the investigator in the "Results" or "Discussion" or "Limitations" section of the study.

EVIDENCE-BASED PRACTICE TIP

Avoiding threats to internal validity when conducting clinical research can be quite difficult at times. Yet this reality does not render studies that have threats useless. Take them into consideration and weigh the total evidence of a study for not only its statistical meaningfulness but also its clinical meaningfulness.

External Validity

External validity deals with possible problems of generalizability of the investigation's findings to additional populations and to other environmental conditions. External validity questions under what conditions and with what types of subjects the same results can be expected to occur. The goal of the researcher is to select a design that maximizes both internal and external validity.

The factors that may affect external validity are related to selection of subjects, study conditions, and type of observations. These factors are termed *effects of selection, reactive effects,* and *effects of testing.* You will notice the similarity in the names of the factors of selection and testing to those of the threats to internal validity. When considering factors as internal threats, you should assesses them as they relate to the testing of *independent* and *dependent* variables within the study, and when assessing them as external threats, you should considers them in terms of the *generalizability* or use outside of the study to other populations and settings. The Critical Thinking Decision Path for threats to validity displays the way threats to internal and external validity can interact with each other. It is important to remember that this decision path is not exhaustive of the type of threats and their interaction. Problems of internal validity are generally easier to control. Generalizability issues are more difficult to deal with because it means that the researcher is assuming that other populations are similar to the one being tested. External validity factors include effect of selection, reactivity effects, and effect of testing.

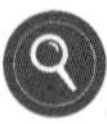

EVIDENCE-BASED PRACTICE TIP

Generalizability depends on who actually participates in a study. Not everyone who is approached actually participates, and not everyone who agrees to participate completes a study. As you review studies, think about how well this group reflects the population of interest.

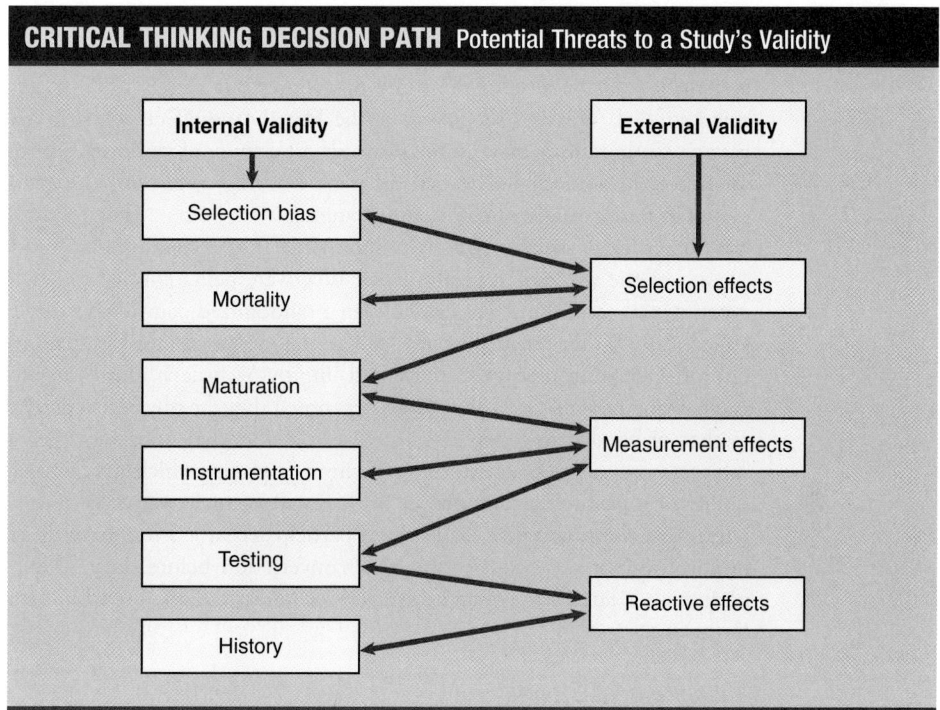

Selection Effects

Selection refers to the generalizability of the results to other populations. An example of the effects of selection occurs when the researcher cannot attain the ideal sample population. At times, numbers of available subjects may be low or not accessible to the researcher; the researcher may then need to choose a nonprobability method of sampling over a probability method (see Chapter 10). Therefore the type of sampling method used and how subjects are assigned to research conditions affect the generalizability to other groups, the external validity.

Examples of selection effects are depicted when researchers note any of the following:

- "Limitations of this study include a relatively small sample of culturally deaf adults and non-randomized assignment to groups, precluding meaningful analysis of interactions between multiple demographic characteristics. Without a control group, investigators can not conclude with certainty that the benefits reported were actually the result of the information counseling session" (Jones et al., 2007; see Appendix B).
- "The use of a small convenience sample of primarily White, English speaking, well-educated mothers of pre-schoolers, most of whom were connected with community services, limits the generalizability of findings to those of similar characteristics" (Sgarbossa & Ford-Gilboe, 2004).
- "The relatively small sample size of Chinese youth and low variability of peer risky behaviors may account for the nonsignificant findings" (Wilgerodt, 2008).

These remarks caution you about potential error of generalizing beyond the type of sample in a study but also point out the usefulness of the findings for practice and future research aimed at building the research in these areas.

Reactive Effects

Reactivity is defined as the subjects' responses to being studied. Subjects may respond to the investigator not because of the study procedures but merely as an independent response to being studied. This is also known as the Hawthorne effect, which is named after Western Electric Corporation's Hawthorne plant, where a study of working conditions was conducted. The researchers developed several different working conditions (i.e., turning up the lights, piping in music loudly or softly, and changing work hours). They found that no matter what was done, the workers' productivity increased. They concluded that production increased as a result of the workers' realization that they were being studied rather than because of the experimental conditions. For example, in a randomized controlled study by Bennett and colleagues (2007) that tested the effect of a telephone-based motivational interviewing intervention on increasing physical activity and improving fitness, improving health self-efficacy in adults living in rural areas, the researchers noted that the physical activity counselors were not masked or blinded to group assignments. Therefore the counselors knew to which group the subjects were assigned, control or experimental group, which may have allowed for the possibility of introducing components of the experimental treatment to the control group. The researchers also noted that each subject participated in a 6-minute walk test that used a strict protocol, but it was also possible that conversation before the test might have influenced performance rate. The researchers made recommendations for future studies to avoid such threats.

Measurement Effects

Administration of a pretest in a study affects the generalizability of the findings to other populations and is known as measurement effects. Just as pretesting affects the posttest results within a study, pretesting affects the posttest results and generalizability outside the study. For example, suppose a researcher wants to conduct a study with the aim of changing attitudes toward acquired immunodeficiency syndrome (AIDS). To accomplish this, an education program on the risk factors for AIDS is incorporated. To test whether the education program changes attitudes toward AIDS, tests are given before and after the teaching intervention. The pretest on attitudes allows the subjects to examine their attitudes regarding AIDS. The subjects' responses on follow-up testing may differ from those of individuals who were given the education program and did not see the pretest. Therefore when a study is conducted and a pretest is given, it may "prime" the subjects and affect the researcher's ability to generalize to other situations.

HELPFUL HINT

When reviewing a study, be aware of the internal and external threats to validity. These threats do not make a study useless—but actually more useful—to you. Recognition of the threats allows researchers to build on data and you to think through what part of the study can be applied to practice. Specific threats to validity depend on the type of design and generalizations the researcher hopes to make.

There are other threats to external validity that depend on the type of design and methods of sampling used by the researcher, but these are beyond the scope of this text. Campbell and Stanley (1966) offer detailed coverage of the issues related to internal and external validity.

APPRAISING THE EVIDENCE

Quantitative Research

Critiquing the design of a study requires you to first have knowledge of the overall implications that the choice of a particular design may have for the study as a whole (see Critiquing Criteria box below). When reading a study, first consider the level of evidence provided by the design and how the potential strength and quality of findings can be used to improve or change practice. When researchers design a study, but before the study begins, they decide how they will collect data, what instruments will be used, what the inclusion and exclusion criteria will be, and who and how large the sample will be to diminish bias or threats to the study's validity. These choices are based on the nature of the research question or hypothesis. Minimizing threats to internal and external validity of a study enhances the strength of evidence for any quantitative design. The concept of the research design is an all-inclusive one that parallels the concept of the theoretical framework. The research design is similar to the study's theoretical framework in that it deals with a piece of the research study that affects the whole. For you to knowledgeably appraise the design in light of the entire study, it is important to understand the factors that influence the choice and the implications of the design. In this chapter, the meaning, purpose, and important factors of design choice, as well as the vocabulary that accompanies these factors, have been introduced.

Several criteria for evaluating the design related to maximizing control, minimizing threats to internal and external validity and as a result sources of bias, can be drawn from this chapter. You should remember that the criteria are applied differently with various designs. Different application does not mean that you will find a haphazard approach to design. It means that each design has particular criteria that allow you to classify the design by type (e.g., experimental or nonexperimental). These criteria must be met and addressed in conducting a study. The particulars of specific designs are addressed in Chapters 8 and 9. The following discussion primarily pertains to the overall appraisal of a quantitative research design.

The research design should reflect that an objective review of the literature and establishment of a theoretical framework guided the development of the research question and hypothesis and the choice of the design. When reading a study there is no explicit statement regarding how the design was chosen, but the literature reviewed will provide clues as to why the researcher chose the design of the study. You can evaluate this by critiquing the study's framework and literature review (see Chapter 3). Is the question new and not extensively researched? Has a great deal been done on the question, or is it a new or different way of looking at an old question? Depending on the level of the question, the investigators make certain choices. For example, in the Meneses and colleagues (2007) study, the researchers wanted to test a controlled intervention; thus they developed a randomized controlled trial (Level II design). However, the purpose of the Horgas and colleagues (2008) study was much different. The Horgas study examined the relationship between pain and functional disability in older black and white adults. The study did not test an intervention but explored how variables of health related to each other in specific populations (Level IV design). The choice of question and design allowed the researchers to assess different types of questions that are a part of nursing practice.

CRITIQUING CRITERIA: *Quantitative Research*

1. Is the type of design employed appropriate?
2. Does the researcher use the various concepts of control that are consistent with the type of design chosen?
3. Does the design used seem to reflect consideration of feasibility issues?
4. Does the design used seem to flow from the proposed research question, theoretical framework, literature review, and hypothesis?
5. What are the threats to internal validity or sources of bias?
6. What are the controls for the threats to internal validity?
7. What are the threats to external validity or generalizability?
8. What are the controls for the threats to external validity?
9. Is the design appropriately linked to the evidence hierarchy?

You should be alert for the means investigators use to maintain control (e.g., homogeneity in the sample, consistent data-collection procedures, how or if the independent variable was manipulated, and whether randomization was used). As you can see in Chapter 8, all of these criteria must be met for an experimental design. As you begin to understand the types of designs (i.e., experimental, quasi-experimental, and nonexperimental designs such as survey and relationship designs), you will find that control is applied in varying degrees, or—as in the case of a survey study—the independent variable is not manipulated at all (see Chapter 9). The level of control and its applications presented in Chapters 8 and 9 provide the remaining knowledge to fully critique the aspects of a study's design.

Once it has been established whether the necessary control or uniformity of conditions has been maintained, you must determine whether the study is feasible and the findings valid. You should ask whether the findings are the result of the variables tested—and thus internally valid—or whether there could be another explanation. To assess this aspect, the threats to internal validity should be reviewed. If the investigator's study was systematic, well grounded in theory, and followed the criteria for each of the processes, you will probably conclude that the study is internally valid. No study is perfect; there is always the potential for bias or threats to validity. This is not because the research was poorly conducted or the researcher did not think through the process completely; rather, it is that when conducting research with human subjects there is always some potential for error. Subjects can drop out of studies, and data collectors can make errors and be inconsistent. Sometimes errors cannot be controlled by the researcher. If there are policy changes during a study an intervention can be affected. As you read studies, note how every facet of the study was conducted, what potential errors could have arisen, and how the researcher addressed the sources of bias in the limitations section of the study. As nurses build a body of science, it is important that we learn from each other to avoid potential pitfalls in future research and its application to practice.

In addition, you must know whether a study has external validity or generalizability to other populations or environmental conditions. External validity can be claimed only after internal validity has been established. If the credibility of a study (internal validity) has not been established, a study cannot be generalized (external validity) to other populations. Determination of external validity of the findings goes hand-in-hand with the sampling frame (see Chapter 10). If the study is not representative of any one group or one phenomenon of interest, external validity may be limited or not present at all. You will find that establishment of internal and external validity requires not only knowledge of the threats to internal and external validity but also knowledge of the phenomenon being studied. Knowledge of the phenomenon being studied allows critical judgments to be made about the linkage of theories and variables for testing. As you appraise studies you should find that the design follows from the theoretical framework, literature review, research question, and hypotheses. You should feel, on the basis of clinical knowledge and knowledge of the research process, that the investigators are not comparing apples to oranges.

CRITICAL THINKING CHALLENGES

- How do the three criteria for an experimental design, manipulation, randomization, and control, minimize bias and decrease threats to internal validity?
- Argue your case for supporting or not supporting the following claim: "A study that does not use an experimental design does not decrease the value of the study even though it may influence the applicability of the findings in practice." Include examples to support your rationale.
- Why do researchers state that randomized clinical trials provide the strongest evidence for an individual study when using an evidence-based practice model?
- As you critically appraise a research study that uses an experimental or quasi-experimental design, why is it important for you to look for evidence of intervention fidelity? How does intervention fidelity increase the strength and qulaity of the evidence provided by the findings of a study using these types of designs?

KEY POINTS

- The purpose of the design is to provide the master plan for a research study.
- There are many types of designs. No matter which type of design the researcher uses, the purpose always remains the same.
- You should be able to locate within the study a sense of the question that the researcher wished to answer. The question should be proposed with a plan for the accomplishment of the investigation. Depending on the question, you should be able to recognize the steps taken by the investigator to ensure control, eliminate bias, and increase generalizability.
- The choice of the specific design depends on the nature of the question. Specification of the nature of the research question requires that the design reflects the investigator's attempts to maintain objectivity, accuracy, pragmatic considerations, and, most important, control.
- Control affects not only the outcome of a study but also its future use. The design should also reflect how the investigator attempted to control threats to both internal and external validity.
- Internal validity must be established before external validity can be established.
- No matter which design the researcher chooses, it should be evident to the reader that the choice was based on a thorough examination of the research question within a theoretical framework.

- The design, research question, literature review, theoretical framework, and hypothesis should all interrelate to demonstrate a woven pattern.
- The choice of the design is affected by pragmatic issues. At times, two different designs may be equally valid for the same question.
- The choice of design affects the study's level of evidence.

REFERENCES

Bennett JA, Lyons KS, Winters-Stone K, et al: Motivational interviewing to increase physical activity in long-term cancer survivors: a randomized controlled trial, *Nurs Res* 56(1):18-27, 2007.

Budin WC, Hoskins CN, Haber J, et al: Breast cancer education, counseling and adjustment among patients and partners: a randomized clinical trial, *Nurs Res* 57(3):199-213, 2008.

Bull MJ, Hansen HE, Gross CR: A professional-patient partnership model of discharge planning with elders hospitalized with heart failure, *Appl Nurs Res* 13(1):19-28, 2000.

Campbell D, Stanley J: *Experimental and quasi-experimental designs for research*, Chicago, 1966, Rand-McNally.

Chang SH, Wung SF, Crogan NL: Improving activities of daily living for nursing home elder persons in Taiwan, *Nurs Res* 57(3):191-198, 2008.

Horgas AL, Yoon S, Nichols AL, et al: The relationship between pain and functional disability in black and white older adults, *Res Nurs Health* 31:1-14, 2008.

Howie-Esquivel J, Dracup K: Does oxygen saturation or distance walked predict rehospitalization in heart failure? *J Cardiovasc Nurs* 23(4):349-356, 2008.

Jones EC, Renger R, Kang Y: Self efficacy for health related behaviors among deaf adults, *Res Nurs Health* 30:185-192, 2007.

Koniak-Griffin D, Verzeminieks IL, Anderson NLR, et al: Nursing visitation for adolescent mothers two-year infant health and maternal outcomes, *Nurs Res* 52(2):127-135, 2004.

Meneses KD, McNees P, Loerzel VW, et al: Transition from treatment to survivorship: effects of a psychoeducational intervention on quality of life in breast cancer survivors, *Oncol Nurs Forum* 34(5):1007-1016, 2007.

Newlin K, Melkus GD, Tappen R, et al.: Relationships of religion and spirituality to glycemic control in Black women with Type 2 diabetes, *Nurs Res* 7(5):331-339, 2008.

Santacroce SJ, Maccarelli LM, Grey M: Intervention fidelity, *Nurs Res* 53(1):63-66, 2004.

Sgarbossa RN, Ford-Gilboe M: Mother's friendship quality, parental support, quality of life, and family health led by adolescent mothers with preschool children, *J Family Nurs* 10:212-232, 2004.

Thompson C, Dalgleish L, Bucknell T, et al: The effects of time pressure and experience on nurses risk assessment decisions, *Nurs Res* 57:302-311, 2008.

Whitmer K, Sweeney C, Slivjak A, et al: Strategies for maintaining integrity of a behavioral intervention, *West J Nurs Res* 27(3):338-345, 2005.

Wilgerodt MA: Family and peer influences on adjustment among Chinese, Filipino and white youth, *Nurs Res* 57(6):395-405, 2008.

FOR FURTHER STUDY

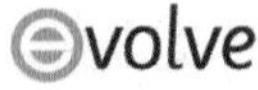

Go to Evolve at http://evolve.elsevier.com/LoBiondo/ for review questions, critiquing exercises, and additional research articles for practice in reviewing and critiquing.

8

Experimental and Quasi-Experimental Designs

Susan Sullivan-Bolyai and Carol Bova

KEY TERMS

a priori
after-only design
after-only nonequivalent control group design
antecedent variable
attention control
control
dependent variable
design
experiment
experimental design
independent variable
intervening variable
intervention fidelity
manipulation
mortality
nonequivalent control group design
one group (pretest-posttest) design
power analysis
quasi-experimental design
randomization (random assignment)
randomized controlled trial (RCT)
Solomon four-group design
testing
time series design
treatment effect
true or classic experiment

LEARNING OUTCOMES

After reading this chapter, you should be able to do the following:

- Describe the purpose of experimental and quasi-experimental research.
- Describe the characteristics of experimental and quasi-experimental studies.
- Distinguish the differences between experimental and quasi-experimental designs.
- List the strengths and weaknesses of experimental and quasi-experimental designs.
- Identify the types of experimental and quasi-experimental designs.
- List the criteria necessary for inferring cause-and-effect relationships.
- Identify potential validity issues associated with experimental and quasi-experimental designs.
- Critically evaluate the findings of experimental and quasi-experimental studies.
- Identify the contribution of experimental and quasi-experimental designs to evidence-based practice.

STUDY RESOURCES

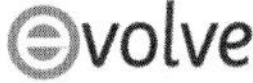

Go to Evolve at http://evolve.elsevier.com/LoBiondo/ for review questions, critiquing exercises, and additional research articles for practice in reviewing and critiquing.

RESEARCH PROCESS

One purpose of scientific research is to determine cause-and-effect relationships. In nursing practice we are concerned with identifying and developing interventions to maintain or improve patient outcomes and base practice on evidence. We test the effectiveness of nursing interventions by using **experimental** and **quasi-experimental designs.** These **designs** differ from nonexperimental designs in one important way: the researcher actively intervenes to bring about the desired effect and does not passively observe behaviors or actions. Experimental and quasi-experimental studies are also important to consider in relation to evidence-based practice because they provide Level II and Level III evidence, which are the two highest level levels of evidence for a single study (see Chapter 1).

Experimental designs are particularly suitable for testing cause-and-effect relationships because they help eliminate potential alternative explanations (also referred to as threats to internal validity; see Chapter 7). To infer causality requires that the following three criteria be met:

- The causal (independent) and effect (dependent) variables must be associated with each other.
- The cause must precede the effect.
- The relationship must not be explainable by another variable.

When you critique studies that use experimental and quasi-experimental designs, the primary focus is on the validity of the conclusion that the experimental treatment, or **independent variable,** caused the desired effect on the outcome, or **dependent variable.** The validity of the conclusion depends on just how well the researcher has controlled the other variables that may explain the relationship studied.

The purpose of this chapter is to acquaint you with the issues involved in interpreting and applying to practice the findings of studies that use **experimental** and **quasi-experimental designs.** These designs are listed in Box 8-1. The Critical Thinking Decision Path shows an algorithm that influences a researcher's choice of experimental or quasi-experimental design. In the literature, studies that use an experimental or quasi-experimental design are often referred to as therapy or intervention articles.

BOX 8-1 Summary of Experimental and Quasi-Experimental Research Designs

EXPERIMENTAL DESIGNS

- True experiment (pretest-posttest control group) design
- Solomon four-group design
- After-only design

QUASI-EXPERIMENTAL DESIGNS

- Nonequivalent control group design
- After-only nonequivalent control group design
- One group (pretest-posttest) design
- Time series design

CRITICAL THINKING DECISION PATH Experimental and Quasi-Experimental Design

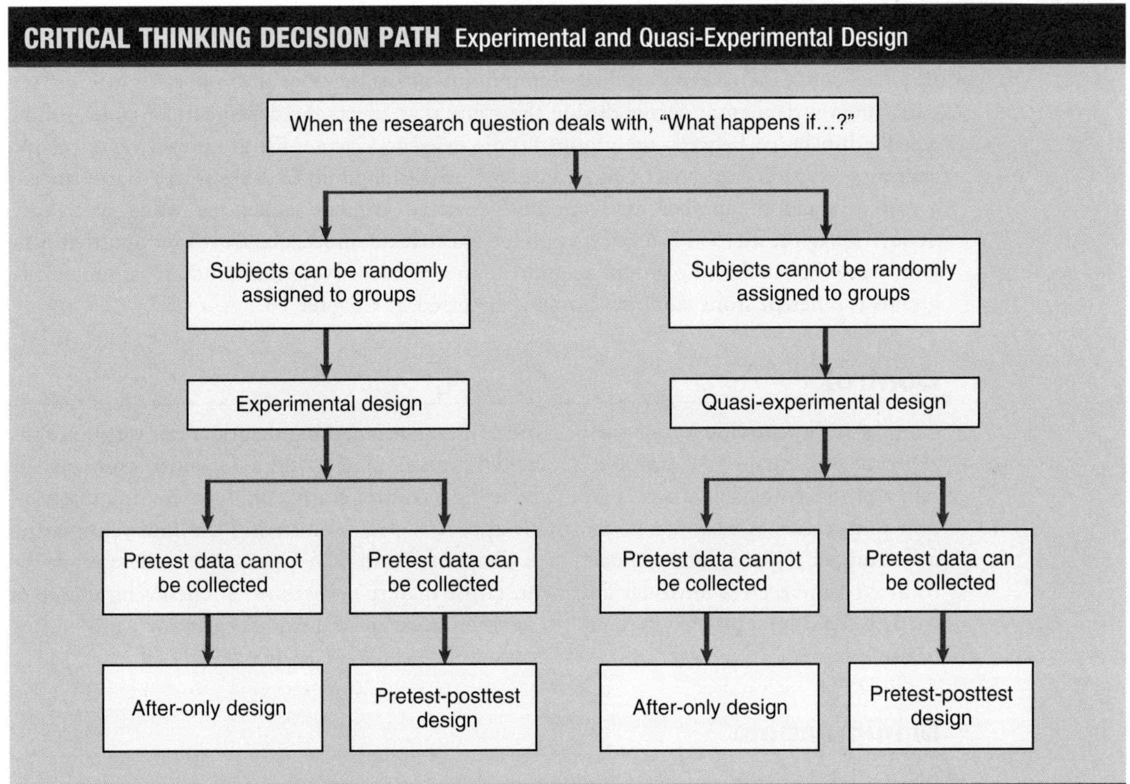

TRUE EXPERIMENTAL DESIGN

An experiment is a scientific investigation that makes observations and collects data according to explicit criteria. A **true** experimental design has three identifying properties:

- Randomization
- Control
- Manipulation

A research study using a true experimental design is commonly called a randomized controlled trial (RCT). In hospital and clinic settings it may be referred to as a "clinical trial" and is commonly used in drug trials. An RCT is considered to be the best research design, the "gold standard," for providing information about cause-and-effect relationships. An individual RCT generates Level II evidence (see Chapter 1) because of the minimal bias introduced by this design through the use of randomization, control, and manipulation. The higher a well-controlled design is on the hierarchy, the more confident you are that the intervention will be effective and produce the same results over time (see Chapters 1 and 7).

Randomization

Randomization, or random assignment, is required for a study to be considered a true experimental design. It involves the distribution of subjects to either the experimental or the control group on a purely random basis. That is, each subject has an equal chance of being assigned to any group. Randomization may be done individually or by groups (Duffy, 2006). Random assignment to experimental or control groups reduces systematic bias that may affect the dependent variable being studied. Randomization assumes that any important **intervening variable** (a variable that occurs during the study that affects the dependent variable) will be equally distributed between the groups (as discussed in Chapter 7), minimizes variance, and decreases selection bias. Several procedures are used to randomize subjects to groups, such as a table of random numbers or computer-generated number sequences (Wang & Bakhai, 2006). Whatever method is used, it is important that the process be truly random, that it be tamperproof, and that the group assignment is concealed. Note that random assignment to groups is different from random sampling discussed in Chapter 10.

Control

Control is the introduction of one or more constants (something that does not vary) into the experimental situation. Control is acquired by manipulating the independent variable, by randomly assigning subjects to a group, by using a control group, and by preparing intervention protocols that maintain a consistent approach to administering the intervention and collecting data (procedure manuals—see Chapters 7 and 12). In experimental research the control group receives the usual treatment, rather than the experimental one (Whittemore & Melkus, 2008) or a placebo (a sham intervention in behavioral studies or an inert pill in drug trials).

Manipulation

Manipulation is the process of "doing something" to at least some of the involved subjects. The independent variable is manipulated by giving the experimental treatment to some participants in the study and not to others or by giving different amounts of it to different groups. The independent variable might be a treatment, a teaching plan, or a medication. It is the effect of this manipulation that is measured to determine the result of the experimental treatment on the dependent variable compared to those who did not receive the treatment.

Box 8-2 provides an illustration of how the three major properties of true experimental design (randomization, control, and manipulation) are used in an intervention study and how the researchers ruled out other potential explanations or bias (threats to internal validity) for the results. This information will help you decide if the study may be helpful in your own clinical setting.

The description in Box 8-2 is also a clear example of the control property (along with randomization and manipulation) that the researchers have placed on the intervention (Barkauskas et al., 2005). This control also helped rule out potential threats to the study's internal validity (see Chapter 7, not to be confused with instrument threats to validity, described in Chapter 13) of the findings such as the following:

- *Selection:* The representativeness of the sample
- *History:* Events that may have contributed to the results versus the intervention
- *Maturation:* Developmental processes that can occur that potentially could alter the results versus the intervention

However, if any of these threats occurred, the researchers (who implemented random assignment) tested statistically for differences between the groups and found that there were none, reassuring the reader that the randomization process worked.

BOX **8-2** Properties of an Experimental Study

- This RCT examined the efficacy of a psychoeducational support intervention (independent variable, variable that is being manipulated) on women breast cancer survivors' quality of life (dependent variable) during their posttreatment recovery phase.
- Figure 2 (Appendix A) illustrates how women (*N* = 261) were randomly assigned to one of two groups. All women who met the study criteria had an equal and known chance of being assigned to either the control or experimental group. The criteria ensured that the two study groups were comparable on **preexisting factors** (sometimes referred to as **antecedent variables**) that might affect the results, such as age, educational level, and marital status.
- The researchers also checked statistically whether random assignment produced groups that were similar and under *results* stated that no significant differences were found between the two groups and that both groups were equivalent at baseline, thus the randomization process was successful.
- The experimental group (*N* = 129) (see Figure 1, Appendix A) received a combination of structured face-to-face and telephone educational support, written, and audiotaped reinforcement on a monthly basis over a 6-month period.
- The control group (*N* = 132) received what is referred to as **attention control,** operationalized as the control group receiving the same amount of "attention" as the experimental group.
- All subjects received an equivalent amount of time and the same number of unstructured interactions (telephone calls and face-to-face nurse interaction) as the intervention group.
- However, the control group interactions did not include the breast cancer education intervention components (see Appendix A). Figure 1 (Appendix A) displays how the control group at the end of the study (in month 6) received structured education and support sessions, as did the experimental group during month 1. It was important to give both groups of women psychoeducational support because the existing empirical literature reported that this type of intervention positively affects quality of life for cancer patients.
- Thus, ethically it was important to provide both groups with psychoeducational support. The difference is that the researchers provided the control group with attention control until the study's end so they could measure the psychoeducational group differences before providing them with the same educational sessions (see the last two boxes under wait control group in Appendix A, Figure 1, compared to the experimental group boxes).
- The experimental group receiving the educational sessions at the beginning allowed for reinforcement of information over the course of the 6 months. Compared to the control group, they reported better quality of life at both the 3- and 6-month data points, suggesting that the intervention as designed (refer again to Figure 1) is effective over the 6-month posttreatment time.

Meneses DK, McNees P, Loerzel W, et al: Transition from treatment to survivorship: effects of a psychoeducational intervention on quality of life in breast cancer survivors, *Oncol Nurs Forum* 34:1007-1016, 2007. (see Appendix A).

We have briefly discussed RCTs and how they precisely use control, manipulation, and randomization to test the effectiveness of an intervention. RCTs:

- Use an experimental and control group (illustrated in Meneses et al., 2007), sometimes referred to as experimental and control arms.
- Have a very specific sampling plan, using clear-cut *inclusion* and *exclusion* criteria (who will be allowed into the study, who will not).
- Administer the intervention in a consistent way, called *intervention fidelity*
- Typically carry out statistical comparisons to determine any differences between groups.
- Pay important attention to the sample size.

It is important that the researchers ensure that the sample size chosen is large enough to make sure there are enough subjects in both study groups to statistically detect differences between those receiving the intervention and those who did not. This is called the ability to statistically detect the **treatment effect.** The mathematical procedure to determine the number for each arm (group) of the study is referred to as a **power analysis** (see Chapter 10). You will generally find power analysis information in the sample section of the research article. For example, you will know there was an appropriate plan for an adequate sample size when the following type of statement is included, "A total sample of 244 patient partners (61 per group) would be required to achieve at least an 80% power for an effect size of this magnitude (f= 0.25)" (Budin, 2008).

It is not necessary for you to learn how to calculate the power, but you are looking for assurances from the researchers that they thought about an adequate sample for the study. Many considerations are determined by the researcher regarding the intervention before the study regarding power. This information is critical to assess because with a small sample size differences may not be statistically evident, thus creating the potential for a *type II error* (accepting the null hypothesis when it is false) (see Chapter 14).

Carefully read the intervention and control group section of the article to see exactly what each group received and what the differences between groups were. In Appendix A, Meneses and colleagues (2007) provide the reader with a detailed description and illustration of the intervention. In a study that tested the effectiveness of an enhanced prostate cancer screening decision aid, Weinrich and colleagues (2007) reported that there were differences in length and content of educational materials between the intervention and control groups. That is the kind of inconsistency that should make you wonder if either of the characteristics of the materials (length and content) might have influenced the findings.

Another important feature of an RCT is the need to carefully design **intervention fidelity** procedures. **Intervention fidelity** involves the process of enhancing internal validity by ensuring that the intervention is actually delivered systematically to all subjects in the intervention group (Santacroce et al., 2004). To enhance intervention fidelity the researcher develops a system for evaluating how consistently the intervention was carried out by those delivering the intervention. Meneses and colleagues (2007) described specific activities that maintained the integrity of the intervention and control sessions. These activities include development of a procedure manual that provides for *consistent* training of the interventionists and other involved research staff, intervention delivery protocols, *standardized* data-collection procedures, and/or supervision which consists of *frequent review* of the intervention either by observation, videotaping, or audiotaping of sessions.

Types of Experimental Designs

There are many different experimental designs (Campbell & Stanley, 1966). Each is based on the classic design called the **true experiment** or RCT diagrammed in Figure 8-1, *A*. The **classic** RCT is conducted as follows:

1. The researcher recruits a sample from the population.
2. Baseline preintervention demographic, personal characteristics, and measurement of the intended study concepts or dependent variables (sometimes referred to as empirical indicators as these are the outcomes that the researcher wishes to assess for change) are collected from the entire sample.
3. Subjects are then randomized to either the intervention or the control group.
4. After each group receives either the experimental intervention (usual care, or standard treatment, education or placebo), both groups complete postintervention measures to see if any changes have occurred in the dependent variables.

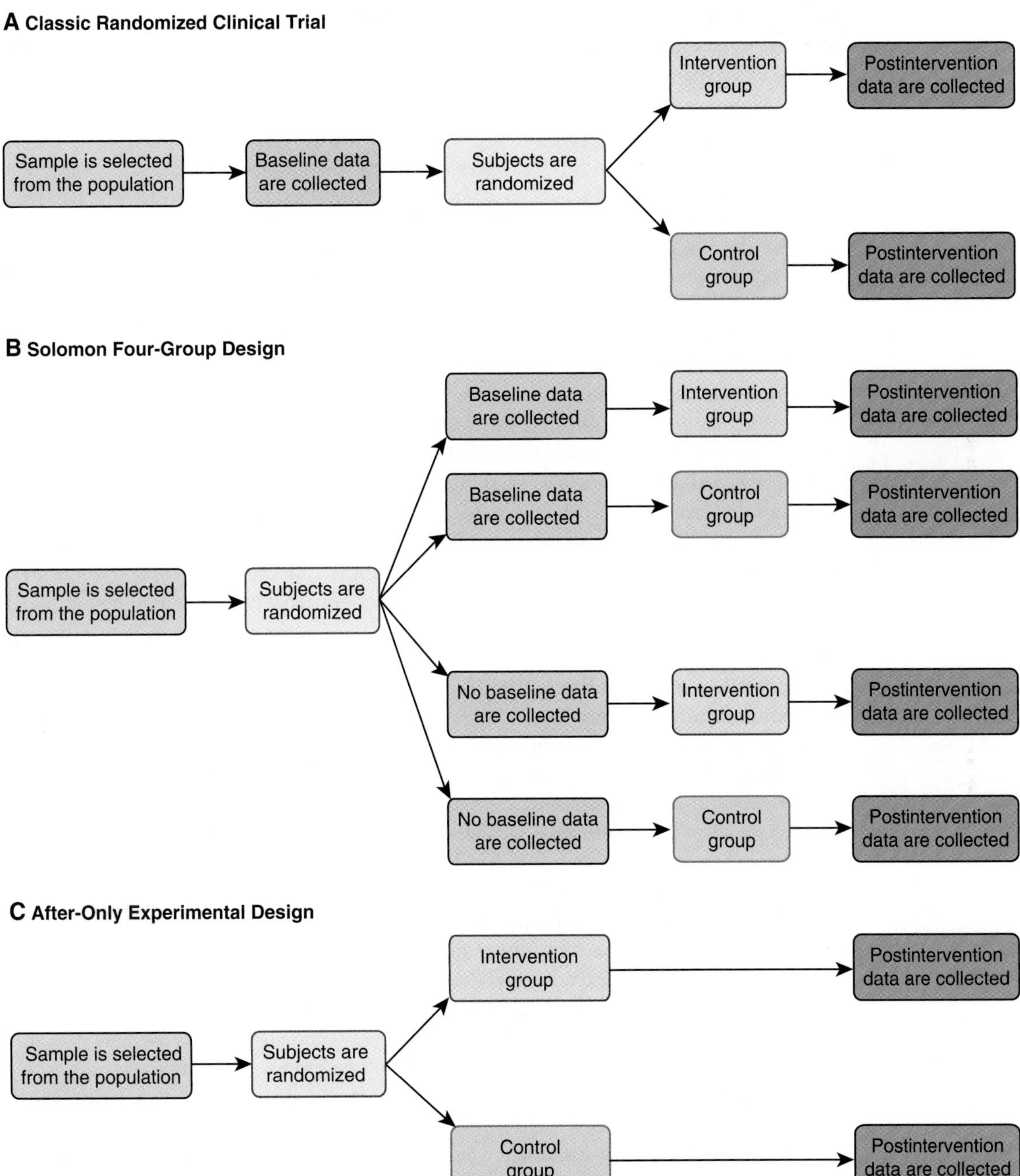

Figure 8-1 Experimental designs. **A,** Classic randomized clinical trial. **B,** Solomon four-group design. **C,** After-only experimental design.

Thus all true experimental designs have subjects randomly assigned to groups, have an experimental treatment introduced to some of the subjects, have a comparison control group, and have the differential effects of the treatment observed.

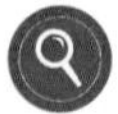

EVIDENCE-BASED PRACTICE TIP

The term *randomized controlled trial (RCT)* is often used to refer to a true experimental design in health care research and is frequently used in nursing research as the gold standard design because it minimizes bias or threats to validity. Because of ethical issues, rarely is "no treatment" acceptable. Typically either "standard treatment" or another version or dose of "something" is provided to the control group. Only when there is no standard or comparable treatment available is a no-treatment control group appropriate.

It is important to note that the control group occasionally gets no treatment (see the Evidence-Based Practice Tip), some other form of standard treatment, or a different dose of the intervention. The dependent variable or variables are measured later for comparison with the experimental group, as illustrated by Meneses and colleagues (2007). The degree of difference between the two groups at the end of the study indicates the confidence the researcher has that a causal link exists (i.e., that the intervention caused the differences in group responses) between the independent and dependent variables. Because random assignment and the control inherent in this design minimize the effects of many threats to internal study validity or bias (see Chapter 7), it is a strong design for testing cause-and-effect relationships. However, the design is not perfect. Some study threats to internal validity cannot be controlled in true experimental studies. For example:

- *Mortality:* People tend to drop out of studies, especially those that require their participation over an extended period of time. When reading experimental studies, it is important to examine the sample and the results carefully to see if excessive dropouts or deaths occurred or occurred in one group more than the other, which can affect the study findings.
- *Testing* also can be a problem, especially if the same measurement is given twice. Subjects tend to score better the second time just by remembering the items on the test. Researchers can avoid this problem in one of two ways: they might use different or equivalent forms of the same test for the two measurements (see Chapter 13), or they might use a more complex experimental design called the Solomon four-group design.

The **Solomon four-group design,** shown in Figure 8-1, *B,* has two groups that are identical to those used in the classic experimental design, plus two additional groups: an experimental after-group and a control after-group. As the diagram shows, subjects are randomly assigned to one of four groups before baseline data are collected (compared to after baseline data collection as in the classic RCT). This design results in two groups that only receive a posttest (rather than pretest and posttest), which provides an opportunity to rule out result distortions that may have occurred (testing is a threat to internal validity) due to exposure to the pretest. Common sense tells us that this design would require a larger sample size, which also means this type of study would be more costly. For example, Weinrich and colleagues (2007) used the Solomon four-group design to test an enhanced prostate cancer screening decision aid versus standard education with middle-aged men.

- They hypothesized that those who received the pretest would have higher posttest knowledge.
- The men were first randomly assigned to one of four groups with experimental and control groups receiving pretest and posttest, and the other experimental and control groups receiving posttest only.

- As in the Meneses article, they also tested and found no differences across the four groups in demographics, family history of prostate cancer, or previous history of screening prostate examinations, thus ensuring that the randomization process was successful.
- The findings revealed that outcomes varied depending on group assignment (those with pretest and posttest had significantly higher scores vs. the posttest-only intervention group), *but* also varied on whether the men had had previous digital rectal examinations.

This is further discussed below under RCT. Although this design helps evaluate the effects of testing, the threat of mortality (dropout) remains a problem, as with the classic experimental design.

A less frequently used experimental design is the **after-only design,** shown in Figure 8-1, *C.* This design, which is sometimes called the posttest-only control group design, is composed of two randomly assigned groups, but unlike the true experimental design, neither group is pretested or measured. Again, the independent variable is introduced to the experimental group and not to the control group. The process of randomly assigning the subjects to groups is assumed to be sufficient to ensure a lack of bias so that the researcher can still determine whether the intervention created significant differences between the two groups. This design is particularly useful when testing effects that are expected to be a major problem, when outcomes cannot be measured beforehand (i.e., postoperative pain management).

Thus, when critiquing experimental research articles in the research literature to help inform your evidence-based decisions, consider what type of design was used; how the groups were formed (i.e., did the researchers use randomization); whether the groups were different at baseline, and if so, how they were different; each of the study threats to internal validity, and what kind of manipulation (i.e., intervention) was given to the experimental group and what the control group received.

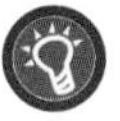

HELPFUL HINT

Look for evidence of preestablished inclusion and exclusion criteria for the study participants.

Strengths and Weaknesses of the Experimental Design

Experimental designs are the most powerful for testing cause-and-effect relationships due to the control, manipulation, and randomization components. Therefore the design offers a better chance of measuring if the intervention caused the change or difference in the two groups. For example, Meneses and associates (2007) were able to conclude from their findings that the psychoeducational intervention for breast cancer survivors was effective in improving subjects' quality of life. If you were working in an oncology clinic and wanted to start a similar intervention, you could use the strength and quality of evidence provided by the findings in this study as a starting point for putting research findings into clinical practice.

Still, experimental designs have some weaknesses as well. They are complicated to design and can be costly to implement. For example, there may not be an adequate number of potential study participants in the accessible population. Another problem with experimental designs is that they may be difficult or impractical to carry out in a particular clinical setting. An example might be trying to randomly assign patients from one hospital unit to different groups when nurses might talk to each other about the different treatments. Experimental procedures also may be disruptive to the usual routine of the setting. If several nurses are involved in administering the experimental program, it may be impossible to ensure that the program is administered in the same way to each subject. Another problem is that many important variables that are related to patient care outcomes are not amenable to manipulation for ethical reasons. For example, cigarette smoking is known to be related to lung cancer but you could not randomly assign people to smoking or non-smoking groups. Health status varies with age and socioeconomic status. No matter how careful a researcher is, no one can assign subjects randomly by age or by a certain income level.

Because of these problems in carrying out true experiments, researchers frequently turn to another type of research design to evaluate cause-and-effect relationships. Such designs, because they look like experiments but lack some of the control of the true experimental design, are called quasi experimental studies.

QUASI-EXPERIMENTAL DESIGNS

Quasi-experimental designs are also intended to test cause-and-effect relationships. However, in a quasi-experimental design random assignment to the treatment or control group may not have been undertaken, or there may not be a control group. These characteristics of a true experiment may not be possible because of the nature of the independent variable or the nature of the available subjects.

Without all of the characteristics associated with a true experiment, internal validity may be compromised, and the ability to determine that the treatment resulted in the changes observed in outcomes is weakened. Therefore the basic problem with the quasi-experimental approach is a weakened confidence in making causal assertions that the results occurred because of the intervention. Instead, the findings may be a result of other extraneous variables. Because of the lack of control, quasi-experimental designs are subject to contamination by many, if not all, of the threats to internal validity discussed in Chapter 7. As a result, Level III (versus Level II with experimental studies) evidence is provided by studies that use quasi-experimental designs.

HELPFUL HINT

Remember that researchers often make trade-offs and sometimes use a quasi-experimental design instead of an experimental design because it may be pragmatically impossible to randomly assign subjects to groups. Not using the "purest" design does not decrease the value of the study even though it may decrease the strength of the findings.

Types of Quasi-Experimental Designs

There are many different quasi-experimental designs, but we will limit the discussion to only those most commonly used in nursing research. Refer back to the true experimental design shown in Figure 8-1, *A*, and compare it with the **nonequivalent control group design** shown in Figure 8-2, *A*. Note that this design looks exactly like the true experiment except that subjects are not randomly assigned to groups. Suppose a researcher is interested in the effects of a new diabetes education program on the physical and psychosocial outcomes of newly diagnosed diabetes. Under certain conditions, the researcher might be able to randomly assign subjects to either the group receiving the new program or the group receiving the usual program, but for any number of reasons, that design might not be possible.

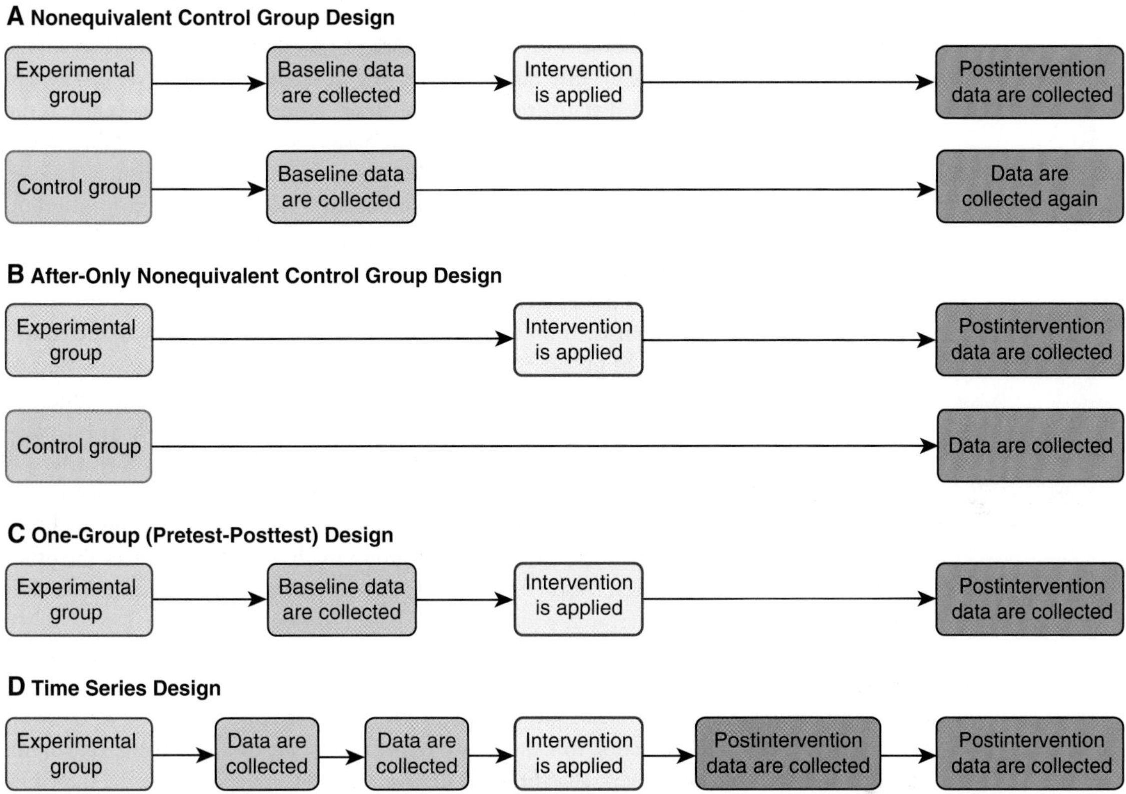

Figure 8-2 Quasi-experimental designs. **A,** Nonequivalent control group design. **B,** After-only nonequivalent control group design. **C,** One-group (pretest-posttest) design. **D,** Time series design.

- For example, nurses on the unit where patients are admitted might be so excited about the new program that they cannot help but include the new information for all patients.
- The researcher has two choices—to abandon the study or to conduct a *quasi experiment.*
- To conduct a quasi experiment, the researcher might use one unit as the intervention group for the new program and find a similar unit that has not been introduced to the new program and study the newly diagnosed patients with diabetes who are admitted to that unit as a comparison group. The study would then involve a quasi-experimental design.

The **nonequivalent control group design** is commonly used in nursing research studies conducted in clinical settings. The basic problem with this design is the weakened confidence the researcher can have in assuming that the experimental and comparison groups are similar at the beginning of the study. Threats to internal validity, such as *selection, maturation, testing,* and *mortality,* are possible with this design. However, the design is relatively strong because by gathering the data at the pretest, the researcher can compare the equivalence of the two groups on important antecedent variables before the independent variable is introduced. In the previous example, the motivation of the patients to learn about their medical condition might be important in determining the effect of the diabetes education program. At the outset of the study the researcher could include some measure of motivation to learn. Then differences between the two groups on this variable could be tested, and if significant differences existed, they could be controlled statistically in the analysis. Nonetheless, the strength of the causal assertions that can be made on the basis of such designs depends on the ability of the researcher to identify and measure or control possible threats to internal validity.

Jones and colleagues (2007) (see Appendix B) conducted a nonequivalent control group (pretest-posttest) quasi-experimental design to determine the effectiveness of the Deaf Heart Health Intervention (DHHI) on improving self-efficacy for preventive cardiovascular disease (CVD) health behaviors for culturally deaf adults.

- Intervention—classes consisted of 2-hour education classes every week over the course of 8 weeks entirely taught in sign language.
- Group assignment—the groups were determined by location: Phoenix became the control group and Tucson the experimental group. The groups were divided for pragmatic reasons. The researchers were worried that the deaf community in each city was very close knit and small. Thus there was a good chance that the subjects would do what is referred to as "cross-talk" and share information received from the intervention group (also called "contamination," when one group inadvertently influences the other group). The other practical reason for providing the Tucson group with the intervention was that most of their research educators were based in that city.
- The researchers also tested for group differences at baseline, but unlike the groups in the Meneses and colleagues (2007) study, these researchers found a difference in ethnic composition between the two groups. To control for this issue they used a statistical test that would account for this difference (ANCOVA; see Chapter 14). Controlling for ethnic differences, total self-efficacy scores were significantly higher in the intervention versus the comparison group on posttest.
- Although the lack of randomization resulted in less confidence in the findings, the results still suggest that CVD education among deaf adults can increase their confidence in preventing this disease.

Now suppose that the researcher did not think to measure the subjects before the introduction of the new treatment (or the researcher was hired after the new program began) but later decided that it would be useful to have data demonstrating the effect of the program. Perhaps, for example, a third party, such as an insurance company, asks for such data to determine whether they should pay the extra cost of the new teaching program. Sometimes, the outcomes simply cannot be measured before the intervention, as with prenatal interventions that are expected to affect birth outcomes. The study that could be conducted would look like the **after-only nonequivalent control group design,** shown in Figure 8-2, *B.* This design is similar to the after-only experimental design, but randomization is not used to assign subjects to groups and makes the assumption that the two groups are equivalent and comparable before the introduction of the independent variable. Thus the soundness of the design and the confidence that we can put in the findings depend on the soundness of this assumption of preintervention comparability. Often it is difficult to support the assertion that the two nonrandomly assigned groups are comparable at the outset of the study because there is no way of assessing its validity.

In the example of the teaching program for patients with newly diagnosed diabetes, measuring the subjects' motivation after the teaching program would not tell us whether their motivations differed before they received the program, and it is possible that the teaching program would motivate individuals to learn more about their health problem. Therefore the researcher's conclusion that the teaching program improved physical status and psychosocial outcomes would be subject to the alternative conclusion that the results were an effect of preexisting motivations (selection effect) in combination with greater learning in those so motivated (selection-maturation interaction). Nonetheless, this design is frequently used in nursing research because opportunities for data collection may be limited related to when potential subjects come into a setting and because it is particularly useful with testing effects that may be problematic.

A study by Hall and colleagues (2004) used an after-only quasi-experimental design to test the preliminary efficacy of an adult learning theory-based training curriculum with adult peritoneal dialysis outpatients:

- New patients starting peritoneal dialysis were trained using the experimental curriculum or a conventional training program.
- Because patients were new to peritoneal dialysis, there were no preintervention data available for comparison (i.e., infection rate), so a quasi-experimental after-only design was used.
- The two groups were compared on outcomes after program completion. Patients who participated in the theory-based training curriculum had fewer exit site infections, better fluid balance, and better adherence to treatment than those in the conventional program.

Thus the researchers were able to demonstrate the preliminary efficacy of this new program in improving patient peritoneal dialysis outcomes.

Another quasi-experimental design is a **one-group (pretest-posttest) design** (Figure 8-2, *C*), which is used by researchers when only one group is available for study. Data are collected before and after an experimental treatment on one group of subjects. In this type of design, there is no control group and no randomization, which are important characteristics that enhance internal validity. Therefore it becomes important that the evidence generated by the findings of this type of quasi-experimental design is interpreted with careful consideration of the design limitations.

Another quasi-experimental approach used by researchers when only one group is available to study over a longer period of time is called a **time series design** (Figure 8-2, *D*). Time series designs are useful for determining trends over time. Data are collected multiple times before the introduction of the treatment to establish a baseline point of reference on outcomes. The experimental treatment is introduced, and data are collected multiple times afterward to determine a change from baseline. The broad range and number of data-collection points helps rule out alternative explanations, such as history effects. However, a testing threat to internal validity is ever present because of multiple data-collection points, and without a control group, the threats of selection and maturation cannot be ruled out (see Chapter 7).

HELPFUL HINT

One of the reasons replication is so important in nursing research is that so many problems cannot be subjected to experimental methods. Therefore the consistency of findings across many populations helps support a cause-and-effect relationship even when an experimental study cannot be conducted.

Strengths and Weaknesses of Quasi-Experimental Designs

Given the problems inherent in interpreting the results of studies using quasi-experimental designs, you may be wondering why anyone would use them. Quasi-experimental designs are used frequently because they are practical, less costly, feasible, and generalizable. These designs are more adaptable to the real-world practice setting than the controlled experimental designs.

In addition, for some hypotheses, these designs may be the only way to evaluate the effect of the independent variable of interest.

The weaknesses of the quasi-experimental approach involve mainly the inability to make clear cause-and-effect statements. However, if the researcher can rule out any plausible alternative explanations for the findings, such studies can lead to increased knowledge about causal relationships. Jones and colleagues (2007) provide a clear example of how statistical analysis can help control for such confounding variables. Researchers have other options for ruling out these alternative explanations as well. They may control extraneous variables (alternative events that could explain the findings) **a priori** (before initiating the intervention) by design. There are also methods to control extraneous variables statistically by using tests such as ANCOVA (see Chapter 14) as Jones and colleagues did. In some cases, commonsense knowledge of the problem and the population can suggest that a particular explanation is not plausible. Nonetheless, it is important to replicate such studies to support and accumulate stronger evidence that the causal assertions developed through the use of quasi-experimental designs.

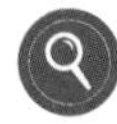

EVIDENCE-BASED PRACTICE TIP

Experimental designs are considered to provide Level II evidence, and quasi-experimental designs are considered to provide Level III evidence. Quasi-experimental designs are lower on the evidence hierarchy because of lack of some research control, which limits the ability to make confident cause-and-effect statements that influence applicability to practice and clinical decision making.

EVIDENCE-BASED PRACTICE

As the science of nursing expands and the cost of health care rises, nurses must become more cognizant of what constitutes best practice for their patient population. Having a basic understanding of the value of intervention studies that use an experimental or quasi-experimental design is critical for improving clinical outcomes. These study designs provide the strongest evidence for making informed clinical decisions. These designs are those most commonly included in studies in systematic reviews (see Chapter 9).

HELPFUL HINT

When reviewing the experimental and quasi-experimental empirical literature, do not limit your search only to your patient population. For example, it is possible that if you are working with adult caregivers, related parent caregiver intervention literature may provide you with strategies as well. Many times with some adaptation, interventions used with one sample might be applicable for other populations.

One cannot assume that because an intervention study has been published it was rigorously done and that the findings apply to your particular practice population. When conducting an evidence-based practice project, the first step after you have identified the clinical question is to collect the strongest, most relevant and current evidence related to your problem. You then need to critically appraise the existing experimental and quasi-experimental literature to evaluate which studies provide the best available evidence. Key points for evaluating the evidence and whether bias has been minimized in experimental and quasi-experimental designs include the following.

- Random assignment to group (experimental or intervention and control or comparison)—how subjects are assigned to groups, equivalence of groups at baseline on key demographic variables
- An adequate sample size—calculated sample size and inclusion and exclusion criteria that are relevant to the clinical problem being studied
- Recruitment of a homogenous sample
- Intervention fidelity or consistent data-collection procedures
- The experimental group is different enough from the control group to detect a clinical and statistical difference (see Chapters 14 and 15)
- Control of intervening or extraneous variables
- The likelihood of changing practice based on one study is unlikely unless it is a large clinical RCT that is based on prior research work

The Cochrane Report (see Chapter 3) provides assessments of clinical studies on a wide range of subjects and assesses the studies for their merit.

APPRAISING THE EVIDENCE

Experimental and Quasi-Experimental Designs

As discussed earlier in the chapter, various designs for research studies differ in the amount of control the researcher has over the antecedent and intervening variables that may affect the results of the study. True experimental designs, which provide Level II evidence, offer the most possibility for control, and nonexperimental designs (Levels IV, V, or VI) offer the least. Quasi-experimental designs, which provide Level III evidence, fall somewhere in between. When conducting an evidence-based practice project, one must always look for studies that provide the highest level of evidence. At times for a specific PICO question (see Chapter 2) you will find both Level II and Level III evidence. Research designs must balance the needs for internal validity and external validity to produce useful results. In addition, judicious use of design requires that the chosen design be appropriate to the problem, free of bias, and capable of answering the research question or hypothesis. Therefore using designs of different levels is appropriate.

Questions that you should pose when reading studies that test cause-and-effect relationships are listed in the Critiquing Criteria box. All of these questions should help you judge whether a causal relationship exists.

For studies in which either experimental or quasi-experimental designs are used, first try to determine the type of design that was used. Often a statement describing the design of the study appears in the abstract and in the methods section of the paper. If such a statement is not present, you should examine the paper for evidence of the following three properties: control, randomization, and manipulation. If all are discussed, the design is probably experimental. On the other hand, if the study involves the administration of an experimental treatment but does not involve the random assignment of subjects to groups, the design is

CRITIQUING CRITERIA: *Experimental and Quasi-Experimental Designs*

1. Is the design used appropriate to the research question or hypothesis?
2. Is the design pragmatic for the setting or sample?
3. Is there a detailed description of the intervention?
4. Is there a description of what the intervention group versus control group received and what the differences are?
5. How is intervention fidelity maintained?
6. Is power analysis used to calculate the appropriate sample size for the study?

Experimental Designs

1. What experimental design is used in the study?
2. How are randomization, control, and manipulation applied?
3. Are there any reasons to believe that there are alternative explanations for the findings?
4. Are all threats to internal validity, including mortality, testing, and selection bias addressed in the report?
5. Are the findings generalizable to the larger population of interest?

Quasi-Experimental Designs

1. What quasi-experimental design is used in the study, and is it appropriate?
2. What are the most common threats to internal and external validity of the findings of this design?
3. What are the plausible alternative explanations, and have they been addressed?
4. Are the author's explanations of threats to internal and external validity acceptable?
5. What does the author say about the limitations of the study?
6. To what extent are the study findings generalizable?

quasi-experimental. Next, try to identify which of the experimental and quasi-experimental designs was used. Determining the answer to these questions gives you a head start, because each design has its inherent threats to validity and this step makes it a bit easier to critically evaluate the study. The next question to ask is whether the researcher required a solution to a cause-and-effect problem. If so, the study is suited to these designs. Finally, think about the conduct of the study in the setting. Is it realistic to think that the study could be conducted in a clinical setting without some contamination?

The most important question to ask yourself as you read experimental studies is the following: "What else could have happened to explain the findings?" Thus it is important that the author provide adequate accounts of how the procedures for randomization, control, and manipulation were carried out. The report should include a description of the procedures for random assignment to such a degree that the reader could determine just how likely it was for any one subject to be assigned to a particular group. The description of the independent variable (intervention) and the control group also should be detailed. The inclusion of this information helps you to decide if it is possible that the treatment given to some subjects in the experimental group might be different from what was given to others in the same group (intervention fidelity). In addition, threats to internal validity, such as testing and mortality, should be addressed as should threats to external validity. Otherwise there is the potential for the findings of the study to be in error and less believable to the reader.

This question of potential alternative explanations or threats to internal validity for the findings is even more important when critically evaluating a quasi-experimental study because quasi-experimental designs cannot possibly control many plausible alternative explanations. A well-written report of a quasi-experimental study systematically reviews potential threats to the internal and external validity of the findings. Then your work is to decide if the author's explanations make sense. For either experimental or quasi-experimental studies, you should also check for a reported power analysis that assures you that an appropriate sample size for detecting a treatment effect was planned, a detailed description of the intervention, what both groups received during the trial, and what intervention fidelity strategies were implemented.

CRITICAL THINKING CHALLENGES

- Describe the ethical issues included in a true experimental research design used by a nurse researcher.
- Describe how a true experimental design could be used in a hospital setting with patients.
- How should a nurse go about critiquing experimental research articles in the research literature so that his or her evidence-based practice is enhanced?
- The nurse researcher is considering using a time series design as a research approach. When would this be an appropriate selection for a research project?

KEY POINTS

- Experimental designs or randomized clinical trials provide the strongest evidence (Level II) for a single study in terms of whether an intervention or treatment affects patient outcomes.
- Two types of design commonly used in nursing research to test hypotheses about cause-and-effect relationships are experimental and quasi-experimental designs. Both are useful for the development of nursing knowledge because they test the effects of nursing actions and lead to the development of prescriptive theory.
- True experiments are characterized by the ability of the researcher to control extraneous variation, to manipulate the independent variable, and to randomly assign subjects to research groups.
- Experiments conducted either in clinical settings or in the laboratory provide the best evidence in support of a causal relationship because the following three criteria can be met: (1) the independent and dependent variables are related to each other; (2) the independent variable chronologically precedes the dependent variable; and (3) the relationship cannot be explained by the presence of a third variable.
- Researchers frequently turn to quasi-experimental designs to test cause-and-effect relationships because experimental designs often are impractical or unethical.
- Quasi experiments may lack either the randomization or the comparison group characteristics of true experiments, or both of these factors. Their usefulness in studying causal relationships depends on the ability of the researcher to rule out plausible threats to the validity of the findings, such as history, selection, maturation, and testing effects.
- The level of evidence (Level III) provided by quasi-experimental designs weakens confidence that the findings were the result of the intervention rather than extraneous variables.
- The overall purpose of critiquing such studies is to assess the validity of the findings and to determine whether these findings are worth incorporating into the nurse's personal practice.

REFERENCES

Barkauskas V, Lusk S, Eakin B: Selecting control interventions for clinical outcome studies, *West J Nurs Res* 27:346-363, 2005.

Budin WC, Hoskins CN, Haber J, Sherman DW: Breast cancer: Education, counseling and adjustment among patients and partners: a randomized clinical trial, *Nurs Res* 57(3):199-213, 2008.

Campbell D, Stanley J: *Experimental and quasiexperimental designs for research*, Chicago, 1966, Rand-McNally.

Duffy ME: The randomized controlled trial: basic considerations, *Clin Nurse Spec* 20(2):62-64, 2006.

Hall G, Bogan A, Dreis S, et al: New directions in peritoneal dialysis patient training, *Nephrol Nurs J* 31:159-163, 2004.

Jones EG, Renger R, Youngmi K, et al: Self-efficacy for health-related behaviors among deaf adults, *Res Nurs Health* 30:185-192, 2007.

Meneses DK, McNees P, Loerzel W, et al: Transition from treatment to survivorship: effects of a psychoeducational intervention on quality of life in breast cancer survivors, *Oncol Nurs Forum* 34:1007-1016, 2007.

Santacroce SJ, Marccarelli L, Grey M: Intervention fidelity, *Nurs Res* 53:63-66, 2004.

Wang D, Bakhai A, eds: *Clinical trials: a practical guide to design, analysis and reporting*, Chicago, 2006, Remedica.

Weinrich SP, Seger R, Curtsinger T, et al: Impact of pretest on posttest knowledge scores with a Solomon four research design, *Cancer Nurs* 30:E16-E28, 2007.

Whittemore R, Melkus G: Designing a research study, *Diabetes Educ* 34:201-216, 2008.

FOR FURTHER STUDY

evolve Go to Evolve at http://evolve.elsevier.com/LoBiondo/ for review questions, critiquing exercises, and additional research articles for practice in reviewing and critiquing.

9

Nonexperimental Designs

Geri LoBiondo-Wood and Judith Haber

KEY TERMS

case control study
cohort study
clinical practice guidelines
correlational study
cross-sectional study
developmental study
ex post facto study
integrative review
longitudinal study
meta-analysis
methodological research
prospective study
psychometrics
relationship/difference studies
repeated measures studies
retrospective study
secondary analysis
survey studies
systematic review

LEARNING OUTCOMES

After reading this chapter, you should be able to do the following:

- Describe the overall purpose of nonexperimental designs.
- Describe the characteristics of survey, relationship, and difference designs.
- Define the differences between survey, relationship, and difference designs. List the advantages and disadvantages of surveys and each type of relationship and difference designs.
- Identify methodological and secondary analysis methods of research.
- Identify the purposes of methodological and secondary analysis methods of research.
- Describe the purposes of a systematic review, meta-analysis, integrative review, and clinical practice guidelines.
- Define the differences between a systematic review, meta-analysis, integrative review, and clinical practice guidelines.
- Discuss relational inferences versus causal inferences as they relate to nonexperimental designs.
- Identify the critical appraisal criteria used to critique nonexperimental research designs.
- Apply the critiquing criteria to the evaluation of nonexperimental research designs as they appear in research reports.
- Apply the critiquing criteria to the evaluation of systematic reviews and clinical practice guidelines.
- Evaluate the strength and quality of evidence by nonexperimental designs.
- Evaluate the strength and quality of evidence provided by systematic reviews, meta-analysis, integrative reviews, and clinical practice guidelines.

STUDY RESOURCES

evolve Go to Evolve at http://evolve.elsevier.com/LoBiondo/ for review questions, critiquing exercises, and additional research articles for practice in reviewing and critiquing.

Many phenomena of interest and relevant to nursing do not lend themselves to an experimental design. For example, nurses studying cancer-related fatigue may be interested in the amount of fatigue, variations in fatigue, and patient fatigue in response to chemotherapy. The investigator would not design an experimental study that would potentially intensify an aspect of a patient's fatigue just to study the fatigue experience. Instead, the researcher would examine the factors that contribute to the variability in a patient's cancer-related fatigue experience using a nonexperimental design. Nonexperimental designs are used in studies in which the researcher wishes to construct a picture of a phenomenon; explore events, people, or situations as they naturally occur; or test relationships and differences among variables. Nonexperimental designs may construct a picture of a phenomenon at one point or over a period of time.

In experimental research the independent variable is manipulated; in nonexperimental research it is not. In nonexperimental research the independent variables have naturally occurred, so to speak, and the investigator cannot directly control them by manipulation. In contrast, in an experimental design the researcher actively manipulates one or more variables. In a nonexperimental design the researcher explores relationships or differences among the variables. Nonexperimental research requires a clear, concise research question or hypothesis that is based on a theoretical framework. Even though the researcher does not actively manipulate the variables, the concepts of control and potential sources of bias (see Chapter 7) should be considered as much as possible. Nonexperimental research designs provide Level IV evidence. The strength of evidence provided by nonexperimental designs is not as strong as that for experimental designs because there is a different degree of control within the study; that is, the independent variable is not manipulated, subjects are not randomized, and there is no control group. Yet the information yielded by these types of studies is critical to developing a base of evidence for practice and may represent the best evidence available to answer research or clinical questions.

Researchers are not in agreement on how to classify nonexperimental studies. A continuum of quantitative research design is presented in Figure 9-1. Nonexperimental studies explore the relationships or the differences between variables. This chapter divides nonexperimental designs into survey studies and relationship/difference studies as illustrated in Box 9-1. These categories are somewhat flexible, and other sources may classify nonexperimental studies in a different way. Some studies fall exclusively within one of these categories, whereas many other studies have characteristics of more than one category (Table 9-1). As you read the research

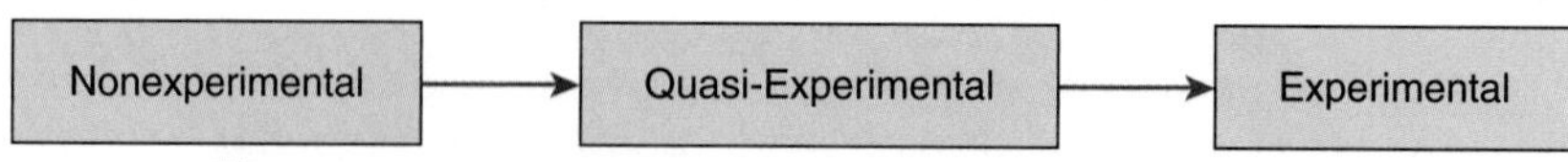

Figure 9-1 Continuum of quantitative research design.

BOX 9-1 Summary of Nonexperimental Research Designs

I. SURVEY STUDIES
A. Descriptive
B. Exploratory
C. Comparative

II. RELATIONSHIP/DIFFERENCE STUDIES
A. Correlational studies
B. Developmental studies
1. Cross-sectional
2. Longitudinal, prospective, and cohort
3. Retrospective, ex post facto, and case control

TABLE 9-1 Examples of Studies with More Than One Design Label

Design Type	Study's Purpose
Descriptive, longitudinal with retrospective, longitudinal with medical records review	To assess patient and provider responses to a computerized symptom assessment system (Carpenter et al., 2008)
Descriptive, exploratory, secondary analysis of a randomized controlled trial	To identify the predictors of fatigue 30 days after completing adjuvant chemotherapy for breast cancer and whether differences are observed between a sleep intervention and a healthy eating attention control group in predicting fatigue (Wielgus et al., 2009)
Correlational, cross-sectional, descriptive	To examine the relations of religion and spirituality to glycemic control in black women with type 2 diabetes (Newlin et al., 2008)
Prospective, cohort	To determine factors predictive of parenting self-efficacy at 12 to 48 hours after childbirth and at 1 month postpartum (Bryanton et al., 2008)
Cross-sectional, predictive correlational	To test theoretically derived relationships between the types and levels of violence exposure and experiences; coping; physical, behavioral, and mental health outcomes (Fredland et al., 2008)

literature you will often find that researchers who are conducting a nonexperimental study use several design classifications for one study. This chapter introduces the various types of nonexperimental designs and discusses their advantages and disadvantages, the use of nonexperimental research, the issues of causality, and the critiquing process as it relates to nonexperimental research. The Critical Thinking Decision Path on the following page outlines the path to the choice of a nonexperimental design.

In addition to nonexperimental studies, there are other types of research methods that contribute to the provision of a practice based on evidence. These methods are: methodological research, secondary analysis, meta-analysis, systematic reviews, integrative reviews, and clinical practice guidelines.

EVIDENCE-BASED PRACTICE TIP

When critically appraising nonexperimental studies, you need to be aware of possible sources of bias that can be introduced at any point in the study.

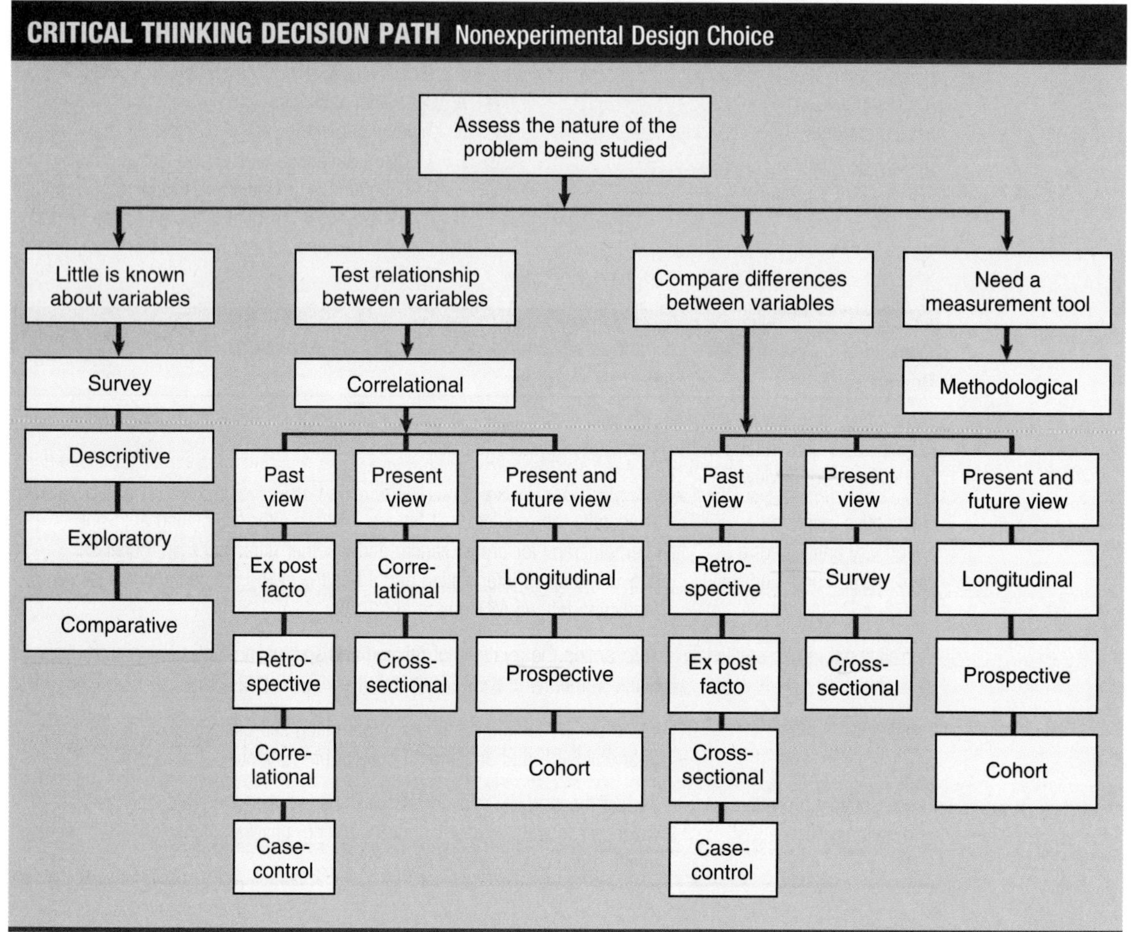

SURVEY STUDIES

The broadest category of nonexperimental designs is the survey study. **Survey studies** are further classified as descriptive, exploratory, or comparative. *Descriptive, exploratory,* or *comparative surveys* collect detailed descriptions of existing variables and use the data to justify and assess current conditions and practices or to make plans for improving health care practices. You will find that the terms *exploratory, descriptive, comparative,* and *survey* are used either alone, interchangeably, or together to describe the design of a study (see Table 9-1).

- Investigators use a descriptive or exploratory survey design to search for accurate information about the characteristics of particular subjects, groups, institutions, or situations or about the frequency of a phenomenon's occurrence, particularly when little is known about the phenomenon. Box 9-2 provides examples of survey studies.
- The types of variables of interest in a survey can be classified as opinions, attitudes, or facts.

BOX 9-2 Survey Design Examples

- Doorenbos and colleagues (2008) conducted a survey of the general Oncology Nurses Society (ONS) membership (with an overall response rate of 713), to determine the priorities of oncology nursing research, including the effect of evidence-based practice resources as identified by the ONS membership.
- Miller and colleagues (2009) conducted a computer-assisted telephone survey of 1,233 adult cancer survivors to assess dietary supplement use and its association with demographic and health-related characteristics. A secondary purpose was to investigate differences in supplement use patterns by cancer site.
- Lopez-McKee and colleagues (2008) conducted a descriptive survey of 68 Mexican-American women who had been identified as regular or infrequent users of mammography for screening based on screening history to examine the relationships between cancer fatalism and other sociocognitive behavioral determinants. Subjects were contacted by phone and invited to participate in a telephone survey.

- Fact variables include attributes of individuals that are a function of their membership in society, such as gender, income level, political and religious affiliations, ethnicity, occupation, and educational level.
- Survey studies provide the basis for further development of programs and interventions. In the ONS survey example (see Box 9-2), fact variables such as gender, age, position, and education were gathered from subjects.
- Surveys are described as comparative when they are used to determine differences between variables. Box 9-2 provides an example of a comparative, descriptive survey by Lopez-McKee and colleagues (2008).
- Data in survey research can be collected through a questionnaire or an interview (see Chapter 12).
- Surveys have either small or large samples of subjects drawn from defined populations, can be either broad or narrow, and can be made up of people or institutions.

For example, if a primary care rehabilitation unit based on a case management model were to be established in a hospital, a survey might be completed on the prospective applicants' attitudes with regard to case management before the unit staff are selected. In a broader example, if a hospital were contemplating converting all patient care units to a case management model, a survey might be conducted to determine attitudes of a representative sample of nurses in the hospital toward case management. The data might provide the basis for projecting in-service needs of nursing regarding case management. The scope and depth of a survey are a function of the nature of the problem.

In surveys investigators attempt only to relate one variable to another, or assess differences between variables, but they do not attempt to determine causation. The two major advantages of surveys are that a great deal of information can be obtained from a large population in a fairly economical manner and that survey research information can be surprisingly accurate. If a sample is representative of the population (see Chapter 10), a relatively small number of subjects can provide an accurate picture of the population.

Survey studies have several disadvantages. First, the information obtained in a survey tends to be superficial. The breadth rather than the depth of the information is emphasized. Second, conducting a survey requires a great deal of expertise in various research areas. The survey investigator must know sampling techniques, questionnaire construction, interviewing, and data analysis to produce a reliable and valid study. Third, large-scale surveys can be time-consuming and costly, although the use of on-site personnel can reduce costs.

HELPFUL HINT
You should recognize that a well-constructed survey can provide a wealth of data about a particular phenomenon of interest, even though causation is not being examined.

EVIDENCE-BASED PRACTICE TIP
Evidence gained from a survey may be coupled with clinical expertise and applied to a similar population to develop an educational program to enhance knowledge and skills in a particular clinical area (e.g., a survey designed to measure the nursing staff's knowledge and attitudes about evidence-based practice where the data are used to develop an evidence-based practice staff development course).

RELATIONSHIP AND DIFFERENCE STUDIES

Investigators also try to trace the relationships or differences between variables that can provide a deeper insight into a phenomenon. These studies can be classified as relationship or difference studies. The following types of relationship/difference studies are discussed: correlational studies and developmental studies.

Correlational Studies

In a correlational study an investigator examines the *relationship* between two or more variables. The researcher

- Is not testing whether one variable causes another variable or how different one variable is from another variable.
- Is testing whether the variables co-vary; that is, as one variable changes, does a related change occur in the other variable.
- Is interested in quantifying the strength of the relationship between variables or in testing a hypothesis or research questions about a specific relationship.

The positive or negative direction of the relationship is also a central concern (see Chapter 14 for an explanation of the correlation coefficient). For example, in their correlational study, Horgas and colleagues (2008) (see Appendix C) examined if there were relationships among race (black and white) and functional disability (physical and social functioning) in older adults. This study tested multiple variables (pain, race, and disability) to assess the relationship among these variables in a sample of community-dwelling black and white older adults. The researchers concluded that having greater functionality-limiting medical diagnoses was associated with increased pain; thus the variables were related to (not causal of) outcomes. Each step of this study was consistent with the aims of exploring the relationship among variables.

It should be remembered that the researchers were not testing a cause-and-effect relationship. All that is known is that the researchers found a relationship and that one variable, pain (pain was significantly associated with or related to greater physical and social functional disability in both physical and social functional domains), varied in a consistent way with the variable of physical and social functional ability for the particular sample studied. When reviewing a correlational study, remember what relationship the researcher tested and notice whether the researcher implied a relationship that is consistent with the theoretical framework and hypotheses being tested. Correlational studies offer researchers and research consumers the following advantages:

- An increased flexibility when investigating complex relationships among variables.
- An efficient and effective method of collecting a large amount of data about a problem.
- A potential for evidence-based application in clinical settings.
- A potential foundation for future, experimental research studies.
- A framework for exploring the relationship between variables that cannot be inherently manipulated (e.g., pain caused functional disability).

You will find that the correlational design has a quality of realism and is particularly appealing because it suggests the potential for practical solutions to clinical problems. The following are disadvantages of correlational studies:

- The researcher is unable to manipulate the variables of interest.
- The researcher does not employ randomization in the sampling procedures because of dealing with preexisting groups, and therefore generalizability is decreased.
- The researcher is unable to determine a causal relationship between the variables because of the lack of manipulation, control, and randomization.
- The strength and quality of evidence is limited by the associative nature of the relationship between the variables.
- A misuse of a correlational design would be if the researcher concluded that a causal relationship exists between the variables.

Correlational studies may be further labeled as *descriptive correlational* or *predictive correlational.* Given the level of evidence provided by the studies in this category, the ability to generalize the findings has some limitations, but often authors conclude the article with some very thoughtful recommendations for future studies in the specific area. The study by Horgas and colleagues (Appendix C) is a well-presented example of a clinical study that uses a correlational design. The inability to draw causal statements should not lead you to conclude that a nonexperimental correlational study uses a weak design. In terms of evidence for practice, the researchers, based on the literature review and their findings, frame the utility of the results in light of previous research and therefore help to establish the "best available" evidence that, combined with clinical expertise, informs clinical decision of the study's applicability to a specific patient population. A correlational design is a very useful design for clinical research studies because many of the phenomena of clinical interest are beyond the researcher's ability to manipulate, control, and randomize.

EVIDENCE-BASED PRACTICE TIP

Establishment of a strong relationship in predictive correlational studies often lends support for attempting to influence the independent variable in a future intervention study.

Developmental Studies

There are also classifications of nonexperimental designs that use a time perspective. Investigators who use **developmental studies** are concerned not only with the existing status and the relationship and differences among phenomena at one point in time but also with changes that result from elapsed time. The following three types of developmental study designs are discussed: cross-sectional, longitudinal or prospective, and retrospective (also labeled as ex post facto or case control). Remember that in the literature, however, studies may be designated by more than one design name. This practice is accepted because many studies have elements of several nonexperimental designs. Table 9-1 provides examples of studies classified with more than one design label.

Cross-Sectional Studies

A **cross-sectional study** examines data at one point in time, that is, data collected on only one occasion with the same subjects rather than with the same subjects at several time points. For example, Hall, Rayens, and Peden (2008) conducted a cross-sectional study:

- The objectives were to identify maternal predictors of children's internalizing and externalizing behaviors.
- The study explored the impact of mothers' thinking, mothers' stressors, and self-esteem on mothers' depression and, in turn, if there was a direct effect of the mothers' self-perception on the children's behavior.
- Subjects were 205 low-income mothers.
- Age of the mothers ranged from 18 to 45.
- Approximately half were Caucasian and half African American.
- Ages of the children ranged from 2 to 6 years.

In this study, the sample subjects participated on one occasion; that is, data were collected on only one occasion from each subject and represented a cross section of mothers and children rather than the researchers following a group of mothers and children over time. The purpose of this study was not to test causality but to explore the potential relationships between and among variables that can be related to maternal depression and subsequently to children's behavior.

Cross-sectional studies can explore relationships and correlations, or differences and comparisons, or both.

EVIDENCE-BASED PRACTICE TIP

Replication of significant findings in nonexperimental studies, using similar and/or different populations, increases your confidence in the conclusions offered by the researcher and the strength of evidence generated by consistent findings from more than one study.

Longitudinal/Prospective/Cohort Studies

In contrast to the cross-sectional design, **longitudinal, prospective,** or **cohort studies** collect data from the same group at different points in time. Prospective, longitudinal, or cohort studies also explore differences and relationships. Longitudinal, prospective, or cohort studies also are referred to as **repeated measures studies.** These terms are interchangeable. For instance, the investigator conducting a study with diabetic children could elect to use a longitudinal design. In that case the investigator could collect yearly data or follow the same children over a number of years to compare changes in the variables at different ages. By collecting data from each subject at yearly intervals, a longitudinal perspective of the diabetic process is accomplished. An example of a cohort study by Chen and colleagues (2008) collected data from 286 older hospitalized patients to describe their functional trajectory during hospitalization and 6 months after hospitalization. Subjects were measured on multiple variables within 48 hours of admission, before discharge, and 3 months and 6 months after hospitalization. These multiple time measurement periods allowed the researchers to study functional changes over a time period.

Cross-sectional and longitudinal designs have many advantages and disadvantages. When assessing the appropriateness of a cross-sectional study versus a longitudinal study, you should first assess the nature of the research question: What is the researcher's goal in light of the theoretical framework and the strength of evidence that will be provided by the findings? For example, in the Chen and colleagues (2008) study, the researchers wished to explore what changes occurred over time in the functional trajectory of an older hospitalized cohort sample; therefore a prospective (longitudinal or cohort) design seems more appropriate. Longitudinal research allows clinicians to assess the incidence of a problem over time and potential reasons for changes in the variables of study. However, the disadvantages inherent in a longitudinal design also must be considered. Data collection may be of long duration and costs therefore high because of the time it takes for the subjects to progress to each data-collection point. Internal validity threats such as testing and mortality also are ever-present and unavoidable in a longitudinal study. Subject loss to follow-up and attrition, whether due to dropout or death, may lead to unintended sample bias that affects internal validity and external validity or generalizability of the findings.

These realities make a longitudinal design costly in terms of time, effort, and money. There is also a chance of confounding variables that could affect the interpretation of the results. Subjects in such a study may respond in a socially desirable way that they believe is congruent with the investigator's expectations (see Hawthorne effect in Chapter 7). However, despite the pragmatic constraints imposed by a longitudinal study, the researcher should proceed with this design if the theoretical framework supports a longitudinal developmental perspective.

One advantage of a longitudinal study is that each subject is followed separately and thereby serves as his or her own control; other advantages are that increased depth of responses can be obtained and early trends in the data can be analyzed. The researcher can assess changes in the variables of interest over time, and both relationships and differences can be explored between variables. Additional advantages and disadvantage of cross-sectional and longitudinal studies are:

- Cross-sectional studies, when compared to longitudinal studies/prospective/cohort studies, are less time-consuming, less expensive, and thus more manageable for the researcher.
- Large amounts of data can be collected at one point, making the results more readily available.
- The confounding variable of maturation, resulting from the elapsed time, is not present.
- The investigator's ability to establish an in-depth developmental assessment of the interrelationships of the phenomena being studied is lessened.

Thus the researcher is unable to determine whether the change that occurred is related to the change that was predicted because the same subjects were not followed over a period of time. In other words, the subjects are unable to serve as their own controls (see Chapter 7). In summary, longitudinal studies begin in the present and end in the future, and cross-sectional studies look at a broader perspective of a cross section of the population at a specific point in time.

EVIDENCE-BASED PRACTICE TIP

The quality of evidence provided by a longitudinal, prospective, or cohort study is stronger than that from other nonexperimental designs because the researcher can determine the incidence of a problem and its possible causes.

TABLE 9-2 Paradigm for the Ex Post Facto Design

Groups (Not Randomly Assigned)	Independent Variable (Not Manipulated by Investigator)	Dependent Variable
Exposed group: cigarette smokers	X Cigarette smoking	Y_e Lung cancer
Control group: nonsmokers		Y_c No lung cancer

Retrospective/Ex Post Facto/Case Control Studies

A **retrospective study** is essentially the same as an **ex post facto study** and a **case control study.** Epidemiologists primarily use the term *retrospective* or *case control,* whereas social scientists prefer the term *ex post facto* (see Chapter 18). In either case, the dependent variable already has been affected by the independent variable, and the investigator attempts to link present events to events that occurred in the past. When scientists wish to explain causality or the factors that determine the occurrence of events or conditions, they prefer to use an experimental design. However, they cannot always manipulate the independent variable, *X,* or use random assignments. When experimental designs that test the effect of an intervention or condition cannot be employed, ex post facto studies may be used. Ex post facto literally means "from after the fact." Ex post facto, retrospective, or case control studies also are known as *causal-comparative* studies or *comparative* studies. As we discuss this design further, you will see that many elements of ex post facto research are similar to quasi-experimental designs because they explore differences between variables (Campbell & Stanley, 1963).

In retrospective/ex post facto/case control studies, a researcher hypothesizes, for instance,

- That *X* (cigarette smoking) is related to and a determinant of *Y* (lung cancer).
- But *X,* the presumed cause, is not manipulated and subjects are not randomly assigned to groups.
- Rather, a group of subjects who have experienced *X* (cigarette smoking) in a normal situation is located and a control group of subjects who have not experienced *X* is chosen.
- The behavior, performance, or condition (lung tissue) of the two groups is compared to determine whether the exposure to *X* had the effect predicted by the hypothesis.

Table 9-2 illustrates this example. Examination of Table 9-2 reveals that although cigarette smoking appears to be a determinant of lung cancer, the researcher is still not able to conclude that a causal relationship exists between the variables because the independent variable has not been manipulated and subjects were not randomly assigned to groups.

Nannini and colleagues (2008) conducted a retrospective study in which they explored the role of substance abuse (smoking, alcohol, and drug use) and weight gain of 15 pounds during pregnancy as potential mediators of the relationship between recent partner abuse and infant birth weight and to explore the role of demographic factors as moderators for the impact of abuse on infant birth weight. Data on the variables were abstracted from the medical records of 1,969 women who had been screened for domestic abuse during pregnancy. From the data gathered, recent physical or psychological abuse had a small but significant effect on birth weight and single marital status was the strongest demographic predictor of decreased infant weight.

A study by Gregory (2008) is another example of a retrospective, case control study.

- The objective was to improve our understanding of the relationship of clinical predictors of necrotizing enterocolitis (NEC) in premature infants.
- Data were collected from 247 medical records of infants diagnosed with NEC. The researchers also correctly concluded that the model requires further development and testing.

The advantages of the retrospective/ex post facto design are similar to those of the correlational design. The additional benefit of the ex post facto/retrospective/case control design is that it offers a higher level of control than a correlational study, thereby increasing the confidence the research consumer would have in the evidence provided by the findings. For example, in the cigarette smoking study, a group of nonsmokers' lung tissue samples are compared with samples of smokers' lung tissue. This comparison enables the researcher to establish the existence of a differential effect of cigarette smoking on lung tissue. However, the researcher remains unable to draw a causal linkage between the two variables, and this inability is the major disadvantage of the retrospective/ex post facto/case control design.

Another disadvantage of retrospective research is the problem of an alternative hypothesis being the reason for the documented relationship. If the researcher obtains data from two existing groups of subjects, such as one that has been exposed to *X* and one that has not, and the data support the hypothesis that *X* is related to *Y*, the researcher cannot be sure whether *X* or some extraneous variable is the real cause of the occurrence of *Y*. As such, the impact or effect of the relationship cannot be estimated accurately. Finding naturally occurring groups of subjects who are similar in all respects except for their exposure to the variable of interest is very difficult. There is always the possibility that the groups differ in some other way, such as exposure to other lung irritants, such as asbestos, that can affect the findings of the study and produce spurious or unreliable results. Consequently, you need to cautiously evaluate the conclusions drawn by the investigator.

HELPFUL HINT

When reading research reports, you will note that at times researchers classify a study's design with more than one design type label. This is correct because research studies often reflect aspects of more than one design label.

Longitudinal/prospective/cohort studies are less common than retrospective/ex post facto/ case control studies. This may be explained by the fact that it can take a long time for the phenomenon of interest to become evident in a prospective study. For example, if researchers were studying pregnant women who regularly consume alcohol, it would take 9 months for the effect of low birth weight in the subjects' infants to become evident and much longer to collect the data from the total sample size needed. The threats to internal validity or bias that may arise in a prospective study are related to the internal validity threats of mortality, instrumentation, and testing. However, longitudinal/prospective/cohort studies are considered to be stronger than retrospective studies because of the degree of control that can be imposed on extraneous variables that might confound the data and lead to bias.

HELPFUL HINT

Remember that nonexperimental designs can test relationships, differences, comparisons, or predictions, depending on the purpose of the study.

PREDICTION AND CAUSALITY IN NONEXPERIMENTAL RESEARCH

A concern of researchers and research consumers are the issues of prediction and causality. Researchers are interested in explaining cause-and-effect relationships, that is, estimating the effect of one phenomenon on another without bias. Historically, researchers have said that only experimental research can support the concept of causality. For example, nurses are interested in discovering what causes anxiety in many settings. If we can uncover the causes, we could develop interventions that would prevent or decrease the anxiety. Causality makes it necessary to order events chronologically; that is, if we find in a randomly assigned experiment that event 1 (stress) occurs before event 2 (anxiety) and that those in the stressed group were anxious whereas those in the unstressed group were not, we can say that the hypothesis of stress causing anxiety is supported by these empirical observations. If these results were found in a nonexperimental study where some subjects underwent the stress of surgery and were anxious and others did not have surgery and were not anxious, we would say that there is an association or relationship between stress (surgery) and anxiety. But on the basis of the results of a nonexperimental study, we could not say that the stress of surgery caused the anxiety.

Many variables (e.g., anxiety) that nurse researchers wish to study cannot be manipulated, nor would it be wise or ethical to try to manipulate them. Yet there is a need to have studies that can assert a predictive or causal sequence; in light of this need, many nurse researchers are using several analytical techniques that can explain the relationships among variables to establish predictive or causal links. These analytical techniques are called *causal modeling, model testing,* and *associated causal analysis techniques* (Kaplan, 2008; Kline, 2005). The reader of research also will find the terms *path analysis, LISREL, analysis of covariance structures, structural equation modeling (SEM),* and *hierarchical linear modeling (HLM)* used to describe the statistical techniques (see Chapter 14) used in these studies. These terms do not designate the design of a study but are statistical tests that are used in many nonexperimental designs to predict how precisely a dependent variable can be predicted based on an independent variable. The study by Horgas and colleagues (2008) (see Appendix C) used structural equation modeling to assess the relationship of the variables that they tested to assess which variables affected pain and disability. Figure 2 in Appendix C displays a model of how the variables predicted or were related to each other.

Researchers at times want to make a forecast or prediction about how patients will respond to an intervention or a disease process or how successful individuals will be in a particular setting or field of specialty. In this case, a model may be tested to assess which independent variables can best explain the dependent variable(s). For example, Bryanton and colleagues (2008) wanted to determine the factors predictive of parenting self-efficacy at 12 and 48 hours after childbirth and 1 month postpartum.

- The study was based on integrating three theories of self-efficacy.
- Subjects were recruited from one location over the period of October 2004 to December 2005.
- A total sample of 652 subjects met the sample size requirements for testing for the predictors of self-efficacy.
- The research question was addressed by using multiple logistic regression.

Based on the framework, sample size, multiple instruments, and analyses, the researchers had findings about the sample's parenting self-efficacy prospectively, parenting self-efficacy after childbirth, and parenting self-efficacy at 1 month after childbirth. The use of a model allowed for the testing of the independent variables and to predict which of the variables were significant or predictive of self-efficacy at each time period.

As nurse researchers develop their programs of research in a specific area, more studies that test models are available. The statistics used in model-testing studies are advanced, but the beginning reader should be able to read the article and understand the purpose of the study and if the model generated was logical and developed with a solid basis from the literature and past research. This section cites several studies that conducted sound tests of theoretical models. A full description of the techniques and principles of causal modeling is beyond the scope of this text; if you want to read about these advanced techniques, a book such as that by Kaplan (2008) is appropriate to consult.

HELPFUL HINT

Nonexperimental clinical research studies have progressed to the point where prediction models are often used to explore or test relationships between independent and dependent variables.

EVIDENCE-BASED PRACTICE TIP

Research studies that use nonexperimental designs that provide Level IV evidence often precede and provide the foundation for building a program of research that leads to experimental designs that test the effectiveness of nursing interventions.

ADDITIONAL TYPES OF QUANTITATIVE METHODS

Other types of quantitative studies complement the science of research. These additional research methods provide a means of viewing and interpreting phenomena that gives further breadth and knowledge to nursing science and practice. The additional types are methodological research, systematic reviews, including meta-analysis and integrative reviews, as well as clinical practice guidelines and secondary analysis.

Methodological Research

Methodological research is the development and evaluation of data-collection instruments, scales, or techniques. As you will find in succeeding chapters (see Chapters 12 and 13), methodology greatly influences research and the evidence produced.

The most significant and critically important aspect of methodological research addressed in measurement development is called **psychometrics.** Psychometrics deals with the theory and development of measurement instruments (such as questionnaires) or measurement techniques (such as observational techniques) through the research process. Psychometrics thus deals with the measurement of a concept, such as anxiety, quality of life, or caregiver burden, with reliable and valid instruments (see Chapter 13 for a discussion of reliability and validity). Psychometrics is a critical issue for nurse researchers. Nurse researchers have used the principles of psychometrics to develop and test measurement instruments that focus on nursing phenomena. Nurse researchers also use instruments developed by other disciplines such as psychology and sociology. Sound measurement tools are critical to the reliability and validity of a study. Although a study's purpose, problems, and procedures may be clear and the data analysis correct and consistent, if the measurement instrument that was used by the researcher has inherent psychometric problems (e.g., lack reliability and validity) (see Chapter 13), the findings are rendered questionable or limited.

The main problem for nurse researchers is locating appropriate measurement tools. Many of the phenomena of interest to nursing practice and research are intangible, such as interpersonal conflict, resilience, quality of life, coping, and symptom management. The intangible nature of various phenomena, yet the recognition of the need to measure them, places methodological research in an important position. Methodological research differs from other designs of research. First, it does not include all of the research process steps as discussed in Chapter 1. Second, to implement its techniques the researcher must have a sound knowledge of psychometrics or must consult with a researcher knowledgeable in psychometric techniques. The methodological researcher is not interested in the relationship of the independent variable and dependent variable or in the effect of an independent variable on a dependent variable. The methodological researcher is interested in identifying an intangible construct (concept) and making it tangible with a paper-and-pencil instrument or observation protocol.

A methodological study basically includes the following steps:

- Defining the construct/concept or behavior to be measured
- Formulating the tool's items
- Developing instructions for users and respondents
- Testing the tool's reliability and validity

These steps require a sound, specific, and exhaustive literature review to identify the theories underlying the construct. The literature review provides the basis of item formulation. Once the items have been developed, the researcher assesses the tool's reliability and validity (see Chapter 13). Various aspects of these procedures may differ according to the instrument's use, purpose, and stage of development.

As an example of methodological research, Moser and colleagues (2009) identified the concept of perceived control; they defined this concept as "an individual's belief that he or she has the resources required to cope with negative events in a way that positively influence such events" (p. 42). They were specifically interested in the role of perceived control in patients with chronic illness, particularly cardiovascular disease. The researchers defined the concept conceptually and operationally and followed through by testing the instrument for reliability and validity (see Chapter 13). Common considerations that researchers incorporate into methodological research are outlined in Table 9-3. Many more examples of methodological research can be found in nursing research literature and many nursing journals. Psychometric or methodological studies are found primarily in journals that report research. The *Journal of Nursing Measurement* is devoted to the publication of information on instruments, tools, and approaches for measurement of variables. The specific procedures of methodological research are beyond the scope of this book, but you are urged to look closely at the tools used in studies.

TABLE 9-3 Common Considerations in the Development of Measurement Tools

Consideration	Example
The well-constructed scale, test, interview schedule, or other form of index should consist of an objective, standardized measure of samples of a behavior that has been clearly defined. Observations should be made on a small but carefully chosen sampling of the behavior of interest, thus permitting us to feel confident that the samples are representative.	In their report of the Controlled Attitudes Scale—Revised (CAS-R), the researchers discuss the development of the tool and multiple studies in which it was tested first (the Controlled Attitudes Scale [CAS]) and now the updated CAS-R. The CAS-R has evolved to be an eight-item scale. The scale has been tested in different cardiac samples. The scale also was based on a thorough review of the theoretical framework of perceived control and other research literature (Moser et al., 2009).
The tool should be standardized; that is, it should be a set of uniform items and response possibilities that are uniformly administered and scored.	In the study by Moser and colleagues (2009), the items are rated based on a patient's perception or attitude of control. The eight items are completed by the patient, or they can be read to the patient. Each item is scored using a Likert scale ranging from 1 to 5 points. The total score is obtained by summation of the ratings for each response.
The items of a measurement tool should be unambiguous; they should be clear-cut, concise, exact statements with only one idea per item. Negative stems or items with negatively phrased response possibilities result in a double negative and ambiguity in meaning and scoring.	In constructing a tool to measure job satisfaction, a nurse scientist writes the following: "I never feel that I don't have time to provide good nursing care." The response format consists of "Agree,""Undecided," and "Disagree." It is very likely that a response of "Disagree" will not reflect the respondent's true intent because of the confusion that is created by the double negatives. For example, one of the CAS-R items states, "I have considerable ability to control my symptoms" (p. 46).
The type of items used in any one test or scale should be restricted to a limited number of variations. Subjects who are expected to shift from one kind of item to another may fail to provide a true response as a result of the distraction of making such a change.	Mixing true-or-false items with questions that require a yes-or-no response and items that provide a response format of five possible answers is conducive to a high level of measurement error.
Items should not provide irrelevant clues. Unless carefully constructed, an item may furnish an indication of the expected response or answer. Furthermore, the correct answer or expected response to one item should not be given by another item.	An item that provides a clue to the expected answer may contain value words that convey cultural expectations, such as the following: "A good wife enjoys caring for her home and family."
The items of a measurement tool should not be made difficult by requiring unnecessarily complex or exact operations. Furthermore, the difficulty of an item should be appropriate to the level of the subjects being assessed. Limiting each item to one concept or idea helps accomplish this objective.	A test constructed to evaluate learning in an introductory course in research methods may contain an item that is inappropriate for the designated group, such as the following: "A nonlinear transformation of data to linear data is a useful procedure before testing a hypothesis of curvilinearity."

Continued

Common Considerations in the Development of Measurement Tools—cont'd

	Example
lictive, or measurement value of a tool legree to which it serves as an indicator of a ind significant area of behavior, known as the universe of content for the behavior. As already emphasized, a behavior must be clearly defined before it can be measured. The definition is developed from the universe of content, that is, the information and research findings that are available for the behavior of interest. The items should reflect that definition. To what extent the test items appear to accomplish this objective is an indication of the validity of the instrument.	Two nurse researchers, A and B, are studying the construct of quality of life. Each has defined this construct in a different way. Consequently, the measurement tool that each nurse devises will include different questions. The questions on each tool will reflect the universe of content for quality of life as defined by each researcher.
The instrument also should adequately cover the defined behavior. The primary consideration is whether the number and nature of items in the sample are adequate. If there are too few items, the accuracy or reliability of the measure must be questioned.	Very few people would be satisfied with an assessment of such traits as intelligence if the scales were limited to three items. Moser and colleagues (2009) discuss that the CAS had only four items, but based on testing, theoretical considerations, and practical considerations, additional items were added. This resulted in a 19-item scale, which on further testing resulted in the current eight-item scale.
The measure must prove its worth empirically through tests of reliability and validity.	A researcher should demonstrate to the reader that the scale is accurate and measures what it purports to measure (see Chapter 13). Moser and colleagues (2009) provide the data on the reliability and validity testing of the CAS-R scale (pp. 46-49).

Systematic Reviews, Meta-Analyses, and Integrative Reviews

Systematic reviews, meta-analyses, and integrative reviews are not designs per se, but research methods for searching, and integrating the literature related to a specific clinical issue based on a scientific approach that takes the results of many studies in a specific area, assesses the studies critically for reliability and validity (quality, quantity, and consistency) (see Chapters 1, 7, 17, and 18), and synthesizes the findings in order to inform practice. Systematic reviews and meta-analyses also grade the evidence on the design type (see Chapters 1 and 17).

Systematic Review

A **systematic review** is a summary of the quantitative research literature that used similar designs based on a focused clinical question. The goal is to bring together all of the studies concerning a particular clinical question and, using rigorous inclusion and exclusion criteria, assess the strength and quality of evidence provided by the chosen studies in relation to sampling issues, threats to internal validity (bias), external validity, and evaluate their results. The purpose is to report in a consolidated fashion the most current and valid research on intervention effectiveness and clinical knowledge, which will ultimately inform evidence-based decision making about the applicability of findings to clinical practice.

The studies in a systematic review once gathered from a comprehensive literature search (see Chapter 3) are assessed for quality, synthesized according to quality or focus, and practice recommendations are made and presented in an article. Often more than one person independently evaluates the studies to be included or excluded in the review. Generally the articles critically appraised are also presented in a table format, which helps you to easily identify the specific studies gathered for the review and their quality. Statistical methods may or may not be used to analyze the included studies.

Murray and colleagues (2009) conducted a systematic review to describe the determinants of place of end-of-life care for patients with cancer. The components of the report included:

- The clinical question was identified and the significance of the clinical issues were delineated.
- Search terms used were *place of care, place of death, hospice, home, nursing home, institution* or *residence, dying, terminal illness, terminally ill, palliative* or *palliative care, terminal illness, cancer, oncology* or *neoplasm,* and demographic factors.
- Years included in the search: 1997 to 2007.
- Databases searched: MEDLINE, EMBASE, PsycINFO, and CINAHL.
- How the articles were assessed was delineated.
- The findings from the literature were organized, critically appraised, and recommendations were made. The studies reviewed were also presented in an evidence table.

Berry and colleagues (2007) conducted a systematic review of oral hygiene practices for intensive care patients receiving mechanical ventilation. The process they used is as follows:

- The clinical question was identified and the significance to practice was described.
- The goal of the review was described.
- The team described how they formulated the clinical question, conducted the search of the literature, and consulted with experts.
- The method used to critically appraise the literature was outlined. The databases searched, the search terms, types of studies included, and the grading system used to evaluate the literature were presented.
- The methodological issues, results, and discussion of the findings were presented.
- Tables were used to display the studies reviewed.
- Recommendations were made based on the data from the studies retrieved.

Meta-Analysis

If statistical techniques are used to summarize and assess studies of the same design to obtain a precise estimate of effect (impact of the intervention or the association between the variables), the systematic review is called a meta-analysis. **Meta-analysis,** in addition to summarizing and appraising the quality of the literature, also statistically analyzes the data from each of the published studies, treating the studies as one large data set to obtain a precise estimate of the effect (impact) of the results of the studies included in the review. Each study is considered a unit of analysis, but all of the studies are combined for the analysis. Meta-analysis also requires a clear clinical question identification, an exhaustive and thorough search of the literature, a description of the terms used to search the databases, a list of the databases searched, years searched, and what system was used to grade the evidence (see Chapters 17 and 18). Meta-analysis is stronger because it is a rigorous process of evidence summarization rather than an effect estimate derived from a single study alone (see Chapter 10). Meta-analysis provides the most powerful and useful evidence available to guide practice, that is, Level I evidence (see Chapters 1, 17, and 18), to estimate the magnitude of an intervention's effect.

Rice and Stead (2008) conducted a meta-analysis for the Cochrane Collaboration (see Appendix E for the complete report). The objective for this meta-analysis was to determine the effectiveness of nursing-delivered smoking cessation interventions. This review follows the standard steps found in all Cochrane reviews, which are as follows:

- Plain language summary
- Background of the question
- Objectives of the search
- Methods for selecting studies for review
- Type of studies reviewed
- Types of participants, types of intervention, types of outcomes in the studies
- Search methods for finding studies
- Data collection
- Analysis of the located studies, including effect sizes
- References and tables to display the data

Integrative Reviews

You will also find reviews of an area of research or theory synthesis termed **integrative reviews** that critically appraise the literature in an area but without a statistical analysis. An integrative review is the broadest category of review (Whittemore, 2005). It can include either theoretical or research literature or both. An integrative review does not include a statistical analysis. An integrative review may include methodology studies, a theory review, or the results of differing research studies with wide-ranging clinical implications (Whittemore, 2005). An integrative review can include both quantitative or qualitative research. Statistics are not used to summarize and make conclusions about the studies.

Integrative Review: Research. Gatti (2008) conducted a research integrative review to identify research pertaining to perceived milk supply as a factor in successful breastfeeding outcomes, the relationship between perceived insufficient milk (PIM) supply and other variables, and the status of current tools to predict who was at risk for problems with milk supply in postpartum mothers. The process used to accomplish this review is as follows:

- Method: identified databases used were CINAHL, MEDLINE, and PubMed.
- Search was conducted in August, 2007.
- Search term used: *perceived milk supply.*
- Search limits: English language, human research from 1996 to 2007.

The article detailed the findings from the literature, including the type and number of studies, each topic area: effect of perceived insufficient milk and relationship with other variables, breastfeeding behaviors, and screening tools. There was an accompanying evidence table that listed the studies' designs, methods, and samples. Gatti also provided a discussion of the key findings in the literature and the limitations, gaps, and future directions for research and practice.

Integrative Review: Theoretical. Kiefer (2008) conducted a theoretical integrative review to determine how the concept of well-being is defined in the literature. The article included the databases searched, search terms used, years of literature included (1995 to 2007), type of literature used, and criteria for article inclusion.

For each of the review methods described—systematic, meta-analysis, or integrative—think about each method as one that progressively sifts and sorts research studies and the data until the highest quality of evidence is used to arrive at the conclusions. First the researcher combines the results of all the studies that focus on a specific question. The studies considered of lowest quality are then excluded and the data are reanalyzed. This process is repeated sequentially, excluding studies until only the studies of highest quality available are included in the analysis. An alteration in the overall results as an outcome of this sorting and separating process suggests how sensitive the conclusions are to the quality of studies included (Whittemore, 2005). No matter which type of review is completed, it is important to understand that the research studies reviewed still must be examined through your evidence-based practice lens. This means that evidence that you have derived through your critical appraisal and synthesis or derived through other researchers' review must be integrated with an individual clinician's expertise and patients' wishes.

You should note that a researcher who uses any of the systematic review methods of combining evidence does not conduct the original studies or analysis of data in the area, but rather takes the data from already published studies and synthesizes the information by following a set of controlled and systematic steps. Systematic methods for combining evidence are used to synthesize both nonexperimental and experimental research studies.

Finally, evidence-based practice requires that you determine, based on the strength and quality of the evidence provided by the systematic review coupled with your clinical expertise and patient values, whether or not you would consider a change in practice. For example, the meta-analysis by Rice and Stead (2008) in Appendix E details the important findings from the literature, and which of the findings could be used in nursing practice and which need further research.

Systematic reviews that use multiple randomized controlled trials (RCTs) to combine study results offer stronger evidence, Level I, in estimating the magnitude of an effect for an intervention (see Chapter 2, Table 2-3). The strength of evidence provided by systematic reviews is a key component for developing a practice based on evidence. *Meta-synthesis,* the qualitative counterpart to systematic reviews, uses qualitative principles to assess qualitative research and is described in Chapter 5.

EVIDENCE-BASED PRACTICE TIP

Evidence-based practice methods such as meta-analysis increase your ability to manage the ever-increasing volume of information produced to develop the best evidence-based practices.

Clinical Practice Guidelines

Clinical practice guidelines are becoming more readily available as evidence regarding practice grows. **Clinical practice guidelines** are systematically developed statements or recommendations that serve as a guide for practitioners and assist in linking practice and research. Guidelines are developed by professional organizations, government agencies, institutions, or convened expert panels. Practice guidelines provide clinicians with an algorithm for clinical management of, or decision making for specific diseases (e.g., colon cancer) or treatments (e.g., pain management). Not all practice guidelines are well developed or built on strong evidence and, like research, must be assessed before implementation. The research findings in a clinical practice guideline need to be evaluated for quality, quantity, and consistency.

Many organizations develop clinical practice guidelines. It is important to know which one to apply to your patients. For example, there are numerous evidence-based practice guidelines developed for the management of pain. These guidelines are available from organizations such as the American Pain Society, National Comprehensive Cancer Network, National Cancer

Institute, American College of Physicians, and the American Academy of Pain Medicine. You as a consumer of evidence need to be able to evaluate each of the guidelines and decide which is the most appropriate for your patient population.

There are several tools for appraising the quality of clinical practice guidelines. The Appraisal of Guidelines Research and Evaluation (AGREE) instrument is widely used to evaluate the applicability of a guideline to practice (AGREE Collaboration, 2003). The instrument contains six areas with a total of 23 questions rated on a 4-point scale. The AGREE guideline assesses:

1. The scope and purpose of the guideline
2. Stakeholder involvement
3. Rigor of the guideline development
4. Clarity and presentation of the guideline
5. Applicability of the guideline to practice
6. Demonstrated editorial independence of the developers

Clinical practice guidelines, although they are systematically developed and make explicit recommendations for practice, may be formatted differently. Practice guidelines should reflect the components listed. Many organizations such as the National Cancer Institutes, Oncology Nursing Society, and the American Heart Association have developed guidelines for practice. Generally these can be located on the organization's website or MEDLINE (see Chapter 3). Well-developed guidelines are constructed using the principles of a systematic review.

Secondary Analysis

Secondary analysis also is not a design but rather a research method in which the researcher takes previously collected and analyzed data from *one* study and reanalyzes the data or a subset of the data for a *secondary* purpose. The original study may be either an experimental or a nonexperimental design. For example, Anderson (2008) conducted a secondary analysis of data from the Substance Abuse and Mental Health Services Administration, Mentoring and Family Strengthening Prevention Initiative study conducted by Bellamy and colleagues (2004). The aim of the original study (Bellamy et al., 2004) was to determine the efficacy of various family-focused model programs on improving family relationships and decreasing youth problem behaviors. Anderson (2008) used the data to determine (1) the correlates of parenting stress across parents; (2) how stress varies across parent, child, and contextual domains (such as family structure, social support, and parent education); and (3) the relationship of parental stress with single parenting, parental health, family cohesion, and involvement (p. 341). The data from this study allowed further in-depth exploration of parenting stress experiences of traditionally underrepresented parent groups, including parents of adolescents and those parenting in high-risk communities. The data cannot be used to infer causality but do provide information for identifying parents at high risk of parenting stress.

HELPFUL HINT

As you read the literature, you will find labels such as *outcomes research, needs assessments, evaluation research,* and *quality assurance.* These studies are not designs per se. These studies use either experimental or nonexperimental designs. Studies with these labels are designed to test the effectiveness of health care techniques, programs, or interventions. When reading such a research study, the reader should assess which design was used and if the principles of the design, sampling strategy, and analysis are consistent with the study's purpose.

APPRAISING THE EVIDENCE

Nonexperimental Designs

Criteria for appraising nonexperimental designs are presented in the Critiquing Criteria box on the following page. When appraising nonexperimental research designs, you should keep in mind that such designs offer the researcher a lower level of control and an increased risk of bias. As such, the level of evidence provided by nonexperimental designs is not as strong as evidence generated by experimental designs in which manipulation, randomization, and control are used, but there are other important clinical research questions that need to be answered beyond the testing of interventions and experimental or quasi-experimental designs. The first step in critiquing research studies that use nonexperimental designs is to determine which type of design was used in the study. Often a statement describing the design of the study appears in the abstract and in the methods section of the report. If such a statement is not present, you should closely examine the paper for evidence of which type of design was employed. You should be able to discern that either a survey or a relationship design was used, as well as the specific subtype. For example, you would expect an investigation of self-concept development in children from birth to 5 years of age to be a relationship study using a longitudinal design. If a longitudinal study was used, you want to assess for possible threats to internal validity or bias such as mortality, testing, and instrumentation. Potential threats to internal or external validity should be recognized by the researchers at the end of the study and, in particular, the limitations section.

Next, evaluate the theoretical framework and underpinnings of the study to determine if a nonexperimental design was the most appropriate approach to the research question or hypothesis. For example, many of the studies on pain (e.g., intensity, severity, perception) discussed throughout this text are suggestive of a relationship between pain and any of the independent variables (diagnosis, coping style, ethnicity) under consideration where the independent variable cannot be manipulated. As such, these studies suggest a nonexperimental correlational, longitudinal/prospective/cohort, a retrospective/ex post facto, a case control, or a cross-sectional design. Investigators will use one of these designs to examine the relationship between the variables in naturally occurring groups. Sometimes you may think that it would have been more appropriate if the investigators had used an experimental or a quasi-experimental design. However, you must recognize that pragmatic or ethical considerations also may have guided the researchers in their choice of design (see Chapters 7 through 11).

Next you should assess whether the research question or hypothesis is consistent with a design in which the independent variable would be manipulated. Many times researchers merely wish to examine if relationships exist between variables. Therefore when you appraise such studies, the purpose of the study should be determined. If the purpose of the study did not include describing a cause-and-effect relationship, the researcher should not be criticized for not looking for one. However, you should be wary of a nonexperimental study in which the researcher suggests a cause-and-effect relationship in the findings.

Finally, the factor or factors that actually influence changes in the dependent variable can be ambiguous in nonexperimental designs. As with all complex phenomena, multiple factors can contribute to variability in the subjects' responses. When an experimental design is not used for controlling some of these extraneous variables that can influence results, the researcher must strive to provide as much control of them as possible within the context of a nonexperi-

CRITIQUING CRITERIA: *Nonexperimental Designs*

1. Which nonexperimental design is used in the study?
2. Based on the theoretical framework, is the rationale for the type of design evident?
3. How is the design congruent with the purpose of the study?
4. Is the design appropriate for the research question or hypothesis?
5. Is the design suited to the data-collection methods?
6. Does the researcher present the findings in a manner congruent with the design used?
7. Does the research go beyond the relational parameters of the findings and erroneously infer cause-and-effect relationships between the variables?
8. Are there any reasons to believe that there are alternative explanations for the findings?
9. Where appropriate, how does the researcher discuss the threats to internal validity (bias) and external validity (generalizability)?
10. How does the author identify the limitations of the study? That is, are the threats to internal validity (bias) and external validity identified?
11. Does the researcher make appropriate recommendations about the applicability based on the strength and quality of evidence provided by the nonexperimental design and the findings?

mental design, to decrease bias. For example, when it has not been possible to randomly assign subjects to treatment groups as an approach to controlling an independent variable, the researchers will most often use strict inclusion and exclusion criteria and calculate an adequate sample size using power analysis that will support a valid testing of how correlated (or predictive) the independent variable is to the dependent variable (see Chapter 10). Threats to internal and external validity or potential sources of bias represent a major influence when interpreting the findings of a nonexperimental study because they impose limitations to the generalizability of the results and applicability to practice. It is also important to remember that prediction of patient clinical outcomes is of critical value for clinical researchers. Nonexperimental designs can be used to make predictions if the study is designed with an adequate sample size (see Chapter 10), collects data consistently, and uses reliable and valid instruments (see Chapter 13).

When you critically appraise a systematic review, meta-analysis, or integrative review, some of the questions to consider are the following:

- Does the review address a focused question or purpose?
- Are there specific inclusion and exclusion criteria for independently judging whether or not the studies or literature provided (databases used, dates for search inclusion provided, and search terms) meet the eligibility criteria?
- Was there any publication bias in the studies reviewed (requires a critique of each study)?
- Are the studies included homogeneous?
  - Similar design
  - Similar interventions
  - Similar outcome measures
  - Are the studies assessed using a quality index or criteria?

If you are appraising methodological research, you need to apply the principles of reliability and validity (see Chapter 13). A secondary analysis needs to be reviewed from several perspectives. First, you need to understand if the researcher followed sound scientific logic in the secondary analysis completed. Second, you need to review the original study that the data were extracted from to assess the reliability and validity of the original study.

If you are critiquing one of the additional research methods discussed, it is important first to identify the method of research used. Once the research method is identified, its specific purpose and format need to be understood. The format and methods of secondary analysis, methodological research, and systematic reviews vary; knowing how they vary allows you to assess whether the process was applied appropriately. Clinical practice guidelines also have specific methods of appraisal and are often evaluated using the AGREE instrument. Some of the basic principles of these methods were presented in this chapter. The specific criteria for evaluating these methods are beyond the scope of this text, but the references provided will assist in this process. Even though the format and methods vary, it is important to remember that all research has a central goal: to answer questions scientifically and provide the strongest, most consistent evidence possible, while controlling for potential bias.

CRITICAL THINKING CHALLENGES

- The mid-term assignment for your research course is to critique an assigned study on the relationship of perception of pain severity and quality of life in advanced cancer patients. Your first job is to decide what kind of design was used and whether it was appropriate for the overall purpose of the study. You think it is a cross-sectional design, but other students think it is a quasi-experimental design because it has several specific hypotheses. How would you support your argument that you are correct?
- You are completing you senior practicum on a surgical unit, and for preconference your student group has just completed a search for studies related to the effectiveness of handwashing in decreasing the incidence of nosocomial infections, but the studies all use an ex post facto/case control design. You want to approach the nurse manager on the unit to present the evidence you have collected and critically appraised, but you are concerned about the strength of the evidence because the studies all use a nonexperimental design. How would you justify that this is the "best available evidence"?
- You are a member of a journal club at your hospital. Your group is interested in the effectiveness of smoking cessation interventions provided by nurses. An electronic search indicates that 12 individual research studies and one meta-analysis meet your inclusion criteria. Would your group begin with critically appraising the 12 individual studies or the one meta-analysis? Provide rationale for your choice, including consideration of the strength and quality of evidence provided by individual studies versus a meta-analysis.
- A patient in a primary care practice who has a history of a "heart murmur" called his nurse practitioner for a prescription for an antibiotic before having a periodontal (gum) procedure. When she responded that according to the new American Heart Association (AHA) clinical practice guideline, antibiotic prophylaxis is no longer considered appropriate for his heart murmur, the patient got upset, stating, "But I always take antibiotics … I want you to tell me why I should believe this guideline … How do I know my heart will not be damaged by listening to you!" What is the purpose of a clinical practice guideline and how would you as an NP respond to this patient?

KEY POINTS

- Nonexperimental research designs are used in studies that construct a picture or make an account of events as they naturally occur. The major difference between nonexperimental and experimental research is that in nonexperimental designs the independent variable is not actively manipulated by the investigator.
- Nonexperimental designs can be classified as either survey studies or relationship/difference studies.
- Survey studies and relationship/difference studies are both descriptive and exploratory in nature.
- Survey research collects detailed descriptions of existing phenomena and uses the data either to justify current conditions and practices or to make more intelligent plans for improving them.
- Relationship studies endeavor to explore the relationships between variables that provide deeper insight into the phenomena of interest.
- Correlational studies examine relationships.
- Developmental studies are further broken down into categories of cross-sectional studies, longitudinal/prospective/cohort studies, retrospective/ex post facto studies, and case control studies.
- Methodological research, secondary analysis, and systematic reviews are examples of other means of adding to the body of nursing research. Both the researcher and the reader must consider the advantages and disadvantages of each design.
- Systematic reviews are a key method for building evidence-based practice.
- Nonexperimental research designs do not enable the investigator to establish cause-and-effect relationships between the variables. Consumers must be wary of nonexperimental studies that make causal claims about the findings unless a causal modeling technique is used.
- Nonexperimental designs also offer the researcher the least amount of control. Threats to validity represent a major influence on the interpretation of a nonexperimental study because they impose limitations on the generalizability of the results and as such should be fully assessed by the critical reader.
- The critiquing process is directed toward evaluating the appropriateness of the selected nonexperimental design in relation to factors such as the research problem, theoretical framework, hypothesis, methodology, and data analysis and interpretation.
- Though nonexperimental designs do not provide the highest level of evidence (Level I), they do provide a wealth of data that become useful pieces for formulating both Level I and Level II studies that are aimed at developing and testing nursing interventions.

REFERENCES

AGREE Collaboration: Development and validation of an international appraisal instrument for assessing the quality of clinical practice guidelines; the AGREE project, *Qual Saf Health Care* 12:18-23, 2003.

Anderson LS: Predictors of parenting stress in a diverse sample of parents of early adolescents in high-risk communities, *Nurs Res* 57(1):340-350, 2008.

Bellamy ND, Springer UF, Sale EW, et al: Structuring a multi-site evaluation for youth mentoring programs to prevent teen alcohol and drug abuse, *J Drug Educ* 34(2):197-212, 2004.

Berry AM, Davidson P, Masters J, et al: Systematic literature review of oral hygiene practices for intensive care patients receiving mechanical ventilation, *Am J Crit Care* 16(6):552-562, 2007.

Bryanton J, Gagnon AJ, Hatem M, et al: Predictors of parenting self-efficacy, *Nurs Res* 57(4):252-259, 2008.

Campbell DT, Stanley JC: *Experimental and quasi-experimental designs for research*, Chicago, 1963, Rand-McNally.

Carpenter JS, Rawl S, Porter J, et al: Oncology outpatient and provider responses to a computerized symptom assessment system, *Oncol Nurs Forum* 35(4):661-670, 2008.

Chen CC, Wang C, Huang GH: Functional trajectory 6 months posthospitalization, *Nurs Res* 57(2):93-100, 2008.

Doorenbos AZ, Berger AM, Brohard-Holbert C, et al: Oncology Nursing Society report: 2008 research priorities survey, *Oncol Nurs Forum* 35(6):891, 2008.

Fredland NM, Campbell JC, Han H: Effect of violence exposure on health outcomes among young urban adolescents, *Nurs Res* 57(3):157-165, 2008.

Gatti L: Maternal perceptions of insufficient milk supply, *J Nurs Sch* 40(4):355-363, 2008.

Gregory KE: Clinical predictors of necrotizing enterocolitis in premature infants, *Nurs Res* 57:260-270, 2008.

Hall LA, Rayens MK, Peden AR: Maternal factors associated with child behavior, *J Nurs Sch* 40(2):124-130, 2008.

Horgas AL, Yoon SL, Nichols AL, Marsiske M: The relationship between pain and functional disability in black and white older adults, *Res Nurs Health* 31(4):341-354, 2008.

Kaplan DW: *Structure equation modeling: foundations and extensions*, Thousand Oaks, CA, 2008, Sage.

Kiefer RA: An integrative review of the concept of well-being, *Holistic Nurs Pract* 22(5):244-252, 2008.

Kline R: *Principles and practices of structural equation modeling*, ed 2, New York, 2005, Guilford Press.

Lopez-McKee G, McNeill JA, Bader J, et al: Comparison of factors affecting repeat mammography screening of low-income Mexican-American women, *Oncol Nurs Forum* 35(6):941-947, 2008.

Miller PE, Vasey JJ, Short S, et al: Dietary supplement use in adult cancer survivors, *Oncol Nurs Forum* 36(1):61-68, 2009.

Moser DK, Riegel B, McKinley S, et al: The Control Attitude Scale—Revised, *Nurs Res* 58(1):42-51, 2009.

Murray MA, Fiset V, Young S, et al: Where the dying live: a systematic review of determinants of place of end of life cancer care, *Oncol Nurs Forum* 36(1):69-77, 2009.

Nannini A, Nazar J, Berg C, et al: Physical injuries reported on hospital visits for assault during the pregnancy-associated period, *Nurs Res* 57(3):144-149, 2008.

Newlin K, Melkus GD, Tappen, R, et al: Relationships of religion and spirituality to glycemic control in Black women with type 2 diabetes, *Nurs Res* 57(5):331-339, 2008.

Rice VH, Stead LF: Nursing interventions for smoking cessation, *Cochrane Database of Systematic Reviews* Jan 23(10), CD001188, 2008.

Whittemore R: Combing evidence in nursing research, *Nurs Res* 54:56-62, 2005.

Wielgus KK, Berger AM, Hertoz M: Predictors of fatigue 30 days after completing anthracycline plus taxane adjuvant chemotherapy for breast cancer, *Oncol Nurs Forum* 36(1):38-48, 2009.

FOR FURTHER STUDY

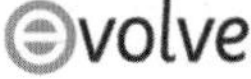

Go to Evolve at http://evolve.elsevier.com/LoBiondo/ for review questions, critiquing exercises, and additional research articles for practice in reviewing and critiquing.

10

Sampling

Judith Haber

KEY TERMS

accessible population
convenience sampling
data saturation
delimitations
element
eligibility criteria
exclusion criteria
inclusion
matching
multistage (cluster) sampling
network (snowball effect) sampling
nonprobability sampling
pilot study
population
probability sampling
purposive sampling
quota sampling
random selection
representative sample
sample
sampling
sampling frame
sampling unit
simple random sampling
snowballing
stratified random sampling
target population

LEARNING OUTCOMES

After reading this chapter, you should be able to do the following:

- Identify the purpose of sampling.
- Define *population, sample,* and *sampling.*
- Compare and contrast a population and a sample.
- Discuss the importance of inclusion and exclusion criteria for sample selection.
- Define *nonprobability* and *probability sampling.*
- Identify the types of nonprobability and probability sampling strategies.
- Compare the advantages and disadvantages of specific nonprobability and probability sampling strategies.
- Discuss the contribution of nonprobability and probability sampling strategies to strength of evidence provided by study findings.
- Discuss the factors that influence determination of sample size.
- Discuss the procedure for drawing a sample.
- Discuss potential threats to internal and external validity as sources of sampling bias
- Use the critiquing criteria to evaluate the "Sample" section of a research report.

STUDY RESOURCES

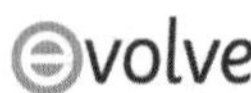

Go to Evolve at http://evolve.elsevier.com/LoBiondo/ for review questions, critiquing exercises, and additional research articles for practice in reviewing and critiquing.

The sampling section of a research study is usually found in the "Methods" section of a research report. It is important for you to understand the sampling process and the ingredients that contribute to a researcher using the most appropriate sampling strategy for the type of research study being conducted. Equally important for you as the research consumer is knowing how to critically appraise the sampling section of a research report to identify how the strengths and weaknesses of the sampling process contributed to the overall strength and quality of evidence provided by the findings of a particular research study.

When you are critically appraising the sampling section of a research study, the threats to internal and external validity as sources of bias need to be considered (see Chapter 7). Your evaluation of the sampling section of a research report is very important in your overall critical appraisal of a research study's findings and their applicability to practice.

Sampling is the process of selecting representative units of a population for study in a research investigation. Although sampling is a complex process, it is a familiar one. In our daily lives, we gather knowledge, make decisions, and formulate predictions based on sampling procedures. For example, nursing students may make generalizations about the overall quality of nursing professors as a result of their exposure to a sample of nursing professors during their undergraduate programs. Patients may make generalizations about a hospital's food or quality of nursing care during a 1-week hospital stay. It is apparent that limited exposure to a limited portion of these experiences forms the basis of our conclusions, and much of our knowledge and decisions are based on our experience with samples.

Researchers also derive knowledge from samples. Many problems in research cannot be solved without employing sampling procedures. For example, when testing the effectiveness of a medication for patients with asthma, the drug is administered to a sample of the population for whom the drug is potentially appropriate. The researcher must come to some conclusions without giving the drug to every known patient with asthma or every laboratory animal in the world. But because human lives are at stake, the researcher cannot afford to arrive casually at conclusions that are based on the first dozen patients available for study.

The impact of arriving at conclusions that are not accurate or making generalizations from a small nonrepresentative sample are much more severe in scientific investigations than in everyday life. Essentially, researchers sample representative segments of the population because it is rarely feasible or necessary to sample the entire population of interest to obtain relevant information.

This chapter will familiarize you with the basic concepts of sampling as they primarily pertain to the principles of quantitative research design, nonprobability and probability sampling, sample size, and the related appraisal process. Sampling issues that relate to qualitative research designs are discussed in Chapter 4, 5, and 6.

SAMPLING CONCEPTS

Population

A **population** is a well-defined set that has certain specified properties. A population can be composed of people, animals, objects, or events. Examples of clinical populations might be all of the female patients admitted to a certain hospital for lumpectomies for treatment of breast cancer during the year 2010, all of the children with asthma in the state of New York, or all of the men and women with a diagnosis of generalized anxiety disorder in the United

States. These examples illustrate that a population may be broadly defined and potentially involve millions of people or narrowly specified to include only several hundred people.

The population criteria establish the **target population,** that is, the entire set of cases about which the researcher would like to make generalizations. A target population might include all undergraduate nursing students enrolled in generic baccalaureate programs in the United States. Because of time, money, and personnel, however, it is often not feasible to pursue a research study using a target population.

An **accessible population,** one that meets the target population criteria and that is available, is used instead. For example, an accessible population might include all full-time generic baccalaureate students attending school in Indiana. Pragmatic factors must also be considered when identifying a potential population of interest.

It is important to know that a population is not restricted to human subjects. It may consist of hospital records; blood, urine, or other specimens taken from patients at a clinic; historical documents; or laboratory animals. For example, a population might consist of all the $HgbA_{1C}$ blood test specimens collected from patients in the Middle City Hospital diabetes clinic or all of the patient charts on file who had been screened during pregnancy for intimate partner abuse. It is apparent that a population can be defined in a variety of ways. The important point to remember is that the basic unit of the population must be clearly defined because the generalizability of the findings will be a function of the population criteria.

Inclusion and Exclusion Criteria

As a reader of a research report, you should consider whether the researcher has identified the population descriptors that form the basis for the inclusion (eligibility) or exclusion (delimitations) criteria that are used to select the sample from the array of all possible units—whether people, objects, or events. These four terms—**inclusion** or **eligibility criteria** and **exclusion criteria** or **delimitations**—are used synonymously when considering subject attributes that would lead a researcher to specify inclusion or exclusion criteria. Insofar as it is possible, the researcher must demonstrate that the exact criteria used to decide whether an individual would be classified as a member of a given population have been specifically delineated. The population descriptors that provide the basis for inclusion (eligibility) criteria should be evident in the sample; that is, the characteristics of the population and the sample should be congruent. The degree of congruence is evaluated to assess the representativeness of the sample.

Think about the concept of inclusion or eligibility criteria applied to a research study where the subjects are patients. For example, participants in a study investigating the effectiveness of a psychoeducational intervention on quality of life in breast cancer survivors in posttreatment survivorship (see Appendix A) had to meet the following inclusion (eligibility) criteria:

1. Age—at least 21 years of age
2. Diagnosis—histologically confirmed Stage 0-II breast cancer
3. Health status—no evidence of local recurrence or metastatic disease
4. Treatment status—received chemotherapy or radiation and may have been on hormonal treatment (e.g., tamoxifen) at study entry
5. Language—English

Inclusion or eligibility criteria may also be viewed as exclusion criteria or delimitations, those characteristics that restrict the population to a homogeneous group of subjects. Examples of exclusion criteria or delimitations include the following: gender, age, marital status, socioeconomic status, religion, ethnicity, level of education, age of children, health status, and diagnosis. In a study examining what patients on hemodialysis perceive about their choice among the three types of renal replacement therapies (transplantation, hemodialysis, and peritoneal dialysis), Landreneau and Ward-Smith (2007) (see Appendix D) established the following exclusion criteria:

- Medical conditions that would make participation in the study a hardship on the individual
- Absence during the usual hemodialysis treatment time
- Comorbid psychiatric conditions

These exclusion criteria or delimitations were selected because of their potential effect of a co-occurring health problem on the patients' perceptions about choice related to treatment of renal failure.

Let us consider the effect of a co-occurring health problem such as dementia on the subject's ability to accurately perceive the differences between three renal replacement therapy options. In patients who had a diagnosis of renal failure, and who also had dementia, the accuracy of that perception would be confounded by their degree of cognitive impairment (e.g., knowledge acquisition, retention, and application). Exclusion criteria were established to decrease the heterogeneity of this sample group because heterogeneity would decrease the strength of the evidence and inhibit the researchers' ability to interpret the findings meaningfully and make generalizations. It is much wiser to study only one homogeneous group or include specific groups as distinct subsets of the sample and study the groups comparatively, as was the case in the study by Landreneau and Ward-Smith (2007).

HELPFUL HINT

Often, researchers do not clearly identify the population under study, or the population is not clarified until the "Discussion" section when the effort is made to discuss the group (population) to which the study findings can be generalized.

For example, in a study investigating the effectiveness of nurse-managed telemonitoring on blood pressure reduction in urban African Americans, the sample consisted of 186 individuals who were recruited through free blood pressure screenings offered at community centers, thrift stores, drug stores, and grocery stores located on the east side of Detroit (Artinian et al., 2007). Because the classification of uncontrolled blood pressure (BP) is based on the average of two or more properly measured seated BP readings on each of two or more visits, participants were screened for study eligibility three times to verify continued uncontrolled BP. The subjects also met the following inclusion criteria, all of which maximized the likelihood of having a homogeneous sample:

- Age 18 years of age or older
- Systolic BP 140 mm Hg or greater
- Diastolic BP 90 mm Hg or greater
- If self-identified as a diabetic or with a history of chronic kidney disease, systolic BP of 130 or greater and diastolic BP of 80 or greater
- Access to a land-based telephone in own residence
- English speaking
- Intent to remain in Detroit for the next year
- Oriented to time, place, and person

Remember that inclusion and exclusion criteria are established to control for extraneous variability or bias that would limit the strength of evidence contributed by the sampling plan in relation to the experimental design of the study. Each inclusion or exclusion criterion should have a rationale, presumably related to a potential contaminating effect on the dependent variable. The careful establishment of sample inclusion or exclusion criteria will increase the precision of the study and strength of evidence, thereby contributing to the accuracy and generalizability of the findings (see Chapter 7).

EVIDENCE-BASED PRACTICE TIP

Consider whether the choice of participants was biased, thereby influencing the strength of evidence provided by the outcomes of the study.

Samples and Sampling

Sampling is a process of selecting a portion or subset of the designated population to represent the entire population. A **sample** is a set of elements that make up the population; an **element** is the most basic unit about which information is collected. The most common element in nursing research is individuals, but other elements (e.g., places or objects) can form the basis of a sample or population. For example, a researcher was planning a study that compared the effectiveness of different nursing interventions on reducing falls in the elderly in long-term care facilities (LTCs). Four LTCs, each using a different falls prevention treatment protocol, were identified as the sampling units rather than the nurses themselves or the treatment alone.

The purpose of sampling is to increase the efficiency of a research study. As a new evaluator of research you must realize that it would not be feasible to examine every element or unit in the population. When sampling is done properly, the researcher can draw inferences and make generalizations about the population without examining each element in the population. Sampling procedures that entail the formulation of specific criteria for selection ensure that the characteristics of the phenomena of interest will be, or are likely to be, present in all of the units being studied. The researcher's efforts to ensure that the sample is representative of the target population strengthens the evidence generated by the sample composition, which puts the researcher in a stronger position to draw conclusions that are generalizable to the population and applicable to practice (see Chapter 7).

After having reviewed a number of research studies, you will recognize that samples and sampling procedures vary in terms of merit. The foremost criterion in appraising a sample is its representativeness. A **representative sample** is one whose key characteristics closely approximate those of the population. If 70% of the population in a study of child-rearing practices consisted of women and 40% were full-time employees, a representative sample should reflect these characteristics in the same proportions.

It must be understood that there is no way to guarantee that a sample is representative without obtaining a database about the entire population. Because it is difficult and inefficient to assess a population, the researcher must use sampling strategies that minimize or control for sample bias. If an appropriate sampling strategy is used, it almost always is possible to obtain a reasonably accurate understanding of the phenomena under investigation by obtaining data from a sample.

TABLE 10-1 Summary of Sampling Strategies

Sampling Strategy	Ease of Drawing Sample	Risk of Bias	Representativeness of Sample
NONPROBABILITY			
Convenience	Easy	Greater than any other sampling strategy	Because samples tend to be self-selecting, representativeness is questionable
Quota	Relatively easy	Contains unknown source of bias that affects external validity	Builds in some representativeness by using knowledge about population of interest
Purposive	Relatively easy	Bias increases with greater heterogeneity of population; conscious bias is also a danger	Very limited ability to generalize because sample is handpicked
PROBABILITY			
Simple random	Laborious	Low	Maximized; probability of nonrepresentativeness decreases with increased sample size
Stratified random	Time-consuming	Low	Enhanced
Cluster	Less time-consuming than simple or stratified	Subject to more sampling errors than simple or stratified	Less representative than simple or stratified

TYPES OF SAMPLES

Sampling strategies are generally grouped into two categories: nonprobability sampling and probability sampling. In **nonprobability sampling,** elements are chosen by nonrandom methods. The drawback of this strategy is that there is no way of estimating each element's probability of being included in the samples. Essentially, there is no way of ensuring that every element has a chance for inclusion in the nonprobability sample.

Probability sampling uses some form of random selection when the sample units are chosen. This type of sample enables the researcher to estimate the probability that each element of the population will be included in the sample. Probability sampling is the more rigorous type of sampling strategy and is more likely to result in a representative sample. The remainder of this section is devoted to a discussion of different types of nonprobability and probability sampling strategies. A summary of sampling strategies appears in Table 10-1. You may wish to refer to this table as the various nonprobability and probability strategies are discussed in the following sections.

EVIDENCE-BASED PRACTICE TIP

Determining whether the sample is representative of the population being studied will influence your interpretation of the evidence provided by the findings and decision making about their relevance to the patient population and practice setting.

HELPFUL HINT

Research articles are not always explicit about the type of sampling strategy that was used. If the sampling strategy is not specified, assume that a convenience sample was used for a quantitative study and a purposive sample was used for a qualitative study.

Nonprobability Sampling

Because of lack of randomization, the findings of studies using a nonprobability sampling strategy are less generalizable than those using a probability sampling strategy, and they tend to produce less representative samples. Such samples are more feasible for the researcher to obtain, however, and many samples—not only in nursing research but also in other disciplines—are nonprobability samples. When a nonprobability sample is carefully chosen to reflect the target population, through the careful use of inclusion and exclusion criteria and adequate sample size, you can have more confidence in the representativeness of the sample and the external validity of the findings. The three major types of nonprobability sampling are the following: convenience, quota, and purposive sampling strategies.

Convenience Sampling

Convenience sampling is the use of the most readily accessible persons or objects as subjects in a study. The subjects may include volunteers, the first 100 patients admitted to hospital X with a particular diagnosis, all of the people enrolled in program Y during the month of September, or all of the students enrolled in course Z at a particular university during 2010. The subjects are convenient and accessible to the researcher and are thus called a *convenience sample.* For example, a researcher studying the relationship between pain and functional disability in black and white older adults recruited a convenience sample of 115 community-dwelling older adults from five senior centers and two churches in a large, racially diverse city in the Midwest who met the eligibility criteria and volunteered to participate in the study (Horgas et al., 2008) (see Appendix C). Another researcher studied the effect of the Deaf Heart Health Intervention (DHHI), which sought to determine its effectiveness in increasing self-efficacy for health behaviors related to risk factors for cardiovascular disease among culturally deaf adults who met the eligibility criteria (Jones et al., 2007) (see Appendix D).

The advantage of a convenience sample is that generally it is easier for the researcher to obtain subjects. The researcher may have to be concerned only with obtaining a sufficient number of subjects who meet the same criteria. Sometimes a convenience sample is the most appropriate sampling strategy to use even though it is not the strongest approach. For example, in the study by Jones and colleagues (2007), participants were not randomly assigned to intervention versus comparison groups because the deaf community in each of the two cities, Tucson and Phoenix, is relatively small and close knit. "Cross-talk" would probably occur between deaf adults assigned to different treatment groups within the same city.

The major disadvantage of a convenience sample is that the risk of bias is greater than in any other type of sample (see Table 10-1). Because convenience samples use voluntary participation, this fact increases the probability of researchers recruiting those people who feel strongly about the issue being studied, which may favor certain outcomes (Sousa et al., 2004). In this case, you can ask yourself the following questions as you think about the strength and quality of evidence contributed by the sampling component of a research study.

TABLE 10-2 Numbers and Percentages of Students in Strata of a Quota Sample of 5,000 Graduates of Nursing Programs in City X

	Diploma Graduates	Associate Degree Graduates	Baccalaureate Graduates
Population	1,000 (20%)	2,000 (40%)	2,000 (40%)
Strata	100	200	200

- What motivated some of the people to participate and others not to participate (self-selection)?
- What kind of data would have been obtained if nonparticipants had also responded?
- How representative are the people who did participate in relation to the population?
- What kind of confidence can you have in the evidence provided by the findings?

Researchers may recruit subjects when they stop people on a street corner to ask their opinion on some issue, place advertisements in the newspaper, or place signs in local churches, community centers, or supermarkets indicating that volunteers are needed for a particular study. To assess the degree to which a convenience sample approximates a random sample, the researcher checks for the representativeness of the convenience sample by comparing the sample to population percentages and, in that way, can assess the extent to which bias is or is not evident (Sousa et al., 2004).

Because acquiring research subjects is a problem that confronts many nurse researchers, innovative recruitment strategies may be used. For example, a researcher may even offer to pay the participants for their time. A unique method of accessing and recruiting subjects is the use of online computer networks (e.g., disease-specific chat rooms, blogs, and bulletin boards). In the evidence hierarchy located in Figure 1-1 (see p. 16), nonprobability sampling is most commonly associated with quantitative nonexperimental or qualitative studies that contribute Level IV through Level VI evidence.

When you appraise a research study you should recognize that the convenience sample strategy, although the most common, is the weakest form of sampling strategy with regard to strength of evidence and generalizability. When a convenience sample is used, caution should be exercised in analyzing and interpreting the data. When critiquing a research study that has employed this sampling strategy, the reviewer should be justifiably skeptical about the external validity of the findings and applicability of the findings (see Chapter 7).

Quota Sampling

Quota sampling refers to a form of nonprobability sampling in which knowledge about the population of interest is used to build some representativeness into the sample (see Table 10-1). A quota sample identifies the strata of the population and proportionally represents the strata in the sample. For example, the data in Table 10-2 reveal that 10% of the 5,000 nurses in city X are diploma graduates, 50% are associate degree graduates, and 40% are baccalaureate graduates. Each stratum of the population should be proportionately represented in the sample. In this case the researcher used a proportional quota sampling strategy and decided to sample 10% of a population of 5,000 (i.e., 500 nurses). Based on the proportion of each stratum in the population, 100 diploma graduates, 200 associate degree graduates, and 200 baccalaureate graduates were the quotas established for the three strata. The researcher recruited subjects who met the eligibility criteria of the study until the quota for each stratum was filled. In other words, once the researcher obtained the necessary 100 diploma graduates, 200 associate degree graduates, and 200 baccalaureate graduates, the sample was complete.

The researcher systematically ensures that proportional segments of the population are included in the sample. The quota sample is not randomly selected (i.e., once the proportional strata have been identified, the researcher recruits and enrolls subjects until the quota for each stratum has been filled) but does increase the representativeness of the sample. This sampling strategy addresses the problem of overrepresentation or underrepresentation of certain segments of a population in a sample.

The characteristics chosen to form the strata are selected according to a researcher's judgment based on knowledge of the population and the literature review. The criterion for selection should be a variable that reflects important differences in the dependent variables under investigation. Age, gender, religion, ethnicity, medical diagnosis, socioeconomic status, level of completed education, and occupational rank are among the variables that are likely to be important stratifying variables in nursing research investigations. For example, McConnell and colleagues (2003) sought to describe patterns of change in physical functioning on a quarterly basis over 1 year among long-term nursing home residents stratified into seven groups according to their level of cognitive impairment on admission.

As you critically appraise a research study, your aim is to determine whether the sample strata appropriately reflect the population under consideration and whether the stratifying variables are homogeneous enough to ensure a meaningful comparison of differences among strata. Establishment of strict inclusion and exclusion criteria and using power analysis to determine appropriate sample size increase the rigor of a quota sampling strategy by creating homogeneous subject categories that facilitate making meaningful comparisons across strata. In cases where the phenomena under investigation are relatively homogeneous within the population, the risk of bias may be minimal.

Purposive Sampling

Purposive sampling is an increasingly common strategy in which the researcher's knowledge of the population and its elements is used to handpick the cases to be included in the sample. The researcher usually selects subjects who are considered to be typical of the population. When a researcher is considering the sampling strategy for a randomized clinical trial focusing on a specific diagnosis or patient population, the sampling strategy is often purposive in nature. For example, Budin and colleagues (2008) explored the differential effect of a phase-specific psychoeducation and telephone counseling intervention on the emotional, social, and physical adjustment of women with breast cancer and their partners. A purposive sample of 249 patient-partner pairs were randomly assigned to one of four groups: one control group and three intervention groups.

HELPFUL HINT

When purposive sampling is used as the first step in recruiting a sample for a randomized clinical trial, as illustrated in Figure 10-1, it is often followed by random assignment of subjects to an intervention or control group, which increases the generalizability of the findings.

Purposive sampling is also commonly used in qualitative research studies. For example, the purpose of a qualitative research study by Fox and Chesla (2008) was to understand the meaning of the patient–health care provider relationship, and how patients believed it affected their health, from the perspective of women with chronic disease. A purposive sample of women between 35 and 55 years of age who had been diagnosed with a chronic disease (e.g., multiple sclerosis, diabetes, asthma, cancer) was recruited through newspaper advertisements, flyers in private practitioner offices, support groups, and word of mouth. These participants were used because they were typical (homogeneous) of the population under consideration, which enhances the representativeness of this nonprobability sampling strategy used to describe a specific, and often underrepresented, minority population.

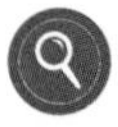

EVIDENCE-BASED PRACTICE TIP

When thinking about applying study findings to your clinical practice, consider whether the participants making up the sample are similar to your own patients.

A purposive sample is used also when a highly unusual group is being studied, such as a population with a rare genetic disease (e.g., Huntington's chorea). In this case, the researcher would describe the sample characteristics precisely to ensure that the reader will have an accurate picture of the subjects in the sample.

This type of sample can also be used to study the differential effect of risk factors in a specific population longitudinally. For example, same-sex monozygotic (MZ) twin pairs who met the eligibility criteria were recruited into a study examining relationships among cardiovascular health indicators and health-promoting behaviors in adult MZ twins. The researchers examined the differential effect of variables potentially influencing cardiovascular health through a health assessment survey that included questions about smoking status, alcohol and caffeine consumption, history of diabetes, and demographic variables such as the degree to which the MZ twins grew up in similar environments. The findings showed that both genetic and behavioral factors contributed to cardiovascular risk and cardiovascular health in participants.

Today, computer networks (e.g., online services) can be of great value in helping researchers access and recruit subjects for purposive samples. One researcher investigating ethnic differences in cancer pain experiences of four ethnic groups in the United States recruited 480 cancer patients (105 Hispanics, 148 whites, 109 African Americans, 118 Asians) through both Internet and community settings, MSN, and Yahoo searches (Im et al., 2007). The Internet settings for recruitment were Internet cancer support groups identified through a Google search convenience sample of staff nurses who were accessible over the Internet. Online support group bulletin boards that facilitate recruitment of subjects for purposive samples exist for people with cancer, rheumatoid arthritis, systemic lupus erythematosus, human immunodeficiency virus/acquired immunodeficiency syndrome (HIV/AIDS), bipolar disorder, Lyme disease, and many others.

The researcher who uses a purposive sample assumes that errors of judgment in overrepresenting or underrepresenting elements of the population in the sample will tend to balance out. There is no objective method, however, for determining the validity of this assumption. You should be aware of the fact that the more heterogeneous the population, the greater the chance of bias being introduced in the selection of a purposive sample. As indicated in Table

BOX 10-1 Criteria for Use of a Purposive Sampling Strategy

- Effective pretesting of newly developed instruments with a purposive sample of divergent types of people
- Validation of a scale or test with a known-group technique
- Collection of exploratory data in relation to an unusual or highly specific population, particularly when the total target population remains an unknown to the researcher
- Collection of descriptive data (e.g., as in qualitative studies) that seek to describe the lived experience of a particular phenomenon (e.g., postpartum depression; caring, hope, or surviving childhood sexual abuse)
- Focus of the study population relates to a specific diagnosis (e.g., type 1 diabetes, multiple sclerosis) or condition (e.g., legal blindness, terminal illness) or demographic characteristic (e.g., same-sex twin pairs)

10-1, conscious bias in the selection of subjects remains a constant danger. Therefore the findings from a study using a purposive sample should be regarded with caution. As with any nonprobability sample, the ability to generalize from the evidence provided by the findings is very limited. Box 10-1 lists several examples of when a purposive sample may be appropriate.

Probability Sampling

The primary characteristic of probability sampling is the random selection of elements from the population. **Random selection** occurs when each element of the population has an equal and independent chance of being included in the sample. In an evidence hierarchy, probability sampling, which is most closely associated with experimental and quasi-experimental designs, represents the strongest type of sampling strategy. The research consumer has greater confidence that the sample is representative rather than biased and more closely reflects the characteristics of the population of interest. Three commonly used probability sampling strategies are simple random sampling, stratified random sampling, and cluster sampling.

Random selection of sample subjects should not be confused with random assignment of subjects. The latter, as discussed in Chapter 8, refers to the assignment of subjects to either an experimental or a control group on a purely random basis.

Simple Random Sampling

Simple random sampling is a carefully controlled process. The researcher defines the population (a set), lists all of the units of the population (a **sampling frame**), and selects a sample of units (a subset) from which the sample will be chosen. For example, in a study investigating the effects of time pressure and experience on nurses' risk assessment decisions, a total of 245 registered nurses from acute care hospital units in the United Kingdom ($N = 95$), Netherlands ($N = 50$), Australia ($N = 50$), and Canada ($N = 50$) participated in the study. The nurses from the United Kingdom were sampled randomly set at approximately 65% of the available nurse population (Thompson et al., 2008).

If American hospitals specializing in the treatment of cancer were the sampling unit, a list of all such hospitals would be the sampling frame. If certified family nurse practitioners (FNPs) constituted the accessible population, a list of those nurses would be the sampling frame.

Once a list of the population elements has been developed, the best method of selecting a random sample is to use a computer program that generates the order in which the random selection of subjects is to be carried out.

The advantages of simple random sampling are as follows:

- Sample selection is not subject to the conscious biases of the researcher.
- Representativeness of the sample in relation to the population characteristics is maximized.
- Differences in the characteristics of the sample and the population are purely a function of chance.
- Probability of choosing a nonrepresentative sample decreases as the size of the sample increases.

Simple random sampling was used in a study examining (1) what proportion of patients treated in an emergency department (ED) for minor injury had a positive psychiatric history or a current psychiatric diagnosis and (2) whether minor injury patients with a positive psychiatric history or current psychiatric disorder differ in demographics, injury characteristics, or screening psychiatric symptom measures compared with injured patients without a psychiatric history or disorder. Men and women who sustained an injury within 24 hours of ED admission, who were 18 years of age and older, and who verbally agreed to release their name and contact information to the study team formed the pool from which participants were randomly selected. Simple random selection was used because of the high flow of injured patients in this ED and because the intensity of diagnostic interviews precluded the use of a consecutive sample (Richmond et al., 2007).

When critically appraising the sample section of a research study, you must remember that despite the use of a carefully controlled sampling procedure that minimizes error, there is no guarantee that the sample will be representative. Factors such as sample heterogeneity and subject dropout may jeopardize the representativeness of the sample despite the most stringent random sampling procedure.

The major disadvantage of simple random sampling is that it is a time-consuming and inefficient method of obtaining a random sample. (For example, consider the task of listing all of the baccalaureate nursing students in the United States.) With random sampling, it may also be impossible to obtain an accurate or complete listing of every element in the population; for example, imagine trying to obtain a list of all completed suicides in New York City for the year 2009. It often is the case that although suicide may have been the cause of death, another cause (e.g., cardiac failure) appears on the death certificate. It would be difficult to estimate how many elements of the target population would be eliminated from consideration. The issue of bias would definitely enter the picture despite the researcher's best efforts. In the final analysis, you, as the evaluator of a research article, must be cautious about generalizing from reported findings, even when random sampling is the stated strategy, if the target population has been difficult or impossible to list completely.

Stratified Random Sampling

Stratified random sampling requires that the population be divided into strata or subgroups as illustrated in Figure 10-1. The subgroups or subsets that the population is divided into are homogeneous. An appropriate number of elements from each subset are randomly selected on the basis of their proportion in the population. The goal of this strategy is to achieve a greater degree of representativeness. Stratified random sampling is similar to the proportional stratified quota sampling strategy discussed earlier in the chapter. The major difference is that stratified random sampling uses a random selection procedure for obtaining sample subjects.

The population is stratified according to any number of attributes, such as age, gender, ethnicity, religion, socioeconomic status, or level of education completed. The variables

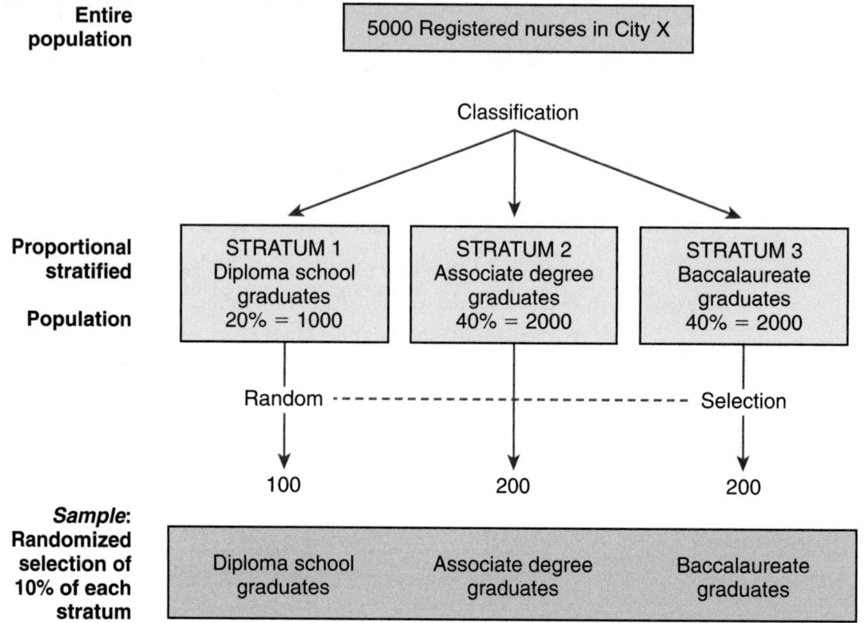

Figure 10-1 Subject selection using a proportional stratified random sampling strategy.

selected to make up the strata should be adaptable to homogeneous subsets with regard to the attributes being studied. The following criteria can be used in the selection of a stratified sample:

- Is there a critical variable or attribute that provides a logical basis for stratifying the sample?
- Does the population list contain sufficient information about the attributes that will be used to divide the sample into subsets?
- Is it appropriate for each subset to be equal in size, or is it more appropriate for each subset to be proportionally stratified based on the proportion of each subset in the population?
- If proportional sampling is being used, is there a sufficient number of subjects in each subset for basing meaningful comparisons?
- Once the subset comparison has been determined, are random procedures used for selection of the sample?

As illustrated in Table 10-1, several advantages to a stratified sampling strategy are the following: (1) the representativeness of the sample is enhanced; (2) the researcher has a valid basis for making comparisons among subsets if information on the critical variables has been available; and (3) the researcher is able to oversample a disproportionately small stratum to adjust for their underrepresentation, statistically weigh the data accordingly, and continue to make legitimate comparisons.

The obstacles encountered by a researcher using this strategy include the following: (1) the difficulty of obtaining a population list containing complete critical variable information; (2) the time-consuming effort of obtaining multiple enumerated lists; (3) the challenge of enrolling proportional strata; and (4) the time and money involved in carrying out a large-scale study using a stratified sampling strategy.

When appraising a study, you must question the appropriateness of this sampling strategy to the problem under investigation. For example, Ulrich and colleagues (2006) conducted a mail survey to identify ethical concerns and conflicts of nurse practitioners (NPs) and physician assistants (PAs) related to managed care in the delivery of primary care to patients and the factors that influence ethical conflict. A self-administered questionnaire was mailed to a stratified sample of 3,900 NPs and PAs practicing in the United States selected from a list provided by Medical Marketing Services, an independent organization that manages medical industry lists. The lists were derived from the American Academy of Physicians Assistants and from the 50 nursing and medical boards in the 50 states. The sample size for each stratum was calculated to detect a correlation of $r = .2$ allowing for a 75% eligibility, 40% response rate, and three different state practice environments (excellent or favorable, acceptable, and limiting or restrictive) allowing for a 10% difference in proportions among strata with 95% confidence and 80% power. This study is a good example of how researchers can mathematically attempt to represent all strata proportionately in the study sample.

HELPFUL HINT

Look for a brief discussion of a study's sampling strategy in the "Methods" section of a research article. Sometimes there is a separate subsection with the heading "Sample," "Subjects," or "Study Participants." A statistical description of the characteristics of the actual sample often does not appear until the "Results" section of a research article. You may also find a table in the Results section that summarizes the sample characteristics using descriptive statistics (see Chapter 14).

Multistage Sampling (Cluster Sampling)

Multistage (cluster) sampling involves a successive random sampling of units (clusters) that progress from large to small and meet sample eligibility criteria. The first-stage **sampling unit** consists of large units or clusters. The second-stage sampling unit consists of smaller units or clusters. Third-stage sampling units are even smaller. For example, if a sample of critical care nurses is desired, the first sampling unit would be a random sample of hospitals, obtained from an American Hospital Association list, that meet the eligibility criteria (e.g., size, type). The second-stage sampling unit would consist of a list of critical care nurses practicing at each hospital selected in the first stage (i.e., the list obtained from the vice president for nursing at each hospital). The criteria for inclusion in the list of critical care nurses were as follows:

1. Certified as a critical care registered nurse (CCRN) with at least 3 years' experience as a critical care nurse
2. At least 75% of the CCRN's time spent in providing direct patient care in a critical care unit
3. Full-time employment at the hospital

The second-stage sampling strategy called for random selection of two CCRNs from each hospital who met the previously mentioned eligibility criteria.

When multistage sampling is used in relation to large national surveys, states are used as the first-stage sampling unit, followed by successively smaller units such as counties, cities, districts, and blocks as the second-stage sampling unit, and finally households as the third-stage sampling unit.

Sampling units or clusters can be selected by simple random or stratified random sampling methods. Suppose that the hospitals, described in the example above, were grouped into four strata according to size (i.e., number of beds), as follows: (1) 200 to 299; (2) 300 to 399; (3) 400 to 499; and (4) 500 or more. Stratum 1 comprised 25% of the population; stratum 2 comprised 30% of the population; stratum 3 comprised 20% of the population; and stratum 4 comprised 25% of the population. This means that either a simple random or a proportional, stratified sampling strategy is used to randomly select hospitals that would proportionately represent the population of hospitals in the American Hospital Association list.

The main advantage of cluster sampling, as illustrated in Table 10-1, is that it is considerably more economical in terms of time and money than other types of probability sampling. There are two major disadvantages: (1) more sampling errors tend to occur than with simple random or stratified random sampling; and (2) the appropriate handling of the statistical data from cluster samples is very complex.

When you are critically appraising a research study, you will need to consider whether the use of cluster sampling is justified in light of the research design, as well as other pragmatic matters, such as economy. For example, in a study investigating relationships among RN staffing adequacy, work environments, and patient outcomes, selection of eligible nurses involved a two-stage sampling strategy (Chang et al., 2006). First, 146 hospitals were randomly selected from all acute care hospitals with at least 99 licensed beds and accredited by the Joint Commission on Accreditation of Healthcare Organizations (JCAHO). Two medical-surgical units in each hospital were identified; nurses and 10 randomly selected patients on each unit were surveyed. Registered nurses employed on each unit for not less than 3 months were eligible to participate. The total sample consisted of 222 nursing units at 126 hospitals.

EVIDENCE-BASED PRACTICE TIP

The sampling strategy, whether probability or nonprobability, must be appropriate to the design and evaluated in relation to the level of evidence provided by the design.

Special Sampling Strategies

Several special sampling strategies are used in nonprobability sampling. **Matching** is a special strategy used to construct an equivalent comparison sample group by filling it with subjects who are similar to each subject in another sample group in relation to preestablished variables such as age, gender, level of education, medical diagnosis, or socioeconomic status. Theoretically, any variable other than the independent variable that could affect the dependent variable should be matched. In reality, the more variables matched, the more difficult it is to obtain an adequate sample size. For example, in a study examining the effect of an ankle strengthening and walking exercise program on improving fall-related outcomes in the elderly, Schoenfelder and Rubenstein (2004) recruited participants from 10 private, urban nursing homes in eastern Iowa. Participants were matched in pairs by Risk Assessment for Falls Scale II scores and then randomly assigned within each pair to the intervention or control group.

Networking sampling, sometimes referred to as **snowballing,** is a strategy used for locating samples that are difficult or impossible to locate in other ways. This sampling strategy takes advantage of social networks and the fact that friends tend to have characteristics in common. When a few subjects with the necessary eligibility criteria are found, the researcher asks for their assistance in getting in touch with others with similar criteria. For example, Berggren

CRITICAL THINKING DECISION PATH Assessing the Relationship Between the Type of Sampling Strategy and the Appropriate Generalizability

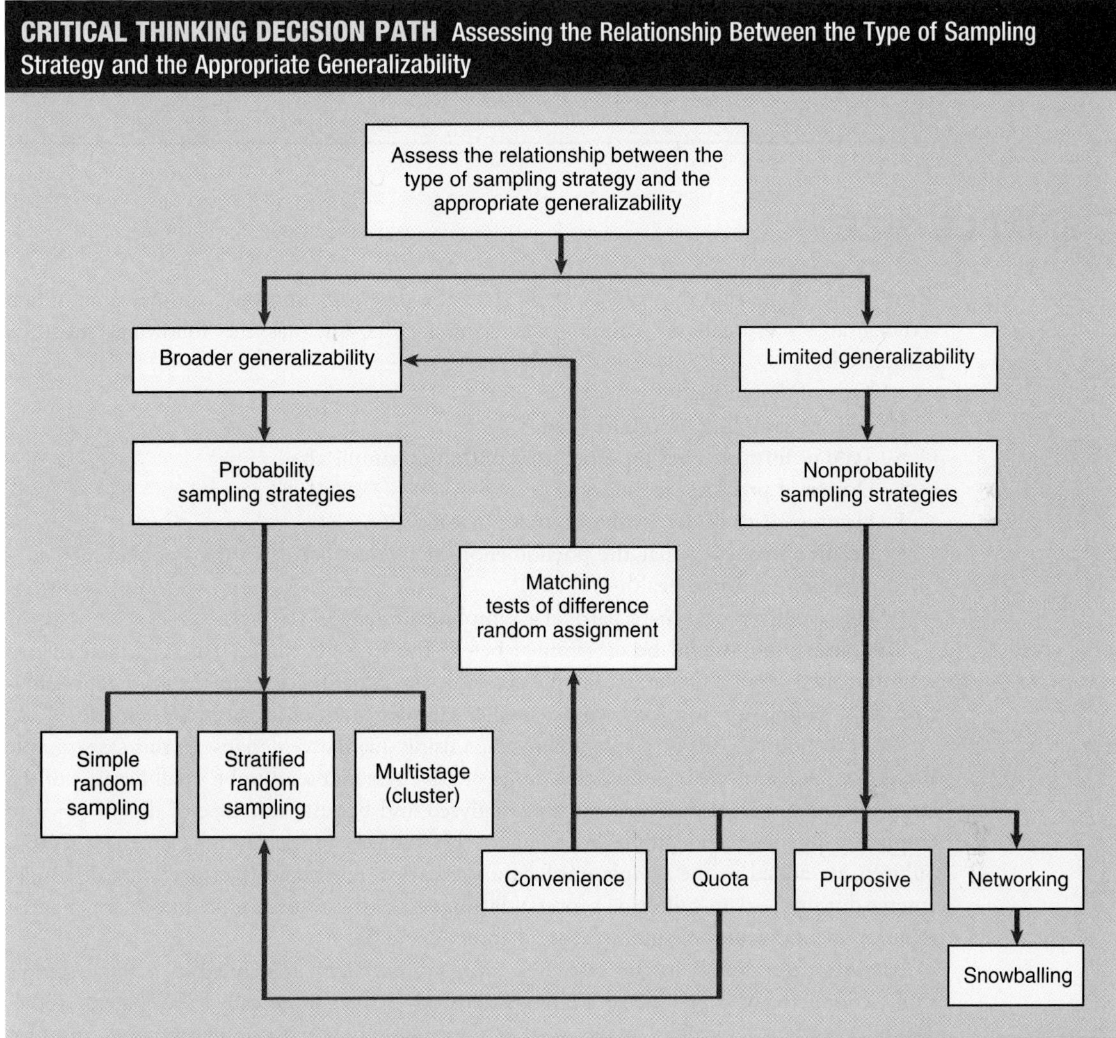

and colleagues (2006) used networking and snowballing to obtain participants for a study exploring the encounters with the health care system for women seeking maternity care in Sweden who were originally from Somalia, Eritrea, and Sudan and had been genitally circumcised. The women were recruited from community groups and by word of mouth referral by interview participants—all of which capture the essence of the **network (snowballing) sampling** strategy that resulted in a sample of 22 women from those countries who met the inclusion criteria.

Today, online computer networks, as described in the section on purposive sampling and in this last example, can be used to assist researchers in acquiring otherwise difficult to locate subjects, thereby taking advantage of the networking or snowball effect.

The Critical Thinking Decision Path illustrates the relationship between the type of sampling strategy and the appropriate generalizability.

HELPFUL HINT

Remember to look for some rationale about the sample size and those strategies the researcher has used (e.g., matching, test of differences on demographic variables) to ascertain or build in sample representativeness.

SAMPLE SIZE

There is no single rule that can be applied to the determination of a sample's size. When arriving at an estimate of sample size, many factors, such as the following, must be considered:

- Type of design used
- Type of sampling procedure used
- Type of formula used for estimating optimum sample size
- Degree of precision required
- Heterogeneity of the attributes under investigation
- Relative frequency that the phenomenon of interest occurs in the population (i.e., a common vs. a rare health problem)
- Projected cost of using a particular sampling strategy

The sample size should be determined before the study is conducted. A general rule of thumb is always to use the largest sample possible. The larger the sample, the more representative of the population it is likely to be; smaller samples produce less accurate results.

One exception to this principle occurs when using qualitative designs. In this case, sample size is not predetermined. Sample sizes in qualitative research tend to be small because of the large volume of verbal data that must be analyzed and because this type of design tends to emphasize intensive and prolonged contact with subjects (Speziale and Carpenter, 2007). Subjects are added to the sample until **data saturation** is reached (i.e., new data no longer emerge during the data-collection process). Fittingness of the data is a more important concern than representativeness of subjects (see Chapters 4 and 5).

Another exception is in the case of a **pilot study,** which is defined as a small sample study, conducted as a prelude to a larger-scale study that is often called the "parent study." The pilot study is typically a smaller scale of the parent study with similar methods and procedures that yield preliminary data that determine the feasibility of conducting a larger-scale study and establish that sufficient scientific evidence exists to justify subsequent, more extensive research.

The principle of "larger is better" holds true for both probability and nonprobability samples. Results based on small samples (under 10) tend to be unstable—the values fluctuate from one sample to the next and it is difficult to apply statistics meaningfully. Small samples tend to increase the probability of obtaining a markedly nonrepresentative sample. As the sample size increases, the mean more closely approximates the population values, thus introducing fewer sampling errors.

An example of this concept is illustrated by a study in which the average monthly sleeping pill consumption is being investigated for patients on a rehabilitation unit after a total knee replacement. The data in Table 10-3 indicate that the population consists of 20 patients whose average consumption of sleeping pills is 15.15 per month. Two simple random samples with sample sizes of 2, 4, 6, and 10 have been drawn from the population of 20 patients. Each

TABLE 10-3 Comparison of Population and Sample Values and Averages in Study of Sleeping Pill Consumption

Number in Group	Group	Number of Sleeping Pills Consumed (Values Expressed Monthly)	Average
20	Population	1, 3, 4, 5, 6, 7, 9, 11, 13, 15, 16, 17, 19, 21, 22, 23, 25, 27, 29, 30	15.15
2	Sample 1A	6, 9	7.5
2	Sample 1B	21, 25	23.0
4	Sample 2A	1, 7, 15, 25	12.0
4	Sample 2B	5, 13, 23, 29	17.5
6	Sample 3A	3, 4, 11, 15, 21, 25	13.3
6	Sample 3B	5, 7, 11, 19, 27, 30	16.5
10	Sample 4A	3, 4, 7, 9, 11, 13, 17, 21, 23, 30	13.8
10	Sample 4B	1, 4, 6, 11, 15, 17, 19, 23, 25, 27	14.8

sample average in the right-hand column represents an estimate of the population average, which is known to be 15.15. In most cases, the population value is unknown to the researchers, but because the population is so small, it could be calculated. As we examine the data in Table 10-3, we note that with a sample size of 2, the estimate might have been wrong by as many as 8 sleeping pills in sample 1B. As the sample size increases, the averages get closer to the population value, and the differences in the estimates between samples A and B also get smaller. Large samples permit the principles of randomization to work effectively (i.e., to counterbalance atypical values in the long run).

It is possible to estimate the sample size needed with the use of a statistical procedure known as power analysis (Cohen, 1988). Power analysis is an advanced statistical technique that is commonly used by researchers and is a requirement for external funding. When it is not used, research consumers will have less confidence provided by the findings because the research study may be based on a sample that is too small. A researcher may commit a type II error of accepting a null hypothesis when it should have been rejected if the sample is too small (see Chapter 14). No matter how high a research design is located on the evidence hierarchy (e.g., Level II—experimental design consisting of a randomized clinical trial), the findings of a study, and their generalizability, are weakened when power analysis is not calculated to ensure an adequate sample size to determine the effect of the intervention.

EVIDENCE-BASED PRACTICE TIP

Research designs and types of samples are often linked. When a nonprobability purposive sampling strategy is used to recruit participants to a study using an experimental design, you would expect random assignment of subjects to an intervention or control group to follow.

It is beyond the scope of this chapter to describe this complex procedure in great detail, but a simple example will illustrate its use. Im and colleagues (2007) wanted to determine ethnic differences in cancer pain among four ethnic groups in the United States. Four hundred eighty cancer patients (105 Hispanics, 148 whites, 109 African Americans, and 118 Asians) were recruited through both Internet (n = 204) and community settings (n = 276).

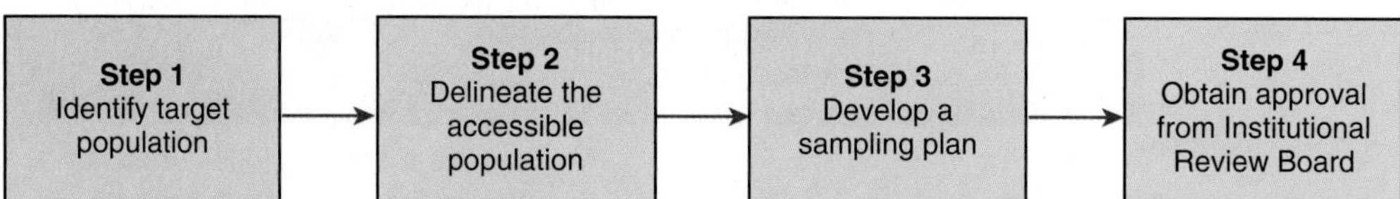

Figure 10-2 Summary of general sampling procedure.

How would a research team such as Im and colleagues know the appropriate number of patients that should be used in the study? When using power analysis, the researcher must estimate how large of a difference will be observed between the four ethnic groups (i.e., to test differences in cancer pain, symptoms accompanying pain, and functional status). If a moderate difference is expected, a conventional effect size of .20 is assumed. With a significance level of .05, a minimum of 68 participants per ethnic group would be needed to detect a statistically significant difference between the groups with a power of .80. The sample in this study ($n = 480$) exceeded the minimum number of 68 per ethnic group.

When calculating sample size using power analysis, the total sample size needs to consider that attrition, or dropouts, will occur and build in approximately 15% extra subjects to make sure that the ability to detect differences between groups or the effect of an intervention remains intact. When expected differences are large, it does not take a very large sample to ensure that differences will be revealed through statistical analysis.

When critically appraising a research study, you should evaluate the sample size in terms of the following: (1) how representative the sample is relative to the target population; and (2) to whom the researcher wishes to generalize the results of the study. The goal of sampling is to have a sample as representative as possible with as little sampling error as possible. Unless representativeness is ensured, all the data in the world become inconsequential.

When an appropriate sample size, including power analysis for calculation of sample size, and sampling strategy have been used, you can feel more confident that the sample is representative of the accessible population rather than biased (Figure 10-2); however, it is more difficult to feel confident that the accessible population is representative of the target population. Are NPs in California representative of all NPs in the United States? It is impossible to be sure about this. Researchers must exercise judgment when assessing typicality. Unfortunately, there are no guidelines for making such judgments, and there is even less basis for you to make such evidence-based decisions. The best rule of thumb to use when evaluating the representativeness of a sample and its generalizability to the target population is to be realistic and conservative about making sweeping claims relative to the findings.

HELPFUL HINT

Remember to evaluate the appropriateness of the generalizations made about the study findings in light of the target population, the accessible population, the type of sampling strategy, and the sample size.

APPRAISING THE EVIDENCE

Sampling

The criteria for critical appraisal of the sampling section of a research study are presented in the Critiquing Criteria box. As the critiquer of a research study, you approach the "Sample" section of a research report with a different perspective than the researcher. You must raise two questions:

1. "If this study were to be replicated, would there be enough information presented about the nature of the population, the sample, the sampling strategy, and sample size of another investigator to carry out the study?"
2. "What are the sampling threats to internal and external validity that are sources of bias?"

The answers to these questions highlight the important link of the sample to the study findings and the strength of the evidence used to make clinical decisions about the applicability of the findings to clinical practice.

Sampling is considered to be one important aspect of the methodology of a research study. Information pertaining to the sample usually appears in the "Methodology" section of the research report. To determine if the study is replicable, you would want to make sure that the sampling section of a research study contained all of the following:

- A brief but complete description of the sample
- Demographic characteristics of the sample
- Inclusion and exclusion criteria
- Sampling strategy used
- Screening, recruitment, and enrollment protocol
- Sample size
- Calculation used to arrive at the appropriate sample size
- Problems encountered in recruiting and/or enrolling the appropriate number of subjects for the study

From these data, you should also be able to decide to what population the findings can be generalized. For example, if a researcher states that 100 subjects were randomly drawn from a population of women 14 years of age or older diagnosed with cervical intraepithelial neoplasia II or III and who were willing to postpone standard ablative therapy and receive topical retinoic acid treatment at affiliated clinics within hospital system X during the year 2010, you can specifically evaluate the parameters of the population. Demographic characteristics of the sample (e.g., age, diagnosis, ethnicity, religion, level of education, socioeconomic status [SES], and marital status) also should be presented in either a tabled or a narrative summary because they provide further explication about the nature of the sample and enable you to appraise the sampling procedure more accurately.

For example, in their study titled "Testing a Nurse-Tailored HIV Medication Adherence Intervention," Holzemer and colleagues (2006) present detailed data summarizing demographic variables of importance. These data are reproduced as follows:

> *The sample was 72.4% African American and 65.4% male, with a mean age of 41.8 years (SD 7.6). In terms of education, 23.9% completed only grade school and 42.0% completed high school. 27.1% had a health literacy level of the sixth grade or below. … Approximately three quarters (75.3%) reported that they were unemployed and 53.1% had no health insurance. Fifty one percent had an AIDS diagnosis and 34.2% and 19.3% reported their*

viral load as undetectable at baseline and 6 months respectively. At baseline, 32.5% reported that they did not know their most recent CD4 count. The average CD4 count at baseline was 394 (SD = 404), and at 6 months 360 (SD = 247). The average viral load at baseline was 66,000 (SD 149,000), and at 6 months, 44,000 (SD 126,000). At baseline, there were no differences between the experimental and control groups on demographic variables, clinical variables, or measures of adherence. There was a significant difference in the number of participants taking an NNRTI in the standard care group (n = 55) compared with the intervention group (n = 40). There were no differences by class of HIV drug (PI < NNRTI < NRTI) with any adherence measures at baseline.

The information that the groups were equivalent on demographic, clinical, or adherence variables at baseline is important because it means that bias related to selection effect is minimized and differences in outcomes related to the effect of the intervention are more likely to be related to the human immunodeficiency virus (HIV) adherence intervention than to differences in the sample groups. It is also helpful if the researcher has presented a rationale for having elected to study one type of population rather than another type of population. In this study testing the effectiveness of an individualized intervention to promote medication adherence, it is appropriate to recruit a sample with low levels of health literacy and medication adherence. This example illustrates how a detailed description of the sample both provides you with a frame of reference for the study population and sample and highlights questions about replicability and bias that need to be raised.

Sampling threats to internal validity that are sources of bias include selection effect and mortality; threats to external validity deal with problems of generalizability of the researcher's findings to additional populations and settings.

In Chapter 7 we talked about how selection effect as a threat to internal validity could occur in studies where a convenience, quota, or purposive sampling strategy was used. In these studies individuals themselves decide whether or not to participate. Suppose a researcher wishes to assess if a new motivational interviewing (MI) telephone counseling intervention contributes to increasing physical activity in adults living in rural settings (Bennett et al., 2008). Assessment of the effectiveness of the program is problematic because the researcher cannot be sure if the new telephone counseling intervention encouraged physical exercise or if only highly motivated individuals volunteered to enroll in the study. To avoid selection bias, the researcher randomly assigned subjects to either the intervention group that received the MI telephone counseling or the control group that only received follow-up phone calls.

Subject mortality or attrition is another threat to internal validity related to sampling (see Chapter 7). Mortality is the loss of subjects from the study, usually from the first data-collection point to the second. If the subjects who remain in the study are different from those who drop out, the results can be affected. When more of the subjects in one group drop out than the other group, the results can also be influenced. It is common for journals to require authors reporting research results to include a flow chart that diagrams the screening, recruitment, enrollment, random assignment, and attrition process and results. For example, see Figure 2 in the study by Meneses and colleagues (2007) that studied the effect of a psycho-educational intervention of the quality of life of breast cancer survivors that appears in Appendix A.

Threats to external validity related to sampling are concerned with generalizability of the results to other populations. Generalizability depends on who actually participates in a study.

CRITIQUING CRITERIA: *Sampling*

1. Have the sample characteristics been completely described?
2. Can the parameters of the study population be inferred from the description of the sample?
3. To what extent is the sample representative of the population as defined?
4. Are the criteria eligibility in the sample specifically identified?
5. Have sample delimitations been established?
6. Would it be possible to replicate the study population?
7. How was the sample selected? Is the method of sample selection appropriate?
8. What kind of bias, if any, is introduced by this sampling method?
9. Is the sample size appropriate? How is it substantiated?
10. Are there indications that rights of subjects have been ensured?
11. Does the researcher identify limitations in generalizability of the findings from the sample to the population? Are they appropriate?
12. Is the sampling strategy appropriate for the design of the study and level of evidence provided by the design?
13. Does the researcher indicate how replication of the study with other samples would provide increased support for the findings?

Not everybody who is approached meets the inclusion criteria, agrees to enroll, or completes the study. At times, numbers of available subjects may be low or not accessible. For example, in the study by Bennett and colleagues (2008), which evaluated whether a telephone-only MI intervention would increase daily physical activity in rural adults, enrollment goals were not met after 5 months of recruitment at rural health clinics. A decision was made to increase enrollment in two ways: (1) by advertising in rural newspapers in other communities with a toll-free number for participants to contact the study staff directly, and (2) by enrolling additional participants during a health and fitness measurement day from among participants in a longitudinal descriptive survey of rural adults. Potential sources of bias included changes in the recruitment plan and recruitment of subjects who were already involved in another study and who were already participating in a health and fitness activity that may reflect individuals who were highly motivated and different from the earlier individuals who enrolled in the study. Generalizability was also limited by the fact that although the eligibility criteria included male and female rural adults, the sample consisted of white females, which reflects a sample that is not representative of the population. As such, the findings cannot be generalized from the study sample to all rural adults.

Bias in sample representativeness and generalizability of findings are important sampling issues that have generated national concern because the presence of these factors decreases confidence in the evidence provided by the findings and limits applicability. Many of the landmark adult health studies (e.g., the Framingham heart study and the Baltimore longitudinal study on aging) historically excluded women as subjects. Despite the all-male samples, the findings of these studies were generalized from males to all adults, in spite of the lack of female representation in the samples. Similarly, the use of largely European-American subjects in clinical trials limits the identification of variant responses to interventions or drugs in ethnic or racially distinct groups (Bailey et al., 2004; Ward, 2003). Findings based on European-American data cannot be generalized to African Americans, Asians, Hispanics, or any other cultural group.

Probability sampling is clearly the ideal sampling procedure for ensuring the representativeness of a study population. Use of random selection procedures (e.g., simple random, stratified, cluster, or systematic sampling strategies) minimizes the occurrence of conscious and unconscious biases, which affect the researcher's ability to generalize about the findings from the sample to the population. You should be able to identify the type of probability strategy used and determine whether the researcher adhered to the criteria for a particular sampling plan.

When a purposive sample is used in experimental and quasi-experimental studies, you should determine whether or how the subjects were assigned to groups. If criteria for random assignment have not been followed, you have a valid basis for being cautious about the strength of evidence provided by the proposed conclusions of the study.

Although random selection is the ideal in establishing the representativeness of a study population, more often realistic barriers (e.g., institutional policy, inaccessibility of subjects, lack of time or money, and current state of knowledge in the field) necessitate the use of nonprobability sampling strategies. Many important research questions that are of interest to nursing do not lend themselves to levels of evidence provided by experimental designs and probability sampling. This is particularly true with qualitative research designs. A well-designed, carefully controlled study using a nonprobability sampling strategy can yield accurate and meaningful evidence that makes a significant contribution to nursing's scientific body of knowledge.

As the evaluator, you must ask a philosophical question: "If it is not possible or appropriate to conduct an experimental or quasi-experimental investigation that uses probability sampling, should the study be abandoned?" The answer usually suggests that it is better to carry out the study and be fully aware of the limitations of the methodology and evidence provided than to lose the knowledge that can be gained. The researcher is always able to move on to subsequent studies that reflect a stronger and more consistent level of evidence either by replicating the study or by using more stringent design and sampling strategies to refine the knowledge derived from a nonexperimental study.

The greatest difficulty in nonprobability sampling stems from the fact that not every element in the population has an equal chance of being represented in the sample. Therefore it is likely that some segment of the population will be systematically underrepresented. If the population is homogeneous on critical characteristics, such as age, gender, socioeconomic status, and diagnosis, systematic bias will not be very important. Few of the attributes that researchers are interested in, however, are sufficiently homogeneous to make sampling bias an irrelevant consideration.

Basically you will decide whether the sample size for a quantitative study is appropriate and its size is justifiable. You want to make sure that the researcher indicated in a research article how the sample size was determined. The method of arriving at the sample size and the rationale should be briefly mentioned. In the study testing the nurse-tailored HIV medication intervention (Holzemer at al., 2006), the power analysis indicated that a sample size of 120 in each of the experimental and control groups was adequate to detect a medium effect size with power greater than 80%.

When appraising qualitative research designs, you also apply criteria related to sampling strategies that are relevant for a particular type of qualitative study. In general, sampling strategies for qualitative studies are purposive because the study of specific phenomena in their natural setting is emphasized; any subject belonging to a specified group is considered to represent that group. For example, when a qualitative study such as "Perceptions of Adult

Patients on Hemodialysis Concerning Choice among Renal Replacement Therapies" (Landreneau & Ward-Smith, 2007) is conducted, the specified group is people on hemodialysis who are asked to discuss their perceptions about their choice among renal replacement therapies. The researcher's goal is to explore what they perceive concerning choice among the three types of renal replacement therapies (hemodialysis, peritoneal dialysis, or renal transplant) and to "grasp and sense" the lived experience of patients on hemodialysis so that nurses can best meet their needs (see Chapters 4, 5, and 6). Keep in mind that qualitative studies will not discuss predetermining sample size or method of arriving at sample size. Rather, sample size will tend to be small and a function of data saturation.

The importance of this example lies not in understanding every technical word cited, but in understanding that this type of statement or some abbreviated form of it meets the criteria stated at the beginning of the paragraph and should be evident in the research report.

Finally, evidence that the rights of human subjects have been protected should appear in the "Sample" section of the research report and probably consists of no more than one sentence. Remember to evaluate whether permission was obtained from an institutional review board that reviewed the study relative to the maintenance of ethical research standards (see Chapter 11). For example, the review board examines the research proposal to determine whether the introduction of an experimental procedure may be potentially harmful and therefore undesirable. You also examine the report for evidence of the subjects' informed consent, as well as protection of their confidentiality or anonymity. It is highly unusual for research studies not to demonstrate evidence of having met these criteria. Nevertheless, you will want to be certain that ethical standards that protect sample subjects have been maintained.

CRITICAL THINKING CHALLENGES

- How do inclusion and exclusion criteria contribute to increasing the strength of evidence provided by the sampling strategy of a research study?
- Why is it important for a researcher to use power analysis to calculate sample size? How does adequate sample size affect subject mortality, representativeness of the sample, the researcher's ability to detect a treatment effect, and your ability to generalize from the study findings to your patient population?
- How does a flowchart such as the one in Figure 2 on p. 470 of the Meneses article in Appendix A contribute to the strength and quality of evidence provided by the findings of research study and their potential for applicability to practice?
- Evaluate the overall strengths and weaknesses of the sampling section of the Meneses research report in Appendix A. What are the sources of bias, if any, that present threats to internal or external validity? How does the sampling strategy contribute to the strength and quality of evidence provided by the findings and their applicability to clinical practice?
- Your research classmate argues that a random sample is always better, even if it is small and represents only one site. Another student counters that a very large convenience sample representing multiple sites can be very significant. Which classmate would you defend and why? How would each scenario affect the strength and quality of evidence provided by the findings?

KEY POINTS

- Sampling is a process that selects representative units of a population for study. Researchers sample representative segments of the population because it is rarely feasible or necessary to sample entire populations of interest to obtain accurate and meaningful information.
- Researchers establish eligibility criteria; these are descriptors of the population and provide the basis for selection of a sample. Eligibility criteria, which are also referred to as delimitations, include the following: age, gender, socioeconomic status, level of education, religion, and ethnicity.
- The researcher must identify the target population (i.e., the entire set of cases about which the researcher would like to make generalizations). Because of the pragmatic constraints, however, the researcher usually uses an accessible population (i.e., one that meets the population criteria and is available).
- A sample is a set of elements that makes up the population.
- A sampling unit is the element or set of elements used for selecting the sample. The foremost criterion in appraising a sample is the representativeness or congruence of characteristics with the population.
- Sampling strategies consist of nonprobability and probability sampling.
- In nonprobability sampling, the elements are chosen by nonrandom methods. Types of nonprobability sampling include convenience, quota, and purposive sampling.
- Probability sampling is characterized by the random selection of elements from the population. In random selection, each element in the population has an equal and independent chance of being included in the sample. Types of probability sampling include simple random, stratified random, and multistage sampling.
- Sample size is a function of the type of sampling procedure being used, the degree of precision required, the type of sample estimation formula being used, the heterogeneity of the study attributes, the relative frequency of occurrence of the phenomena under consideration, and cost.
- Criteria for drawing a sample vary according to the sampling strategy. Systematic organization of the sampling procedure minimizes bias. The target population is identified, the accessible portion of the target population is delineated, permission to conduct the research study is obtained, and a sampling plan is formulated.
- When critically appraising a research report, the sampling plan needs to be evaluated for its appropriateness in relation to the particular research design and level of evidence generated by the design.
- Completeness of the sampling plan is examined in light of potential replicability of the study. The critiquer appraises whether the sampling strategy is the strongest plan for the particular study under consideration.
- An appropriate systematic sampling plan will maximize the efficiency of a research study. It will increase the strength, accuracy, and meaningfulness of the evidence provided by the findings and enhance the generalizability of the findings from the sample to the population.

REFERENCES

Artinian NT, Flack JM, Nordstrom CK, et al: Effects of nurse-managed telemonitoring on blood pressure at 12 month follow-up among urban African-Americans, *Nurs Res* 56(5):312-322, 2007.

Bailey JM, Bieniasz ME, Kmak D, et al: Recruitment and retention of economically underserved women to a cervical cancer prevention trial, *Appl Nurs Res* 17(1):55-60, 2004.

Bennett JA, Young HM, Nail LM, et al: A telephone-only motivational intervention to increase physical activity in rural adults, *Nurs Res* 57(1):24-32, 2008.

Berggren V, Bergstrom S, Edberg AK: Being different and vulnerable: experiences of immigrant African women who have been circumcised and sought maternity care in Sweden, *Transcult Nurs* 17(1):50-57, 2006.

Budin WC, Hoskins CN, Haber J, et al: Breast cancer: Education, counseling, and adjustment among patients and partners: A randomized clinical trial, *Nurs Res* 57(3):199-212, 2008.

Chang Y, Hughes LC, Mark B: Fitting in or standing out: nursing workforce diversity and unit-level outcomes, *Nurs Res* 55(6):373-380, 2006.

Cohen J: *Statistical power analysis for the behavioral sciences*, ed 2, New York, 1988, Academic Press.

Fox S, Chesla C: Living with chronic illness: a phenomenological study of the health effects of the patient-provider relationship, *J Am Acad Nurs Prac* 20:109-117, 2008.

Holzemer WL, Bakken S, Portillo C, et al: Testing a nurse-tailored HIV medication adherence intervention, *Nurs Res* 55(3):189-197, 2006.

Horgas AL, Yoon SL, Nichols AL, et al: The relationship between pain and functional disability in Black and White older adults, *Res Nurs Health* 31(4):341-354, 2008.

Im E, Wonshik C, Guevara E, et al: Gender and ethnic differences in cancer pain experience, *Nurs Res* 56(5):296-306, 2007.

Jones EG, Renger R, Youngmi K: Self-efficacy for health-related behaviors among deaf adults, *Res Nurs Health* 30:185-192, 2007.

Landreneau KJ, Ward-Smith P: Perceptions of adult patients on hemodialysis concerning choice among renal replacement therapies, *Nephrol Nurs J* 34(3):513-525, 2007.

McConnell ES, Branch LG, Sloane RJ, Pieper CF: Natural history of change in physical function among long-stay nursing home residents, *Nurs Res* 52(2):119-126, 2003.

Meneses KD, McNees P, Loerzel VW, et al: Transition from treatment to survivorship: effects of a psychoeducational intervention on quality of life in breast cancer survivors, *Oncol Nurs Forum* 34(5):1007-1016, 2007.

Richmond TS, Hollander JE, Acherson TH, et al: Psychiatric disorders in patients presenting to the emergency department for minor injury, *Nurs Res* 56(4):275-282, 2007.

Schoenfelder DP, Rubenstein LM: An exercise program to improve fall-related outcomes in elderly nursing home residents, *Appl Nurs Res* 17(1):21-31, 2004.

Sousa VD, Zauszniewski JA, Musil CM: How to determine whether a convenience sample represents the population, *Appl Nurs Res* 17(2):130-133, 2004.

Speziale S, Carpenter DR: *Qualitative research in nursing*, ed 3, Philadelphia, 2007, Lippincott.

Thompson C, Dalgeish L, Bucknell T, et al: The effects of time pressure and experience on nurses' risk assessment decisions: a signal detection analysis, *Nurs Res* 57(5):302-311, 2008.

Ulrich CM, Danis M, Ratcliffe SJ, et al: Ethical conflict in nurse practitioners and physician assistants in managed care, *Nurs Res* 55(6):391-401, 2006.

Ward LS: Race as a variable in cross-cultural research, *Nurs Outlook* 51(3):120-125, 2003.

FOR FURTHER STUDY

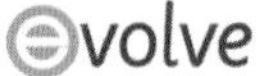

Go to Evolve at http://evolve.elsevier.com/LoBiondo/ for review questions, critiquing exercises, and additional research articles for practice in reviewing and critiquing.

11

Legal and Ethical Issues

Judith Haber

KEY TERMS

anonymity
assent
beneficence
confidentiality
consent
ethics
informed consent
institutional review boards (IRBs)
justice
respect for persons
risk/benefit ratio

LEARNING OUTCOMES

After reading this chapter, you should be able to do the following:

- Describe the historical background that led to the development of ethical guidelines for the use of human subjects in research.
- Identify the essential elements of an informed consent form.
- Evaluate the adequacy of an informed consent form.
- Describe the institutional review board's role in the research review process.
- Identify populations of subjects who require special legal and ethical research considerations.
- Appreciate the nurse researcher's obligations to conduct and report research in an ethical manner.
- Describe the nurse's role as patient advocate in research situations.
- Critique the ethical aspects of a research study.

STUDY RESOURCES

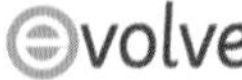

Go to Evolve at http://evolve.elsevier.com/LoBiondo/ for review questions, critiquing exercises, and additional research articles for practice in reviewing and critiquing.

"In the 'court of imagination,' where Americans often play out their racial politics, a ceremony, starring a southern white President of the United States offering an apology and asking for forgiveness from a 94-year-old African-American man, seemed like a fitting close worthy in its tableaux quality of a William Faulkner or Toni Morrison novel. The reason for this drama was the federal government's May 16th formal ceremony of repentance tendered to the aging and ailing survivors of the infamous Tuskegee Syphilis Study. The study is a morality play for many among the African-American public and the scientific research community, serving as our most horrific example of a racist 'scandalous story' … when government doctors played God and science went mad. At the formal White House gathering, when President William J. Clinton apologized on behalf of the American government to the eight remaining survivors of the study, their families, and heirs seemingly a sordid chapter in American research history was closed 25 years after the study itself was forced to end. As the room filled with members of the Black Congressional Caucus, cabinet members, civil rights leaders, members of the Legacy Committee, the Centers for Disease Control (CDC), and five of the survivors, the sense of a dramatic restitution was upon us."

Reverby (2000)

Nurses are in an ideal position to promote patients' awareness of the role played by research in the advancement of science and improvement in patient care. Embedded in our professional Code of Ethics (American Nurses Association [ANA], 2001) is the charge to protect patients from harm; the codes not only are the rules and regulations regarding the involvement of human research subjects to ensure that research is conducted legally and ethically, but also address the conduct of the people who are supposed to be governed by the rules. Researchers themselves and caregivers providing care to patients, who also happen to be research subjects, must be fully committed to the tenets of informed consent and patients' rights. The principle "the ends justify the means" must never be tolerated. Researchers and caregivers of research subjects must take every precaution to protect people being studied from physical or mental harm or discomfort. It is not always clear what constitutes harm or discomfort.

The focus of this chapter is the legal and ethical considerations that must be addressed before, during, and after the conduct of research. Informed consent, institutional review boards, and research involving vulnerable populations—the elderly, pregnant women, children, prisoners, persons with acquired immunodeficiency syndrome (AIDS), are discussed. The nurse's role as patient advocate, whether functioning as researcher, caregiver, or research consumer, is addressed. This focus is consistent with the definition of **ethics,** that is, the theory or discipline dealing with principles of moral values and moral conduct.

ETHICAL AND LEGAL CONSIDERATIONS IN RESEARCH: A HISTORICAL PERSPECTIVE

Past Ethical Dilemmas in Research

Ethical and legal considerations with regard to research first received attention after World War II. When the reigning U.S. Secretary of State and Secretary of War learned that the trials for war criminals would focus on justifying the atrocities committed by Nazi physicians as "medical research," the American Medical Association was asked to appoint a group to develop a code of ethics for research that would serve as a standard for judging the medical atrocities committed by physicians on concentration camp prisoners.

The Nuremberg Code and its definitions of the terms *voluntary, legal capacity, sufficient understanding,* and *enlightened decision* have been the subject of numerous court cases and presidential commissions involved in setting ethical standards in research (Creighton, 1977). The code that was developed requires informed consent in all cases but makes no provisions for any special treatment of children, the elderly, or the mentally incompetent. Several other international standards have followed, the most notable of which was the Declaration of Helsinki, which was adopted in 1964 by the World Medical Assembly and then later revised in 1975 (Levine, 1979).

In the United States, federal guidelines for the ethical conduct of research involving human subjects were not developed until the 1970s. Despite the supposed safeguards provided by the federal guidelines, some of the most atrocious, and hence memorable, examples of unethical research studies took place in the United States as recently as the 1990s. These examples are highlighted in Table 11-1. They are sad reminders of our own tarnished research heritage and illustrate the human consequences of not adhering to ethical research standards.

The conduct of harmful, illegal research made additional controls necessary. In 1973 the Department of Health, Education, and Welfare published the first set of proposed regulations on the protection of human subjects. The most important provision was a regulation mandating that an institutional review board (IRB) functioning in accordance with specifications of

TABLE 11-1 Highlights of Unethical Research Studies Conducted in the United States

Research Study	Year(s)	Focus of Study	Ethical Principle Violated
Hyman vs. Jewish Chronic Disease Hospital case	1965	Doctors injected cancer-ridden aged and senile patients with their own cancer cells to study the rejection response.	Informed consent was not obtained, and there was no indication that the study had been reviewed and approved by an ethics committee. The two physicians claimed that they did not wish to evoke emotional reactions or refusals to participate by informing the subjects of the nature of the study (Hershey & Miller, 1976).
Ivory Coast, Africa, AIDS/AZT case	1994	In clinical trials supported by the U.S. government and conducted in the Ivory Coast, Dominican Republic, and Thailand, some pregnant women infected with the human immunodeficiency virus (HIV) were given placebo pills rather than AZT, a drug known to prevent mothers from passing on the virus to their babies. Babies born to these mothers were in danger of contracting a fatal disease unnecessarily.	Subjects who consented to participate and who were randomized to the control group were denied access to a medication regimen with a known benefit. This violates the subjects' right to fair treatment and protection (French, 1997; Wheeler, 1997).
Midgeville, Georgia, case	1969	Investigational drugs were used on mentally disabled children without first obtaining the opinion of a psychiatrist.	There was no review of the study protocol or institutional approval of the program before implementation (Levine, 1986).

TABLE 11-1 Highlights of Unethical Research Studies Conducted in the United States—cont'd

Research Study	Year(s)	Focus of Study	Ethical Principle Violated
Tuskegee, Alabama, Syphilis Study	1932-1973	For 40 years the U.S. Public Health Service conducted a study using two groups of poor black male sharecroppers. One group consisted of those who had untreated syphilis; the other group was judged to be free of the disease. Treatment was withheld from the group having syphilis even after penicillin became generally available and accepted as effective treatment in the 1950s. Steps were taken to prevent the subjects from obtaining it. The researcher wanted to study the untreated disease.	Many of the subjects who consented to participate in the study were not informed about the purpose and procedures of the research. Others were unaware that they were subjects. The degree of risk outweighed the potential benefit. Withholding of known effective treatment violates the subjects' right to fair treatment and protection from harm (Levine, 1986).
San Antonio Contraceptive Study	1969	In a study examining the side effects of oral contraceptives, 76 impoverished Mexican-American women were randomly assigned to an experimental group receiving birth control pills or a control group receiving placebos. Subjects were not informed about the placebo and attendant risk of pregnancy; 11 subjects became pregnant, 10 of whom were in the placebo control group.	Principles of informed consent were violated; full disclosure of potential risk, harm, results, or side effects was not evident in the informed consent document. The potential risk outweighed the benefits of the study. The subjects' right to fair treatment and protection from harm was violated (Levine, 1986).
Willowbrook Hospital	1972	Mentally incompetent children ($n = 350$) were not admitted to Willowbrook Hospital, a residential treatment facility, unless parents consented to their children being subjects in a study examining the natural history of infectious hepatitis and the effect of gamma globulin. The children were deliberately infected with the hepatitis virus under various conditions; some received gamma globulin; others did not.	Principle of voluntary consent was violated. Parents were coerced to consent to their children's participation as research subjects. Subjects or their guardians have a right to self-determination; that is, they should be free of constraint, coercion, or undue influence of any kind. Many subjects feel pressured to participate in studies if they are in powerless, dependent positions (Rothman, 1982).
UCLA Schizophrenia Medication Study	1983 to present	In a study examining the effects of withdrawing psychotropic medications of 50 patients under treatment for schizophrenia, 23 subjects suffered severe relapses after their medication was stopped. The goal of the study was to determine if some schizophrenics might do better without medications that had deleterious side effects.	Although all subjects signed informed consent documents, they were not informed about how severe their relapses might be, or that they could suffer worsening symptoms with each recurrence. Principles of informed consent were violated; full disclosure of potential risk, harm, results, or side effects was not evident in the informed consent document. The potential risk outweighed the benefits of the study. The subjects' right to fair treatment and protection from harm was violated (Hilts, 1995).

BOX 11-1 Basic Ethical Principles Relevant to the Conduct of Research

RESPECT FOR PERSONS

People have the right to self-determination and to treatment as autonomous agents. Thus they have the freedom to participate or not participate in research. Persons with diminished autonomy are entitled to protection.

BENEFICENCE

Beneficence is an obligation to do no harm and maximize possible benefits. Persons are treated in an ethical manner, their decisions are respected, they are protected from harm, and efforts are made to secure their well-being.

JUSTICE

Human subjects should be treated fairly. An injustice occurs when a benefit to which a person is entitled is denied without good reason or when a burden is imposed unduly.

the department must review and approve all studies. The National Research Act, passed in 1974 (Public Law 93-348), created the National Commission for the Protection of Human Subjects of Biomedical and Behavioral Research. A major charge of the Commission was to identify the basic principles that should underlie the conduct of biomedical and behavioral research involving human subjects and to develop guidelines to ensure that research is conducted in accordance with those principles (Levine, 1986). Three ethical principles were identified as relevant to the conduct of research involving human subjects: the principles of **respect for persons, beneficence,** and **justice.** They are defined in Box 11-1. Included in a report issued in 1979, called the Belmont Report, these principles provided the basis for regulations affecting research sponsored by the federal government. The Belmont Report also served as a model for many of the ethical codes developed by scientific disciplines (National Commission, 1978).

In 1980 the Department of Health and Human Services (DHHS) developed a set of regulations in response to the Commission's recommendations. These regulations were published in 1981 and have been revised several times, with the latest revisions in 2004 (DHHS, 1983, 2003a). These regulations include the following:

- General requirements for informed consent
- Documentation of informed consent
- IRB review of research proposals
- Exempt and expedited review procedures for certain kinds of research
- Criteria for IRB approval of research

The 2001 regulations are part of the Code of Federal Regulations (CFR, 1983) Title 45 Part 46. These regulations are interpreted by the Office for Human Research Protection (OHRP), an agency that is part of the DHHS whose functions are outlined online at http://ohrp.osophs.dhhs.gov. CFR Title 21 Parts 50 and 56 and also CFR Title 45 Part 46 provide guidelines for the protection of human subjects in publicly and privately funded research to ensure privacy and confidentiality of information obtained from research. However, the potential of electronic access and transfer of an individual's health information has led to public concern about the possible abuse of individual health information in all health care contexts, including research. First enacted in 1996 and implemented with regulations on April

13, 2003, the Health Insurance Portability and Accountability Act (HIPAA) (Public Law 104-191) requires the health care profession to protect the privacy of patient information and create standards for electronic data exchange (DHHS, 2003b; Olson, 2003) (see www.hhs.gov/ocr). These regulations will be discussed in detail in the sections on informed consent and institutional review later in this chapter.

In 1992 the National Institutes of Health (NIH) Office of Research Integrity was established to set standards for dealing with allegations of scientific misconduct (Office of Research Integrity, 2000). In 1993 Congress passed the NIH Revitalization Act, which, among other provisions, created a 12-member Commission on Research Integrity to propose new procedures for addressing scientific misconduct. A report, "Integrity and Misconduct in Research," issued by the Commission in 1995 proposed a new definition of scientific misconduct, additional protection for "whistle blowers," and a set of guidelines for handling allegations of scientific misconduct (Commission on Research Integrity, 1995; National Bioethics Advisory Commission, 1998; Ryan, 1996). In 1996 the Office of Research Integrity reviewed and revised the scientific misconduct policy to (1) make a uniform policy that could be used across agencies of the federal government, (2) establish a policy that has the potential to affect the integrity of the research record, and (3) develop a protocol for handling allegations of research misconduct. Concurrently, President Clinton appointed members of the National Bioethics Advisory Commission, which provided guidance to federal agencies on the ethical conduct of current and future human biological and behavioral research related to such controversial issues as cloning, gene transfer, and stem cell research. The Commission concluded its 6-year charge to articulate a set of bioethical research issues in December 2001.

PROTECTION OF HUMAN RIGHTS

Human rights are the claims and demands that have been justified in the eyes of an individual or by a group of individuals. The term refers to the following five rights outlined in the ANA (2001) guidelines:

1. Right to self-determination
2. Right to privacy and dignity
3. Right to anonymity and confidentiality
4. Right to fair treatment
5. Right to protection from discomfort and harm

These rights apply to everyone involved in a research project, including research team members who may be involved in data collection, practicing nurses involved in the research setting, and subjects participating in the study. As you read a research article, you must realize that any issues highlighted in Table 11-2 should have been addressed and resolved before a research study is approved for implementation.

HELPFUL HINT

Recognize that the right to personal privacy may be more difficult to protect when carrying out qualitative studies because of the small sample size and because the subjects' verbatim quotes are often used in the results/findings section of the research report to highlight the findings.

TABLE 11-2 Protection of Human Rights

Definition	Violation of Basic Human Right	Example
RIGHT TO SELF-DETERMINATION		
Based on the ethical principle of respect for persons, people should be treated as autonomous agents who have the freedom to choose without external controls. An autonomous agent is one who is informed about a proposed study and is allowed to choose to participate or not to participate; subjects have the right to withdraw from a study without penalty. Subjects with diminished autonomy are entitled to protection. They are more vulnerable because of age, legal or mental incompetence, terminal illness, or confinement to an institution. Justification for use of vulnerable subjects must be provided.	A subject's right to self-determination is violated through the use of coercion, covert data collection, and deception. • Coercion occurs when an overt threat of harm or excessive reward is presented to ensure compliance. • Covert data collection occurs when people become research subjects and are exposed to research treatments without knowing it. • Deception occurs when subjects are actually misinformed about the purpose of the research. • Potential for violation of the right to self-determination is greater for subjects with diminished autonomy; they have decreased ability to give informed consent and are vulnerable.	Subjects may feel that their care will be adversely affected if they refuse to participate in research. The Jewish Chronic Disease Hospital Study (see Table 11-1) is an example of a study in which patients and their doctors did not know that cancer cells were being injected. In the Milgrim (1963) study, subjects were deceived when asked to administer electric shocks to another person; the person was really an actor who pretended to feel the shocks. Subjects administering the shocks were very stressed by participating in this study, although they were not administering shocks at all. The Willowbrook Study (see Table 11-1) is an example of how coercion was used to obtain parental consent of vulnerable mentally retarded children who would not be admitted to the institution unless the children participated in a study in which they were deliberately injected with the hepatitis virus.
RIGHT TO PRIVACY AND DIGNITY		
Based on the principle of respect, privacy is the freedom of a person to determine the time, extent, and circumstances under which private information is shared or withheld from others.	The Privacy Act of 1974 was instituted to protect subjects from such violations. These occur most frequently during data collection when invasive questions are asked that might result in loss of job, friendships, or dignity or might create embarrassment and mental distress. It also may occur when subjects are unaware that information is being shared with others.	Subjects may be asked personal questions such as the following: "Were you sexually abused as a child?" "Do you use drugs?" "What are your sexual preferences?" When questions are asked using hidden microphones or hidden tape recorders, the subjects' privacy is invaded because they have no knowledge that the data are being shared with others. Subjects also have a right to control access of others to their records.
RIGHT TO ANONYMITY AND CONFIDENTIALITY		
Based on the principle of respect, **anonymity** exists when the subject's identity cannot be linked, even by the researcher, with his or her individual responses (ANA, 1985).	Anonymity is violated when the subjects' responses can be linked with their identity.	Subjects are given a code number instead of using names for identification purposes. Subjects' names are never used when reporting findings.

TABLE 11-2 Protection of Human Rights—cont'd

Definition	Violation of Basic Human Right	Example
RIGHT TO ANONYMITY AND CONFIDENTIALITY—cont'd		
Confidentiality means that individual identities of subjects will not be linked to the information they provide and will not be publicly divulged.	Confidentiality is breached when a researcher, either by accident or by direct action, allows an unauthorized person to gain access to study data that contain information about subject identity or responses that create a potentially harmful situation for subjects.	Breaches of confidentiality with regard to sexual preference, income, drug use, prejudice, or personality variables can be harmful to subjects. Data are analyzed as group data so that individuals cannot be identified by their responses.
RIGHT TO FAIR TREATMENT		
Based on the ethical principle of justice, people should be treated fairly and should receive what they are due or owed. Fair treatment is equitable selection of subjects and their treatment during the research study. This includes selection of subjects for reasons directly related to the problem studied vs. convenience, compromised position, or vulnerability. It also includes fair treatment of subjects during the study, including fair distribution of risks and benefits regardless of age, race, or socioeconomic status.	Injustices with regard to subject selection have occurred as a result of social, cultural, racial, and gender biases in society. Historically, research subjects often have been obtained from groups of people who were regarded as having less "social value," such as the poor, prisoners, slaves, the mentally incompetent, and the dying. Often subjects were treated carelessly, without consideration of physical or psychological harm.	The Tuskegee Syphilis Study (1973), the Jewish Chronic Disease Study (1965), the San Antonio Contraceptive Study (1969), and the Willowbrook Study (1972) (see Table 11-1) all provide examples related to unfair subject selection. Investigators should not be late for data-collection appointments, should terminate data collection on time, should not change agreed-on procedures or activities without consent, and should provide agreed-on benefits such as a copy of the study findings or a participation fee.
RIGHT TO PROTECTION FROM DISCOMFORT AND HARM		
Based on the ethical principle of beneficence, people must take an active role in promoting good and preventing harm in the world around them, as well as in research studies. Discomfort and harm can be physical, psychological, social, or economic in nature. There are five categories of studies based on levels of harm and discomfort: 1. No anticipated effects 2. Temporary discomfort 3. Unusual level of temporary discomfort 4. Risk of permanent damage 5. Certainty of permanent damage	Subjects' right to be protected is violated when researchers know in advance that harm, death, or disabling injury will occur and thus the benefits do not outweigh the risk.	Temporary physical discomfort involving minimal risk includes fatigue or headache; emotional discomfort includes the expense involved in traveling to and from the data-collection site. Studies examining sensitive issues, such as rape, incest, or spouse abuse, might cause unusual levels of temporary discomfort by opening up current and/or past traumatic experiences. In these situations, researchers assess distress levels and provide debriefing sessions during which the subject may express feelings and ask questions. The researcher has the opportunity to make referrals for professional intervention.

Continued

TABLE 11-2 Protection of Human Rights—cont'd

Definition	Violation of Basic Human Right	Example
RIGHT TO PROTECTION FROM DISCOMFORT AND HARM—cont'd		
		Studies having the potential to cause permanent damage are more likely to be medical rather than nursing in nature. A recent clinical trial of a new drug, a recombinant activated protein C (rAPC) (Zovan) for treatment of sepsis, was halted when interim findings from the Phase III clinical trials revealed a reduced mortality rate for the treatment group vs. the placebo group. Evaluation of the data led to termination of the trial to make available a known beneficial treatment to all patients. In some research, such as the Tuskegee Syphilis Study or the Nazi medical experiments, subjects experienced permanent damage or death.

Procedures for Protecting Basic Human Rights

Informed Consent

Elements of informed consent illustrated by the ethical principles of respect and its related right to self-determination are outlined in Box 11-2 and Table 11-2. Nurses need to understand elements of informed consent so that they are knowledgeable participants in obtaining informed consents from patients and/or in critiquing this process as it is presented in research articles. Informed consent is documented by a consent form that is given to prospective subjects and must contain standard elements. It is critical to note that informed consent is not just giving a potential subject a consent form but is a process that must be completed with each subject.

Informed consent is the legal principle that, at least in theory, governs the patient's ability to accept or reject individual medical interventions designed to diagnose or treat an illness. It is also a doctrine that determines and regulates participation in research (Olson, 2003). The Code of Federal Regulations (U.S. Food and Drug Administration [FDA], 1998a) defines the meaning of informed consent as follows:

> *The knowing consent of an individual or his/her legally authorized representative, under circumstances that provide the prospective subject or representative sufficient opportunity to consider whether or not to participate without undue inducement or any element of force, fraud, deceit, duress, or other forms of constraint or coercion.*

No investigator may involve a human as a research subject before obtaining the legally effective informed consent of a subject or legally authorized representative. The study must be explained to all potential subjects, including the study's purpose; procedures; risks, discomforts, and benefits; and expected duration of participation (i.e., when the study's procedures

BOX 11-2 Elements of Informed Consent

1. Title of Protocol
2. Invitation to Participate
3. Basis for Subject Selection
4. Overall Purpose of Study
5. Explanation of Procedures
6. Description of Risks and Discomforts
7. Potential Benefits
8. Alternatives to Participation
9. Financial Obligations
10. Assurance of Confidentiality
11. In Case of Injury Compensation
12. HIPAA Disclosure
13. Subject Withdrawal
14. Offer to Answer Questions
15. Concluding Consent Statement
16. Identification of Investigators

From Code of Federal Regulations: Protection of human subjects, 45 CFR 46, *OPRR Reports,* revised March 8, 1983.

will be implemented, how many times, and in what setting). Potential subjects must also be informed about any appropriate alternative procedures or treatments, if any, that might be advantageous to the subject. For example, in the Tuskegee Syphilis Study, the researchers should have disclosed that penicillin was an effective treatment for syphilis. Any compensation for subjects' participation must be delineated when there is more than minimal risk through disclosure about medical treatments and/or compensation that is available if injury occurs.

Prospective subjects must have time to decide whether to participate in a study. The researcher must not coerce the subject into participating. Nor may researchers collect data on subjects who have explicitly refused to participate in a study. An ethical violation of this principle is illustrated by the halting of eight experiments by the Food and Drug Administration (FDA) at the University of Pennsylvania's Institute for Human Gene Therapy 4 months after the death of an 18-year-old man, Jesse Gelsinger, who received experimental treatment as part of the Institute's research. The Institute could not document that all patients had been informed of the risks and benefits of the procedures. Furthermore, some patients who received the therapy should have been considered ineligible because their illnesses were more severe than allowed by the clinical protocols. Mr. Gelsinger had a non–life-threatening genetic disorder that permits toxic amounts of ammonia to build up in the liver. Nevertheless, he volunteered for an experimental treatment in which normal genes were implanted directly into his liver and he subsequently died of multiple organ failure. The Institute failed to report to the FDA that two patients in Mr. Gelsinger's trial had suffered severe side effects, including inflammation of the liver, as a result of their treatment; this should have triggered a halt to the trial (Brainard & Miller, 2000). Of course, subjects may discontinue participation or withdraw from a study at any time without penalty or loss of benefits.

HELPFUL HINT

Remember that research reports rarely provide readers with detailed information regarding the degree to which the researcher adhered to ethical principles, such as informed consent, because of space limitations in journals that make it impossible to describe all aspects of a study. Failure to mention procedures to safeguard subjects' rights does not necessarily mean that such precautions were not taken.

The language of the consent form must be understandable. For example, the reading level should be no greater than eighth grade for adults, and the use of technical research language should be avoided. Federal guidelines also require that information given to subjects or their representatives must be in a language they can understand (DHHS, 2003b). According to the

Code of Federal Regulations, subjects should in no way be asked to waive their rights or release the investigator from liability for negligence. The elements that need to be contained in an informed consent are listed in Box 11-2.

Investigators obtain **consent** through personal discussion with potential subjects. This process allows the person to obtain immediate answers to questions. However, consent forms, written in narrative or outline form, highlight elements that both inform and remind subjects of the nature of the study and their participation (Dubler & Post, 1998; Haggerty & Hawkins, 2000).

Assurance of anonymity and confidentiality (defined in Table 11-2) is usually conveyed in writing and describes the extent to which confidentiality of the subjects' records will be maintained. The right to privacy is also protected through protection of individually identifiable health information (IIHI). The DHHS developed the following guidelines to help researchers, health care organizations, health care providers, and academic institutions determine when they can use and disclose IIHI:

- The IIHI has to be "de-identified" under the HIPAA Privacy Rule.
- The data are part of a limited data set, and a data use agreement with the researcher is in place.
- The individual who is a potential research subject provides authorization for the researcher to use and disclose his or her protected health information (PHI).
- A waiver or alteration of the authorization requirement is obtained from the IRB.
- The consent form must be signed and dated by the subject. The presence of witnesses is not always necessary but does constitute evidence that the subject concerned actually signed the form. In cases in which the subject is a minor or is physically or mentally incapable of signing the consent, the legal guardian or representative must sign. The investigator also signs the form to indicate commitment to the agreement.

Generally the signed informed consent form is given to the subject. The researcher should keep a copy also. Some research, such as a retrospective chart audit, may not require informed consent—only institutional approval. In some cases when minimal risk is involved, the investigator may have to provide the subject only with an information sheet and verbal explanation. In other cases, such as a volunteer convenience sample, completion and return of research instruments provide evidence of consent. The IRB will help advise on exceptions to these guidelines, cases in which the IRB might grant waivers or amend its guidelines in other ways. The IRB makes the final determination regarding the most appropriate documentation format. Research consumers should note whether and what kind of evidence of informed consent has been provided in a research article.

HELPFUL HINT

Note that researchers often do not obtain written, informed consent when the major means of data collection is through self-administered questionnaires. The researcher usually assumes implied consent in such cases; that is, the return of the completed questionnaire reflects the respondent's voluntary consent to participate.

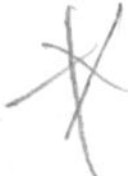

Institutional Review Board

Institutional review boards (IRBs) are boards that review research projects to assess that ethical standards are met in relation to the protection of the rights of human subjects. The National Research Act (1974) requires that such agencies as universities, hospitals, and other health care organizations (e.g., managed care companies) applying for a grant or contract for any project or program that involves the conduct of biomedical or behavioral research involving human subjects must submit with their application assurances that they have established an IRB, sometimes called a human subjects' committee, that reviews the research projects and protects the rights of the human subjects (FDA, 1998b). At agencies where no federal grants or contracts are awarded, there is usually a review mechanism similar to an IRB process, such as a research advisory committee. The National Research Act requires that the IRB have at least five members of various backgrounds to promote complete and adequate project review. The members must be qualified by virtue of their expertise and experience and reflect professional, gender, racial, and cultural diversity. Membership must include one member whose concerns are primarily nonscientific (lawyer, clergy, ethicist) and at least one member from outside the agency. Members of IRBs often have mandatory training in scientific integrity and prevention of scientific misconduct, as do the principal investigator of a research study and his or her research team members. In an effort to protect research subjects, the HIPAA Privacy Rule has made IRB requirements much more stringent for researchers to meet (Clinical Research Resources, 2004).

The IRB is responsible for protecting subjects from undue risk and loss of personal rights and dignity. The **risk-benefit ratio,** the extent to which the benefits of the study are maximized and the risks are minimized such that the subjects are protected from harm during the study is always a major consideration for the researcher. For a research proposal to be eligible for consideration by an IRB, it must already have been approved by a departmental review group such as a nursing research committee that attests to the proposal's scientific merit and congruence with institutional policies, procedures, and mission. The IRB reviews the study's protocol to ensure that it meets the requirements of ethical research that appear in Box 11-3.

Most boards provide guidelines or instructions for researchers that include steps to be taken to receive IRB approval. For example, guidelines for writing a standard consent form or criteria for qualifying for an expedited rather than a full IRB review may be made available. The IRB has the authority to approve research, require modifications, or disapprove a research study. A researcher must receive IRB approval before beginning to conduct research. Institutional review boards have the authority to suspend or terminate approval of research that is not conducted in accordance with IRB requirements or that has been associated with unexpected serious harm to subjects (Pallikkathayll et al., 1998).

BOX 11-3 Code of Federal Regulations for IRB Approval of Research Studies

To approve research, the IRB must determine that the following Code of Federal Regulations has been satisfied:

1. The risks to subjects are minimized.
2. The risks to subjects are reasonable in relation to anticipated benefits.
3. The selection of the subjects is equitable.
4. Informed consent, in one of several possible forms, must be and will be sought from each prospective subject or the subject's legally authorized representative.
5. The informed consent form must be properly documented.
6. Where appropriate, the research plan makes adequate provision for monitoring the data collected to ensure subject safety.
7. Where appropriate, there are adequate provisions to protect the privacy of subjects and the confidentiality of data.
8. Where some or all of the subjects are likely to be vulnerable to coercion or undue influence, such as persons with acute or severe physical or mental illness or persons who are economically or educationally disadvantaged, appropriate additional safeguards are included.

For example, in 2006, researchers at Johns Hopkins University published the results of a program that implemented a simple five-step checklist in nearly every intensive care unit (ICU) in Michigan that was designed to prevent specific hospital-acquired infections. Among the items on the checklist was a reminder to wash hands and don a sterile gown and gloves before inserting large intravenous (IV) lines. The results were remarkable. Within 3 months, the infection rate of bloodstream infections from IV lines fell by two thirds. The average ICU cut its infection rate from 4% to 0%. Over 18 months, the program saved more than 1,500 lives and nearly $200 million. Yet, in 2007, the Office of Human Research protections shut the program down. The agency issued a notice to the researchers and the Michigan Health and Hospital Association that, by introducing a checklist and tracking the results without written informed consent from each patient and health care provider, they had violated scientific ethics regulations and should have sought IRB approval for the program. The logic to what may seem like an illogical decision is that a checklist is an alteration in medical care no less than an experimental drug. They proposed that studying the effect of an experimental drug in people without federal monitoring and explicit written permission from each patient is unethical and illegal. Therefore it is no less unethical and illegal to do the same with a checklist (Miller & Emanuel, 2008; Pronovost et al., 2006). However, a corrective IRB action plan has been instituted and the program will continue when that process is completed.

IRBs also have mechanisms for reviewing research in an expedited manner when the risk to research subjects is minimal (Code of Federal Regulations, 1983). An expedited review usually shortens the length of the review process. Keep in mind that although a researcher may determine that a project involves minimal risk, the IRB makes the final determination, and the research may not be undertaken until then. A full list of research categories eligible for expedited review is available from any IRB office. It includes the following:

- Collection of hair and nail clippings in a nondisfiguring manner
- Collection of excreta and external secretions, including sweat
- Recording of data on subjects 18 years or older, using noninvasive procedures routinely employed in clinical practice
- Voice recordings
- Study of existing data, documents, records, pathological specimens, or diagnostic data

An expedited review does not automatically exempt the researcher from obtaining informed consent.

Health Insurance Portability and Accountability Act of 1996 (HIPAA)

The subject's right to privacy is protected by the Health Insurance Portability and Accountability Act of 1996 (HIPAA), which describes federal standards to protects patients' medical records and other health information (DHHS, 2003b), Compliance with these regulations (known as the Privacy Rule) was required as of April 2003. The HIPAA Privacy Rule expanded a person's privacy to protect his or her IIHI and described the ways in which covered entities can use or disclose this information. Covered entities include the person's (1) health provider, (2) health insurance plan, (3) employer, and (4) health care clearinghouse (public or private entity that processes or facilitates the processing of health information). According to the HIPAA Privacy Rule, IIHI is protected health information. Covered entities such as health care providers and health care agencies can allow researchers access to health care information if the information has been "de-identified," which involves removing the following 17 elements that could be used to identify a person, his or her employer, or his or her relatives.

- Names
- Geographic indicators smaller than a state
- All elements of dates (except year) for dates directly related to an individual (e.g., birth date, discharge date, etc.)
- Telephone numbers
- Facsimile (fax) numbers
- E-mail addresses
- Social Security numbers
- Health plan beneficiary numbers
- Account numbers
- Certificate/license numbers
- Vehicle identification and serial numbers
- Device identifiers and serial numbers
- Web universal resource locators (URLs)
- Internet protocol (IP) address numbers
- Biometric identifiers (e.g., fingerprints)
- Full-face photographic images
- Any other unique identifying number, characteristic, or code

As you can see, researchers are affected by the HIPAA Privacy Rule so that they must follow a proscribed protocol for accessing and communicating research subject information to protect patients' right to privacy.

IRBs can act on requests for a waiver or alteration of the authorization requirement for a research project. An altered authorization requirement occurs when an IRB approves a request that some, but not all, of the de-identification elements (e.g., name or address) be removed from the health information that is to be used in research. The researcher can also request a partial waiver of authorization, which allows the researcher to obtain personal health information (PHI) to contact and recruit potential subjects for a study. It is important to note that all institutions are guided by HIPAA guidelines in developing their informed consent procedures, but they also require additional elements.

The *Federal Register* is a publication that contains updated information about federal guidelines for research involving human subjects. Every researcher should consult an agency's research office to ensure that the application being prepared for IRB approval adheres to the most current requirements. Nurses who are critiquing published research should be conversant with current regulations to determine whether ethical standards have been met. The Critical Thinking Decision Path illustrates the ethical decision-making process an IRB might use in evaluating the risk/benefit ratio of a research study.

Protecting Basic Human Rights of Vulnerable Groups

Researchers are advised to consult their agency's IRB for the most recent federal and state rules and guidelines when considering research involving vulnerable groups who may have diminished autonomy, such as the elderly, children, pregnant women, the unborn, those who are emotionally or physically disabled, prisoners, the deceased, students, and persons with AIDS (Baskin et al., 1998; Dobratz, 2003; Haggerty & Hawkins, 2000; National Bioethics Advisory Commission, 1998; Tigges, 2003). In addition, researchers should consult the IRB before planning research that potentially involves an oversubscribed research population, such as organ transplantation patients or AIDS patients, or "captive" and convenient populations,

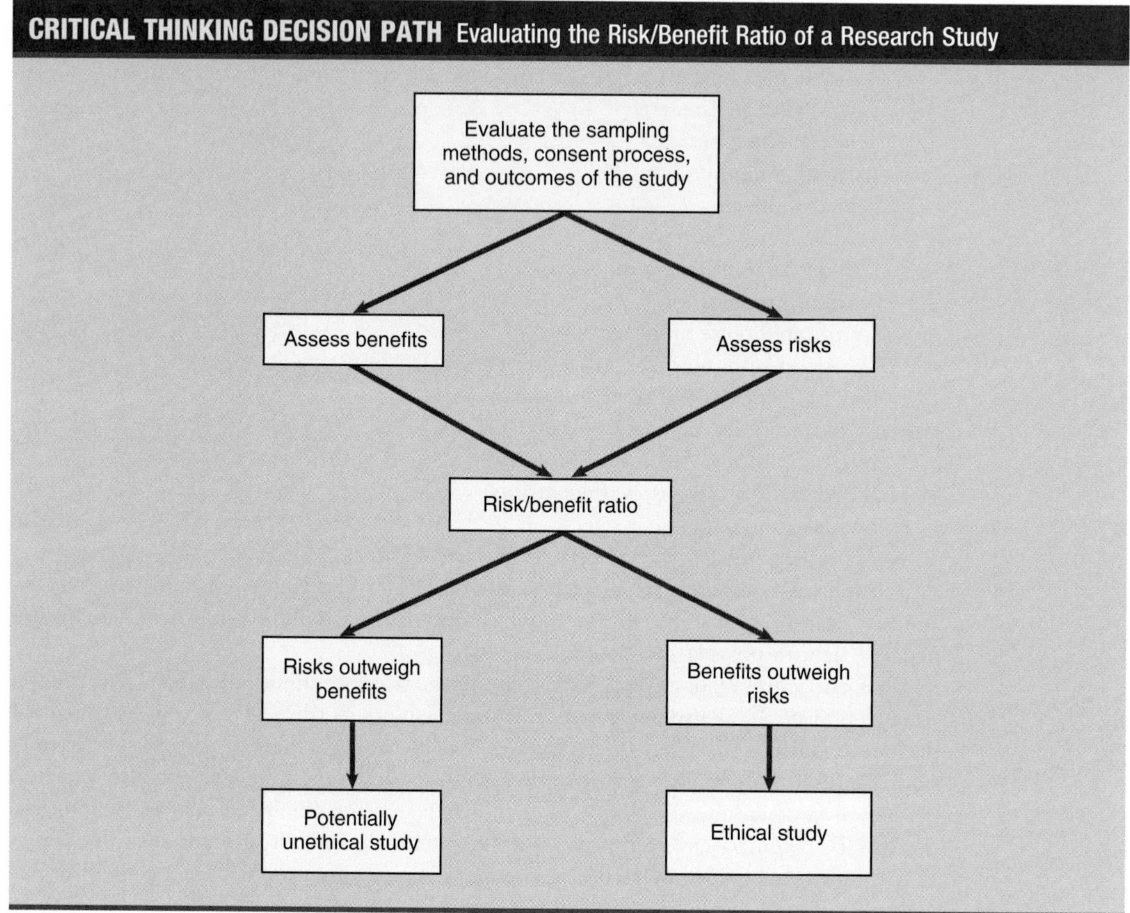

such as prisoners. It should be emphasized that use of special populations does not preclude undertaking research; extra precautions must be taken, however, to protect their rights (Levine, 1995). Davis (1981) reminds us that a society can be judged by the way it treats its most vulnerable people—a point worth remembering in research that involves children, the elderly, and other vulnerable groups.

Mitchell discussed the National Commission's concept of assent versus consent in regard to pediatric research. **Assent** contains the following three fundamental elements:

1. A basic understanding of what the child will be expected to do and what will be done to the child
2. A comprehension of the basic purpose of the research
3. An ability to express a preference regarding participation

In contrast to assent, **consent** OK requires a relatively advanced level of cognitive ability. Informed consent reflects competency standards requiring abstract appreciation and reasoning regarding the information provided. The issue of assent versus consent is an interesting one when one determines at what age children can make meaningful decisions about participating in research. In terms of the work by Piaget regarding cognitive ability, children at age 6 and older can participate in giving assent. Children at age 14 and older, although not legally authorized to give sole consent unless they are emancipated minors, can make such decisions as capably as adults (Mitchell, 1984).

Federal regulations require parental permission whenever a child is involved in research unless otherwise specified, for example, in cases of child abuse or mature minors at minimal risk (Tigges, 2003). If the research involves more than minimal risk and does not offer direct benefit to the individual child, both parents must give permission. When individuals reach maturity, usually at 18 years of age in cases of research, they may render their own consent. They may do so at a younger age if they have been legally declared emancipated minors. Questions regarding this should be addressed by the IRB and/or research administration office and not left to the discretion of the researcher to answer.

The American Geriatrics Society Ethics Committee (1998), as an advocate for the vulnerable elderly who are of increasing dependence and declining cognitive ability, states that elders are precisely the class of persons who were historically and are potentially vulnerable to abuse and for whom the law must struggle to fashion specific protections. The issue of the legal competence of elders is often raised (Flaskerud & Winslow, 1998). There is no issue if the potential subject can supply legally effective informed consent. Competence is not a clear "black or white" situation. The complexity of the study may affect one's ability to consent to participate. The capacity to obtain informed consent should be assessed in each individual for each research protocol being considered (American Geriatrics Society Ethics Committee, 1998). For example, an elderly person may be able to consent to participate in a simple observation study but not in a clinical drug trial.

The issue of the necessity of requiring the elderly to provide consent often arises. Dubler (1993) refers to research requirements for which some or all of the elements of informed consent may be waived:

1. The research involves no more than minimal risk to the subjects.
2. The waiver or alteration will not adversely affect the rights and welfare of the subjects.
3. The research could not feasibly be carried out without the waiver or alteration.
4. Whenever appropriate, the subjects will be provided with additional pertinent information after participation.

No vulnerable population may be singled out for study because it is simply convenient. For example, neither people with mental illness nor prisoners may be studied simply because they are an available and convenient group. Prisoners may be studied if the study pertains to them, that is, studies concerning the effects and processes of incarceration. Similarly, people with mental illness may participate in studies that focus on expanding knowledge about psychiatric disorders and treatments. Students also are often a convenient group. They must not be singled out as research subjects because of convenience; the research questions must have some bearing on their status as students.

Researchers and patient caregivers involved in research with vulnerable people are well advised to seek advice from appropriate IRBs, clinicians, lawyers, ethicists, and others. In all cases, the burden should be on the investigator to show the IRB that it is appropriate to involve vulnerable subjects in research.

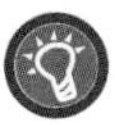

HELPFUL HINT

Keep in mind that researchers rarely mention explicitly that the study participants were vulnerable subjects or that special precautions were taken to appropriately safeguard the human rights of this vulnerable group. Research consumers need to be attentive to the special needs of groups who may be unable to act as their own advocates or are unable to adequately assess the risk/benefit ratio of a research study.

APPRAISING THE EVIDENCE

Legal and Ethical Aspects of a Research Study

Research articles and reports often do not contain detailed information regarding the degree to which or all of the ways in which the investigator adhered to the legal and ethical principles presented in this chapter. Space considerations in articles preclude extensive documentation of all legal and ethical aspects of a research study. Lack of written evidence regarding the protection of human rights does not imply that appropriate steps were not taken.

The Critiquing Criteria box provides guidelines for evaluating the legal and ethical aspects of a research report. When reading a research report, due to space constraints, you will not see all areas explicitly addressed in the research article; however, you should be aware of them and should determine that the researcher has addressed them before gaining IRB approval to conduct the study. A nurse who is asked to serve as a member of an IRB will find the critiquing criteria useful in evaluating the legal and ethical aspects of the research proposal. Box 11-4 provides examples of statements in research articles that illustrate the brevity with which the legal and ethical component of a research study is reported.

Information about the legal and ethical considerations of a study is usually presented in the methods section of a research report. The subsection on the sample or data-collection methods is the most likely place for this information. The author most often indicates in a few sentences that informed consent was obtained and that approval from an IRB or similar committee was granted. It is likely that a paper will not be accepted for publication without such a discussion. This also makes it almost impossible for unauthorized research to be published. Therefore when a research article provides evidence of having been approved by an external review committee, the reader can feel confident that the ethical issues raised by the study have been thoroughly reviewed and resolved.

To protect subject and institutional privacy, the locale of the study frequently is described in general terms in the sample subsection of the report. For example, the article might state that data were collected at a 1,000-bed tertiary care center in the Southwest, without mentioning its name. Protection of subject privacy may be explicitly addressed by statements indicating that anonymity or confidentiality of data was maintained or that grouped data were used in the data analysis.

Determining whether participants were subjected to physical or emotional risk is often accomplished indirectly by evaluating the study's methods section. The reader evaluates the **risk/benefit ratio,** that is, the extent to which the benefits of the study are maximized and the risks are minimized such that subjects are protected from harm during the study (Dubler & Post, 1998; Pruchino & Hayden, 2000).

For example, the study by Melkus and colleagues (2004) compared the effect of a 6-week, cognitive-behavioral (CB), culturally competent diabetes mellitus (DM) intervention program for African-American women (n = 25) with type 2 DM, led by advanced practice registered nurses trained in DM care and certified as DM educators on glycemic control, weight, body mass, and diabetes-related emotional distress. Results from this pilot study, using a one-group, pretest-posttest, quasi-experimental design, demonstrate that women who participated in the CB intervention for 3 months had improved psychosocial and metabolic outcomes as measured by a significant decrease in diabetes-related distress, body mass index, and weight, as well as decreased HbA1c levels to below 8%. The findings related to the outcomes of this low-cost intervention have implications for significant cost savings, at no risk and with poten-

BOX 11-4 Examples of Legal and Ethical Content in Published Research Reports

- "Permission to conduct this project was obtained from the institutional review board, and data collection ensued" (Novotny & Anderson, 2008, p. 408).
- "Permission was received from the university health sciences institutional review board to use the existing anonymous SAMSHA data" (Anderson, 2008, p. 342).
- "The investigators' university and the metropolitan cancer center approved the study. Informed consent was obtained from all participants. Confidentiality was ensured through a coding system with numbers replacing participants' names. Data were collected in private settings" (Fu et al., 2008, p. 342).
- "The study was approved by the university's human subjects committee" (Hall et al., 2008, p. 126).

tial significant benefit to both patients and health care institutions that treat community-residing minority women with type 2 DM.

In another example, a study by LoBiondo-Wood and associates (2000) investigated the relationship between family stress, family coping, social support, perception of stress, and family adaptation in families of children undergoing liver transplants. The benefits to the participants were increased knowledge about the family stressors, strains, and resources needed by families during the long-term process of seeking a transplant for a chronically ill child. Risk was minimized because subjects were mothers of children being evaluated for a liver transplant; the children's usual regimen was not being altered in any way. LoBiondo-Wood and colleagues (2000) state that before interventions can be developed to assist such families during this crisis, clinicians need to understand how aspects of family life are affected. You could infer from a description of the method that the benefits were greater than the risks and subjects were protected from harm. The findings of the study highlighted the need to understand the impact of transplantation on the family as a whole. As health care providers move to cost containment and documentation of outcomes that affect the child's family and that family's ability to cope and care for a member with chronic health care needs, research needs to focus on what aspects of the child's care are compromised if the family's needs are not addressed. The obligation to balance the risks and benefits of a study is the responsibility of the researcher. However, when you read a research report, you also should be confident that subjects have been protected from harm.

When considering the special needs of vulnerable subjects, you should be sensitive to whether the special needs of groups, unable to act on their own behalf, have been addressed. For instance, has the right of self-determination been addressed by the informed consent

CRITIQUING CRITERIA: *Legal and Ethical Issues*

1. Was the study approved by an IRB or other agency committee members?
2. Is there evidence that informed consent was obtained from all subjects or their representatives? How was it obtained?
3. Were the subjects protected from physical or emotional harm?
4. Were the subjects or their representatives informed about the purpose and nature of the study?
5. Were the subjects or their representatives informed about any potential risks that might result from participation in the study?
6. Is the research study designed to maximize the benefit(s) to human subjects and minimize the risks?
7. Were subjects coerced or unduly influenced to participate in this study? Did they have the right to refuse to participate or withdraw without penalty? Were vulnerable subjects used?
8. Were appropriate steps taken to safeguard the privacy of subjects? How have data been kept anonymous and/or confidential?

protocol identified in the research report? For example, in a study by Koenes and Karshmer (2000) comparing whether the incidence of depression was greater among blind adolescents than a sighted comparison group, the study was approved by the institutional committee for review of research involving human subjects, as well as the school administrators and parents or guardians, who had to provide written consent for subject participation. Actual student participation was entirely voluntary; students were invited to participate in a study designed to "explore stress and its impact on adolescence." All students were individually recruited, and 22 adolescents who had been legally blind since birth and 29 sighted adolescents participated in the study.

When qualitative studies are reported, verbatim quotes from informants often are incorporated into the findings section of the article. In such cases, you will evaluate how effectively the author protected the informant's identity, either by using a fictitious name or by withholding information such as age, gender, occupation, or other potentially identifying data (see Chapters 4, 5, and 6 for special ethical issues related to qualitative research).

It should be apparent from the preceding sections that although the need for guidelines for the use of human and animal subjects in research is evident and the principles themselves are clear, there are many instances when you must use your best judgment both as a patient advocate and as a research consumer when evaluating the ethical nature of a research project. In any research situation, the basic guiding principle of protecting the patient's human rights must always apply. When conflicts arise, you must feel free to raise suitable questions with appropriate resources and personnel. In an institution these may include contacting the researcher first and then, if there is no resolution, the director of nursing research and the chairperson of the IRB. In cases when ethical considerations in a research article are in question, clarification from a colleague, agency, or IRB is indicated. You should pursue your concerns until satisfied that the patient's rights and your rights as a professional nurse are protected.

CRITICAL THINKING CHALLENGES

- A state government official interested in determining the number of infants infected with the human immunodeficiency virus (HIV) has approached your hospital to participate in a state-wide funded study. The protocol will include the testing of all newborns for HIV, but the mothers will not be told that the test is being done, nor will they be told the results. Using the basic ethical principles found in Box 11-2, defend or refute the practice. How will the findings of the proposed study be affected if the protocol is carried out?
- As a research consumer, what kind of information related to the legal and ethical aspects of a research study would you expect to see written about in a published research study? How does that differ from the data the researcher would have to prepare for an IRB submission?
- A randomized clinical trial (RCT) testing the effectiveness of a new Lyme disease vaccine is being conducted as a multi-site RCT. There are two vaccine intervention groups, each of which is receiving a different vaccine, and one control group that is receiving a placebo. Using the information in Table 11-2, identify the conditions under which the RCT is halted due to potential legal and ethical issues to subjects.
- What does risk/benefit ratio mean and how does it influence the strength and quality of evidence required for clinical decision making?

KEY POINTS

- Ethical and legal considerations in research first received attention after World War II during the Nuremberg Trials, from which developed the Nuremberg Code. This became the standard for research guidelines protecting the human rights of research subjects.
- The National Research Act, passed in 1974, created the National Commission for the Protection of Human Subjects of Biomedical and Behavioral Research. The findings, contained in the Belmont Report, discuss three basic ethical principles (respect for persons, beneficence, and justice) that underlie the conduct of research involving human subjects. Federal regulations developed in response to the Commission's report provide guidelines for informed consent and IRB protocols.
- The ANA's Commission on Nursing Research published *Human Rights Guidelines for Nurses in Clinical and Other Research* in 1985, for protection of human rights of research subjects. It is relevant to nurses as researchers as well as caregivers. The ANA's *Code for Nurses* (ANA, 2001) is integral with the research guidelines.
- The Health Insurance Portability and Accountability Act (HIPAA), implemented in 2003, includes privacy rules to protect an individual's health information that affect health care organizations and the conduct of research.
- Protection of human rights includes (1) right to self-determination, (2) right to privacy and dignity, (3) right to anonymity and confidentiality, (4) right to fair treatment, and (5) right to protection from discomfort and harm.
- Procedures for protecting basic human rights include gaining informed consent, which illustrates the ethical principle of respect, and obtaining IRB approval, which illustrates the ethical principles of respect, beneficence, and justice.
- Special consideration should be given to studies involving vulnerable populations, such as children, the elderly, prisoners, and those who are mentally or physically disabled.
- Nurses as consumers of research must be knowledgeable about the legal and ethical components of a research study so they can evaluate whether a researcher has ensured appropriate protection of human or animal rights.

REFERENCES

American Geriatrics Society Ethics Committee: Informed consent for research on human subjects with dementia, *J Am Geriatr Soc* 46(10):1308-1310, 1998.

American Nurses Association: *Human rights guidelines for nurses in clinical and other research*, Kansas City, MO, 1985, Author.

American Nurses Association: *Code for nurses with interpretive statements*, Kansas City, MO, 2001, Author.

Anderson LS: Predictors of parenting stress in a diverse sample of parents of early adolescents in high-risk communities, *Nurs Res* 57(5):340-350, 2008.

Baskin SA, Morris J, Ahronheim JC, et al: Barriers to obtaining consent in dementia research: implications for surrogate decision-making, *J Am Geriatr Soc* 46(3):287-290, 1998.

Brainard J, Miller DW: U.S. regulators suspend medical studies at two universities, *Chronicle of Higher Education,* A30, February 4, 2000.

Clinical Research Resources: *Regulations and guidance on clinical investigator and IRB responsibilities*, Philadelphia, 2004, Author.

Code of Federal Regulations: Protection of human subjects, 45 CFR 46, *OPRR Reports,* revised March 8, 1983.

Commission on Research Integrity: *Integrity and misconduct in research*, Washington, DC, 1995, USDHHS.

Creighton H: Legal concerns of nursing research, *Nurs Res* 26(4):337-340, 1977.

Davis A: Ethical issues in gerontological nursing research, *Geriatr Nurs* 2:267-272, 1981.

Department of Health and Human Services: Department of Health and Human Services rules and regulations, 45CF46, Title 45, Part 46, *Fed Regul,* March 8, 1983.

Department of Health and Human Services: Standards for privacy of individually identifiable health information: final rule, *Code Fed Regul,* Title 45, Parts 160 and 164, April 17, 2003a. Retrieved January 3, 2005, from www.hhs.gov/ocr/hipaa/finalreg.html.

Department of Health and Human Services: Institutional review boards and the HIPAA privacy rule: information for researchers, September 25, 2003b. Retrieved January 3, 2005, from http://privacy rule and research.nih.gov/irbandprivacyrule.asp.

Dobratz MC: Issues and dilemmas in conducting research with vulnerable home hospice patients, *J Nurs Sch* 35(4):371-376, 2003.

Dubler NN: Personal communication, 1993.

Dubler NN, Post LF: Truth telling and informed consent. In Holland JC, editor: *Textbook of psycho-oncology,* New York, 1998, Oxford Press.

Flaskerud JH, Winslow BJ: Conceptualizing vulnerable populations health-related research, *Nurs Res* 47(2):69-78, 1998.

Food and Drug Administration: A guide to informed consent, *Code Fed Regul,* Title 21, Part 50, 1998a. Retrieved January 3, 2005, from www.fda.gov/oc/ohrt/irbs/informedconsent.html.

Food and Drug Administration: Institutional review boards, *Code Fed Regul,* Title 21, Part 56, 1998b. Retrieved January 6, 2005, from www.fda.gov/oc/ohrt/irbs/appendixc.html.

French HW: AIDS research in Africa: juggling risks and hopes, *New York Times,* A1, A12, October 9, 1997.

Fu MR, Axelrod D, Haber J: Breast-cancer–related lymphedema: information, symptoms, and risk-reduction behaviors, *J Nurs Sch* 40(4):341-348, 2008.

Haggerty LA, Hawkins J: Informed consent and the limits of confidentiality, *West J Nurs Res* 22(4):508-514, 2000.

Hall LA, Rayens MK, Peden AR: Maternal factors associated with child behavior, *J Nurs Sch* 40(2):124-130, 2008.

Hershey N, Miller RD: *Human experimentation and the law*, Germantown, MD, 1976, Aspen.

Hilts PJ: Agency faults a UCLA study for suffering of mental patients, *New York Times,* A1, A11, March 9, 1995.

Koenes SG, Karshmer JF: Depression: a comparison study between blind and sighted adolescents, *Issues Ment Health Nurs* 21:269-279, 2000.

Levine RJ: Clarifying the concepts of research ethics, *Hastings Cent Rep* 93(3):21-26, 1979.

Levine RJ: *Ethics and regulation of clinical research,* ed 2, Baltimore-Munich, 1986, Urban & Schwartzenberg.

Levine RJ: Consent for research on children, *Chronicle of Higher Education*, B1-B2, November 10, 1995.

LoBiondo-Wood G, Williams L, Kouzekanani K, et al: Family adaptation to a child's transplant: pre-transplant phase, *Prog Transplant* 10(2):1-6, 2000.

Melkus GD, Spollett G, Jefferson V, et al: A culturally competent intervention of education and care for black women with type 2 diabetes, *Appl Nurs Res* 17(1):10-20, 2004.

Miller FG, Emanuel EJ: Quality-improvement research and informed consent, *N Engl J Med* 358(8):765-767, 2008.

Mitchell K: Protecting children's rights during research, *Pediatr Nurs* 10:9-10, 1984.

National Commission for the Protection of Human Subjects of Biomedical and Behavioral Research: *Belmont report: ethical principles and guidelines for research involving human subjects,* DHEW Pub No 05, Washington, DC, 1978, US Government Printing Office, 78-0012.

Novotny NL, Anderson MA: Prediction of readmission in medical inpatients using the probability of repeated admission instrument, *Nurs Res* 57(6):406-415, 2008.

Office of Research Integrity Web site: http://ori.dhhs.gov, 2000.

Olson DP: HIPAA privacy regulations and nursing research, *Nurs Res* 52(5):344-348, 2003.

Pallikkathayll L, Crighton F, Aaronson LS: Balancing ethical quandaries with scientific rigor: part I, *West J Nurs Res* 20(3):388-393, 1998.

Pronovost P, Needham D, Berenholtz S, et al: An intervention to decrease catheter-related bloodstream infections in the ICU, *N Engl J Med* 355(26):2725-2732, 2006.

Pruchino RA, Hayden JM: Interview modality: effects on costs and data quality in a sample of older women, *J Aging Health* 12(1):3-24, 2000.

Reverby SM: History of an apology: from Tuskegee to the White House, *Res Pract* (8):1-12, 2000.

Rothman DJ: Were Tuskegee and Willowbrook studies in nature? *Hastings Cent Rep* 12(2):5-7, 1982.

Ryan K: Scientific misconduct in perspective: the need to improve accountability, *Chronicle of Higher Education,* B1-B2, July 19, 1996.

Tigges BB: Parental consent and adolescent risk behavior research, *J Nurs Sch* 35(3):283-289, 2003.

Wheeler DL: Three medical organizations embroiled in controversy over use of placebos in AIDS studies abroad, *Chronicle of Higher Education,* A15-A16, August 13, 1997.

FOR FURTHER STUDY

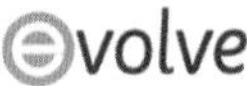

Go to Evolve at http://evolve.elsevier.com/LoBiondo/ for review questions, critiquing exercises, and additional research articles for practice in reviewing and critiquing.

12

Data-Collection Methods

Susan Sullivan-Bolyai and Carol Bova

KEY TERMS

anecdotes
closed-ended questions
concealment
consistency
content analysis
debriefing
demographic data
existing data
field notes
intervention
intervention fidelity
interview guide
interviews
Likert-type scales
measurement
measurement error
objective
open-ended questions
operational definition
participant observation
questionnaires
random error
reactivity
respondent burden
scale
scientific observation
self-report
systematic
systematic error

LEARNING OUTCOMES

After reading this chapter, you should be able to do the following:

- Define the types of data-collection methods used in nursing research.
- List the advantages and disadvantages of each data-collection method.
- Compare how specific data-collection methods contribute to the strength of evidence in a research study.
- Identify potential sources of bias related to data collection.
- Discuss the importance of intervention fidelity in data collection.
- Critically evaluate the data-collection methods used in published research studies.

STUDY RESOURCES

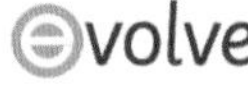

Go to Evolve at http://evolve.elsevier.com/LoBiondo/ for review questions, critiquing exercises, and additional research articles for practice in reviewing and critiquing.

Nurses are always collecting information (or data) from patients. We collect data on blood pressure, age, weight, height, and laboratory values as part of our daily work. Data collected for practice purposes and data collected for research have several key differences. Data-collection procedures in research must be objective and systematic. By **objective,** we mean that the data collected are free from the researchers' personal biases, beliefs, values, or attitudes. By **systematic,** we mean that the data are collected in a uniform, consistent, or standard way from each subject by everyone who is involved in the data-collection process. When reading a study, the data-collection methods should be identifiable and repeatable. Thus, when reading the research literature to inform your evidence-based practice, there are several issues to consider regarding study data-collection descriptions.

It is important that researchers carefully define the *concepts* or *variables* they are interested in measuring. The process of translating a concept into a measurable variable for data collection requires the development of an **operational definition.** An operational definition is how the researcher will measure each variable. For example, Horgas and colleagues (2008) (see Appendix C) defined *disability* as including both physical and social functional limitations and operationally measured the variables using the Sickness Impact Profile. Meneses and colleagues (2007) (see Appendix A) defined *quality of life* as including the four domains of physical, psychological, social, and spiritual well-being and measured quality of life with the Quality of Life–Breast Cancer Survivors Scale.

Ultimately, the degree to which the researcher is able to clearly define the variables of interest and measure them in an unbiased and consistent way is an important determinant of how useful the data will be to guide practice. The purpose of this chapter is to familiarize you with the various ways that researchers collect data from and about subjects. The chapter provides you with the tools for evaluating the types of data-collection procedures commonly used in research publications, their strengths and weaknesses, and how consistent data-collection operations can increase rigor (intervention fidelity) and decrease bias that affects the internal and external validity of a study and how useful each technique is for providing evidence for nursing practice. This information will help you critique the research literature and decide whether the findings provide evidence that is applicable to your practice setting.

MEASURING VARIABLES OF INTEREST

To a large extent, the success of a study depends on the quality of the data-collection methods chosen and employed. Researchers have many types of methods available for collecting information from subjects in research studies. Determining what **measurement** to use in a particular investigation may be the most difficult and time-consuming step in study design. Thus the process of evaluating and selecting the available instruments to measure variables of interest is of critical importance to the potential success of the study.

As you read research articles you should find that, regardless of which data-collection technique was used, it was consistent with the study's aim, hypotheses, setting, and population. Data-collection methods may be viewed as a two-step process. First, the researcher chooses the method or methods to be used in a study. In this chapter the selection of measures and the implementation of the data-collection process are discussed. An algorithm that influences a researcher's choice of data-collection methods is diagrammed in the Critical Thinking

CRITICAL THINKING DECISION PATH Consumer of Research Literature Review

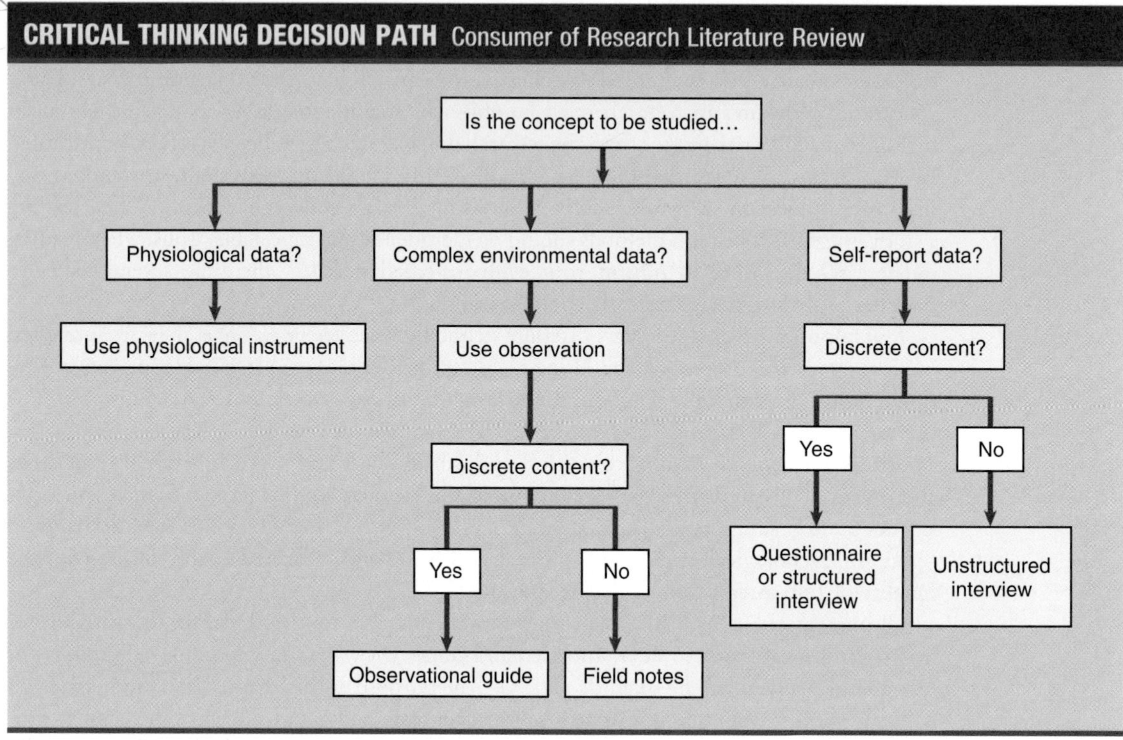

Decision Path. The next important step is deciding if these methods are reliable and valid. Reliability and validity of instruments used to collect data are discussed in Chapter 13.

DATA-COLLECTION METHODS

When reading a research article, be aware that investigators must decide early in the research process whether they need to collect their own data or whether data already exist in the form of records or databases. This decision is based on a thorough review of the literature and the availability of existing data. If the researcher determines that no data exist, new data can be collected through observation, through self-report (interviewing or questionnaires), or by collecting physiological data using standardized instruments or testing procedures (e.g., laboratory tests, x-rays). **Existing data** can be collected for research purposes by extracting data from medical records or databases using standardized procedures. Each of these methods has a specific purpose, as well as certain pros and cons inherent in its use. It is also important to remember that all data-collection methods rely on the ability of the researcher to standardize these procedures to increase data accuracy and reduce measurement error.

Measurement error is the difference between what really exists and what is measured in a given study. Every study has some amount of measurement error. Measurement error can be random or systematic (see Chapter 13). **Random error** occurs when scores vary in a random way. Random error occurs when data collectors do not use standard procedures to collect data consistently among all subjects in a study. **Systematic error** occurs when scores are incorrect but they are incorrect in the same direction. An example of systematic error occurs when all subjects were weighed using a weight scale that is under by 3 pounds for all subjects in the study. Researchers attempt to design data-collection methods that will be consistently applied across all subjects and time points to increase **intervention fidelity** so that measurement error leading to study bias is decreased. **Consistency** and intervention fidelity are used interchangeably and mean that data are collected from each subject in exactly the same manner with the same method by carefully trained data collectors (see Chapter 8). To help you decipher the quality of the data-collection section in an empirical article, we will next discuss the three main methods used for collecting data: observation, self-report, and physiological measurement.

HELPFUL HINT

Remember that the researcher may not always present complete information about the way the data were collected, especially when established tools were used. To learn about the tool that was used in greater detail, you may need to consult the original article describing the tool.

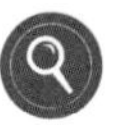

EVIDENCE-BASED PRACTICE TIP

It is difficult to place confidence in a study's findings if the data-collection methods are not consistent.

Observational Methods

Observation is an important method for collecting data on how people behave under certain conditions. Observation can take place in a natural setting (e.g., in the home, in the community, or on a nursing unit) or laboratory setting and often includes collecting data on communication (verbal, nonverbal), behavior, and environmental conditions. Observation is also useful for collecting data that may have cultural or contextual connotations. For example, if a nurse researcher wanted to understand the emergence of obesity among immigrants to the United States, it might be useful to observe food preparation, exercise patterns, and shopping practices among specific immigrant groups.

Although observing the environment is a normal part of living, **scientific observation** places a great deal of emphasis on the objective and systematic nature of the observation. The researcher is not merely looking at what is happening, but rather is watching with a trained eye for specific events. To be scientific, observations must fulfill the following four conditions:

1. The observations undertaken are consistent with the study's aims/objectives.
2. There is a standardized and systematic plan for the observation and the recording of data.
3. All of the observations are checked and controlled.
4. The observations are related to scientific concepts and theories.

		Concealment	
		Yes	No
Intervention	Yes	Researcher hidden An intervention	Researcher open An intervention
	No	Researcher hidden No intervention	Researcher open No intervention

Figure 12-1 Types of observational roles in research.

Observational methods may be structured or unstructured. Unstructured observation methods are not characterized by a total absence of structure but usually involve collecting descriptive information about the topic of interest. In **participant observation,** the observer keeps field notes to record the activities, as well as the observer's interpretations of these activities. **Field notes** are a short summary of observations made during data collection. *Field notes* usually are not restricted to any particular type of action or behavior; rather, they represent a narrative set of written notes intended to paint a picture of a social situation in a more general sense. Another type of unstructured observation is the use of anecdotes. **Anecdotes** are summaries of a particular observation that usually focus on the behaviors of interest and frequently add to the richness of research reports by illustrating a particular point. For example, Hamilton and Manias (2007) studied the observation methods of psychiatric nurses and their invisibility in an active inpatient psychiatric setting. Fieldwork data (field notes, including anecdotes that provided examples) were generated by participant observation, individual interviews, and two focus groups.

Structured observations involve specifying in advance what behaviors or events are to be observed. Typically, standardized forms are used for record keeping and include categorization systems, checklists, or rating scales. Structured observation relies heavily on the formal training and standardization of the observers (see earlier discussion and Chapter 13 for an explanation of interrater reliability).

Observational methods can be distinguished also by the role of the observer. The observer's role is determined by the amount of interaction between the observer and those being observed. These methods are illustrated in Figure 12-1. **Concealment** refers to whether the subjects know they are being observed, and **intervention** deals with whether the observer provokes actions from those who are being observed. Box 12-1 describes the four basic types of observational roles implemented by the observer(s). These are distinguishable by the amount of concealment or intervention implemented by the observer.

Observing subjects without their knowledge may violate assumptions of informed consent, and therefore researchers face ethical problems with this approach. However, sometimes there is no other way to collect such data, and the data collected are unlikely to have negative consequences for the subject; in these cases, the disadvantages of the study are outweighed by the advantages. Further, the problem is often handled by informing subjects after the observa-

BOX 12-1 Basic Types of Observational Roles

1. *Concealment without intervention.* The researcher watches the subjects without their knowledge of the observation, and does not provoke the subject into action. Often such concealed observations use hidden television cameras, audiotapes, or one-way mirrors. This method is often used in observational studies of children. You may be familiar with rooms with one-way mirrors in which a researcher can observe the behavior of the occupants of the room without being observed by them. Such studies allow for the observation of children's natural behavior and are often used in developmental research.
2. *Concealment with intervention.* Concealed observation with intervention involves staging a situation and observing the behaviors that are evoked in the subjects as a result of the intervention. Because the subjects are unaware of their participation in a research study, this type of observation has fallen into disfavor and rarely is used in nursing research.
3. *No concealment without intervention.* The researcher obtains informed consent from the subject to be observed and then simply observes his or her behavior. This was the type of observation done in a study by Aitken and colleagues (2009); nurses providing sedation management for a critically ill patient were observed and asked to think aloud during two occasions for 2 hours of care to examine the decision-making processes that nurses use when assessing and managing sedation needs of critically ill patients. This study included no concealment without an intervention.
4. *No concealment with intervention.* No concealment with intervention is employed when the researcher is observing the effects of an intervention introduced for scientific purposes. Because the subjects know they are participating in a research study, there are few problems with ethical concerns, but *reactivity* is also a problem with this type of study.

tion, allowing them the opportunity to refuse to have their data included in the study, and discussing any questions they might have. This process is called **debriefing.**

When the observer is neither concealed nor intervening, the ethical question is not a problem. Here the observer makes no attempt to change the subjects' behavior and informs them that they are to be observed. Because the observer is present, this type of observation allows a greater depth of material to be studied than if the observer is separated from the subject by an artificial barrier, such as a one-way mirror. **Participant observation** is a commonly used observational technique in which the researcher functions as a part of a social group to study the group in question. The problem with this type of observation is **reactivity** (also referred to as the Hawthorne effect), or the distortion created when the subjects change behavior because they are being observed.

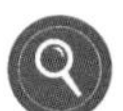

EVIDENCE-BASED PRACTICE TIP

When reading a research report that uses observation as a data-collection method, you want to note evidence of consistency across data collectors through use of interrater reliability (see Chapter 13) data. When that is present, it increases your confidence that the data were collected systematically.

Scientific observation has several advantages as a data-collection method, the main one being that observation may be the only way for the researcher to study the variable of interest. For example, what people say they do often is not what they really do. Therefore, if the study is designed to obtain substantive findings about human behavior, observation may be the only way to ensure the validity of the findings. In addition, no other data-collection method can match the depth and variety of information that can be collected when using these techniques. Such techniques also are quite flexible in that they may be used in both experimental and nonexperimental designs and in laboratory and field studies.

As with all data-collection methods, observation also has its disadvantages. Data obtained by observational techniques are vulnerable to observer bias. Emotions, prejudices, and values can influence the way that behaviors and events are observed and recorded. In general, the more the observer needs to make inferences and judgments about what is being observed, the more likely it is that distortions will occur. Thus in judging the adequacy of observation methods, it is important to consider how observation forms were constructed and how observers were trained and evaluated.

Ethical issues can also occur when observation is used to collect data. This occurs most often when research subjects are not fully aware that they are being observed. For the most part, it is best to fully inform research subjects of the purpose of the study and the fact that they are being observed. But in certain circumstances, informing the subjects will change behaviors (Hawthorne effect; see Chapter 7). For example, if a nurse researcher wanted to study hand-washing frequency on a nursing unit, telling the nurses that they were being observed for their rate of hand washing would likely increase the hand-washing rate and thereby make the study results less valid. Therefore researchers must carefully balance full disclosure of all research procedures with the ability to obtain valid data through observational methods.

HELPFUL HINT

Sometimes a researcher may carefully train and supervise observers or data collectors, but the research report does not address this. Often the length of research reports dictates that certain information cannot be included. Readers can often assume that if reliability data are provided, appropriate training and supervision occurred.

Self-Report Methods

Self-report data-collection methods require subjects to respond directly to either **interviews** or structured **questionnaires** (often called paper-and-pencil instruments) about their experiences, behaviors, feelings, or attitudes. Self-report methods are commonly used in nursing research and are most useful for collecting data on variables that cannot be directly observed or measured by physiological instruments. Some of the variables commonly measured by self-report in nursing research studies include quality of life, satisfaction with nursing care, social support, pain, uncertainty, and functional status.

When evaluating self-report methods there are several considerations:

- *Social desirability.* There is no way to know for sure if a subject is telling the truth. People are known to respond to questions in a way that makes a favorable impression. For example, if a nurse researcher asks patients to describe the positive and negative aspects of nursing care received on a nursing unit, the patient may want to please the researcher and respond with all positive responses, thus introducing bias into the data-collection process. There is no way to tell whether the respondent is telling the truth or responding in a socially desirable way, so the accuracy of self-report measures is always open for scrutiny.
- *Respondent burden* is another concern for researchers who use a self-report (Ulrich et al., 2005). **Respondent burden** occurs when the length of the questionnaire or interview is too long or the questions too difficult for respondents to answer in a reasonable amount of time considering their age, health condition, or mental status. Respondent burden can result in incomplete or erroneous answers, as well as missing data, which may jeopardize the validity of the study findings.

BOX 12-2 Open-Ended and Closed-Ended Questions Uses

- **Open-ended questions** are used when the researcher wants the subjects to respond in their own words or when the researcher does not know all of the possible alternative responses. Interviews that use open-ended questions often use a list of questions and probes called an **interview guide.** Responses to the interview guide are often audio-recorded to accurately capture the subject's responses. An example of an open-ended question is used for the interview in Appendix D.
- **Closed-ended questions** are structured, fixed-response items with a fixed number of responses. Closed-ended questions are best used when the question has a finite number of responses and the respondent is to choose the one closest to the correct response. Fixed-response items have the advantage of simplifying the respondent's task and the researcher's analysis, but they may miss some important information about the subject. Interviews that use closed-ended questions typically record a subject's responses directly on the questionnaire. An example of a closed-ended item is found in Box 12-3.

Interviews and Questionnaires

Interviews are a method of data collection where a data collector asks subjects to respond to a set of open-ended or closed-ended questions as described in Box 12-2. Interviews are used in both quantitative and qualitative research. Interviews are best used when the researcher may need to clarify the task for the respondent or is interested in obtaining more personal information from the respondent.

Open-ended questions allow more varied information to be collected and require a qualitative or content analysis method to analyze responses (see Chapter 5). **Content analysis** is a method of analyzing narrative or word responses to questions and either counting similar responses or grouping the responses into themes or categories (also used in qualitative research). Interviews may take place face-to-face, over the telephone, or online via a Web-based format.

Questionnaires are paper-and-pencil instruments designed to gather data from individuals about knowledge, attitudes, beliefs, and feelings. Questionnaires, like interviews, may be open-ended or closed-ended as presented in Box 12-2. Questionnaires are most useful when there is a finite set of questions. Individual items in a questionnaire must be clearly written so that the intent of the question and the nature of the response options are clear to the respondent. Questionnaires may be composed of individual items that measure different variables or concepts (e.g., age, race, ethnicity, and years of education) or scales. Survey researchers rely almost entirely on questionnaires for data collection.

Questionnaires can be referred to as instruments, scales, or tools. When multiple items are used to measure a single concept such as quality of life or anxiety and the scores on those items are combined mathematically to obtain an overall score, the questionnaire or measurement instrument is called a **scale.** The important issue is that each of the items must be measuring the same concept or variable. An intelligence test is an example of a scale that combines individual item responses to determine an overall quantification of intelligence.

In the study by Jones and colleagues (2007) (see Appendix B), the physical activity subscale had seven items that measured the single concept "beliefs about a person's ability to perform physical activity or exercise." Subjects were asked to respond to a five-point scale, ranging from 0 (not at all) to 4 (completely) for each of the seven physical activity items. Thus the range of scores for physical activity would be 0 to 28. In the Jones and colleagues (2007)

BOX 12-3 Examples of Open-Ended and Closed-Ended Questions

OPEN-ENDED QUESTIONS

Please list the three most important reasons why you chose to stay in your current job:

1. ______________________
2. ______________________
3. ______________________

CLOSED-ENDED QUESTIONS (LIKERT SCALE)

How satisfied are you with your current position?

1	2	3	4	5
Very satisfied	Moderately satisfied	Undecided	Moderately dissatisfied	Very dissatisfied

CLOSED-ENDED QUESTIONS

On average, how many patients do you care for in one day?

1. 1 to 3
2. 4 to 6
3. 7 to 9
4. 10 to 12
5. 13 to 15
6. 16 to 18
7. 19 to 20
8. More than 20

study, the average physical activity score was 13.89, indicating an average level of physical activity among the study subjects. The response options for scales are typically lists of statements on which respondents indicate, for example, whether they "strongly agree," "agree," "disagree," or "strongly disagree." This type of response option is called a **Likert-type scale.** "True" or "false" may also be a response option.

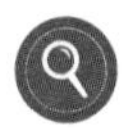

EVIDENCE-BASED PRACTICE TIP

Scales used in research should have evidence of adequate reliability and validity so that you feel confident that the findings reflect what the researcher intended to measure (see Chapter 13).

Box 12-3 shows three items from a survey of nursing job satisfaction. The first item is closed-ended and uses a Likert scale response format. The second item is also closed-ended, and it forces respondents to choose from a finite number of possible answers. The third item is open-ended and allows respondents to use their own words to answer the question, and therefore there are an unlimited number of possible answers. Often, researchers use a combination of Likert-type, closed-ended, and open-ended questions when collecting data in nursing research.

HELPFUL HINT

Remember, sometimes researchers make trade-offs when determining the measures to be used. For example, a researcher may want to learn about an individual's attitudes regarding job satisfaction; practicalities may preclude using an interview, so a questionnaire may be used instead.

Horgas and associates (2008) (see Appendix C) used self-report methods (paper-and-pencil questionnaire) to measure the relationship between pain and disability in urban older adults. They used multiple items to measure the presence, intensity, duration, and location of pain and were careful to make sure that the data-collection measures were reliable and valid for use with both older adult African Americans and white Americans. To measure disability, the researchers chose three subscales from the Sickness Impact Profile Short Form (SIP68) (de

Bruin et al., 1994), which measured physical functioning and social functioning. They also collected **demographic data.** Demographic data include information that describes important characteristics about the subjects in a study (e.g., age, gender, race, ethnicity, education, marital status). It is important to collect demographic data in order to describe and compare different study samples so you can evaluate how similar the sample is to patients you care for in your community. Finally, the researchers collected data from the subjects about health conditions using the Older Americans Resources and Services (OARS) Multidimensional Assessment (George & Fillenbaum, 1985). Data collected using this instrument was then categorized by an expert panel to evaluate the medical conditions that often resulted in physical or social disability. Therefore this data-collection method required that subjects self-report their health conditions, and then the researchers applied a scoring system to rate the degree of functional limitation for each of the subjects. Horgas and colleagues (2008) also provided important information about the potential *respondent burden* associated with the questionnaire. For example, they reported the following:

- Reading level (eighth grade)
- Questionnaire font size (14-point font)
- Need to read and assist some subjects
- Time it took to complete the questionnaire (30 minutes)

This information is very important for judging the respondent burden associated with study participation. It is important to examine the benefits and caveats associated with using interviews and questionnaires as self-report data-collection methods. Interviews offer some advantages over questionnaires. The response rate is almost always higher with interviews and there are fewer missing data, which helps reduce bias.

Another advantage of the interview is that some people, such as children, the blind, and those with low literacy, could not fill out a questionnaire, but they could participate in an interview. With an interview, the data collector knows who is giving the answers. When questionnaires are mailed, for example, anyone in the household could be the person who supplies the answers. Interviews also allow for some safeguards to be built into the interview situation. Interviewers can clarify misunderstood questions and observe the level of the respondent's understanding and record these observations in a uniform way. In addition, the researcher has strict control over the order of the questions.

With questionnaires, the respondent can answer questions in any order. Sometimes changing the order of the questions can change the response. Finally, interviews allow for richer and more complex data to be collected. This is particularly so when open-ended responses are sought. Even when closed-ended response items are used, interviewers can probe to understand why a respondent answered in a particular way.

Questionnaires also have certain advantages. They are much less expensive to administer than interviews because interviews require hiring and thoroughly training interviewers. Thus if a researcher has a fixed amount of time and money, a larger and more diverse sample can be obtained with questionnaires. Questionnaires also allow for confidentiality and anonymity, which may be important if the study deals with sensitive issues. Finally, the fact that no interviewer is present assures the researcher and the reader that there will be no interviewer bias. *Interviewer bias* occurs when the interviewer unwittingly leads the respondent to answer in a certain way. This problem can be especially pronounced in studies that use open-ended questions. A subtle nod of the head, for example, could lead a respondent to change an answer to correspond with what the researcher wants to hear.

Finally, the use of Internet-based self-report data collection (both interviewing and questionnaire delivery) has gained momentum. The use of an online format is economical and can capture subjects from different geographic areas without the expense of travel or mailings. Open-ended questions are already typed and do not require transcription, and closed-ended questions can often be imported directly into statistical analysis software and therefore reduce data entry mistakes. The main concerns with Internet-based data-collection procedures involve the difficulty of ensuring informed consent (is checking a box indicating agreement to participate the same thing as signing an informed consent form?) and the protection of subject anonymity, which is difficult to guarantee with any Internet-based venue. In addition, the requirement that subjects have computer access limits the use of this method in certain age-groups and populations. However, the advantages of increased efficiency and accuracy make Internet-based data collection a growing trend among nurse researchers.

Physiological Measurement

Physiological data collection involves the use of specialized equipment to determine the physical and biological status of subjects. Such measures can be *physical,* such as weight or temperature; *chemical,* such as blood glucose level; *microbiological,* as with cultures; or *anatomical,* as in radiological examinations. What separates these data-collection procedures from others used in research is that they require special equipment to make the observation.

Physiological or biological measurement is particularly suited to the study of many types of nursing problems. For example, examining different methods for taking a patient's temperature or blood pressure or monitoring blood glucose levels may yield important information for determining the effectiveness of certain nursing monitoring procedures or interventions. But it is important that the data-collection method be applied consistently to all subjects in the study. For example, nurses are quite familiar with taking blood pressures. However, for research studies that involve blood pressure measurement, the process must be standardized (Bern et al., 2007; Pickering et al., 2005). The subject must be positioned (sitting or lying down) the same way for a specified period of time, the same blood pressure instrument must be used, and often multiple blood pressures are taken under the same conditions and an average is taken of the multiple readings.

The advantages of using physiological data-collection methods include the objectivity, precision, and sensitivity associated with these measures. Such methods are generally quite objective because unless there is a technical malfunction, two readings of the same instrument taken at the same time by two different nurses are likely to yield the same result. Because such instruments are intended to measure the variable being studied, they offer the advantage of being precise and sensitive enough to pick up subtle variations in the variable of interest. It is also unlikely that a subject in a study can deliberately distort physiological information.

Physiological measurements are not without inherent disadvantages. Disadvantages to consider include the following:

- Some instruments may be quite expensive to obtain and use.
- Physiological instruments often require specialized knowledge and training to be used accurately.
- Another problem is that simply by using them, the variable of interest may be changed. For example, an individual's blood pressure may increase just because a health care professional enters the room (termed *white coat syndrome*).

- Although some researchers think of these instruments as being nonintrusive, the presence of some types of devices might change the measurement. For example, the presence of a heart rate monitoring device might make some patients anxious and increase their heart rate.
- Additionally, nearly all types of measuring devices are affected in some way by the environment. Even a simple thermometer can be affected by the subject drinking something hot or smoking a cigarette immediately before the temperature is taken. Thus it is important to consider whether the researcher controlled such environmental variables in the study.

Existing Data

All of the data-collection methods discussed thus far concern the ways that nurse researchers gather new data to study phenomena of interest. Not all studies, though, require a researcher to acquire new information. Sometimes existing data can be examined in a new way to study a problem. The use of records (e.g., medical records, care plans, hospital records, death certificates) and databases (e.g., U.S. Census, National Cancer Data Base, Minimum Data Set for Nursing Home Resident Assessment and Care Screening) are frequently used to answer research questions about clinical problems. Typically, this type of research design is referred to as *secondary analysis.*

The use of available data has certain advantages. First, data are already collected, thus eliminating subject burden and recruitment problems. Second, most databases contain large populations; therefore sample size is rarely a problem and random sampling is possible. Larger samples allow the researcher to do more sophisticated analytic procedures, and random sampling enhances generalizability of findings. Some records and databases collect standardized data in a uniform way and allow the researcher to examine trends over time. Finally, the use of available records has the potential to save significant time and money.

On the other hand, institutions may be reluctant to allow researchers to have access to their records. If the records are kept so that an individual cannot be identified (known as de-identified data), this is usually not a problem. However, the Health Insurance Portability and Accountability Act (HIPAA), a federal law, protects the rights of individuals who may be identified in records (Olsen, 2003) (see Chapter 11). Recent interest in computerization of health records has led to discussion about the desirability of access to such records for research. At this point, it is not clear how much computerized health data will be readily available for research purposes.

Another problem that affects the quality of available data is that the researcher has access only to those records that have survived. If the records available are not representative of all of the possible records, the researcher may have a problem with bias. Often there is no way to tell whether the records have been saved in a biased manner, and the researcher has to make an intelligent guess as to their accuracy. For example, a researcher might be interested in studying socioeconomic factors associated with the suicide rate. These data frequently are underreported because of the stigma attached to suicide, so the records would be biased.

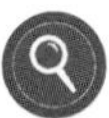

EVIDENCE-BASED PRACTICE TIP

Critical appraisal of any data-collection method includes evaluating the appropriateness, objectivity, and consistency of the method employed.

CONSTRUCTION OF NEW INSTRUMENTS

Sometimes researchers cannot locate an instrument or scale with acceptable reliability and validity to measure the variable of interest. This often is the case when testing a part of a nursing theory or when evaluating the effect of a clinical intervention. In this situation, a new instrument or scale must be developed. For example, Upton and Upton (2006) used instrument development procedures to develop a scale that measured nurses' knowledge, practice, and attitudes toward evidence-based practice.

Instrument development is complex and time consuming. It consists of the following steps:
- Define the concept to be measured
- Clarify the target population
- Develop the items
- Assess the items for content validity
- Develop instructions for respondents and users
- Pretest and pilot test the items
- Estimate reliability and validity

Defining the concept to be measured requires that the researcher develop an expertise in the concept. This requires an extensive review of the literature and of all existing tests and measurements that deal with related concepts. The researcher will use all of this information to synthesize the available knowledge so that the construct can be defined.

Once defined, the individual items measuring the concept can be developed. The researcher will develop many more items than are needed to address each aspect of the concept. The items are evaluated by a panel of experts in the field called content validity judges, so that the researcher is assured that the items measure what they are intended to measure (content validity) (see Chapter 13). Eventually the number of items will be decreased because some items will not work as they were intended and they will be eliminated from the scale. In this phase, the researcher needs to ensure consistency among the items, as well as consistency in testing and scoring procedures.

Finally, the researcher administers or pilot tests the new instrument by giving it to a group of people who are similar to those who will be studied in the larger investigation. The purpose of this analysis is to determine the quality of the instrument as a whole (reliability and validity), as well as the ability of each item to discriminate individual respondents (variance in item response). Pilot testing a new instrument also yields important evidence about the reading level (too low or too high), length of the instrument (too short or too long), directions (clear or not clear), and response rate (the percent of potential subjects who return a completed scale). Pilot testing allows one to assess if the instrument is appropriate for the target population in terms of culture or context. The researcher also may administer a related instrument to see if the new instrument is sufficiently different from the older one. Instrument development and testing is an important part of nursing science because our ability to evaluate evidence related to practice depends on measuring nursing phenomena in a clear, consistent, and reliable way.

Data-Collection Methods

Assessing the adequacy of data-collection methods is an important part of evaluating the results of studies that provide evidence for clinical practice. The data-collection procedures provide a snapshot of how the study was conducted. From an evidence-based practice perspective you can judge if the data-collection procedures would fit within your clinical environment and with your population of interest. The manner in which the data were collected affects the study's internal and external validity. A well-developed methods portion of a study assists with the avoidance of any bias in the findings. A key element for evidence-based practice is if the procedures were consistently completed. In addition to the procedures being consistent, also assess the following:

- If observation was used, was an observation guide developed and were the observers trained and supervised until there was a high level of interrater reliability? How was the training confirmed periodically throughout the study to maintain fidelity and avoid bias?
- Was a data-collection procedure manual developed and used during the study?
- If the study tested an intervention, was there training evident for the interventionists and the data collectors?
- If a physiological instrument was used, what measures were taken to ensure that the instrument was properly calibrated throughout the study and the data were collected in the same manner from each subject?
- If there were missing data, how were the data accounted for?

Evaluating the adequacy of data-collection methods from written research reports can be problematic because some research articles provide minimal information about the details of data-collection methods. Typically, the interview guide, questionnaires, or scales are not available for review. However, research articles should indicate the following:

- Type(s) of data-collection method used (self-report, observation, physiological measurement, or use of existing data)
- Evidence of training and supervision for the data collectors and interventionists
- Consistency with which data-collection procedures were applied across subjects
- Any threats to internal validity or bias related to issues of instrumentation or testing
- Any sources of bias related to external validity issues, such as the Hawthorne effect
- Scale reliability and validity discussed
- Interrater reliability across data collectors and time points (if observation was used)

When you review the data-collection methods section of a research study, it is important to think about the strength and quality of the evidence contributed by the data-collection components of the study. To the extent you have confidence that:

- An appropriate data-collection method was used
- Data collectors were appropriately trained and supervised
- Data were collected consistently by all data collectors
- Respondent burden, reactivity, and social desirability was avoided

you can critically appraise a study in terms of data-collection bias being minimized, thereby strengthening potential applicability of the evidence provided by the findings. Because a research article does not always provide all of the details, it is not uncommon to contact the researcher to obtain added information that may assist you in using results in practice. These questions are listed in the Critiquing Criteria box.

CRITIQUING CRITERIA: *Data-Collection Methods*

1. Are all of the data-collection instruments clearly identified and described?
2. Are operational definitions provided and clear?
3. Is the rationale for their selection given?
4. Is the method used appropriate to the problem being studied?
5. Were the methods used appropriate to the clinical situation?
6. Was a standardized manual used to guide data collection?
7. Were all data collectors adequately trained and supervised?
8. Are the data-collection procedures the same for all subjects?

Observational Methods

1. Who did the observing?
2. Were the observers trained to minimize any bias?
3. Was there an observational guide?
4. Were the observers required to make inferences about what they saw?
5. Is there any reason to believe that the presence of the observers affected the behavior of the subjects?
6. Were the observations performed using the principles of informed consent?
7. Was interrater agreement between observers established?

Self-Report: Interviews

1. Is the interview schedule described adequately enough to know whether it covers the topic?
2. Is there clear indication that the subjects understood the task and the questions?
3. Who were the interviewers, and how were they trained?
4. Is there evidence of any interviewer bias?

Self-Report: Questionnaires

1. Is the questionnaire described well enough to know whether it covers the topic?
2. Is there evidence that subjects were able to answer the questions?
3. Are the majority of the items appropriately closed-ended or open-ended?

Physiological Measurement

1. Is the instrument used appropriate to the research question or hypothesis?
2. Is a rationale given for why a particular instrument was selected?
3. Is there a provision for evaluating the accuracy of the instrument?

Existing Data: Records and Databases

1. Are the existing data used appropriately considering the research question and hypothesis being studied?
2. Are the data examined in such a way as to provide new information?
3. Is there any indication of selection bias in the available records?

CRITICAL THINKING CHALLENGES

1. When a researcher opts to use observation as the data-collection method. What steps must be taken must be taken to minimize bias ?
2. In a randomized clinical trial (RCT) investigating the differential effect of an educational video intervention in comparison to a telephone counseling intervention, data were collected at four different hospitals by four different data collectors. What steps should the researcher take to insure intervention fidelity?
3. What are the strengths and weaknesses of collecting data using existing sources such as records, charts, and data bases?
4. A journal club just finished reading the research report by Horgas and colleagues in Appendix C. As part of their critical appraisal of this study, they needed to identify the strengths and weaknesses of the data-collection section of this research study.
5. How does a training manual decrease the possibility of introducing bias in to the data-collection process, thereby increasing intervention fidelity?

KEY POINTS

- Data-collection methods are described as being both objective and systematic. The data-collection methods of a study provide the operational definitions of the relevant variables.
- Types of data-collection methods include observational, self-report, physiological, and existing data. Each method has advantages and disadvantages.
- Physiological measurement involves the use of technical instruments to collect data about patients' physical, chemical, microbiological, or anatomical status. They are suited to studying patient clinical outcomes and how to improve the effectiveness of nursing care. Physiological measurements are objective, precise, and sensitive. Expertise, training, and consistent application of these tests or procedures is needed to reduce measurement error associated with this data-collection method.
- Observational methods are used in nursing research when the variables of interest deal with events or behaviors. Scientific observation requires preplanning, systematic recording, controlling the observations, and providing a relationship to scientific theory. This method is best suited to research problems that are difficult to view as a part of a whole. Observational methods have several advantages: they provide flexibility to measure many types of situations, and they allow for depth and breadth of information to be collected. Observation has disadvantages as well: data may be distorted as a result of the observer's presence, and observations may be biased by the person who is doing the observing.
- Interviews are commonly used data-collection methods in nursing research. Either open-ended or closed-ended questions may be used when asking the subject questions. The form of the question should be clear to the respondent, free of suggestion, and grammatically correct.
- Questionnaires, or paper-and-pencil tests, are useful when there are a finite number of questions to be asked. Questions need to be clear and specific. Questionnaires are less costly in time and money to administer to large groups of subjects, particularly if the sub-

jects are geographically widespread. Questionnaires also can be completely anonymous and prevent interviewer bias.

- Existing data in the form of records or large databases are an important source for research data. The use of available data may save the researcher considerable time and money when conducting a study. This method reduces problems with subject recruitment, access, and ethical concerns. However, records and available data are subject to problems of authenticity and accuracy.

REFERENCES

Aitken LM, Marshall AP, Elliott R, et al: Critical care nurses decision making: sedation and management in intensive care, *J Clin Nurs* 18(1):36-45, 2009.

Bern L, Brandt M, Mbelu N, et al: Differences in blood pressure values obtained with automated and manual methods in medical inpatients, *Medsurg Nurs* 16:356-361, 2007.

de Bruin AF, de Witte LP, Diedriks JPM: The Sickness Impact Profile: SIP68 a short generic version: first evaluation of the reliability and reproducibility, *J Clin Epidemiol* 47:863-871, 1994.

George LK, Fillenbaum GG: OARS methodology: a decade of experience in geriatric assessment, *J Am Geriatr Soc* 33:607-615, 1985.

Hamilton BE, Manias E: Rethinking nurses' observations: psychiatric nursing skills and invisibility in an acute inpatient setting, *Social Science Medicine* 65(2):331-343, 2007.

Horgas AL, Yoon SL, Nichols AL, et al: The relationship between pain and functional status in black and white older adults, *Res Nurs Health* 31(4):341-354, 2008.

Jones EG, Renger R, Kang Y: Self-efficacy for health related behaviors among deaf adults, *Res Nurs Health* 30:185-192, 2007.

Meneses KD, McNees P, Loerzel VW, et al: Transition from treatment to survivorship: effects of a psychoeducational intervention on quality of life in breast cancer survivors, *Oncol Nurs Forum* 34(5):1007-1016, 2007.

Olsen DP: HIPAA privacy regulations and nursing research, *Nurs Res* 52:344-348, 2003.

Pickering T, Hall J, Appel L, et al: Recommendations for blood pressure measurement in humans and experimental animals. Part 1: Blood pressure measurement in humans: a statement for professionals from the subcommittee of professional and public education of the American Heart Association Council on High Blood Pressure Research, *Hypertension* 45:142-161, 2005.

Ulrich CM, Wallen GR, Feister A, et al: Respondent burden in clinical research: when are we asking too much of subjects? *Ethics and Human Research* 27:17-20, 2005.

Upton D, Upton P: Development of an evidence-based practice questionnaire for nurses, *J Adv Nurs* 54:454-458, 2006.

FOR FURTHER STUDY

Evolve

Go to Evolve at http://evolve.elsevier.com/LoBiondo/ for review questions, critiquing exercises, and additional research articles for practice in reviewing and critiquing.

13

Reliability and Validity

Geri LoBiondo-Wood and Judith Haber

KEY TERMS

- chance (random) errors
- concurrent validity
- constructs
- construct validity
- content validity
- content validity index
- contrasted-groups (known-groups) approach
- convergent validity
- criterion-related validity
- Cronbach's alpha
- divergent/discriminant validity
- equivalence
- error variance
- face validity
- factor analysis
- homogeneity
- hypothesis-testing approach
- internal consistency
- interrater reliability
- item to total correlations
- kappa
- Kuder-Richardson (KR-20) coefficient
- multitrait-multimethod approach
- observed test score
- parallel or alternate form reliability
- predictive validity
- reliability
- reliability coefficient
- split-half reliability
- stability
- systematic (constant) error
- test-retest reliability
- validity

LEARNING OUTCOMES

After reading this chapter, you should be able to do the following:

- Discuss how measurement error can affect the outcomes of a research study.
- Discuss the purposes of reliability and validity.
- Define *reliability.*
- Discuss the concepts of stability, equivalence, and homogeneity as they relate to reliability.
- Compare and contrast the estimates of reliability.
- Define *validity.*
- Compare and contrast content, criterion-related, and construct validity.
- Identify the criteria for critiquing the reliability and validity of measurement tools.
- Use the critiquing criteria to evaluate the reliability and validity of measurement tools.
- Discuss how evidence related to reliability and validity contributes to the strength and quality of evidence provided by the findings of a research study and applicability to practice.

STUDY RESOURCES

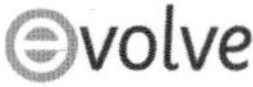

Go to Evolve at http://evolve.elsevier.com/LoBiondo/ for review questions, critiquing exercises, and additional research articles for practice in reviewing and critiquing.

Measurement of nursing phenomena is a major concern of nursing researchers. Unless measurement instruments validly and reliably reflect the concepts of the theory being tested, conclusions drawn from a study will be invalid or biased and will not advance the development of evidence-based practice. Issues of reliability and validity are of central concern to the researcher, as well as to you as an appraiser of research. From either perspective, the measurement instruments that are used in a research study must be evaluated. Many new instruments relevant to nursing practice, and a growing number of established measurement instruments, are available to researchers. Researchers often face the challenge of developing new instruments and, as part of that process, establishing the reliability and validity of those instruments. The growing importance of measurement issues, instrument development, and related issues (e.g., reliability and validity) is evident in the issues of the *Journal of Nursing Measurement* and other nursing research journals.

Nurse investigators use instruments that have been developed by researchers in nursing and other disciplines. When reading research studies and reports, you must assess the reliability and validity of the instruments used in the study to determine the soundness of these selections in relation to the concepts (concepts are often called **constructs** in instrument development studies) or variables under investigation. The appropriateness of the instruments and the extent to which reliability and validity are demonstrated have a profound influence on the strength of the findings, the extent to which bias is present, and the internal and external validity of the study. Invalid measures produce invalid estimates of the relationships between variables, thus introducing bias, which affects internal validity. The use of invalid measures produces inaccurate generalizations to the populations being studied, thus introducing a source of bias that affects external validity and the confidence with which we decide to apply or not apply research findings in clinical practice. As such, the assessment of reliability and validity is an extremely important critical appraisal skill for assessing the strength and quality of evidence provided by the design and findings of a research study and their applicability to practice.

Regardless of whether a new or already developed measurement instrument is used in a research study, evidence of reliability and validity is of crucial importance. This chapter examines the major types of reliability and validity and demonstrates the applicability of these concepts to the development, selection, and evaluation of measurement instruments in nursing research and evidence-based practice.

RELIABILITY, VALIDITY, AND MEASUREMENT ERROR

Reliability is the ability of an instrument to measure the attributes of a concept or construct consistently. **Validity** is the extent to which an instrument measures the attributes of a concept accurately. Each of these properties of an instrument will be discussed later in the chapter. To understand reliability and validity, you need to understand potential errors related to measurement instruments. Researchers may be concerned about whether the scores that were obtained for a sample of subjects were consistent, true measures of the behaviors and thus an accurate reflection of the differences between individuals. The extent of variability in test scores that is attributable to error rather than a true measure of the behaviors is the **error variance.** Error in measurement can occur in multiple ways during data collection.

An **observed test score** that is derived from a set of items actually consists of the true score plus error (Figure 13-1). The error may be either chance error or random error, or it may be

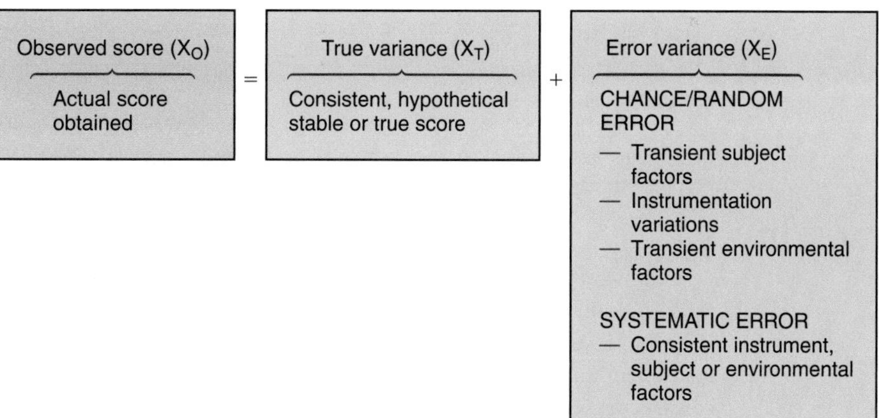

Figure 13-1 Components of observed scores.

systematic or constant error. Validity is concerned with systematic error, whereas reliability is concerned with random error. **Chance** or **random errors** are errors that are difficult to control (e.g., a respondent's anxiety level at the time of testing). Random errors are unsystematic in nature. Random errors are a result of a transient state in the subject, the context of the study, or the administration of the instrument. For example, perceptions or behaviors that occur at a specific point in time (e.g., anxiety) are known as a state or transient characteristic and are often beyond the awareness and control of the examiner. Another example of random error is in a study that measures blood pressure. Random error resulting in different blood pressure readings could occur by misplacement of the cuff, not waiting for a specific time period before taking the blood pressure, or placing the arm randomly in relationship to the heart while measuring blood pressure.

Systematic or **constant error** is measurement error that is attributable to relatively stable characteristics of the study population that may bias their behavior and/or cause incorrect instrument calibration. Such error has a systematic biasing influence on the subjects' responses and thereby influences the validity of the instruments. For instance, level of education, socio-economic status, social desirability, response set, or other characteristics may influence the validity of the instrument by altering measurement of the "true" responses in a systematic way.

For example, a subject is completing a survey about attitudes about caring for elderly patients. If he or she wants to please the investigator, items may constantly be answered in a socially desirable way rather than how the individual actually feels, thus making the estimate of validity inaccurate. Systematic error occurs also when an instrument is improperly calibrated. Consider a scale that consistently gives a person's weight at 2 pounds less than the actual body weight. The scale could be quite reliable (i.e., capable of reproducing the precise measurement), but the result is consistently invalid.

The concept of error is important when appraising instruments found in a study. The information regarding the instruments' reliability and validity is found in the instrument or measures section of a research study, which can be separately titled or appear as a subsection of the methods section of a research report, unless the study is a psychometric or instrument development study (see Chapter 9).

HELPFUL HINT

Research articles vary considerably in the amount of detail included about reliability and validity. When the focus of a study is tool development, psychometric evaluation—including extensive reliability and validity data—is carefully documented and appears throughout the article rather than briefly in the "Instruments" or "Measures" section, as in articles reporting on the results of individual studies.

VALIDITY

Validity is the extent to which an instrument measures the attributes of a concept accurately. When an instrument is valid, it truly reflects the concept it is supposed to measure. A valid instrument that is supposed to measure anxiety does so; it does not measure some other construct, such as stress. A reliable measure can consistently rank participants on a given concept or variable (e.g., anxiety), but a valid measure correctly measures the concept of interest. A measure can be reliable but not valid. Let us say that a researcher wanted to measure anxiety in patients by measuring their body temperatures. The researcher could obtain highly accurate, consistent, and precise temperature recordings, but such a measure could not be a valid indicator of anxiety. Thus the high reliability of an instrument is not necessarily congruent with evidence of validity. A valid instrument, however, is reliable. An instrument cannot validly measure the attribute of interest if it is erratic, inconsistent, and inaccurate. There are three major kinds of validity that vary according to the kind of information provided and the purpose of the investigator (i.e., *content, criterion-related,* and *construct validity*). As you appraise research articles you will want to evaluate whether sufficient evidence of validity is present and whether the type of validity is appropriate to the design of the study and instruments used in the study.

As you read the instruments or measures sections of research studies, you will notice that validity data are reported much less frequently than reliability data. DeVon and colleagues (2007) note that adequate validity is frequently claimed, but rarely is the method specified. This lack of reporting, largely due to publication space constraints, shows the importance of critiquing the quality of the instruments and the conclusions (see Chapters 14 and 15).

EVIDENCE-BASED PRACTICE TIP

Selecting measurement instruments that have strong evidence of validity increases your confidence in the study findings—that the researcher actually measured what she or he intended to measure.

Content Validity

Content validity represents the universe of content, or the domain of a given construct. The universe of content provides the framework and basis for developing the items that will adequately represent the content. When an investigator is developing an instrument and issues of content validity arise, the concern is whether the measurement instrument and the items it contains are representative of the content domain that the researcher intends to measure. The researcher begins by defining the concept and identifying the attributes or dimensions that are the components of the concept. The items that reflect the concept and its dimensions are developed.

When the researcher has completed this task, the items are submitted to a panel of judges considered to be experts about this concept. For example, researchers typically request that the

BOX 13-1 Published Examples of Content Validity and Content Validity Index

The following text from various articles describes how content and content validity index can be determined in an article:

CONTENT VALIDITY

A study by Wu and colleagues (2008) tested the psychometric properties of the 32-item Medication Adherence Scale (MAS) that was designed to measure factors influencing adherence to the prescribed medication regimen for patients with heart failure. "Content validity was achieved by having the instrument reviewed by four experts in the field of heart failure who commented on the appropriateness, completeness and wording of the items. Items on which there was not 100% agreement were deleted, or in the case that wording only was a concern, the wording was changed" (Wu et al., 2008, p. 335).

CONTENT VALIDITY INDEX

"Each of the(se) ratings was done using the four-point scale described by Waltz et al. (2005). Each of the four content raters rated each of the 10 symptoms on the following 4-point scale: 1 = relevant to the domain, 2 = somewhat relevant to the domain, 3 = quite relevant and 4 = very relevant to the domain. Percent agreement (PO) and content validity index (CVI) coefficients were then calculated between each possible pair of content experts. ... Desirable criteria for PO and CVI were set at .80" (Nieveen et al., 2008).

CONTENT VALIDITY AND CONTENT VALIDITY INDEX

"Content validity for The Quality of Care for Assisted Living (OIQ-AL) was supported by two expert panels of people experienced in the assisted-living field, and a content validity index calculated for the first version of the scale is high (3.43 on a four-point scale) with only 5 items having average ratings less than 3.0 and none were less than 2.0. The Quality of Care for Assisted Living (OIQ-AL) gives reliable and valid scores for researchers, and may be useful for consumers, providers, and others interested in measuring quality of care in assisted-living facilities" (Rantz et al., 2008).

judges indicate their agreement with the scope of the items and the extent to which the items reflect the concept under consideration. Box 13-1 provides an example of content validity.

Another method frequently used to establish content validity is the **content validity index** (CVI). The content validity index moves beyond the level of agreement of a panel of expert judges and calculates an index of interrater agreement or relevance. This calculation gives a researcher more confidence or evidence that the instrument truly reflects the concept or construct. When reading the instrument section of a research article, note that the authors will comment if a CVI was used to assess the content validity for an instrument. When you are reading a psychometric study that reports the development of an instrument, you will find great detail and a much longer section of how exactly the researchers calculated the CVI and the acceptable cut-offs for the items. In the scientific literature there has been discussion of accepting a CVI of .78 to 1.0 depending on the number of experts (DeVon et al., 2007; Lynn, 1986; Schilling et al., 2007). An example from a study that tested content validity using the CVI is presented in Box 13-1. When reading a study in which an instrument was used that had established content validity, you may or may not see any detail beyond the simple statement that content validity was established.

A subtype of content validity is **face validity,** which is a rudimentary type of validity that basically verifies that the instrument gives the appearance of measuring the concept. It is an intuitive type of validity in which colleagues or subjects are asked to read the instrument and evaluate the content in terms of whether it appears to reflect the concept the researcher intends to measure.

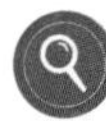

EVIDENCE-BASED PRACTICE TIP

If face and/or content validity, the most basic types of validity, was (were) the only type(s) of validity reported in a research article, you would not appraise the measurement instruments(s) as having strong psychometric properties, which would negatively influence your confidence about the study findings.

BOX 13-2 Published Examples of Reported Criterion-Related Validity

CONCURRENT VALIDITY

Actigraphy as an objective measure of sleep has been validated using concurrent validity with polysomnography, wrist actigraphy (a wrist motion sensor), and sleep diaries in the home environment. Wrist actigraphy has been validated with electroencephalograph measures of sleep and awakenings on men and women and on healthy and disturbed sleepers. Moderate to high correlations are documented between polysomnographic laboratory measures (gold standard for measuring sleep-wake patterns) and wrist actigraphy measures in various groups of research participants (Hudson et al., 2008).

PREDICTIVE VALIDITY

Predictive validity of the Alzheimer's Disease and Related Dementia Mood Scale (AD-RD) was established by assessing the relationship between the five subscales of the AD-RD, which were the predictors, and a criterion event, the score on the AD-RD. Participants were divided into depressed and not depressed groups based on their CSDD scores of greater than 7 or less than 7, respectively. Significant differences in scores between the depressed and not depressed groups were found on all five AD-RD Mood Scale subscales (Tappen & Williams, 2008).

Criterion-Related Validity

Criterion-related validity indicates to what degree the subject's performance on the measurement instrument and the subject's actual behavior are related. The criterion is usually the second measure, which assesses the same concept under study.

Two forms of criterion-related validity are concurrent and predictive. Concurrent validity refers to the degree of correlation of one test with the scores of another more established instrument of the same concept when both are administered at the same time. A high correlation coefficient indicates agreement between the two measures and evidence of concurrent validity.

Tse and colleagues (2008) assessed concurrent validity of the Harris Infant Neuromotor Test (HINT), a newer instrument, by administering it with the similar Alberta Infant Motor Scale (AIMS), a well-established instrument, to measure neuromotor profiles in 121 typical and at-risk infants at two time periods during the first year of life. The researchers administered both instruments at each time period. The calculated correlation coefficients for the two instruments at both time periods exceeded .80. The researchers thus were able to say that the newer instrument had a good to excellent concurrent validity.

Predictive validity refers to the degree of correlation between the measure of the concept and some future measure of the same concept. Because of the passage of time, the correlation coefficients are likely to be lower for predictive validity studies. Steinke and colleagues (2008) used the Charleson Comorbidity Index to determine the effect of clinical conditions (current condition) on the patient's prognosis or outcomes (future measure). They noted that numerous studies have established the reliability and validity of the Charleson Comorbidity Index and it has been significantly correlated with mortality, disability, readmission, and length of stay, therefore providing strong evidence of predictive validity (Steinke et al., 2008, p. 326). Examples of concurrent and predictive validity as they appear in research articles are illustrated in Box 13-2.

Construct Validity

Construct validity is based on the extent to which a test measures a theoretical construct, attribute, or trait. It attempts to validate a body of theory underlying the measurement by testing of the hypothesized relationships. Empirical testing confirms or fails to confirm the

BOX 13-3 Published Examples of Reported Construct Validity

The following text from various articles describes how construct validity can be determined in an article.

CONSTRUCT, CONVERGENT, DIVERGENT, AND PREDICTIVE VALIDITY

In a study by Steinke and others (2008) exploring sexual self-concept, anxiety, and self-efficacy as predictors of sexual activity in heart failure and healthy elders, anxiety and depression were assessed using the anxiety and depression subscales of the Brief Symptom Inventory. "Construct, convergent, divergent (discriminant) **and** predictive validity of the instrument have been established in a series of studies" (Steinke et al., 2008, p. 326).

CONTRASTED GROUPS (KNOWN GROUPS)

In a study by Weiss and colleagues (2006) that adapted the Perceived Readiness for Discharge after Birth Scale (PRDBS), the contrasted groups or known groups approach to establishing construct validity was used. They compared several groups of mothers hypothesized to differ in their perceived readiness for discharge (e.g., breast-feeding versus bottle-feeding mothers, primiparas versus multiparas, and those with and without clinical variances during their postpartum stay in the hospital).

CONVERGENT VALIDITY

"Convergent construct validity of the Self-Efficacy Relocation Scale (SERS) was assessed by comparison with the PRO and EM subscales which are part of the Psychological Well-Being Scale (Ryff & Keyes, 1995). Because self-efficacy is essential to well-being, it was hypothesized that fair to moderate positive correlations would exist with scores on these two measures of psychological well-being" (Rossen & Gruber, 2007).

DIVERGENT (DISCRIMINANT) VALIDITY

Divergent validity of the Purposeful Action Medication-Taking Questionnaire (MTQ: Purposeful Action), an instrument designed to assess the reasons people decide to accept medication treatment, was confirmed by a low correlation between the MTQ: Purposeful Action and the Lifestyle Business Questionnaire (LBQ). The LBQ is used to measure a patient's consistency in keeping to general routines or level of busyness, and its contrast with a purposeful action (Johnson & Rogers, 2006).

FACTOR ANALYSIS

"Exploratory factor analysis and hypothesis testing were used to evaluate the validity of the subscales. Factor analysis of the MAS was performed using the principal component analysis extraction method with varimax rotation. Eigenvalues greater than one, scree plot, and total variance explained were the criteria for factor extraction" (Wu et al., 2008, p. 337).

HYPOTHESIS TESTING

"The following **hypotheses,** which are based on previous findings in the literature demonstrating that patients with more knowledge related to medication adherence, fewer barriers and better attitudes were more adherent, were tested to further investigate the construct validity of the MAS. Hypothesis 1: Patients who have higher knowledge and attitude score and lower barrier scores will have a higher medication adherence assessed by the MEMS. Hypothesis 2: Patients who self-report greater adherence to their prescribed medication will have higher knowledge and attitude scores and lower barrier scores" (Wu et al., 2008, p. 337).

relationships that are predicted between and/or among concepts and, as such, provides more or less support for the construct validity of the instruments measuring those concepts. The establishment of construct validity is a complex process, often involving several studies and approaches. The hypothesis-testing, factor analytical, convergent and divergent, and contrasted-groups approaches are discussed. Box 13-3 provides examples of different types of construct validity as it is reported in published research articles.

Hypothesis-Testing Approach

When the hypothesis-testing approach is used, the investigator uses the theory or concept underlying the measurement instruments to validate the instrument. The investigator does this by developing hypotheses regarding the behavior of individuals with varying scores on the measurement instrument, collecting data to test the hypotheses, and making inferences on the basis of the findings concerning whether the rationale underlying the instrument's construction is adequate to explain the findings and thereby provide support for evidence of construct validity.

Convergent, Divergent, and Multitrait-Multimethod Approaches

Strategies for assessing construct validity include convergent, divergent, and multitrait-multimethod approaches. **Convergent validity** refers to a search for other measures of the construct. Sometimes two or more instruments that theoretically measure the same construct are identified, and both are administered to the same subjects. A correlational analysis (i.e., test of relationship; see Chapter 14) is performed. If the measures are positively correlated, convergent validity is said to be supported.

Divergent validity, sometimes called **discriminant validity,** uses measurement approaches that differentiate one construct from others that may be similar. Sometimes researchers search for instruments that measure the opposite of the construct. If the divergent measure is negatively related to other measures, validity for the measure is strengthened. Crncec, Barnett, and Matthey (2008) tested the psychometric properties of a new instrument, the Karitane Parenting Confidence Scale (KPCS), which was developed to measure parental self-efficacy for both convergent and discriminant validity. In their study, in addition to the new instrument, they used four other established instruments as measures to test the KPSC against. The instruments were the Parenting Sense of Competence Scale (PSOC), which measures parents' self-esteem; the Maternal Efficacy Questionnaire (MEQ), which asks mothers to rate how good they perceive themselves to be at performing different parenting tasks; the Parenting Stress Index—Short Form (PSI-SF), which measures stress in the parent-child system; and the Edinburgh Postnatal Depression Scale (EPDS), which screens for postpartum depression. The subjects were divided into four groups: women who expressed interest in participating in infant research, and three groups of women experiencing various levels of difficulty in parenting and who were receiving varying levels of interventions for parenting or mood difficulties.

Convergent validity was established by exploring the correlations between the KPCS and selected subscales of the four other measures. The KPCS scores were associated (correlated) in the appropriate direction, demonstrating sound convergent validity. **Discriminant validity** was established by analyzing the KPSC scores for the four groups with a one-way analysis (ANOVA) and post hoc tests (see Chapter 14). Additional comparisons found that the control group scored significantly higher than the three clinical groups, as expected, thereby supporting evidence of discriminant validity. Discriminant validity was further tested by exploring preintervention and postintervention KPCS scores; the results indicated that there was a statistically significant difference between the preintervention and postintervention scores, thus supporting the instrument's ability to discriminate between different types of groups. Thus the difference found among the divergent groups supported the discriminant validity for the measure.

HELPFUL HINT

When validity data about the measurement instruments used in a study are not included in a research article, you have no way of determining whether the intended concept is actually being captured by the measurement instrument. Before you use the results in such a case, it is important to go back to the original primary source to check the instrument's validity.

A specific method of assessing convergent and divergent validity is the **multitrait-multimethod approach.** Similar to the approach described, this method, proposed by Campbell and Fiske (1959), also involves examining the relationship between instruments that should measure the same construct (convergent validity) and between those that should measure different constructs (discriminant validity). A variety of measurement strategies, however, are used. For example, anxiety could be measured by the following:

- Administering the State-Trait Anxiety Inventory
- Recording blood pressure readings
- Asking the subject about anxious feelings
- Observing the subject's behavior

The results of one of these measures should then be correlated with the results of each of the others in a multitrait-multimethod matrix (Waltz et al., 2005).The use of multiple measures of a concept decreases *systematic error*. A variety of data-collection methods (e.g., self-report, observation, interview, and collection of physiological data) will also diminish the effect of systematic error.

Contrasted-Groups Approach

When the **contrasted-groups approach** (sometimes called the **known-groups approach**) is used to test construct validity, the researcher identifies two groups of individuals who are suspected to score extremely high or low in the characteristic being measured by the instrument. The instrument is administered to both the high-scoring and the low-scoring group, and the differences in scores are examined. If the instrument is sensitive to individual differences in the trait being measured, the mean performance of these two groups should differ significantly and evidence of construct validity would be supported. A *t* test or analysis of variance could be used to statistically test the difference between the two groups. In the study by Weiss and colleagues (2006), the researchers adapted the Perceived Readiness for Discharge after Birth Scale and assessed the instrument using known groups by comparing several groups of mothers hypothesized to differ in their readiness for discharge. The differing groups included were new mothers (primiparas) and multiparas, bottle-feeding and breast-feeding mothers, and vaginal birth and cesarean birth mothers.

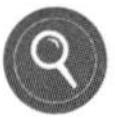

EVIDENCE-BASED PRACTICE TIP

When the instruments used in a study are presented, note whether the sample(s) used to develop the measurement instrument(s) is (are) similar to your patient population.

Factor Analytical Approach

A final approach to assessing construct validity is **factor analysis.** This is a procedure that gives the researcher information about the extent to which a set of items measures the same underlying construct or dimension of a construct. Factor analysis assesses the degree to which the individual items on a scale truly cluster together around one or more dimensions. Items designed to measure the same dimension should load on the same factor; those designed to measure different dimensions should load on different factors (Anastasi & Urbina, 1997; Nunnally & Bernstein, 1993). This analysis will also indicate whether the items in the instrument reflect a single construct or several constructs.

Crncec and colleagues (2008) performed a factor analysis to determine the factor structure of the Karitane Parenting Confidence Scale (KPCS). They found with testing that the factor analysis suggested a three-factor solution or three components of parenting. Variables (items) loading on component one focused on perceptions of parenting; component two, available parenting support; and component three, perceptions about child development. These three factor components (parenting, support, and child development) became the subscales of the instruments.

The Critical Thinking Decision Path will help you assess the appropriateness of the type of validity and reliability selected for use in a particular research study.

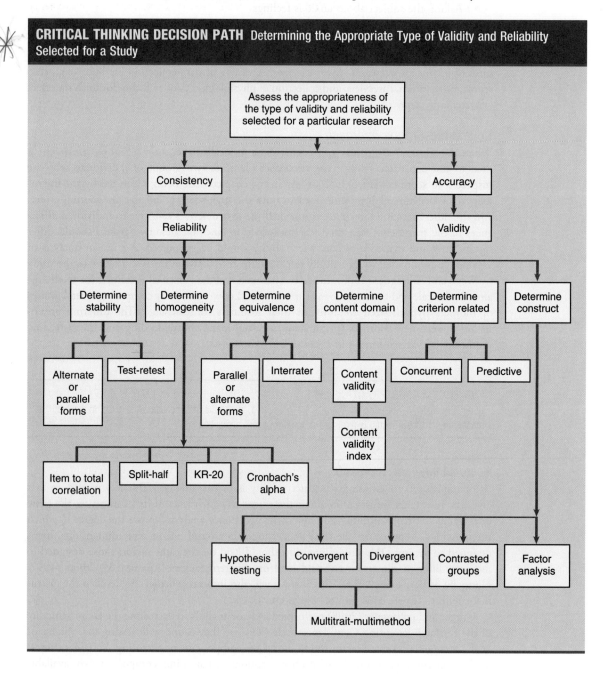

CRITICAL THINKING DECISION PATH Determining the Appropriate Type of Validity and Reliability Selected for a Study

RELIABILITY

Reliable people are those whose behavior can be relied on to be consistent and predictable. Likewise, the **reliability** of a research instrument is defined as the extent to which the instrument yields the same results on repeated measures. Reliability is concerned with consistency, accuracy, precision, stability, equivalence, and homogeneity. Concurrent with the questions of validity or after they are answered, you ask how reliable the instrument is. A reliable measure is one that can produce the same results if the behavior is measured again by the same scale. Reliability then refers to the proportion of consistency to inconsistency in measurement. In other words, if we use the same or comparable instruments on more than one occasion to measure a set of behaviors that ordinarily remains relatively constant, we would expect similar results if the instruments are reliable.

The three main attributes of a reliable scale are stability, homogeneity, and equivalence. The **stability** of an instrument refers to the instrument's ability to produce the same results with repeated testing. The **homogeneity** of an instrument means that all of the items in an instrument measure the same concept or characteristic. An instrument is said to exhibit **equivalence** if it produces the same results when equivalent or parallel instruments or procedures are used. Each of these attributes and the means to estimate them will be discussed. Before these are discussed, an understanding of how to interpret reliability is essential.

Reliability Coefficient Interpretation

Because all of the attributes of reliability are concerned with the degree of consistency between scores that are obtained at two or more independent times of testing, they often are expressed in terms of a correlation coefficient. The reliability coefficient ranges from 0 to 1. The **reliability coefficient** expresses the relationship between the error variance, the true variance, and the observed score. A zero correlation indicates that there is no relationship. When the error variance in a measurement instrument is low, the reliability coefficient will be closer to 1. The closer to 1 the coefficient is, the more reliable the instrument. For example, a reliability coefficient of an instrument is reported to be 0.89. This tells you that the error variance is small and the instrument has little measurement error. On the other hand, if the reliability coefficient of a measure is reported to be 0.49, the error variance is high and the instrument has a problem with measurement error. For a instrument to be considered reliable, a level of 0.70 or higher is considered to be an acceptable level of reliability. The interpretation of the reliability coefficient depends on the proposed purpose of the measure.

There are five major tests of reliability that can be used to calculate a reliability coefficient. The tests used depend on the nature of the instrument. They are known as **test-retest, parallel or alternate form, item to total correlation, split-half, Kuder-Richardson (KR-20), Cronbach's alpha,** and **interrater reliability.** These tests are discussed as they relate to the attributes of stability, equivalence, and homogeneity (Box 13-4). There is no best means to assess reliability in relationship to stability, homogeneity, and equivalence. You should be aware that the method of reliability that the researcher uses should be consistent with the study's aim.

BOX 13-4 Measures Used to Test Reliability

STABILITY	HOMOGENEITY	EQUIVALENCE
Test-retest reliability	Item to total correlation	Parallel or alternate form
Parallel or alternate form	Split-half reliability	Interrater reliability
	Kuder-Richardson coefficient	
	Cronbach's alpha	

Stability

An instrument is thought to be stable or to exhibit stability when the same results are obtained on repeated administration of the instrument. Researchers are concerned with an instrument's stability when they expect the instrument to measure a concept consistently over a period of time. Measurement over time is important when an instrument is used in a longitudinal study and therefore will be used on several occasions. Stability is also a consideration when a researcher is conducting an intervention study that is designed to effect a change in a specific variable. In this case, the instrument is administered once and then again later, after the alteration or change intervention has been completed. The tests that are used to estimate stability are test-retest and parallel or alternate form.

Test-Retest Reliability

Test-retest reliability is the administration of the same instrument to the same subjects under similar conditions on two or more occasions. Scores from repeated testing are compared. This comparison is expressed by a correlation coefficient, usually a Pearson *r* (see Chapter 14). The interval between repeated administrations varies and depends on the concept or variable being measured. For example, if the variable that the test measures is related to the developmental stages in children, the interval between tests should be short. The amount of time over which the variable was measured should also be recorded in the report. An example of an instrument that was assessed for test-retest reliability is the Quality of Life–Breast Cancer Survivor instrument that was used in the Meneses (2007) study (see Appendix A). In this case, the interval was adequate (2 weeks) between testing and the coefficient was above .70 (Nunnally & Bernstein, 1993). Box 13-5 provides other examples of test-retest reliability.

HELPFUL HINT

When a longitudinal design with multiple data-collection points is being conducted, look for evidence of test-retest or parallel form reliability.

Parallel or Alternate Form

Parallel or alternate form reliability is applicable and can be tested only if two comparable forms of the *same* instrument exist. Not many instruments have a parallel form. It is similar to test-retest reliability in that the same individuals are tested within a specific interval, but it differs because a *different* form of the *same* test is given to the subjects on the second testing. **Parallel forms** or tests contain the same types of items that are based on the same concept, but the wording of the items is different. The development of parallel forms is desired if the

BOX 13-5 Published Examples of Reported Reliability

RELIABILITY

Internal Consistency, Item Correlations, Inter-Item Correlations Reliability

A study by Wu and colleagues (2008, p. 337) tested the reliability of the subscales of the Medication Adherence Scale (MAS) by examining internal consistency, item correlations, and inter-item correlations of the subscales: "A Cronbach's alpha of .70 was considered acceptable support for the internal consistency of the MAS subscales. Item-total correlations and inter-item correlations were conducted to examine the homogeneity of the MAS. Coefficients greater than .30 were considered acceptable for item-total correlations. Inter-item correlations between .30 and .70 were considered acceptable." "Cronbach's alpha for the MAS was.85, which supported the internal consistency reliability of the MAS" (p. 338).

TEST-RETEST AND INTERNAL CONSISTENCY RELIABILITY

In a study investigating the effect of a psychoeducational intervention on quality of life (QOL) in breast cancer survivors, the Quality of Life–Breast Cancer Survivors scale was adapted from the QOL–Cancer Survivors Scale. "Test-retest reliability of the original QOL–Cancer Survivors Scale was .89 and Cronbach's alpha was .93. Alpha coefficients for the current study were .93 for the total QOL score, .99 for the physical domain, .96 for the psychological domain, and .85 for both the social and spiritual domains" (Meneses et al., 2007).

Test-Retest Reliability

The Karitane Parenting Confidence Scale (KPCS) is designed to assess perceived self-efficacy in the parents of infants. "Participants in the control group completed a 4 week follow-up to determine the test-retest reliability of the KPCS. A 4 week period was selected as this was deemed sufficiently large to reduce the likelihood that parents would remember their previous KPCS responses, yet not so large as to introduce infant maturational effects in parents' KPCS ratings" (Crncec et al., 2008).

Kuder-Richardson Internal Consistency Reliability

In a study exploring the effect of providing lymphedema information on breast cancer survivors' symptoms and practice of risk reduction behaviors, Fu and colleagues (2008) used the Lymphedema and Breast Cancer Questionnaire (LBCQ) to assess lymphedema symptoms. Because the response format was "Yes" or "No" regarding whether a symptom is currently present, the Kuder-Richardson-20 test was used to establish the internal consistency reliability. "Previous studies have shown an acceptable internal consistency using Kuder-Richardson-20. Kuder-Richardson-20 for this sample was $r = 0.82$ indicating appropriate internal consistency."

Split-Half Reliability

The Edinburgh Postnatal Depression Scale (EPDS) is used for community screening for postnatal depression and reports a split-half reliability of .88.

Interrater Reliability and Kappa

In a study examining the interrater and intrarater reliability of classifying pressure ulcers from photographs of pressure ulcers and incontinence lesions the following was information was presented. There are only a limited number of studies that evaluate the interrater reliability of pressure ulcer grading according to the European Pressure Ulcer Advisory Panel Classification. The study consisted of two phases. In the first phase 56 photos, together with a random selection of 9 photos from the same set, were presented twice to 473 nurses. In the second phase, the 56 photos were presented twice to 86 other nurses with an interval of 1 month and in a different order. All of the nurses were familiar with the classification system. They did not receive additional training on classification and were asked to classify the lesions as normal skin, blanchable erythema, pressure ulcers, or incontinence lesions. Results indicated that in the first phase, the multirater kappa for the 473 participating nurses was 0.37 ($p < .001$). Nonblanchable erythema was often confused with blanchable erythema and incontinence lesions. In the second phase, the interrater agreement was not significantly different in both sessions. The intrarater agreement was 0.52. The authors concluded that differentiating between and among lesions using this classification system is difficult (Defloor et al., 2006).

instrument is intended to measure a variable for which a researcher believes that "test-wiseness" will be a problem (see Chapter 7). For example, the randomized controlled trial" "Breast Cancer: Education, Counseling, and Adjustment" (Budin et al., 2008) studied the differential effect of a phase-specific standardized educational video intervention in comparison to a telephone counseling intervention on physical, emotional, and social adjustment in women with breast cancer and their partners. The use of repeated measures over the four data-collection points—"Coping with Your Diagnosis," "Recovering from Surgery," "Understanding Adjuvant Therapy," and "Ongoing Recovery"—made it appropriate to use two alternate forms of the Partner Relationship Inventory (Hoskins, 1988) to measure emotional adjustment in partners. An item on one scale ("I am able to tell my partner how I feel") is consistent with the paired item on the second form ("My partner tries to understand my feelings"). Practically speaking, it is difficult to develop alternate forms of an instrument when one considers the many issues of reliability and validity of an instrument. If alternate forms of a test exist, they should be highly correlated if the measures are to be considered reliable.

Internal Consistency/Homogeneity

Another attribute of an instrument related to reliability is the **internal consistency** or **homogeneity** with which the items within the scale reflect or measure the same concept. This means that the items within the scale correlate or are complementary to each other. This also means that a scale is unidimensional. A unidimensional scale is one that measures one concept, such as self-efficacy. Box 13-5 provides several examples of how internal consistency is reported in the literature. Internal consistency can be assessed by using one of four methods: item to total correlations, split-half reliability, Kuder-Richardson (KR-20) coefficient, or Cronbach's alpha (see Box 13-5).

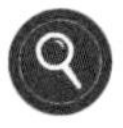

EVIDENCE-BASED PRACTICE TIP

When the characteristics of a study sample differ significantly from the sample in the original study, check to see if the researcher has reestablished the reliability of the instrument with the current sample.

Item to Total Correlations

Item to total correlations measure the relationship between each of the items and the total scale. When item to total correlations are calculated, a correlation for each item on the scale is generated (Table 13-1). Items that do not achieve a high correlation may be deleted from the instrument. Usually in a research study, all of the item to total correlations are not reported unless the study is a report of a methodological study. The lowest and highest correlations are typically reported. An example of an item to total correlation report is illustrated in the study by Gary and Yarandi (2004) in which item to total correlations were computed for the 21-item Beck Depression Inventory II (BDI II), which measures depression in three dimensions: cognition, somatization, and motivation. The individual items range from .34 (loss of interest in sex) to .63 (sadness). The authors report that all of the corrected item to total correlations were significant after a "Bonferroni adjustment (alpha/21) was used to control for the overall error rate." They also determined that the coefficient alpha of the BDI II for the current sample

TABLE 13-1 Means, Standard Deviations, and Corrected Item-Total Correlations (Cronbach's Alpha = 0.90)

Variable	Mean	SD	[illegible]
Sadness	0.21	0.46	0.63
Pessimism	0.12	0.39	0.47
Past failure	0.25	0.57	0.44
Loss of pleasure	0.33	0.59	0.61
Guilty feelings	0.33	0.50	0.53
Punishment feelings	0.19	0.56	0.57
Self-dislike	0.17	0.54	0.51
Self-criticalness	0.30	0.63	0.52
Suicidal thoughts or wishes	0.05	0.28	0.40
Crying	0.38	0.89	0.52
Agitation	0.43	0.85	0.52
Loss of interest	0.26	0.57	0.58
Indecisiveness	0.24	0.58	0.54
Worthlessness	0.11	0.40	0.51
Loss of energy	0.62	0.58	0.47
Changes in sleeping patterns	0.84	0.95	0.58
Irritability	0.31	0.62	0.59
Changes in appetite	0.64	0.82	0.45
Concentration difficulty	0.54	0.75	0.60
Tiredness or fatigue	0.74	0.81	0.61
Loss of interest in sex	0.64	0.87	0.34

of rural southern African-American women was 0.91, suggesting a high level of internal consistency for the study sample and thus supporting the reliability of the scale (Nunnally & Bernstein, 1993).

Cronbach's Alpha

The fourth and most commonly used test of internal consistency is **Cronbach's alpha.** Many scales used to measure psychosocial variables and attitudes have a Likert scale response format. A Likert scale format asks the subject to respond to a question on a scale of varying degrees of intensity between two extremes. The two extremes are anchored by responses ranging from "strongly agree" to "strongly disagree" or "most like me" to "least like me." The points between the two extremes may range from 1 to 4, 1 to 5, or 1 to 7. Subjects are asked to circle the response closest to how they feel. In Appendix B, the Jones and colleagues (2007) study, the researchers report the internal consistency for the instruments they used: "The Cronbach's alpha for the total scale was .94 in two samples." Figure 13-2 provides examples of items from a instrument that uses a Likert scale format. Cronbach's alpha simultaneously compares each item in the scale with the others. A total score is then used in the analysis of data as illustrated in Table 13-2. When alphas were above .70, it was sufficient evidence for supporting the internal consistency of the instrument. Examples of reported Cronbach's alpha are provided in Box 13-6.

I trust that life events happen to fit a plan that is larger and more gentle than I can know.
1 2 3 4 5
Never Always
I am aware of an inner source of comfort, strength, and security.
1 2 3 4 5
Never Always

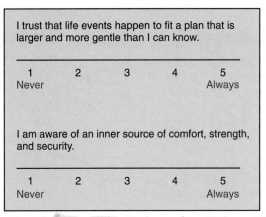

Figure 13-2 Examples of a Likert scale. (Redrawn from Roberts KT, Aspy CB: Development of the serenity scale, *J Nurs Meas* 1[2]:145-164, 1993.)

TABLE 13-2 Examples of Cronbach's Alpha

Dimensions	Original	Sample 1	Sample 2	Sample 3
Negative reactivity	.90	.89	.90	.92
Task persistence	.90	.89	.91	.92
Approach/withdrawal	.88	.84	.86	.92
Activity	.85	.80	.86	.92

BOX 13-6 Examples of Reported Cronbach's Alpha

- "Alpha coefficients for the current study were .93 for the total QOL score, .99 for the physical domain and .85 for both the social and spiritual domain" (Meneses et al., 2007, p. 1010).
- "Adequate internal consistency has been reported with the original scale (α = .82) and was demonstrated with the modified scale in this study (α = .86)" (Whittemore et al., 2009).
- "Perceived health status was measured with the General Health Rating Index (Davies & Ware, 1981), which contains 22 Likert type items with a 4-point response set. Cronbach's alpha estimates of reliability for this sample were: sexual awareness, α = .83; sexual motivation α = .79; sexual assertiveness , α = .67; sexual esteem, α = .86" (Rew et al., 2008, p. 111).

Split-Half Reliability

Split-half reliability involves dividing a scale into two halves and making a comparison. The halves may be odd-numbered and even-numbered items or may be a simple division of the first from the second half, or items may be randomly selected into halves that will be analyzed opposite one another. The split-half method provides a measure of consistency in terms of sampling the content. The two halves of the test or the contents in both halves are assumed to be comparable, and a reliability coefficient is calculated. If the scores for the two halves are approximately equal, the test may be considered reliable. A formula called the Spearman-Brown formula is one method used to calculate the reliability coefficient. In a study by Anderson (2008) investigating predictors of parenting stress in a diverse sample of parents of early adolescents in high-risk communities, social support was assessed with the 15-item

Family Support Scale, which asks parents to report, on a scale of 1 to 5, how often they received help or support in raising their child from other parents, friends, spouse or partner's parents, and professional services. Split-half reliability for the Family Support Scale was reported to be .75, demonstrating consistency between the items and satisfactory reliability.

Kuder-Richardson (KR-20) Coefficient

The **Kuder-Richardson (KR-20) coefficient** is the estimate of homogeneity used for instruments that have a dichotomous response format. A dichotomous response format is one in which the question asks for a "yes/no" or "true/false" response. The technique yields a correlation that is based on the consistency of responses to all the items of a single form of a test that is administered one time. In a study investigating the effectiveness of a randomized support group intervention for African-American women with breast cancer, breast cancer knowledge was assessed with a 25-item true/false scale developed for the study. Items were obtained from the American Cancer Society's publication entitled *Cancer Facts and Figures* and comprised the following categories: knowledge of risk factors for developing breast cancer; symptoms of breast cancer; side effects of treatment; treatment efficacy; and methods of treatment. Because the scale was a binary format (true/false), Kuder-Richardson reliability for the entire scale was calculated at 0.75, which is acceptable, having exceeded the minimum acceptable KR-20 score of 0.70.

HELPFUL HINT

If a research article provides information about the reliability of a measurement instrument but does not specify the type of reliability, it is probably safe to assume that internal consistency reliability was assessed using Cronbach's alpha.

Equivalence

Equivalence either is the consistency or agreement among observers using the same measurement instrument or is the consistency or agreement between alternate forms of a instrument. An instrument is thought to demonstrate equivalence when two or more observers have a high percentage of agreement of an observed behavior or when alternate forms of a test yield a high correlation. There are two methods to test equivalence: interrater reliability and alternate or parallel form.

Interrater Reliability

Some measurement instruments are not self-administered questionnaires but are direct measurements of observed behavior. Instruments that depend on direct observation of a behavior that is to be systematically recorded must be tested for **interrater reliability.** To accomplish interrater reliability, two or more individuals should make an observation or one observer should examine the behavior on several occasions. The observers should be trained or oriented to the definition and operationalization of the behavior to be observed. In the method of direct observation of behavior, the consistency or reliability of the observations between observers is extremely important. In the instance of interrater reliability, the reliability or consistency of the observer is tested rather than the reliability of the instrument. Interrater reliability is expressed as a percentage of agreement between scorers or as a correlation coefficient of the scores assigned to the observed behaviors.

In a study by Rantz and colleagues (2008) that field tested and refined the psychometric evaluation of a new measure of quality of care for assisted living, interrater reliability of the final 34-item Observable Indicators of Nursing Home Care Quality–Assisted Living (OIQ-AL was established using the simultaneous interrater observations made by two registered nurses (RNs) in 73 assisted living/residential care facilities. Five of the six subscales of the OIQ-AL and the total scale had very good interrater reliability ranging from .68 to .94, but one subscale showed substandard interrater reliability.

Santacroce, Maccarelli, and Grey (2004) note that consistency in observation or intervention delivery is key to concluding that the evidence provided by the study findings is valid and reliable. Another type of interrater reliability is Cohen's kappa, a coefficient of agreement between two raters that is considered to be a more precise estimate of interrater reliability. Kappa (K) expresses the level of agreement observed beyond the level that would be expected by chance alone. K ranges from +1 (total agreement) to 0 (no agreement). A K of .80 or better indicates good interrater reliability. K between .80 and .68 is considered acceptable/substantial agreement; less than .68 allows tentative conclusions to be drawn at times when lower levels are accepted (McDowell & Newell, 1996).

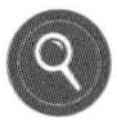

EVIDENCE-BASED PRACTICE TIP

Interrater reliability is an important approach to minimizing bias.

Parallel or Alternate Form

Parallel or alternate form was described in the discussion of stability in this chapter. Use of parallel forms is a measure of stability and equivalence. The procedures for assessing equivalence using parallel forms are the same.

HOW VALIDITY AND RELABILITY ARE REPORTED

When reading a research article that tests research questions or hypotheses, a lengthy discussion of how the different types of reliability and validity were obtained will not be found. What is found in the methods section of a research report is the title of the instrument, a definition of the concept/construct that it measures, and a sentence or two of the data that support the reliability and validity assessed previously. This level of discussion is appropriate. Examples of what the reader will see include the following:

- "Construct, convergent discriminate and predictive validity of the instrument have been established in a series of studies" (Steinke et al., 2008, p. 326).
- "The Jalowiec Coping Scale (JCS) has good reliability and validity from previous studies (Jalowiec, 2003). Alpha reliability for the total effectiveness score from the present sample was .92" (Jalowiec et al., 2007).
- "Psychosocial data were collected on depressive symptoms as measured by the Center for Epidemiological Studies—Depression Scale (CES-D). High internal consistency, acceptable test-retest reliability and good construct validity have been demonstrated" (Whittemore et al., 2009, p. 6).

APPRAISING THE EVIDENCE

Reliability and Validity

Reliability and validity are two crucial aspects in the critical appraisal of a measurement instrument. Criteria for critiquing reliability and validity are presented in the Critiquing Criteria box. When reviewing a research article you need to appraise each instrument's level of reliability and validity. In a research report, the reliability and validity for each measure should be presented or a reference given where it was described in more detail. If these data have not been presented at all, you must seriously question the merit and use of the instrument and the evidence provided by the study's results.

The amount of information provided for each instrument will vary depending on the study type and the instrument. In a psychometric study (an instrument development study) you will find great detail regarding how the researchers established the reliability and validity of the instrument. When reading a research article in which the instruments are used to test a research question or hypothesis, you may find only brief reference to the type of reliability and validity of the instrument. If the instrument is a well-known, reliable, and valid instrument, it is not uncommon that only a passing comment may be made, which is appropriate. For example, in a study that measured anxiety and depression, the researchers (Steinke et al., 2008) used the subscale of anxiety and depression from the Brief Symptom Inventory (BSI) and stated that "the BSI has well-established validity and reliability" (p. 326). Sometimes, the authors will cite a reference that you can go to if you are interested in detailed data about the instrument's reliability or validity. For example, in a study examining the use of the Pra, a instrument for identifying and predicting adult medical inpatients at risk for early readmission, Novotny and Anderson (2008) state that "the instrument's validity was supported in a national sample of Medicare beneficiaries (Boult et al., 1995)."

If a study does not use reliable and valid questionnaires, you need to consider the sources of bias that may exist as threats to internal or external validity. It is very difficult to place confidence in the evidence generated by a study's findings if the measures used did not have established validity and reliability. The following discussion highlights key areas related to reliability and validity that should be evident to you as you read a research article.

Appropriate reliability tests should have been performed by the developer of the measurement instrument and should then have been included by the current researcher in the research report. If the initial standardization sample and the current sample have different characteristics (e.g., age, gender, ethnicity, race, geographic location, etc.), you would expect the following: (1) that a pilot study for the present sample would have been conducted to determine if the reliability was maintained, or (2) that a reliability estimate was calculated on the current sample. For example, if the standardization sample for a instrument that measures "satisfaction in an intimate heterosexual relationship" comprises undergraduate college students and if an investigator plans to use the instrument with married couples, it would be advisable to establish the reliability of the instrument with the latter group.

CRITIQUING CRITERIA: *Reliability and Validity*

1. Was an appropriate method used to test the reliability of the instrument?
2. Is the reliability of the instrument adequate?
3. Was an appropriate method(s) used to test the validity of the instrument?
4. Is the validity of the measurement instrument adequate?
5. If the sample from the developmental stage of the instrument was different from the current sample, were the reliability and validity recalculated to determine if the instrument is appropriate for use in a different population?
6. Have the strengths and weaknesses related to the reliability and validity of each instrument been presented?
7. What kinds of threats to internal and/or external validity are presented by weaknesses in reliability and/or validity?
8. Are strengths and weaknesses of the reliability and validity appropriately addressed in the "Discussion," "Limitations," or "Recommendations" sections of the report?
9. How do the reliability and/or validity affect the strength and quality of the evidence provided by the study findings?

The investigator determines which type of reliability procedures are used in the study, depending on the nature of the measurement instrument and how it will be used. For example, if the instrument is to be administered twice, you would expect to read that test-retest reliability was used to establish the stability of the instrument. If an alternate form has been developed for use in a repeated-measures design, evidence of alternate form reliability should be presented to determine the equivalence of the parallel forms. If the degree of internal consistency among the items is relevant, an appropriate test of internal consistency should be presented. In some instances, more than one type of reliability will be presented, but as you assess the instruments section of a research report, you should determine whether all are appropriate. For example, the Kuder-Richardson formula implies that there is a single right or wrong answer, making it inappropriate to use with scales that provide a format of three or more possible responses. In such cases, another formula is applied, such as Cronbach's coefficient alpha formula. Another important consideration is the acceptable level of reliability, which varies according to the type of test. Reliability coefficients of 0.70 or higher are desirable. The validity of an instrument is limited by its reliability; that is, less confidence can be placed in scores from tests with low reliability coefficients.

Satisfactory evidence of validity will probably be the most difficult item for you to ascertain. It is this aspect of measurement that is most likely to fall short of meeting the required criteria. Page count limitations often account for this brevity. Detailed validity data usually are only reported in studies focused on instrument development; therefore validity data are only mentioned briefly or, sometimes, not at all. For example, in a study examining the relationship of religion and spirituality to glycemic control in black women with type 2 diabetes, diabetes-specific social support (DSSC) was measured using a subscale of the Diabetes Care Profile. Validity data are only mentioned in one sentence (Newlin et al., 2008): "Concurrent validity has been established between the Diabetes Care Profile and other measures of social support (Fitzgerald & Davis, 1996)."

The most common type of reported validity is content validity. When reviewing a study, you want to find evidence of content validity. Once again, you will find the detailed reporting of content validity and the CVI in psychometric studies; Box 13-2 provides a good example of how content validity is reported in that kind of article. Such procedures provide you with assurance that the instrument is psychometrically sound and that the content of the items is consistent with the conceptual framework and construct definitions. In research studies where several instruments are used, the reporting of content validity is either absent or very brief. For example, in a study investigating the relationship between pain and functional disability in black and white older adults, a 24-item medical conditions checklist from the Older Americans Resources and Services (OARS) Multidimensional Assessment was used as an indicator of health status. "An expert panel of four advanced practice nurses reviewed the checklist and identified 12 medical conditions often associated with disability" (Horgas et al., 2008) (see Appendix C).

Construct validity and criterion-related validity are some of the more precise statistical tests of whether the instrument measures what it is supposed to measure. Ideally, an instrument should provide evidence of content validity, as well as criterion-related or construct validity, before one invests a high level of confidence in the instrument. You can expect to see evidence that the reliability and validity of a measurement instrument are reestablished periodically, as Jones and colleagues (2007) (see Appendix B) discuss.

You would also expect to see the strengths and weaknesses of instrument reliability and validity presented in the "Discussion," "Limitations," and/or "Recommendations" sections of a research article. In this context, the reliability and validity might be discussed in terms of bias, that is, threats to internal and/or external validity, that affect the study findings. For example, in a research study testing the effectiveness of a Web-based asthma education program, test-retest reliability of the Asthma Knowledge Questionnaire (AKQ), including time intervals and correlations, need to be reported in order for you to know that the change in knowledge scores was due to the education program, rather than instability of the AKQ. The findings of any study are not credible if the measurement instruments are not credible. This means that satisfactory reliability and validity that attest to the consistency and accuracy of the instruments used in a study must be evident and interpreted by the author(s) if the findings are to be applicable and generalizable. Finally, recommendations for improving future studies in relation to instrument reliability and validity should be proposed.

As you can see, the area of reliability and validity is complex. These aspects of research reports can be evaluated to varying degrees. You should not feel inhibited by the complexity of this topic but may use the guidelines presented in this chapter to systematically assess the reliability and validity aspects of a research study. Collegial dialogue is also an approach to evaluating the merits and shortcomings of an existing, as well as a newly developed, instrument that is reported in the nursing literature. Such an exchange promotes the understanding of methodologies and techniques of reliability and validity, stimulates the acquisition of a basic knowledge of psychometrics, and encourages the exploration of alternative methods of observation and use of reliable and valid instruments in clinical practice.

CRITICAL THINKING CHALLENGES

- Discuss the types of validity that must be established before you invest a high level of confidence in the measurement instruments used in a research study.
- What are the major tests of reliability? Why is it important to establish the appropriate type of reliability for a measurement instrument?
- A journal club just finished reading the research report by Meneses and colleagues in Appendix A. As part of their critical appraisal of this study, they needed to identify the strengths and weaknesses of the reliability and validity section of this research report. If you were a member of this journal club, how would you assess the reliability and validity of the instruments used in this study?
- How does the strength and quality of evidence related to reliability and validity influence applicability of findings to clinical practice?
- When a researcher does not report reliability or validity data, which threats to internal and/or external validity should you consider? How would these threats affect the strength and quality of evidence provided by the findings of the study?

KEY POINTS

- Reliability and validity are crucial aspects of conducting and critiquing research.
- Validity is the extent to which an instrument measures the attributes of a concept accurately. Three types of validity are content validity, criterion-related validity, and construct validity.
- The choice of a method for establishing reliability or validity is important and is made by the researcher on the basis of the characteristics of the measurement device in question and its intended use.
- Reliability is the ability of an instrument to measure the attributes of a concept or construct consistently. The major tests of reliability are as follows: test-retest, parallel or alternate form, split-half, item to total correlation, Kuder-Richardson, Cronbach's alpha, and interrater reliability.
- The selection of a method for establishing reliability or validity depends on the characteristics of the instrument, the testing method that is used for collecting data from the sample, and the kinds of data that are obtained.
- Critical appraisal of instrument reliability and validity in a research report focuses on internal and external validity as sources of bias that contribute to the strength and quality of evidence provided by the findings.

REFERENCES

Anastasi A, Urbina S: Psychological testing, ed 7, New York, 1997, Macmillan.

Anderson LS: Predictors of parenting stress in a diverse sample of parents of early adolescents in high-risk communities, *Nurs Res* 57(5):340-350, 2008.

Budin WC, Hoskins CN, Haber J, et al: Education, counseling, and adjustment among patient and partners: a randomized clinical trial, *Nurs Res* 57:199-213, 2008.

Campbell D, Fiske D: Convergent and discriminant validation by the matrix, *Psychol Bull* 53:273-302, 1959.

Crncec R, Barnett B, Matthey S: Development of an instrument to assess perceived efficacy in the parents of infants, *Res Nurs Health* 31:442-453, 2008.

Defloor T, Schoonhoven L, Katrien V, et al: Reliability of the European pressure ulcer advisory panel classification system, *J Adv Nurs* 54(2):189-198, 2006.

DeVon FA, Block ME, Moyle-Wright P, et al: A psychometric toolbox for testing validity and reliability, *J Nurs Sch* 39(2):155-164, 2007.

Fu MR, Axelrod D, Haber J: Breast-cancer-related lymphedema: information, symptoms, and risk-reduction behaviors, *J Nurs Sch* 40(4):341-348, 2008.

Gary FA, Yarandi HN: Depression among southern rural African American women. *Nurs Res* 53(4):251-259, 2004.

Horgas AL, Yoon SL, Nichols AL, Marsiske M: The relationship between pain and functional disability in black and white older adults, *Res Nurs Health* (40):341-354, 2008.

Hoskins CN: *The partner relationship inventory*, Palo Alto, CA, 1988, Consulting Psychologists Press.

Hudson AL, Portillo CJ, Lee KL: Sleep disturbances in women with HIV or AIDS, *Nurs Res* 57(5):360-366, 2008.

Jalowiec A, Grady KL, White-Williams C: Predictors of perceived coping effectiveness in patients awaiting a heart transplant, *Nurs Res* 56(4):260-268, 2007.

Johnson MJ, Rogers S: Development of the purposeful action medication questionnaire, *West J Nurs Res* 28(3):335-351, 2006.

Jones EC, Renger R, Kang Y: Self efficacy for health related behaviors among deaf adults, *Res Nurs Health* 30:185-192, 2007.

Lynn MR: Determination and quantification of content validity, *Nurs Res* 35:382-385, 1986.

McDowell I, Newell C: *Measuring health: a guide to rating scales and questionnaires*, New York, 1996, Oxford Press.

Meneses KD, McNees P, Loerzel VW, et al: Transition from treatment to survivorship: effects of a psychoeducational intervention on quality of life in breast cancer survivors, *Oncol Nurs Forum* 34(5):1007-1016, 2007.

Newlin K, Melkus GD, Tappen R, et al: Relationships of religion and spirituality to glycemic control in black women with type 2 diabetes, *Nurs Res* 57(5):331-339, 2008.

Nieveen JL, Zimmerman LM, Barnason SA, Yates BC: Development and content validity testing of the cardiac symptom survey in patients after coronary artery bypass grafting, *Heart Lung* 37(1):17-27, 2008.

Novotny NL, Anderson MA: Prediction of early readmission in medical inpatients using the probability of repeated admission instrument, *Nurs Res* 57(6):406-415, 2008.

Nunnally JC, Bernstein IH: *Psychometric theory*, ed 3, New York, 1993, McGraw-Hill.

Rantz MJ, Aud MA, Zwygart-Stauffacher M, et al: Field testing, refinement, and psychometric evaluation of a new measure of quality of care for assisted living, *J Nurs Meas* 16(1):16-29, 2008.

Rew L, Grady M, Whittaker TA, et al: Interaction of duration of homelessness and gender on adolescent sexual health indicators, *J Nurs Sch* 40(2):109-115, 2008.

Rossen EK, Gruber KJ: Development and psychometric testing of the relocation self-efficacy scale, *Nurs Res* 56(4):244-251, 2007.

Santacroce SJ, Maccarelli LM, Grey M: Intervention fidelity, *Nurs Res* 53(10):63-66, 2004.

Schilling LS, Dixon JK, Knafl KA, et al: Determining content validity of a self-report instrument for adolescents using a heterogeneous expert panel, *Nurs Res* 56(6):361-366, 2007.

Steinke EE, Wright DW, Chung ML, et al: Sexual self-concept, anxiety, and self-efficacy predict sexual activity in heart failure and healthy elders, *Heart Lung* 37(5):323-333, 2008.

Tappen RM, Williams CL: Development and testing of the Alzheimer's disease and related dementia's mood scale, *Nurs Res* 57(6):426-435, 2008.

Tse L, Mayson TA, Leo S, et al: Concurrent validity of the harris infant neuromotor test and the Alberta infant motor scale, *J Pediatr Nurs* 23(1):28-36, 2008.

Waltz C, Strickland O, Lenz E: *Measurement in nursing research*, ed 3, Philadelphia, 2005, FA Davis.

Weiss M, Ryan P, Lokken L: Validity and reliability of the perceived readiness for discharge after birth scale, *J Obstet Gynecol Neonat Nurs* 35(1):34-45, 2006.

Whittemore R, Melkus G, Wagner J, et al: Translating the diabetes prevention program to primary care, *Nurs Res* 58(1):2-12, 2009.

Wu J, Chung M, Lennie TA, et al: Testing the psychometric properties of the medication adherence scale in patients with heart failure, *Heart Lung* 37(5):334-343, 2008.

FOR FURTHER STUDY

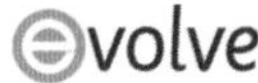

Go to Evolve at http://evolve.elsevier.com/LoBiondo/ for review questions, critiquing exercises, and additional research articles for practice in reviewing and critiquing.

14

Data Analysis: Descriptive and Inferential Statistics

Susan Sullivan-Bolyai and Carol Bova

KEY TERMS

- analysis of covariance (ANCOVA)
- analysis of variance (ANOVA)
- categorical variable
- chi-square (χ^2)
- continuous variable
- correlation
- degrees of freedom
- descriptive statistics
- dichotomous variable
- factor analysis
- Fisher's exact probability test
- frequency distribution
- inferential statistics
- interval measurement
- levels of measurement
- level of significance (alpha level)
- mean
- measures of central tendency
- measures of variability
- median
- measurement
- modality
- mode
- multiple analysis of variance (MANOVA)
- multiple regression
- multivariate statistics
- nominal measurement
- nonparametric statistics
- normal curve
- null hypothesis
- ordinal measurement
- parameter
- parametric statistics
- Pearson correlation coefficient (Pearson *r*; Pearson product moment correlation coefficient)
- percentile
- probability
- range
- ratio measurement
- sampling error
- scientific hypothesis
- semiquartile range
- standard deviation (SD)
- statistic
- *t* statistic
- type I error
- type II error
- Z score

LEARNING OUTCOMES

After reading this chapter, you should be able to do the following:

- Differentiate between descriptive and inferential statistics.
- State the purposes of descriptive statistics.
- Identify the levels of measurement in a research study.
- Describe a frequency distribution.
- List measures of central tendency and their use.
- List measures of variability and their use.
- Identify the purpose of inferential statistics.
- Explain the concept of probability as it applies to the analysis of sample data.
- Distinguish between a type I and type II error and its effect on a study's outcome.
- Distinguish between parametric and nonparametric tests.

- List some commonly used statistical tests and their purposes.
- Critically appraise the statistics used in published research studies.
- Evaluate the strength and quality of the evidence provided by the findings of a research study and determine their applicability to practice.

STUDY RESOURCES

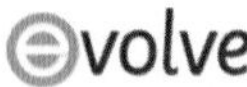

Go to Evolve at http://evolve.elsevier.com/LoBiondo/ for review questions, critiquing exercises, and additional research articles for practice in reviewing and critiquing.

It is important for you to understand the principles underlying statistical methods used in quantitative nursing research. This understanding allows you to critically analyze the results of research that may be useful to practice. Researchers link the statistical analyses they choose with the type of research question, design, and level of data collected. Ultimately, statistical procedures are used to provide organization and meaning to data.

As you read a research article you will find a discussion of the statistical procedures used in both the methods and results sections. In the methods section, you will find the planned statistical analyses. In the results section, you will find the data generated from testing the hypotheses or research questions. These data are the analyses using both descriptive and inferential **statistics.**

Procedures that allow researchers to describe and summarize data are known as **descriptive statistics.** Often researchers use the demographic and clinical data collected to *describe* the sample using descriptive statistics. Descriptive techniques include measures of central tendency, such as mean, median, and mode; measures of variability, such as range and standard deviation (SD); and some correlation techniques, such as scatter plots. For example, Meneses and associates (2007) (see Appendix A) used descriptive statistics to inform the reader about the subjects' personal characteristics (mean age = 54.5 years, 82% Caucasian, 48% with a college education) and clinical characteristics (90% had not participated in a cancer support group, 60% had breast-conserving surgery, 69% received radiation therapy, and 54% received chemotherapy).

Data-collection procedures that allow researchers to estimate how reliably they can make *predictions* and *generalize* findings based on the data are known as **inferential statistics.** Inferential statistics are used to analyze the data collected, test hypotheses, and answer the research questions in a research study. With inferential statistics, the researcher is trying to draw conclusions that extend beyond the immediate data of the study.

This chapter describes how researchers use descriptive and inferential statistics in nursing research studies. This will help you to determine the appropriateness of the statistics used and to interpret the strength and quality of the reported findings, as well as the clinical significance and applicability of the research results for your evidence-based practice.

LEVELS OF MEASUREMENT

Measurement is the process of assigning numbers to variables or events according to rules. Every variable in a research study that is assigned a specific number must be similar to every other variable assigned that number. In other words, if you decide to assign the number 1 to represent all male subjects in a sample and the number 2 to represent all female subjects, you must use this same numbering scheme throughout your study.

The measurement level is determined by the nature of the object or event being measured. Understanding the different **levels of measurement** is an important first step when you evaluate the statistical analyses used in a study. There are four levels of measurement: nominal, ordinal, interval, or ratio (Table 14-1). The level of measurement of each variable determines the type of statistic that can be used to answer a research question or test a hypothesis. The higher the level of measurement, the greater the flexibility the researcher has in choosing statistical procedures. Every attempt should be made to use the highest level of measurement possible so that the maximum amount of information will be obtained from the data. The following Critical Thinking Decision Path illustrates the relationship between levels of measurement and appropriate choice of descriptive statistics.

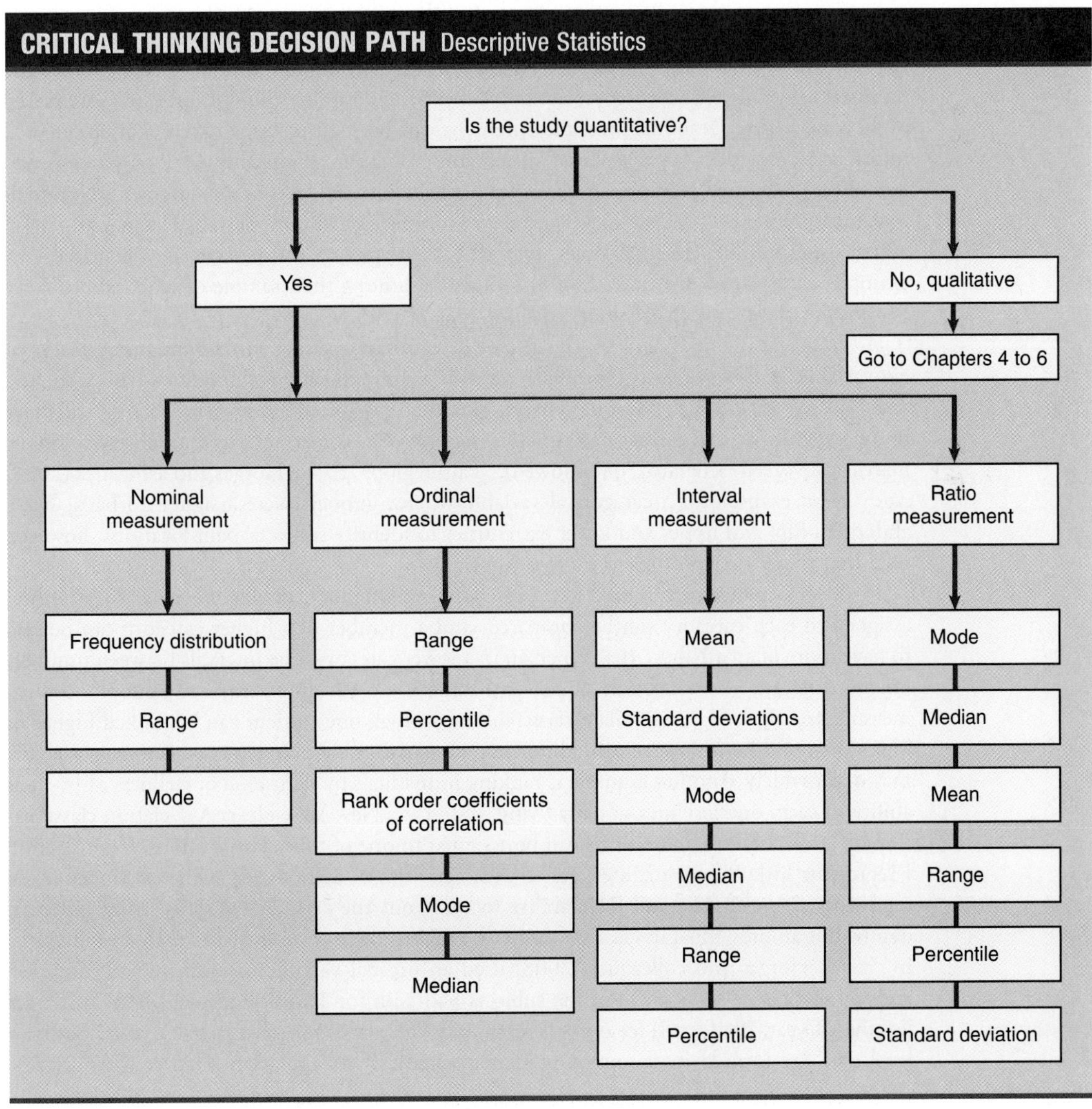

TABLE 14-1 Level of Measurement Summary Table

Measurement	Description	Measures of Central Tendency	Measures of Variability
Nominal	Classification	Mode	Modal percentage, range, frequency distribution
Ordinal	Relative rankings	Mode, median	Range, percentile, semiquartile range, frequency distribution
Interval	Rank ordering with equal intervals	Mode, median, mean	Range, percentile, semiquartile range, standard deviation
Ratio	Rank ordering with equal intervals and absolute zero	Mode, median, mean	All

Nominal measurement is used to classify variables or events into categories. The categories are mutually exclusive; the variable or event either has or does not have the characteristic. The numbers assigned to each category are only labels; such numbers do not indicate more or less of a characteristic. Nominal-level measurement can be used to categorize a sample on such information as gender, marital status, or religious affiliation. For example, Horgas and associates (2008) measured pain presence (yes/no) using a nominal level of measurement. Nominal-level measurement is the lowest level and allows for the least amount of statistical manipulation. When using nominal-level variables, typically the frequency and percent are calculated. For example, Horgas and associates (2008) found that among their sample of older adults, 50% (n = 69) of their subjects experienced some type of pain.

A variable at the nominal level can also be categorized as either a ***dichotomous*** or ***categorical*** variable. A *dichotomous* (nominal) variable is one that has *only two true values,* such as true/false or yes/no. On the other hand, nominal variables that are *categorical* still have mutually exclusive categories but have *more than two true values,* such as marital status (single, married, divorced, separated, or widowed). "Pain regions" in the Horgas and associates (2008) study is an example of a categorical variable where numbers were assigned to back, head, abdomen, hip, and upper and lower extremities to identify subjects' pain locations; however, note that there was no order to these categories.

Ordinal measurement is used to show relative rankings of variables or events. The numbers assigned to each category can be compared, and a member of a higher category can be said to have more of an attribute than a person in a lower category. The intervals between numbers on the scale are not necessarily equal, and there is no absolute zero. For example, ordinal measurement is used to formulate class rankings, where one student can be ranked higher or lower than another. However, the difference in actual grade point average between students may differ widely. Another example is ranking individuals by their level of wellness or by their ability to carry out activities of daily living. Using the New York Heart Association classification of cardiac failure, individuals can be assigned to one of four classifications. Classification I represents little disease or interference with activities of daily living, while classification IV represents severe disease and little ability to carry out the activities of daily living independently, but an individual in class IV cannot be said to be four times sicker than an individual in class I. Horgas and colleagues (2008) used an ordinal variable to measure pain duration and found that 27% (n = 31) of the subjects had pain for 1 to 5 years, 19.1% (n = 22) for less than 1 year, 7% (n = 8) for 6 to 10 years, and 7% (n = 8) for more than 11 years. Ordinal-level data are limited in the amount of mathematical manipulation possible. Frequencies, percents, medians, percentiles, and rank order coefficients of correlation can be calculated for ordinal-level data.

Interval measurement shows rankings of events or variables on a scale with equal intervals between the numbers. The zero point remains arbitrary and not absolute. For example, interval measurements are used in measuring temperatures on the Fahrenheit scale. The distances between degrees are equal, but the zero point is arbitrary and does not represent the absence of temperature. Test scores also represent interval data. The differences between test scores represent equal intervals, but a zero does not represent the total absence of knowledge.

In many areas in the social sciences, including nursing, the classification of the level of measurement of scales that use Likert-type response options to measure concepts such as quality of life, depression, functional status, or social support is controversial, with some regarding these measurements as ordinal and others as interval. You need to be aware of this controversy and to look at each study individually in terms of how the data are analyzed. Interval-level data allow more manipulation of data, including the addition and subtraction of numbers and the calculation of means. This additional manipulation is why many argue for classifying behavioral scale data as interval level. For example, Horgas and colleagues (2008) used two scales to measure physical (scale = 0 to 21) and social (scale = 0 to 11) limitations and reported the means and standard deviations (SD) for these interval-level data.

Ratio measurement shows rankings of events or variables on scales with equal intervals and absolute zeros. The number represents the actual amount of the property the object possesses. Ratio measurement is the highest level of measurement, but it is most often used in the physical sciences. Examples of ratio-level data that are commonly used in nursing research are height, weight, pulse, and blood pressure. All mathematical procedures can be performed on data from ratio scales. Therefore the use of any statistical procedure is possible as long as it is appropriate to the design of the study.

HELPFUL HINT
The term **continuous data** is also used to represent a measure that contains a range of values along a continuum and may include ordinal-, interval-, and ratio-level data (Munro, 2005). An example is heart rate.

HELPFUL HINT
Descriptive statistics assist in summarizing data. The descriptive statistics calculated must be appropriate to both the purpose of the study and the level of measurement.

DESCRIPTIVE STATISTICS

Frequency Distribution

One way of organizing descriptive data is by using a frequency distribution. In a **frequency distribution** the number of times each event occurs is counted. The data can also be grouped and the frequency of each group is reported. Table 14-2 shows the results of an examination given to a class of 51 students. The results of the examination are reported in several ways. The columns on the left give the raw data tally and the frequency for each grade, and the columns on the right give the grouped data tally and grouped frequencies.

TABLE 14-2 Frequency Distribution

INDIVIDUAL			GROUP		
Score	**Tally**	**Frequency**	**Score**	**Tally**	**Frequency**
90	I	1	>89	I	1
88	I	1			
86	I	1	80-89	IIIII IIIII IIIII	15
84	IIIII I	6			
82	II	2	70-79	IIIII IIIII IIIII IIIII III	23
80	IIIII	5			
78	IIIII	5			
76	I	1	60-69	IIIII IIIII	10
74	IIIII II	7			
72	IIIII IIII	9	<59	II	2
70	I	1			
68	III	3			
66	II	2			
64	IIII	4			
62	I	1			
60		0			
58	I	1			
56		0			
54	I	1			
52		0			
50		0			
Total		51			51

Mean, 73.1; standard deviation, 12.1; median, 74; mode, 72; range, 36 (54-90).

When data are grouped, it is necessary to define the size of the group or the interval width so that no score will fall into two groups and each group will be mutually exclusive. The grouping of the data in Table 14-2 prevents overlap; each score falls into only one group. The grouping should allow for a precise presentation of the data without serious loss of information. Jones and colleagues (2007) reported frequency data in Table 1 (p. 190) of their study among deaf adults. They chose to represent the data according to groups (intervention and comparison groups).

Information about frequency distributions may be presented in the form of a table, such as Table 14-2, or in graphic form. Figure 14-1 illustrates the most common graphic forms: the histogram and the frequency polygon. The two graphic methods are similar in that both plot scores or percentages of occurrence against frequency. The greater the number of points plotted, the smoother the resulting graph. The shape of the resulting graph allows for observations that further describe the data.

Measures of Central Tendency

Measures of central tendency are used to describe the pattern of responses among a sample. Measures of central tendency include the mean, median, and mode. They yield a single number that describes the middle of the group and summarize the members of a sample. Each

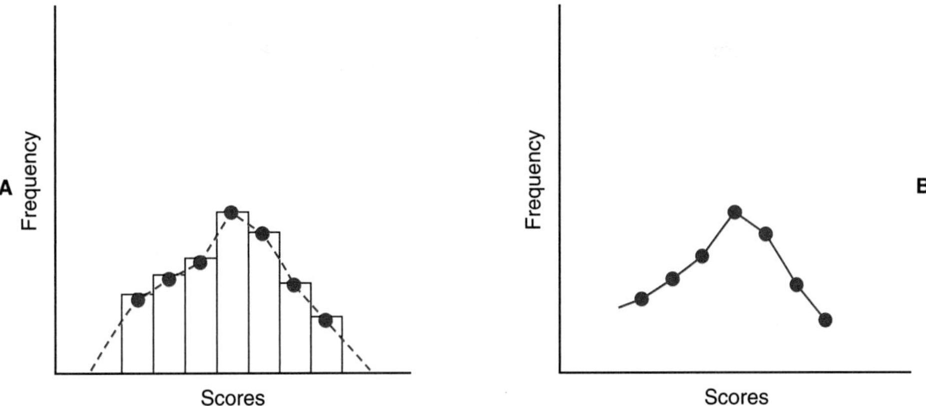

Figure 14-1 Frequency distributions. **A,** Histogram. **B,** Frequency polygon.

measure of central tendency has a specific use and is most appropriate to specific kinds of measurement and types of distributions.

The **mean** is the arithmetical average of all the scores (add all of the values in a distribution and divide by the total number of values) and is used with interval or ratio data. The mean is the most widely used measure of central tendency. Most statistical tests of significance use the mean. The mean is affected by every score and can change greatly with extreme scores, especially in studies that have a limited sample size. The mean is generally considered the single best point for summarizing data when using interval- or ratio-level data. You can find the mean in research reports by looking for the symbols M = or $\overline{x}$.

The **median** is the score where 50% of the scores are above it and 50% of the scores are below it. The median is not sensitive to extremes in high and low scores. It is best used when the data are skewed (see Normal Distribution in this chapter), and the researcher is interested in the "typical" score. For example, if age is a variable and there is a wide range with extreme scores that may affect the mean, it would be appropriate to also report the median. The median is easy to find either by inspection or by calculation and can be used with ordinal-, interval-, and ratio-level data.

The **mode** is the most frequent value in a distribution. The mode is determined by inspection of the frequency distribution (not by mathematical calculation). For example, in Table 14-2 the mode would be a score of 72 because nine students received this score and it represents the score that was attained by the greatest number of students. It is important to note that a sample distribution can have more than one mode. The number of modes contained in a distribution is called the **modality** of the distribution. It is also possible to have no mode when all scores in a distribution are different. The mode is most often used with nominal data but can be used with all levels of measurement. The mode cannot be used for calculations, and it is unstable; that is, the mode can fluctuate widely from sample to sample from the same population.

HELPFUL HINT

Of the three measures of central tendency, the mean is the most stable, the least affected by extremes, and the most useful for other calculations. The mean can only be calculated with interval and ratio data.

When you examine a research report, the measures of central tendency provide you with important information about the distribution of scores in a sample. If the distribution is symmetrical and unimodal, the mean, median, and mode will coincide. If the distribution is skewed (asymmetrical), the mean will be pulled in the direction of the long tail of the distribution and will differ from the median. With a skewed distribution, all three statistics should be reported. It is also helpful to report the mean and median for interval- and ratio-level data so the reader knows whether or not the distribution was symmetrical.

HELPFUL HINT

Measures of central tendency are descriptive statistics that describe the characteristics of a sample.

Normal Distribution

The concept of the **normal distribution** is based on the observation that data from repeated measures of interval- or ratio-level data group themselves about a midpoint in a distribution in a manner that closely approximates the normal curve illustrated in Figure 14-2. The normal curve is one that is symmetrical about the mean and is unimodal. The mean, median, and mode are equal. An additional characteristic of the normal curve is that a fixed percentage of the scores falls within a given distance of the mean. As shown in Figure 14-2, about 68% of the scores or means will fall within 1 SD of the mean, 95% within 2 SD of the mean, and 99.7% within 3 SD of the mean.

However, not all data approximate the normal curve. Some samples are nonsymmetrical and the peak is off-center. The distribution of scores is called a positive skew when the mean is to the right of the median and a negative skew when the mean is to the left of the median. Figure 14-3 illustrates positive and negative skew. In each diagram the peak is off-center and

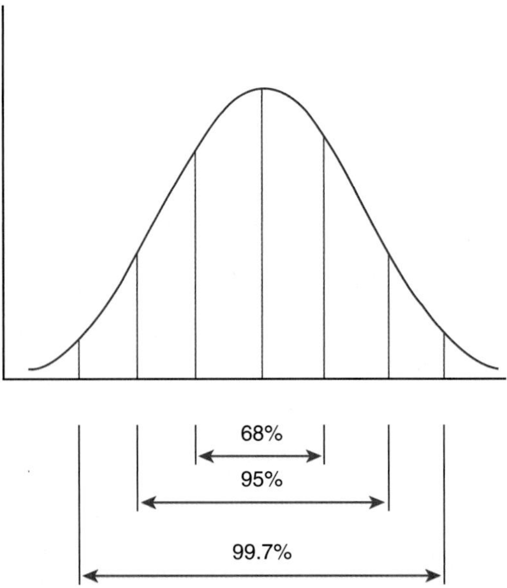

Figure 14-2 The normal distribution and associated standard deviations.

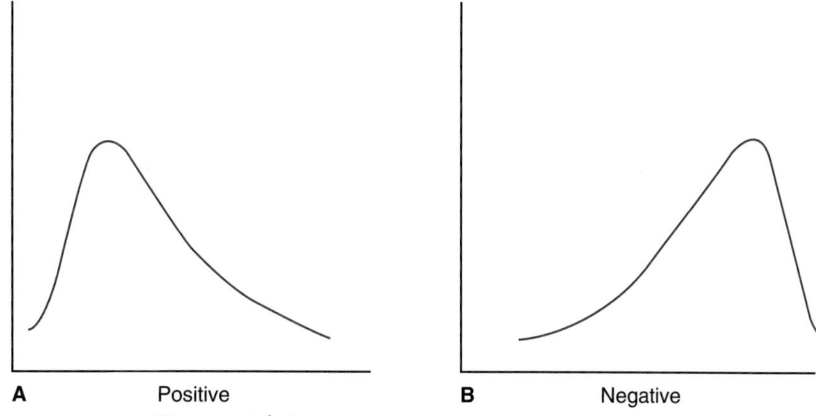

Figure 14-3 **A,** Positive skew. **B,** Negative skew.

one tail is longer. The presence or absence of a normal distribution is a fundamental issue when examining the appropriate use of inferential statistical procedures.

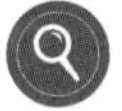

EVIDENCE-BASED PRACTICE TIP

Inspection of descriptive statistics for the sample will indicate whether or not the sample data are skewed.

Interpreting Measures of Variability

Variability or dispersion is concerned with the spread of data. Measures of variability answer questions such as the following: "Is the sample homogeneous or heterogeneous?" "Is the sample similar or different?" If a researcher measures oral temperatures in two samples, one sample drawn from a healthy population and one sample from a hospitalized population, it is possible that the two samples will have the same mean. However, it is likely that there will be a wider range of temperatures in the hospitalized sample than in the healthy sample. Measures of variability are used to describe these differences in the dispersion of data. As with measures of central tendency, the various measures of variability are appropriate to specific kinds of measurement and types of distributions.

HELPFUL HINT

Remember that descriptive statistics related to variability will enable you to evaluate the homogeneity or heterogeneity of a sample.

The range is the simplest but most unstable measure of variability. Range is the difference between the highest and lowest scores. A change in either of these two scores would change the range. The range should always be reported with other measures of variability. The range in Table 14-2 is 36, but this could easily change with an increase or decrease in the high score of 90 or the low score of 54. Jones and associates (2007) reported the range of ages among their sample by group. For the intervention group the mean age was 51.3 years with a range of 18 to 83 years, and for the comparison group the mean age was 50.6 years with a range of 22 to 85 years. This information lets you know that the groups were very similar by age.

The semiquartile range **(semiinterquartile range)** indicates the range of the middle 50% of the scores. It is more stable than the range, because it is less likely to be changed by a single extreme score. It lies between the upper and lower quartiles, the upper quartile being the point below which 75% of the scores fall and the lower quartile being the point below which 25% of the scores fall. The middle 50% of the scores in Table 14-2 lies between 68 and 78, and the semiquartile range is 10.

A percentile represents the percentage of cases a given score exceeds. The median is the 50% percentile, and in Table 14-2 it is a score of 74. A score in the 90th percentile is exceeded by only 10% of the scores. The zero percentile and the 100th percentile are usually dropped.

The standard deviation (SD) is the most frequently used measure of variability, and it is based on the concept of the normal curve (see Figure 14-2). It is a measure of average deviation of the scores from the mean and as such should always be reported with the mean. The SD takes all scores into account and can be used to interpret individual scores. The SD is used in the calculation of many inferential statistics. One limitation of the SD is that it is expressed in terms of the units used in the measurement and cannot be used to compare means that have different units. If researchers were interested in the relationship between height measured in inches and weight measured in pounds, it would be necessary for them to convert the height and weight measurements to standard units or Z scores.

The Z score is used to compare measurements in standard units. Each of the scores is converted to a Z score, and then the Z scores are used to examine the relative distance of the scores from the mean. A Z score of 1.5 means that the observation is 1.5 SD above the mean, whereas a Z score of −2 means that the observation is 2 SD below the mean. By using Z scores, a researcher can compare results from scales that use different measurement units, such as height and weight.

HELPFUL HINT

Many measures of variability exist. The SD is the most stable and useful because it helps you to visualize how the scores disperse around the mean.

INFERENTIAL STATISTICS

Inferential statistics combine mathematical processes and logic and allow researchers to test hypotheses about a population using data obtained from probability samples. Statistical inference is generally used for two purposes—to estimate the probability that the statistics in the sample accurately reflect the population parameter and to test hypotheses about a population.

A parameter is a characteristic of a *population,* whereas a statistic is a characteristic of a *sample.* We use statistics to estimate population parameters. Suppose we randomly sample 100 people with chronic lung disease and use an interval-level scale to study their knowledge of the disease. If the mean score for these subjects is 65, the mean represents the sample statistic. If we were able to study every subject with chronic lung disease, we could calculate an average knowledge score and that score would be the parameter for the population. As you know, a researcher rarely is able to study an entire population, so inferential statistics provide evidence that allow the researcher to make statements about the larger population from studying the sample.

The example given alludes to two important qualifications of how a study must be conducted so that inferential statistics may be used. First, it was stated that the sample was selected using probability methods (see Chapter 10). Because you are already familiar wi tages of probability sampling, it should be clear that if we wish to make statem population from a sample, that sample must be representative. All procedures fo statistics are based on the assumption that the sample was drawn with a known Second, the scale used has to be at either an interval or a ratio level of measurem ... This is because the mathematical operations involved in doing inferential statistics require this higher level of measurement. It should be noted that in studies that use nonprobability methods of sampling, inferential statistics are also used. To compensate for the use of nonprobability sampling methods, researchers employ such techniques as sample size estimation using power analysis. The following two Critical Thinking Decision Paths examine inferential statistics and provide matrices that researchers use for statistical decision making.

EVIDENCE-BASED PRACTICE TIP

Try to figure out whether the statistical test chosen was appropriate for the design, the type of data collected, and the level of measurement.

CRITICAL THINKING DECISION PATH Inferential Statistics—Difference Questions

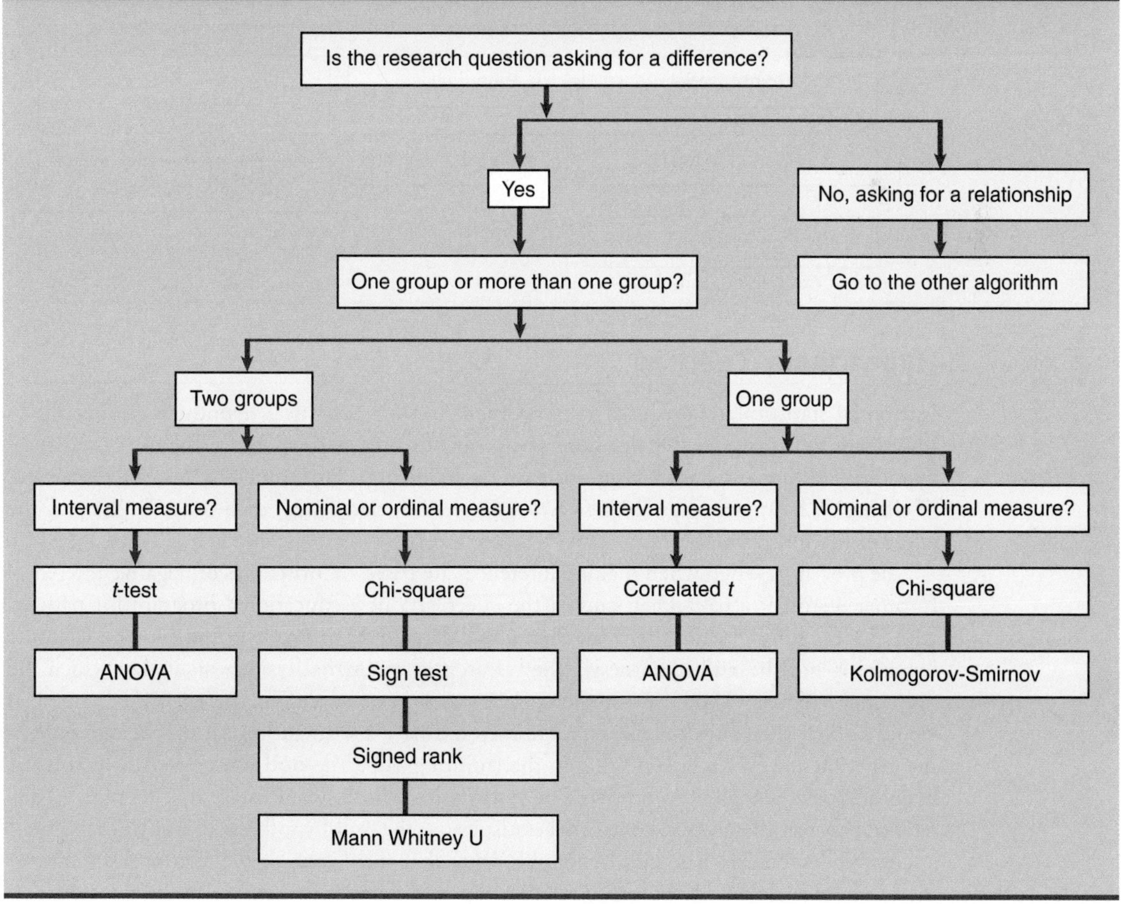

Is the research question asking for a difference?

- Yes
  - One group or more than one group?
    - Two groups
      - Interval measure?
        - *t*-test
        - ANOVA
      - Nominal or ordinal measure?
        - Chi-square
        - Sign test
        - Signed rank
        - Mann Whitney U
    - One group
      - Interval measure?
        - Correlated *t*
        - ANOVA
      - Nominal or ordinal measure?
        - Chi-square
        - Kolmogorov-Smirnov
- No, asking for a relationship
  - Go to the other algorithm

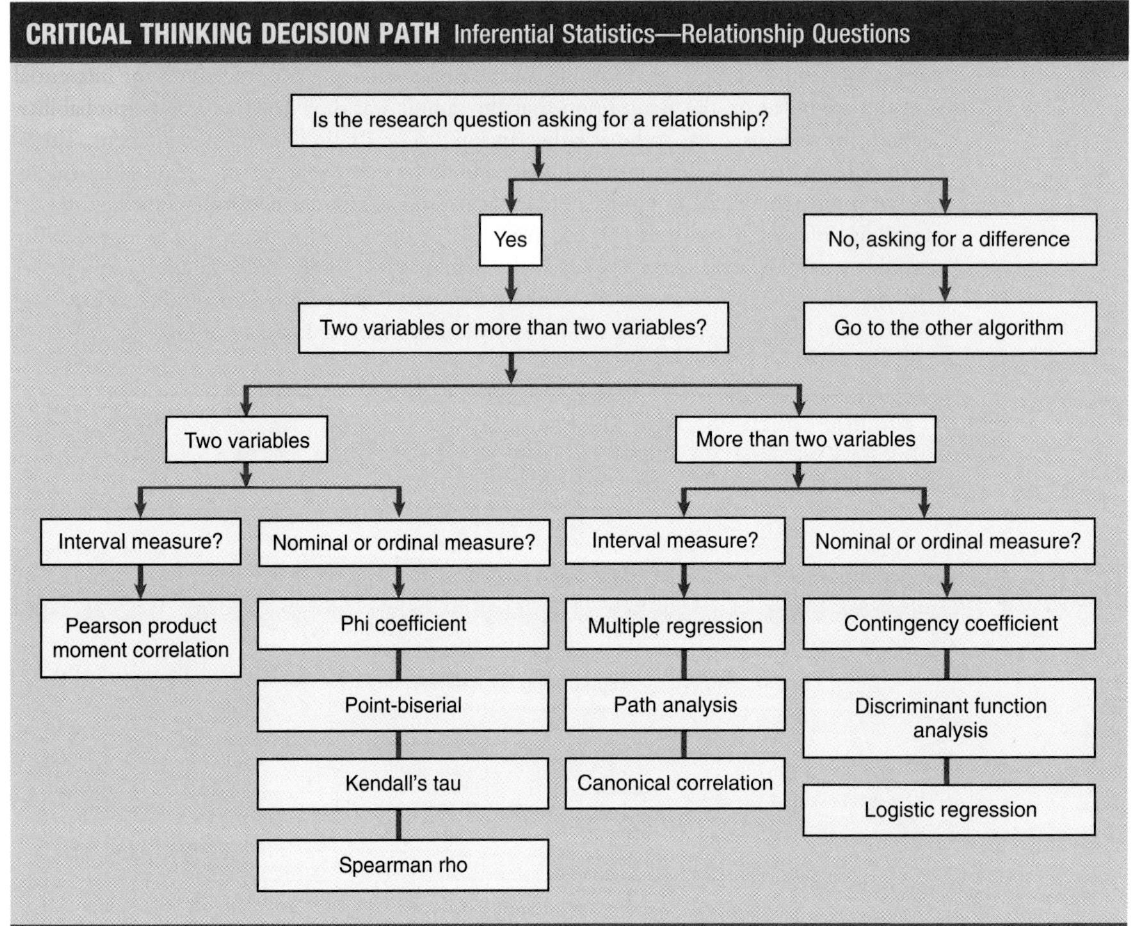

Hypothesis Testing

Inferential statistics are also used for hypothesis testing. Statistical hypothesis testing allows researchers to make objective decisions about the outcome of their study. The use of statistical hypothesis testing answers such questions as the following: "How much of this effect is a result of chance?" "How strongly are these two variables associated with each other?" "What is the effect of the intervention?"

The procedures used when making inferences are based on principles of negative inference. In other words, if a researcher studied the effect of a new educational program for patients with chronic lung disease, the researcher would actually have two hypotheses—the scientific hypothesis and the null hypothesis. The research or **scientific hypothesis** is that which the researcher believes will be the outcome of the study. In our example, the scientific hypothesis would be that the educational intervention would have a marked impact on the outcome in the experimental group beyond that in the control group. The **null hypothesis,** which is the hypothesis that actually can be tested by statistical methods, would state that there is no difference between the groups. Inferential statistics use the null hypothesis to test the validity of a scientific hypothesis. The null hypothesis states that there is no actual relationship between the variables and that any observed relationship or difference is merely a function of chance.

HELPFUL HINT

Remember that most samples used in clinical research are samples of convenience, but often researchers use inferential statistics. Although such use violates one of the assumptions of such tests, the tests are robust enough to not seriously affect the results unless the data are skewed in unknown ways.

Probability

Probability theory underlies all of the procedures discussed in this chapter. The **probability** of an event is its long-run relative frequency (0% to 100%) in repeated trials under similar conditions. In other words, what are the chances of obtaining the same result from a study that can be carried out many times under identical conditions? It is the notion of repeated trials that allows researchers to use probability to test hypotheses.

Statistical probability is based on the concept of **sampling error.** Remember that the use of inferential statistics is based on random sampling. However, even when samples are randomly selected, there is always the possibility of some error in sampling. Therefore the characteristics of any given sample may be different from those of the entire population. The tendency for statistics to fluctuate from one sample to another is known as sampling error.

EVIDENCE-BASED PRACTICE TIP

Remember that the strength and quality of evidence are enhanced by repeated trials that have consistent findings, thereby increasing generalizability of the findings and applicability to clinical practice.

Type I and Type II Errors

Statistical inference is always based on incomplete information about a population, and it is possible for errors to occur. There are two types of errors in statistical inference—type I and type II errors. A **type I error** occurs when a researcher rejects a null hypothesis when it is actually true (e.g., accepts the premise that there is a difference when actually there is no difference between groups). A **type II error** occurs when a researcher accepts a null hypothesis that is actually false (e.g., accepts the premise that there is no difference between the groups when a difference actually exists). The relationship of the two types of errors is shown in Figure 14-4.

When critiquing a study to see if there is a possibility of a type I error having occurred (rejecting the null hypothesis when it is actually true), one should consider the reliability and validity of the instruments used. For example, if the instruments did not accurately measure

	REALITY	
Conclusion of test of significance	Null hypothesis is true	Null hypothesis is not true
Not statistically significant	Correct conclusion	Type II error
Statistically significant	Type I error	Correct conclusion

Figure 14-4 Outcome of statistical decision making.

the intervention variables, one could conclude that the intervention made a difference when in reality it did not. It is critical to consider the reliability and validity of all the measurement instruments reported (see Chapter 13). For example, Jones and colleagues (2007) reported that they reassessed the reliability of the Self-Rated Abilities for Health Practices (SRAHP) scale in their sample and found that it was reliable as evidenced by a Cronbach's alpha of .92 (refer to Chapter 13 to review scale reliability). This gives the reader greater confidence in the results of the study, which found a significant difference on the SRAHP scale between the intervention and comparisons groups.

In a practice discipline, type I errors usually are considered more serious because if a researcher declares that differences exist where none are present, the potential exists for patient care to be affected adversely. Type II errors (accepting the null hypothesis when it is false) often occur when the sample is too small, thereby limiting the opportunity to measure *the treatment effect,* a true difference between two groups. A larger sample size improves the ability to *detect the treatment effect,* that is, differences between two groups. If no significant difference is found between two groups with a large sample, it provides stronger evidence (than with a small sample) not to reject the null hypothesis.

Level of Significance

The researcher does not know when an error in statistical decision making has occurred. It is possible to know only that the null hypothesis is indeed true or false if data from the total population are available. However, the researcher can control the risk of making type I errors by setting the level of significance before the study begins (a priori).

The **level of significance (alpha level)** is the probability of making a type I error, the probability of rejecting a true null hypothesis. The minimum level of significance acceptable for nursing research is 0.05. If the researcher sets alpha, or the level of significance, at 0.05, the researcher is willing to accept the fact that if the study were done 100 times, the decision to reject the null hypothesis would be wrong 5 times out of those 100 trials. If, as is sometimes done, the researcher wants to have a smaller risk of rejecting a true null hypothesis, the level of significance may be set at 0.01. In this case the researcher is willing to be wrong only once in 100 trials.

The decision as to how strictly the alpha level should be set depends on how important it is to not make an error. For example, if the results of a study are to be used to determine whether a great deal of money should be spent in an area of nursing care, the researcher may decide that the accuracy of the results is so important that an alpha level of 0.01 is needed. In most studies, however, alpha is set at 0.05.

Perhaps you are thinking that researchers should always use the lowest alpha level possible to keep the risk of both types of errors at a minimum. Unfortunately, decreasing the risk of making a type I error increases the risk of making a type II error. Therefore the researcher always has to accept more of a risk of one type of error when setting the alpha level.

HELPFUL HINT

Decreasing the alpha level acceptable for a study increases the chance that a type II error will occur. Remember that when a researcher is doing many statistical tests, the probability of some of the tests being significant increases as the number of tests increases. Therefore when a number of tests are being conducted, the researcher will often decrease the alpha level to 0.01.

Clinical and Statistical Significance

It is important for you to realize that there is a difference between statistical significance and clinical significance (LeFort, 1993). When a researcher tests a hypothesis and finds that it is statistically significant, this means that the finding is unlikely to have happened by chance. For example, if a study was designed to test an intervention to help a large sample of obese patients lose weight and the researchers found that a change in weight of 1.02 pounds was statistically significant, this would be questionable, because few would say that a change in weight of just over 1 pound would represent a clinically significant difference. Therefore as a consumer of research it is important for you to evaluate the clinical significance of findings, as well as the statistical significance.

Some people believe that if findings are not statistically significant, they have no practical value. However, knowing that something does not work is important information to share with the scientific community. Nonsupported hypotheses provide as much information about the intervention as do supported hypotheses. Nonsignificant results (sometimes called negative findings) force the researcher to return to the literature and consider alternative explanations for why the intervention did not work as planned.

EVIDENCE-BASED PRACTICE TIP

You will study the results to determine whether the new treatment is effective, the size of the effect, and whether the effect is clinically important.

Parametric and Nonparametric Statistics

Tests of significance may be parametric or nonparametric. Many studies in nursing research use parametric tests that have the following three attributes:

1. They involve the estimation of at least one population parameter.
2. They require measurement on at least an interval scale.
3. They involve certain assumptions about the variables being studied.

One important assumption is that the variable is normally distributed in the overall population.

In contrast to parametric tests, **nonparametric statistics** are not based on the estimation of population parameters, so they involve less restrictive assumptions about the underlying distribution. Nonparametric tests usually are applied when the variables have been measured on a nominal or ordinal scale or when the distribution of scores is severely skewed.

HELPFUL HINT

Just because a researcher has used nonparametric statistics does not mean that the study is not useful. The use of nonparametric statistics is appropriate when measurements are not made at the interval level or the variable under study is not normally distributed.

There has been some debate about the relative merits of the two types of statistical tests. The moderate position taken by most researchers and statisticians is that nonparametric statistics are best used when data are not at the interval level of measurement, when the sample

TABLE 14-3 Tests of Differences Between Means

Level of Measurement	One Group	TWO GROUPS Related	Independent	More Than Two Groups
NONPARAMETRIC				
Nominal	Chi-square	Chi-square Fisher exact probability	Chi-square	Chi-square
Ordinal	Kolmogorov-Smirnov	Sign test Wilcoxon matched pairs Signed rank	Chi-square Median test Mann-Whitney U	Chi-square
PARAMETRIC				
Interval or ratio	Correlated *t* ANOVA (repeated measures)	Correlated *t*	Independent *t* ANOVA	ANOVA ANCOVA MANOVA

TABLE 14-4 Tests of Association

Level of Measurement	Two Variables	More Than Two Variables
NONPARAMETRIC		
Nominal	Phi coefficient Point-biserial	Contingency coefficient
Ordinal	Kendall's tau Spearman rho	Discriminant function analysis
PARAMETRIC		
Interval or ratio	Pearson *r*	Multiple regression Path analysis Canonical correlation

is small and data do not approximate a normal distribution. However, most researchers prefer to use **parametric statistics** whenever possible (as long as data meet the assumptions) because they are more powerful and more flexible than nonparametric statistics.

Tables 14-3 and 14-4 show the most commonly used inferential statistics. The test used depends on the level of the measurement of the variables in question and the type of hypothesis being studied. Basically, these statistics test two types of hypotheses—that there is a difference between groups (see Table 14-3) or that there is a relationship between two or more variables (see Table 14-4).

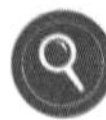

EVIDENCE-BASED PRACTICE TIP

Try to discern whether the test chosen for analyzing the data was chosen because it gave a significant *p* value. A statistical test should be chosen on the basis of its appropriateness for the type of data collected, not because it gives the answer that the researcher hoped to obtain.

Tests of Difference

The type of test used for any particular study depends primarily on whether the researcher is examining differences in one, two, or three or more groups and whether the data to be analyzed are nominal, ordinal, or interval (see Table 14-3). Suppose a researcher has conducted an experimental study using an after-only design (see Chapter 8). What the researcher hopes to determine is that the two randomly assigned groups are different after the introduction of the experimental treatment. If the measurements taken are at the interval level, the researcher would use the *t* test to analyze the data. If the *t* statistic was found to be high enough as to be unlikely to have occurred by chance, the researcher would reject the null hypothesis and conclude that the two groups were indeed more different than would have been expected on the basis of chance alone. In other words, the researcher would conclude that the experimental treatment had the desired effect.

EVIDENCE-BASED PRACTICE TIP

Tests of difference are most commonly used in experimental and quasi-experimental designs that provide Level II and Level III evidence.

The *t* statistic is commonly used in nursing research. This statistic tests whether two group means are different. Thus this statistic is used when the researcher has two groups, and the question is whether the mean scores on some measure are more different than would be expected by chance. To use this test, the dependent variable must have been measured at the interval or ratio level, and the two groups must be independent. By independent we mean that nothing in one group helps determine who is in the other group. If the groups are related, as when samples are matched, and the researcher also wants to determine differences between the two groups, a paired or correlated *t* test would be used. The degrees of freedom (represents the freedom of a score's value to vary given what is known about the other scores and the sum of scores; often $df = N - 1$) that are reported with the *t* statistic and the probability value (*p*). Degrees of freedom is usually abbreviated as *df.*

The *t* statistic illustrates one of the major purposes of research in nursing—to demonstrate that there are differences between groups. Groups may be naturally occurring collections, such as gender, or they may be experimentally created, such as the treatment and control groups. Sometimes a researcher has more than two groups, or measurements are taken more than once, and then analysis of variance (ANOVA) is used. ANOVA is similar to the *t* test. Like the *t* statistic, ANOVA tests whether group means differ, but rather than testing each pair of means separately, ANOVA considers the variation between groups and within groups.

HELPFUL HINT

A research report may not always contain the test that was done. You can find this information by looking at the tables. For example, a table with *t* statistics will contain a column for "*t*" values, and an ANOVA table will contain "*F*" values.

Analysis of covariance (ANCOVA) is used to measures difference among group means, but it also uses a statistical technique to equate the groups under study on an important variable. Jones and colleagues (2007) used ANCOVA to compare the intervention and control group on the major outcome variable but to also control for the different scores on the SRAHP scale at baseline. Another expansion of the notion of analysis of variance is **multiple analysis of variance (MANOVA),** which also is used to determine differences in group means, but it is used when there is more than one dependent variable.

Nonparametric Statistics

When data are at the nominal level and the researcher wants to determine whether groups are different, the researcher uses the **chi-square (χ^2).** Chi-square is a nonparametric statistic used to determine whether the frequency in each category is different from what would be expected by chance. As with the *t* test and ANOVA, if the calculated chi-square is high enough, the researcher would conclude that the frequencies found would not be expected on the basis of chance alone, and the null hypothesis would be rejected. Although this test is quite robust and can be used in many different situations, it cannot be used to compare frequencies when samples are small and expected frequencies are less than 6 in each cell. In these instances the **Fisher's exact probability test** is used.

When the data are ranks, or are at the ordinal level, researchers have several other nonparametric tests at their disposal. These include the *Kolmogorov-Smirnov test,* the *sign test,* the *Wilcoxon matched pairs test,* the *signed rank test for related groups,* the *median test,* and the *Mann-Whitney U test for independent groups.* Explanation of these tests is beyond the scope of this chapter; those readers who desire further information should consult a general statistics book.

HELPFUL HINT

Chi-square is the test of difference commonly used for nominal level demographic variables such as gender, marital status, religion, ethnicity, and others.

EVIDENCE-BASED PRACTICE TIP

You will often note that in the Results or Findings section of a research report parametric (e.g., *t*-tests, ANOVA) and nonparametric (e.g., chi-square, Fisher's exact probability test) will be used to test differences between and among variables depending on their level of measurement. For example, chi-square may be used to test differences between nominal level demographic variables, *t*-tests will be used to test the hypotheses or research questions about differences between two groups, and ANOVA will be used to test differences between and among groups when there are multiple comparisons.

Tests of Relationships

Researchers often are interested in exploring the *relationship* between two or more variables. Such studies use statistics that determine the **correlation,** or the degree of association, between two or more variables. Tests of the relationships between variables are sometimes considered to be descriptive statistics when they are used to describe the magnitude and direction of a relationship of two variables in a sample and the researcher does not wish to make statements about the larger population. Such statistics also can be inferential when they are used to test hypotheses about the correlations that exist in the target population.

Null hypothesis tests of the relationships between variables assume that there is no relationship between the variables. Thus when a researcher rejects this type of null hypothesis, the conclusion is that the variables are in fact related. Suppose a researcher is interested in the relationship between the age of patients and the length of time it takes them to recover from

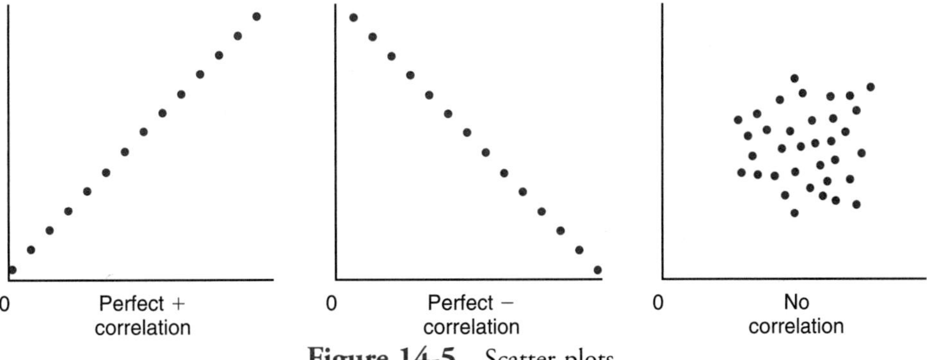

Figure 14-5 Scatter plots.

surgery. As with other statistics discussed, the researcher would design a study to collect the appropriate data and then analyze the data using measures of association. In the example, age and length of time until recovery can be considered interval-level measurements. The researcher would use a test called the **Pearson correlation coefficient, Pearson *r*,** or **Pearson product moment correlation coefficient.** Once the Pearson *r* is calculated, the researcher consults the distribution for this test to determine whether the value obtained is likely to have occurred by chance. Again, the research reports both the value of the correlation and its probability of occurring by chance.

Correlation coefficients can range in value from −1.0 to +1.0 and also can be zero. A zero coefficient means that there is no relationship between the variables. *A perfect positive correlation* is indicated by a +1.0 coefficient, and a *perfect negative correlation* by a −1.0 coefficient. We can illustrate the meaning of these coefficients by using the example from the previous paragraph. If there were no relationship between the age of the patient and the time required for the patient to recover from surgery, the researcher would find a correlation of zero. However, if the correlation was +1.0, this would mean that the older the patient, the longer the recovery time. A negative coefficient would imply that the younger the patient, the longer the recovery time. Figure 14-5 illustrates a perfect positive correlation, a perfect negative correlation, and no correlation.

Of course, relationships are rarely perfect. The magnitude of the relationship is indicated by how close the correlation comes to the absolute value of 1. Thus a correlation of −0.76 is just as strong as a correlation of +0.76, but the direction of the relationship is opposite. In addition, a correlation of 0.76 is stronger than a correlation of 0.32. When a researcher tests hypotheses about the relationships between two variables, the test considers whether the magnitude of the correlation is large enough not to have occurred by chance. This is the meaning of the probability value or the *p* value reported with correlation coefficients. As with other statistical tests of significance, the larger the sample, the greater the likelihood of finding a significant correlation. Therefore researchers also report the degrees of freedom *(df)* associated with the test performed.

Nominal and ordinal data also can be tested for relationships by nonparametric statistics. When two variables being tested have only two levels (e.g., male/female; yes/no), the *phi coefficient* can be used to express relationships. When the researcher is interested in the relationship between a nominal variable and an interval variable, the *point-biserial correlation* is used. *Spearman rho* is used to determine the degree of association between two sets of ranks, as is *Kendall's tau.* All of these correlation coefficients may range in value from −1.0 to +1.0. These tests are shown in Table 14-4.

EVIDENCE-BASED PRACTICE TIP

Tests of relationship are usually associated with nonexperimental designs that provide Level IV evidence. Establishment of a strong statistically significant relationship between variables often lends support for replicating the study to increase the consistency of the findings and provide a foundation for developing an intervention study.

Advanced Statistics

Nurse researchers are often interested in health problems that are very complex and require that we analyze many different variables at once using advanced statistical procedures called **multivariate statistics.** Computer software has made the use of multivariate statistics quite accessible to researchers. When researchers are interested in understanding more about a problem than just the relationship between two variables, they often use a technique called **multiple regression,** which measures the relationship between one interval-level–dependent variable and several independent variables. Multiple regression is the expansion of correlation to include more than two variables, and it is used when the researcher wants to determine what variables contribute to the explanation of the dependent variable and to what degree. For example, a researcher may be interested in determining what factors help women decide to breast-feed their infants. A number of variables, such as the mother's age, previous experience with breast-feeding, number of other children, and knowledge of the advantages of breast-feeding, might be measured and then analyzed to see whether they, separately and together, predict the length of breast-feeding. Such a study would require the use of multiple regression. The results of a study such as this might help nurses know that a younger mother with only one other child might be more likely to benefit from a teaching program about breast-feeding than an older mother with several other children.

Another advanced technique often used in nursing research is **factor analysis.** There are two types of factor analysis, exploratory and confirmatory factor analysis. Exploratory factor analysis is used to reduce a set of data so that it may be easily described and used. It is also used in the early phases of instrument development and theory development. Factor analysis is used to determine whether a scale actually measured the concepts that it is intended to measure. Confirmatory factor analysis resembles structural equation modeling and is used in instrument development to examine construct validity and reliability and to compare factor structures across groups (Aroian & Norris, 2005).

Many nursing studies use statistical modeling procedures to answer research questions. Causal modeling is used most often when researchers want to test hypotheses and theoretically derived relationships. *Path analysis, structured equation modeling (SEM),* and *linear structural relations analysis (LISREL)* are different types of modeling procedures used in nursing research. For example, Horgas and colleagues (2008) used SEM to explain the role of pain as a moderator of race on disability.

Many other statistical techniques are available to nurse researchers. It is beyond the scope of this chapter to review all statistical analyses available. You should consider having several statistical texts available to you as you sort through the evidence reported in studies that are important to your clinical practice (e.g., Field, 2005; Munro, 2005).

APPRAISING THE EVIDENCE

Descriptive and Inferential Statistics

Nurses are challenged to understand the results of research studies that use sophisticated statistical procedures. Understanding the principles that guide statistical analysis is the first step in this process. Statistics are used in nursing research to describe the samples of research studies and to test for hypothesized differences or associations in the sample. Knowing the characteristics of the sample of a research study allows you to determine whether the results are potentially useful for the patients you take care of on a day-to-day basis. For example, if a study sample was primarily white with a mean age of 42 years (SD 2.5), the findings may not be applicable if your patients are mostly elderly and African-American. Cultural, demographic, or clinical factors of an elderly population of a different ethnic group may contribute to different results. Thus understanding the descriptive statistics of a study assists you in determining the applicability of findings to your practice setting.

Statistics are also used to test hypotheses. Inferential statistics used to analyze data and the associated significance level (p values) indicate the likelihood that the association or difference found in any study is due to chance or to a true difference between groups. The closer the p value is to zero, the less likely the association or difference of a study is due to chance. Thus inferential statistics provide an objective way to determine if the results of the study are likely to be a true representation of reality. However, it is still important for you to judge the clinical significance of the findings. Was there a big enough effect (difference between the experimental and control group) to warrant changing current practice?

The Cochrane Report by Stead and Rice (2008) (see Appendix E) provides an excellent example of the summarization of many studies (meta-analysis) that can help direct an evidence based practice geared to choosing the most appropriate nursing delivered smoking cessation interventions to improve health.

EVIDENCE-BASED PRACTICE TIP

A basic understanding of statistics will improve your ability to think about the effect of the independent variable (IV) on the dependent variable (DV) and related patient outcomes for your patient population and practice setting.

There are a few steps to follow when critiquing the statistics used in nursing studies (see Critiquing Criteria box). It is important for you to remember that the procedures for summarizing and analyzing data should make sense in light of the purpose of the study. Before a decision can be made as to whether the statistics employed make sense, it is important to return to the beginning of the research study and review the purpose of the study. Just as the hypotheses or research questions should flow from the purpose of a study, so should the hypotheses or research questions suggest the type of analysis that will follow. The hypotheses or the research questions should indicate the major variables that are expected to be presented in summary form. Each of the variables in the hypotheses or research questions should be followed in the "Results" section with appropriate descriptive information.

After reviewing the hypotheses or research questions, you should proceed to the "Methods" section. Next, try to determine the level of measurement for each variable. From this informa-

CRITIQUING CRITERIA: *Descriptive and Inferential Statistics*

1. Were appropriate descriptive statistics used?
2. What level of measurement is used to measure each of the major variables?
3. Is the sample size large enough to prevent one extreme score from affecting the summary statistics used?
4. What descriptive statistics are reported?
5. Were these descriptive statistics appropriate to the level of measurement for each variable?
6. Are there appropriate summary statistics for each major variable, for example, demographic variables, and any other relevant data?
7. Does the hypothesis indicate that the researcher is interested in testing for differences between groups or in testing for relationships? What is the level of significance?
8. Does the level of measurement permit the use of parametric statistics?
9. Is the size of the sample large enough to permit the use of parametric statistics?
10. Has the researcher provided enough information to decide whether the appropriate statistics were used?
11. Are the statistics used appropriate to the hypothesis, the research question, the method, the sample, and the level of measurement?
12. Are the results for each of the research questions or hypotheses presented clearly and appropriately?
13. If tables and graphs are used, do they agree with the text and extend it, or do they merely repeat it?
14. Are the results understandable?
15. Is a distinction made between clinical significance and statistical significance? How is it made?

tion it is possible to determine the measures of central tendency and variability that should be used to summarize the data. For example, you would not expect to see a mean used as a summary statistic for the nominal variable of gender. In all likelihood, gender would be reported as a frequency distribution. But you would expect to find a mean and SD for a variable that used a scale. The means and SD should be provided for measurements performed at the interval level. The sample size is another aspect of the "Methods" section that is important to review when evaluating the researcher's use of descriptive statistics. The sample is usually described using descriptive summary statistics. Remember, the larger the sample, the less chance that one outlying score will affect the summary statistics. It is also important to note whether the researchers indicated that they did a power analysis to estimate the sample size needed to conduct the study.

If tables or graphs are used, they should agree with the information presented in the text. Evaluate whether the tables and graphs are clearly labeled. If the researcher presents grouped frequency data, the groups should be logical and mutually exclusive. The size of the interval in grouped data should not obscure the pattern of the data, nor should it create an artificial pattern. Each table and graph should be referred to in the text, but each should add to the text—not merely repeat it.

The following are some simple steps for reading a table:

1. Look at the title of the table and see if it matches the purpose of the table.
2. Review the column headings and assess whether the headings follow logically from the title.
3. Look at the abbreviations used. Are they clear and easy to understand? Are any nonstandard abbreviations explained?
4. Evaluate whether the statistics contained in the table are appropriate to the level of measurement for each variable.

After evaluating the descriptive statistics, inferential statistics can then be evaluated. The place to begin appraising the inferential statistical analysis of a research report is with the hypothesis or research question. If the hypothesis or research question indicates that a relationship will be found, you should expect to find indices of correlation. If the study is experimental or quasi-experimental, the hypothesis or research question would indicate that the author is looking for significant differences between the groups studied, and you would expect to find statistical tests of differences between means that test the effect of the intervention. Then as you read the "Methods" section of the paper, again consider what level of measurement the author has used to measure the important variables. If the level of measurement is interval or ratio, the statistics most likely will be parametric statistics. On the other hand, if the variables are measured at the nominal or ordinal level, the statistics used should be nonparametric. Also consider the size of the sample, and remember that samples have to be large enough to permit the assumption of normality. If the sample is quite small, for example, 5 to 10 subjects, the researcher may have violated the assumptions necessary for inferential statistics to be used. Thus the important question is whether the researcher has provided enough justification to use the statistics presented.

Finally, consider the results as they are presented. There should be enough data presented for each hypothesis or research question studied to determine whether the researcher actually examined each hypothesis or research question. The tables should accurately reflect the procedure performed and be in harmony with the text. For example, the text should not indicate that a test reached statistical significance while the tables indicate that the probability value of the test was above 0.05. If the researcher has used analyses that are not discussed in this text, you may want to refer to a statistics text to decide whether the analysis was appropriate to the hypothesis or research question and the level of measurement.

There are two other aspects of the data analysis section that you should appraise. The results of the study in the text of the paper should be clear. In addition, the author should attempt to make a distinction between clinical and statistical significance of the evidence related to the findings. Some results may be statistically significant, but their clinical importance may be doubtful in terms of applicability for a patient population or clinical setting. If this is so, the author should note it. Alternatively, you may find yourself reading a research report that is elegantly presented, but you come away with a "so what?" feeling. From an evidence-based practice perspective, a significant hypothesis or research question should contribute to improving patient care and clinical outcomes. The important question to ask is "What is the strength and quality of the evidence provided by the findings of this study and their applicability to practice?"

Note that the critical analysis of a research paper's statistical analysis is not done in a vacuum. It is possible to judge the adequacy of the analysis only in relationship to the other important aspects of the paper: the problem, the hypotheses, the research question, the design, the data-collection methods, and the sample. Without consideration of these aspects of the research process, the statistics themselves have very little meaning.

CRITICAL THINKING CHALLENGES

- When reading a research study, what is the significance of applying findings if a nurse researcher made a type I error in statistical inference?
- What is the relationship between the level of measurement a researcher uses and the choice of statistics used? As you read a research study, identify the statistics, level of measurement, and the associated level of evidence provided by the design.
- When reviewing a study the sample size provided does not seem adequate. Before you make this final decision, think about how the design type (i.e., pilot study, intervention study), data collection methods, the number of variables, and the sensitivity of the data collection instruments can affect your decision.
- When reading a study you find that the findings were not significant statistically. Consider what the application of such findings could possibly offer your practice.

KEY POINTS

- Descriptive statistics are a means of describing and organizing data gathered in research.
- The four levels of measurement are nominal, ordinal, interval, and ratio. Each has appropriate descriptive techniques associated with it.
- Measures of central tendency describe the average member of a sample. The mode is the most frequent score, the median is the middle score, and the mean is the arithmetical average of the scores. The mean is the most stable and useful of the measures of central tendency, and with the standard deviation it forms the basis for many of the inferential statistics.
- The frequency distribution presents data in tabular or graphic form and allows for the calculation or observations of characteristics of the distribution of the data, including skewness, symmetry, and modality.
- In nonsymmetrical distributions, the degree and direction of the off-center peak are described in terms of positive or negative skew.
- The range reflects differences between high and low scores.
- The standard deviation is the most stable and useful measure of variability. It is derived from the concept of the normal curve. In the normal curve, sample scores and the means of large numbers of samples group themselves around the midpoint in the distribution, with a fixed percentage of the scores falling within given distances of the mean. This tendency of means to approximate the normal curve is called the sampling distribution of the means. A Z score is the standard deviation converted to standard units.
- Inferential statistics are a tool to test hypotheses about populations from sample data.
- Because the sampling distribution of the means follows a normal curve, researchers are able to estimate the probability that a certain sample will have the same properties as the total population of interest. Sampling distributions provide the basis for all inferential statistics.
- Inferential statistics allow researchers to estimate population parameters and to test hypotheses. The use of these statistics allows researchers to make objective decisions about the outcome of the study. Such decisions are based on the rejection or acceptance of the null hypothesis, which states that there is no relationship between the variables.

- If the null hypothesis is accepted, this result indicates that the findings are likely to have occurred by chance. If the null hypothesis is rejected, the researcher accepts the scientific hypothesis that a relationship exists between the variables that is unlikely to have been found by chance.
- Statistical hypothesis testing is subject to two types of errors—type I and type II.
- Type I error occurs when the researcher rejects a null hypothesis that is actually true.
- Type II error occurs when the researcher accepts a null hypothesis that is actually false.
- The researcher controls the risk of making a type I error by setting the alpha level, or level of significance. Unfortunately, reducing the risk of a type I error by reducing the level of significance increases the risk of making a type II error.
- The results of statistical tests are reported to be significant or nonsignificant. Statistically significant results are those whose probability of occurring is less than 0.05 or 0.01, depending on the level of significance set by the researcher.
- Commonly used parametric and nonparametric statistical tests include those that test for differences between means, such as the *t* test and ANOVA, and those that test for differences in proportions, such as the chi-square test.
- Tests that examine data for the presence of relationships include the Pearson *r*, the sign test, the Wilcoxon matched pairs, signed rank test, and multiple regression.
- The most important aspect of critiquing statistical analyses is the relationship of the statistics employed to the problem, design, and method used in the study. Clues to the appropriate statistical test to be used by the researcher should stem from the researcher's hypotheses. The reader also should determine if all of the hypotheses have been presented in the paper.
- A basic understanding of statistics will improve your ability to think about the level of evidence provided by the study design and findings and their relevance to patient outcomes for your patient population and practice setting.

REFERENCES

Aroian KJ, Norris AE: Confirmatory factor analysis. In Munro BH: *Statistical methods for health care research*, ed 5, Philadelphia, 2005, Lippincott Dixon.

Field A: *Discovering statistics using SPSS*, ed 2, Thousand Oaks, CA, 2005, Sage.

Horgas AL, Yoon S, Nichols AL, et al: The relationship between pain and functional disability in black and white older adults, *Res Nurs Health* 31:1-14, 2008.

Jones EG, Renger R, Kang Y: Self-efficacy for health related behaviors among deaf adults, *Res Nurs Health* 30:185-192, 2007.

LeFort SM: The statistical versus clinical significance debate, *Image J Nurs Sch* 25:57-62, 1993.

Meneses KD, McNees P, Loerzel VW, et al: Transition from treatment to survivorship: effects of a psychoeducational intervention on quality of life in breast cancer survivors, *Oncol Nurs Forum* 34(5):1007-1016, 2007.

Munro BH: *Statistical methods for health care research*, ed 5, Philadelphia, 2005, Lippincott.

FOR FURTHER STUDY

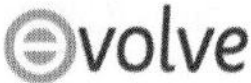

Go to Evolve at http://evolve.elsevier.com/LoBiondo/ for review questions, critiquing exercises, and additional research articles for practice in reviewing and critiquing.

15

Understanding Research Findings

Geri LoBiondo-Wood

KEY TERMS

confidence interval
findings
generalizability
limitations
recommendations

LEARNING OUTCOMES

After reading this chapter, you should be able to do the following:

- Discuss the difference between the "Results" and the "Discussion" sections of a research article.
- Identify the format and components of the "Results" section.
- Determine if both statistically supported and statistically unsupported findings are appropriately discussed.
- Determine whether the results are objectively reported.
- Describe how tables and figures are used in a research report.
- List the criteria of a meaningful table.
- Identify the format and components of the "Discussion" section.
- Determine the purpose of the "Discussion" section.
- Discuss the importance of including generalizability and limitations of a study in the report.
- Determine the purpose of including recommendations in the study report.
- Discuss how the strength, quality, and consistency of evidence provided by the findings are related to a study's results, limitations, generalizability, and applicability to practice.

STUDY RESOURCES

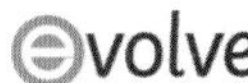

Go to Evolve at http://evolve.elsevier.com/LoBiondo/ for review questions, critiquing exercises, and additional research articles for practice in reviewing and critiquing.

The ultimate goals of nursing research are to develop nursing knowledge and evidence-based nursing practice, thereby supporting the scientific basis of nursing. From a clinical application perspective, the analysis of the results, discussion of the results, interpretations, and generalizability that a researcher generates from a study becomes a highly important piece of the research study. After the analysis of the data, the researcher puts the final pieces of the jigsaw puzzle together to view the total picture with a critical eye. This process is analogous to evaluation, the last step in the nursing process. You may view these last sections as an easier step for the investigator, but it is here that a most critical and creative process comes to the forefront. In the final sections of the report, after the statistical procedures have been applied, the researcher relates the statistical or numerical findings to the research question, hypotheses, theoretical framework, literature, methods, and analyses and begins the task of reviewing the study for any potential bias and formulates the application of the study's findings to practice.

The final sections of published research reports are generally titled "Results" and "Discussion," but other topics, such as conclusions, limitations of findings, implications for future research and nursing practice, recommendations, and application to practice, may be separately addressed or subsumed within these sections. The presentation format of these areas is a function of the author's and the journal's stylistic considerations. The function of these final sections is to relate all aspects of the research process, as well as to discuss, interpret, and identify the limitations, the threats related to bias, and generalizability relevant to the investigation, thereby furthering evidence-based practice. The process that both an investigator and you use to assess the results of a study is depicted in the Critical Thinking Decision Path.

The goal of this chapter is to introduce the purpose and content of the final sections of a research study where data are presented, interpreted, discussed, and generalized. An understanding of what an investigator presents in these sections will help the research consumer to critically analyze an investigator's findings.

FINDINGS

The **findings** of a study are the results, conclusions, interpretations, recommendations, and implications for future research and nursing practice, which are addressed by separating the presentation into two major areas. These two areas are the results and the discussion of the results. The "Results" section focuses on the results or statistical findings of a study, and the "Discussion" section focuses on the remaining topics. For both sections, the rule applies—as it does to all other sections of a report—that the content must be presented clearly, concisely, and logically.

EVIDENCE-BASED PRACTICE TIP

Evidence-based practice is an active process that requires you to consider how, and if, research findings are applicable to your patient population and practice setting.

Results

The "Results" section of a research report is considered to be the data-bound section of the report and is where the quantitative data or numbers generated by the descriptive and inferential statistical tests are presented. Other headings that may be used for the results section

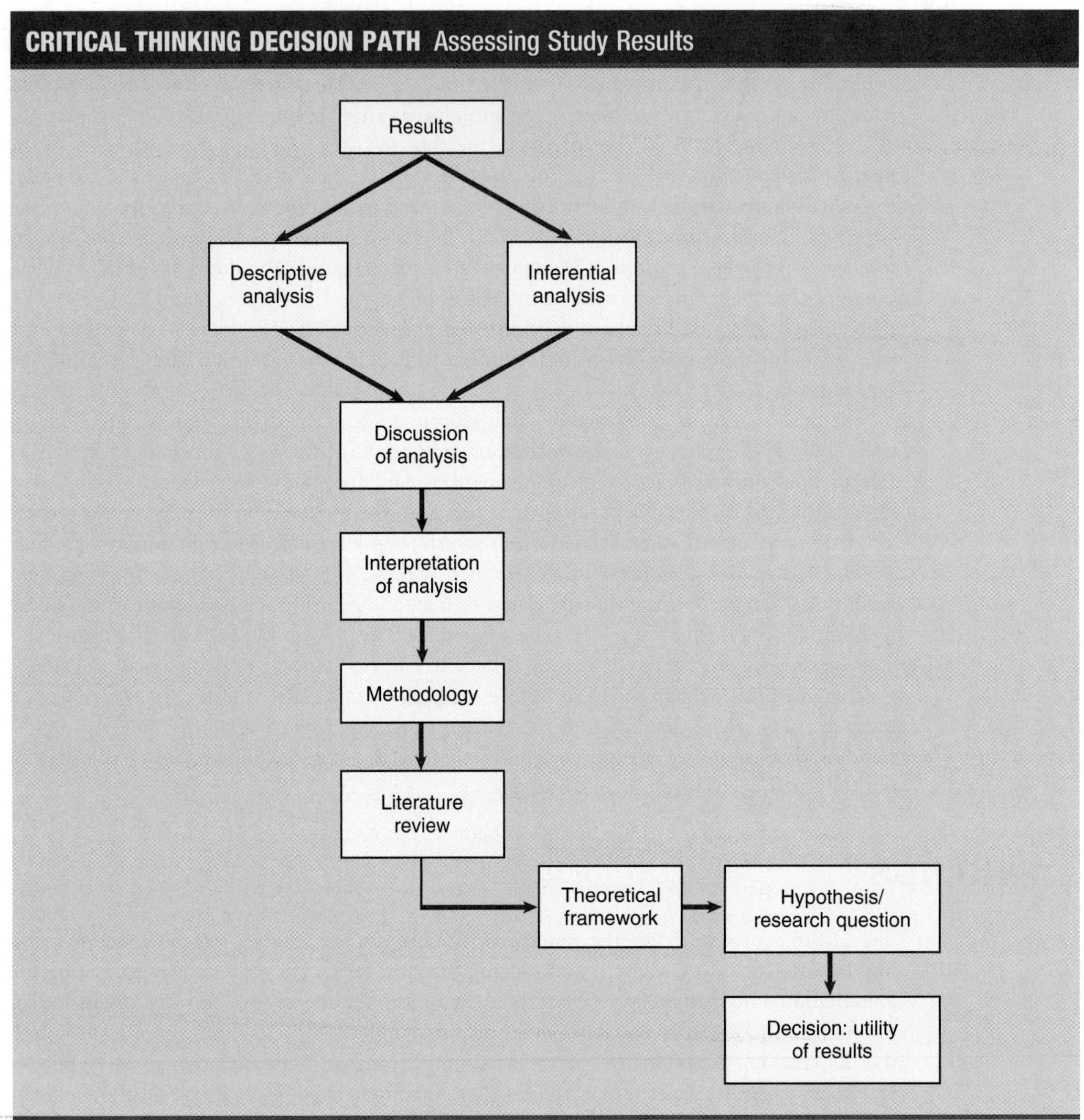

are "Statistical Analyses," "Data Analysis," or "Analysis." The results of the data analysis set the stage for the interpretations or discussion and the limitations sections that follows the results. The "Results" section should reflect analysis of each research question and/or hypothesis tested. The information from each hypothesis or research question should be sequentially presented. The tests used to analyze the data should be identified. If the exact test that was used is not explicitly stated, the values obtained should be noted. The researcher does this by providing the numerical values of the statistics and stating the specific test value and probability level achieved (see Chapter 14). Examples of these statistical results can be found in Table

TABLE 15-1 Examples of Reported Statistical Results

Statistical Test	Examples of Reported Results
Mean	$m = 118.28$
Standard deviation	SD = 62.5
Pearson correlation	$r = 0.49$, $P < 0.01$
Analysis of variance	$F = 3.59$, $df = 2, 48$, $P < 0.05$
t test	$t = 2.65$, $P < 0.01$
Chi-square	$\chi^2 = 2.52$, $df = 1$, $P < 0.05$

15-1. These numbers and their signs should not frighten you. The numbers are important, but there is much more to the research process than the numbers. They are one piece of the whole. Chapter 14 conceptually presents the meanings of the numbers found in studies. Whether you only superficially understand statistics or have an in-depth knowledge of statistics, it should be obvious that the results are clearly stated, and the presence or lack of statistically significant results should be noted.

HELPFUL HINT

In the "Results" section of a research report, the descriptive statistics results are generally presented first; then the inferential results of each of hypothesis or research question that was tested are presented.

At times at the beginning of the "Results" section the researchers will often begin by identifying the name of the statistical software program they used to analyze the data. This is not a statistical test but a computer program specifically designed to analyze a variety of statistical tests. For example, Jones and colleagues (2007) (see Appendix B) state that "data were analyzed using SPSS 12.0" (p. 189). SPSS was the statistical program and the statistical tests used were chi-square, *t* tests, and ANOVA (see Chapter 14).

The researcher is bound to present the data for all of the hypotheses posed or research questions asked (e.g., whether the hypotheses were accepted, rejected, supported, partially supported, or not supported). If the data supported the hypotheses, it may be assumed that the hypotheses were *proven,* but this is not true. It does not necessarily mean that the hypotheses were proven; it only means that the hypotheses were supported and the results suggest that the relationships or differences tested, which were derived from the theoretical framework, were probably logical in that study's sample. You may think that if a researcher's results are not supported statistically or are only partially supported, the study is irrelevant or possibly should not have been published, but this also is not true. If the data are not supported, you should not expect the researcher to bury the work in a file. It is as important for you to review and understand unsupported studies as it is for the researcher. Information obtained from unsupported studies can often be as useful as data obtained from supported studies.

Unsupported studies can be used to suggest **limitations** (problems with the study's validity, bias, or study weaknesses) of particular aspects of a study's design and procedures. Data from unsupported studies may suggest that current modes of practice or current theory in an area may not be supported by research evidence and therefore must be reexamined, researched further, and not at this time be used to support changes in practice. Data help generate new knowledge and evidence, as well as prevent knowledge stagnation. Generally, the results are

BOX 15-1 Examples of Results Section

- "Blacks and Whites did not differ significantly in intensity ($t = -1.14$, $df = 44$, $p = .26$) or duration of self-reported pain ($\chi^2 = 3.68$, $df = 3$, $p = .30$) or in the number of pain locations reported ($t = -1.12$, $df = 67$, $p = .23$)" (Horgas et al., 2008).
- "GEE analysis showed significance differences in overall and psychological and social well-being scores between the two groups" ($p < .001$) (Meneses et al., 2007).
- "Total self-efficacy scores were significantly higher in the intervention group after the Deaf Heart Health Intervention (DHHI), controlling for the total self-efficacy score at baseline ($F[1,81]) = 26.02$, $p < .05$" (Jones et al., 2007).

interpreted in a separate section of the report. At times, you may find that the "Results" section contains the results and the researcher's interpretations, which are generally found in the "Discussion" section. Integrating the results with the discussion in a report is the author's or journal editor's decision. Both sections may be integrated when a study contains several segments that may be viewed as fairly separate subproblems of a major overall problem.

The investigator should also demonstrate objectivity in the presentation of the results. For example, a quote by Jones and colleagues (2007) (see Appendix B) is the appropriate way to express results: "The hypothesis was supported. The mean score SRAHP for the total sample ($n = 84$) was 77.87 (range 38-107, SD = 17.85) at Time 1 were significantly higher in the comparison group ($p < .05$) than in the intervention group." The investigators would be accused of lacking objectivity if they had stated the results in the following manner: "The results were not surprising as we found that the mean scores were significantly higher in the comparison group, as we expected." Opinions or reactionary statements about the data in the "Results" section are therefore avoided. Box 15-1 provides examples of objectively stated results. As you appraise a study, you should consider the following points when reading the "Results" section:

- The investigators responded objectively to the results in the discussion of the results.
- In the discussion of the results, the investigator interpreted the evidence provided by the results, with a careful reflection on all aspects of the study that preceded the results.
- The data presented are summarized. Much data are generated, but only the critical summary numbers for each test are presented. Examples of summarized demographic data are the means and standard deviations of age, education, and income. Including all data is too cumbersome. The results can be viewed as a summary.
- The reduction of data is done both in the written text and through the use of tables and figures. Tables and figures facilitate the presentation of large amounts of data.
- Results for the descriptive and inferential statistics for each hypothesis or research question are presented. No data should be omitted even if they are not significant.
- Any untoward events during the course of the study should be reported.

In their study, Jones and associates (2007) developed tables to present the results visually. Table 15-2 provides descriptive results about the subjects' demographics. Table 15-3 provides the pretest and posttest scores of the intervention and comparison groups on the self-rated abilities scale for health practices. Tables allow researchers to provide a more visually thorough explanation and discussion of the results. If tables and figures are used, they must be concise. Although the text is the major mode of communicating the results, the tables and figures serve a supplementary but independent role. The role of tables and figures is to report results with some detail that the investigator does not explore in the text. This does not mean that tables and figures should not be mentioned in the text. The amount of detail that the author uses

TABLE 15-2 Demographic Characteristics of Participants

Variable	Intervention Group ($n = 32$)	Comparison Group ($n = 52$)
Age	51.3 ± 15.4 (18-83)	50.6 ± 20.1 (22-85)
M ± SD (range)		
Education	11.8 ± 2.9 (5-18)	11.9 ± 3.5 (4-20)
M ± SD (range)		
Sex		
Men	14 (43.8%)	21 (40.4%)
Women	18 (57.2%)	31 (59.6%)
Ethnicity		
White (NH)	20 (62.5%)	45 (86.5%)
Hispanic (MA)	10 (31.3%)	2 (3.8%)
African American	0 (0.0%)	2 (3.8%)
Other	2 (6.2%)	2 (3.8%)
Missing	0	1 (2.1%)
Living situation		
Married/partnered	15 (46.9%)	17 (32.7%)
Single	16 (50.0%)	34 (65.4%)
Missing	1 (3.1%)	1 (1.9%)

Jones EG, Renger R, Kang Y: Self-efficacy for health-related behaviors among deaf adults, *Res Nurs Health* 30:185-192, 2007.

MA, Mexican American; *NH*, non-Hispanic.

TABLE 15-3 The Self-Rated Abilities Scale for Health Practices: Intervention versus Comparison Groups

	PRETEST		POSTTEST	
	Mean (SD)	Range	Corrected Mean (SE)	Range
Intervention group ($n = 32$)				
Total	65.85 (18.06)	38-99	83.90 (2.17)	59-104
Nutrition	16.34 (5.60)	5-26	22.00 (0.58)	12-26
Psychological well-being	17.23 (5.01)	4-26	20.55 (0.69)	10-27
Physical activity	13.89 (7.13)	2-26	20.26 (0.79)	9-27
Responsible health practices	18.39 (4.76)	4-27	20.84 (0.71)	9-27
Comparison group ($n = 52$)				
Total	85.27 (13.20)	59-107	80.78 (1.64)	60-112
Nutrition	20.89 (3.84)	12-28	19.94 (0.44)	12-28
Psychological well-being	20.83 (3.89)	12-28	20.29 (0.53)	13-28
Physical activity	21.00 (5.53)	5-28	20.07 (4.86)	7-28
Responsible health practices	22.55 (4.07)	14-28	21.71 (0.54)	13-28

Jones EG, Renger R, Kang Y: Self-efficacy for health-related behaviors among deaf adults, *Res Nurs Health* 30:185-192, 2007.

in the text to describe the specific tabled data varies with the needs of the researcher. A good table is one that meets the following criteria:

- Supplements and economizes the text
- Has precise titles and headings
- Does not repeat the text

Tables are found in each of the studies in the Appendices. Each one of these tables helps to economize and supplement the text clearly with precise data that help you to visualize the variables quickly and to assess the results.

HELPFUL HINT

A well-written "Results" section is systematic, logical, concise, and drawn from all of the analyzed data. All that is written in the "Results" section should be geared to letting the data reflect the testing of the research questions and hypotheses. The length of this section depends on the scope and breadth of the analysis.

Discussion

In the final section of the report, the investigator interprets and discusses the results of the study. In the "Discussion" section, a skilled researcher makes the data come alive. The researcher gives the numbers in quantitative studies or the concepts in qualitative studies meaning and interpretation. The "Discussion" section will contain the discussion of the findings, the study's **limitations,** and **recommendations** for practice and future research. At times these topics are separated as stand-alone sections of the research report, or they may be integrated under the title of "Discussion." You may ask where the investigator extracted the meaning that is applied in this section. If the researcher does the job properly, you will find a return to the beginning of the study. The researcher returns to the earlier points in the study where a purpose, objective and research question and/or a hypothesis was identified and independent and dependent variables were related on the basis of a theoretical framework and literature review (see Chapter 3). It is in this section that the researcher discusses the following:

- Both the supported and nonsupported data
- The limitations or weaknesses (threats to internal or external validity) of a study in light of the design, the sample, instruments, or data-collection procedures
- How the theoretical framework was supported or not supported
- How the data may suggest additional or previously unrealized findings
- The strength and quality of the evidence provided by the study and its findings interpreted in relation to its applicability to practice and future research

Even if the data are supported, you should not believe it to be the final word. It is important to remember that statistical significance is not the endpoint of a researcher's thinking and low *p* values may not be indicative of research breakthroughs. It is important to think beyond statistical significance to clinical significance. This means that statistical significance in a research study does not always indicate that the results of a study are clinically significant. As the body of nursing research grows, so does the profession's ability to critically analyze beyond the test of significance and assess a research study's applicability to practice. Chapters 17 and 18 review methods used to analyze the usefulness and applicability of research findings. Within nursing and health care literature, discussion of clinical significance and evidence-based practice has become a focal point (Gold & Taylor, 2007; Titler, 2008). As indicated throughout this text, many important pieces in the research puzzle must fit together for a study to be evaluated as a well-done study. The evidence generated by the findings of a research study is appraised in order to validate current practice and/or support the need for a change in practice. Results of nonsupported hypotheses do not require the investigator to go on a fault-finding tour of each piece of the project—this can become an overdone process. All research has weakness. The final discussion is an attempt to identify the strengths as well as the weaknesses or bias of the study.

Therefore researchers and appraisers should accept statistical significance with prudence. Statistically significant findings are not the sole means of establishing the study's merit. Remember that accepting statistical significance solely means that one is accepting that the sample mean is the same as the population mean, which may not be true (see Chapter 10). Another method to assess if the findings from one study can be generalized is to calculate a **confidence interval.** A confidence interval quantifies the uncertainty of a statistic or the probable value range within which a population parameter is expected to lie (see Chapter 18). The process used to calculate a confidence interval is beyond the scope of this text, but references are provided for further explanation (Gardner & Altman, 1986; Gardner & Altman, 1989; Wright, 1997). Other aspects, such as the sample, instruments, and data-collection methods, must also be considered.

EVIDENCE-BASED PRACTICE TIP

As you reflect on the results of a study, think about how the results fit with previous research on the topic and the strength and quality of available evidence on which to base clinical practice decisions.

Whether the results are or are not statistically supported, in the "Discussion" section the researcher returns to the conceptual/theoretical framework and analyzes each step of the research process to accomplish a discussion of the following issues:

- Suggest what the possible or actual problems were in the study.
- Whether findings are supported or not supported, the researcher is obliged to review the study's processes.
- Was the theoretical thinking correct? (see Chapter 3)
- Was the chosen design correct? (see Chapters 8 and 9)
- Sampling methods (see Chapter 10): Was the sample size adequate? Were the inclusion and exclusion criteria delineated well?
- Did any bias arise during the conduct of the study, that is, threats to internal and external validity? (see Chapter 7)
- Was data collection consistent and did it exhibit fidelity? (see Chapter 12)
- Instruments: Were they sensitive to what was being testing? Were they reliable and valid? (see Chapters 12 and 13)
- Discuss the analysis choices (see Chapter 14).

Whether the results are or are not supported, the investigator attempts to go on a fact-finding tour rather than a fault-finding one. The purpose of the "Discussion" section, then, is not to show humility or one's technical competence but rather to enable you to judge the validity of the interpretations drawn from the data and the general worth of the study. It is in the "Discussion" section of the report that the researcher ties together all the loose ends of the study and returns to the beginning to assess if the findings support, extend, or counter the theoretical framework of the study. It is from this point that you can begin to think about clinical relevance, the need for replication, or the germination of an idea for further research. The researcher also includes generalizability and recommendations for future research, as well as a summary or a conclusion. For example, Bennett and colleagues (2007), in a randomized controlled trial (RCT) that tested motivational interviewing as a method to increase physical activity in long-term cancer patients, acknowledged one of the study's limitation as the physical activity counselor's lack of masking to group assignments, which presented the possibility of introducing components of the motivational intervention to not only the experimental group but also the control group.

Generalizations (**generalizability**) are inferences that the data are representative of similar phenomena in a population beyond the study's sample. Reviewers of research findings are cautioned not to generalize beyond the population on which a study is based. Rarely, if ever, can one study be a recommendation for action. Beware of research studies that may overgeneralize. Generalizations that draw conclusions and make inferences for a specific group within a particular situation and at a particular time are appropriate. An example of such a limitation is drawn from the study conducted by Horgas and associates (2008) (see Appendix C). The researchers appropriately noted the following:

> *"Several limitations of this study should be noted. First, we examined the role of race, measured by racial category, not ethnicity. Our convenience sample of modest size, recruited from churches and senior centers in one urban metropolitan area in the Midwest, limited to those able to participate in community-based activities, may have excluded housebound or more functionally impaired adults. The non-randomly selected sample was not fully representative of the older adult population. Finally, several variables might have been overlooked in this cross-sectional study."*

This type of statement is important for reviewers of research. It helps to guide thinking in terms of a study's clinical relevance and also suggests areas for further research. One study does not provide all of the answers, nor should it. In fact, the risk versus the benefit of the potential change in practice must be considered in terms of the strength and quality of the evidence. The greater the risk involved in making a change in practice, the stronger the evidence needs to be to justify the merit of implementing a practice change. The final steps of evaluation are critical links to the refinement of practice and the generation of future research. Evaluation of research, like evaluation of the nursing process, is not the last link in the chain but a connection between the strength of the evidence that may serve to improve nursing care and inform clinical decision-making and support an evidence-based practice.

HELPFUL HINT

It has been said that a good study is one that raises more questions than it answers. So you should not view an investigator's review of limitations, generalizations, and implications of the findings for practice as lack of research skills but as the beginning of the next step in the research process.

BOX 15-2 Examples of Research Recommendations and Practice Implications

RESEARCH RECOMMENDATIONS

- "The Deaf Heart Health Intervention (DHHI) was effective in increasing culturally deaf adults self-efficacy for targeted health behaviors related to modifiable CVD risk factors. A clinical trial of the DHHI will be necessary to evaluate the theoretical correlations between self-efficacy and targeted behaviors and the effectiveness of the DHHI in decreasing risk for CVD among culturally deaf communities" (Jones et al., 2007).
- "Researchers seeking to use information documented in the medical record as study data should consider a prospective research design that allows for review of the medical record and data collection while the patient is being cared for by the clinical team documenting on the patient status" (Gregory, 2008).
- "First this randomized trial adds to a very small but growing body of psychoeducational interventions to improve QOL in post-treatment survivorship. Differential aspects of QOL contributed to overall improvement in QOL, notably psychological and social interventions. Determining what proportion of education or emotional support contributed to improved outcomes is important in future cancer survivorship research" (Meneses et al., 2007).

PRACTICE IMPLICATIONS

- "From a clinical perspective, translation of research findings into practice can be accomplished in several venues—through established and new cancer survivorship clinics, in comprehensive breast health and breast cancer programs, and in individual practice. The study also demonstrates that oncology nurses with their strong background in education and support are well positioned to lead the translation of research findings into practice" (Meneses et al., 2007).
- "Findings from this study indicate that race, reflected by Black or White identification did not influence characteristics of pain in a general, non clinical population of older adults. Pain had negative consequences for daily functioning of this population. A finding more apparent in whites than Blacks" (Horgas et al., 2008).
- "Results of the current study provided information regarding variables prior to treatment that predicted higher fatigue 30 days after completing treatment. The finding assists with identifying those most in need of early and intensive teaching on strategies to manage fatigue" (Wielgus et al., 2009).

The final area that the investigator integrates into the "Discussion" section is the recommendations. The **recommendations** are the investigator's suggestions for the study's application to practice, theory, and further research. This requires the investigator to reflect on the following questions:

- "What contribution to clinical practice does this study make?"
- "What are the strength, quality, and consistency of the evidence provided by the findings?"
- "Does the evidence provided in the findings validate current practice or support the need for change in practice?"

Box 15-2 provides examples of recommendations for future research and implications for nursing practice. This evaluation places the study into the realm of what is known and what needs to be known before being used. Nursing knowledge and evidence-based practice have grown tremendously over the last century through the efforts of many nurse researchers and scholars.

APPRAISING THE EVIDENCE

Research Findings

The "Results" and the "Discussion of the Results" sections are the researcher's opportunity to examine the logic of the hypothesis(es) or research question(s) posed, the theoretical framework, the methods, and the analysis (see the following Critiquing Criteria box). This final section requires as much logic, conciseness, and specificity as employed in the preceding steps of the research process. You should be able to identify statements of the type of analysis that was used and whether the data statistically supported the hypothesis(es) or research question(s). These statements should be straightforward and not reflect bias (see Tables 15-2 and 15-3). Auxiliary data or serendipitous findings also may be presented. If such auxiliary findings are presented, they should be as dispassionately presented as were the hypothesis and research question data. The statistical test used also should be noted. The numerical value of the obtained data also should be presented (see Tables 15-1, 15-2, and 15-3). The presentation of the tests, the numerical values found, and the statements of support or nonsupport should be clear, concise, and systematically reported. For illustrative purposes that facilitate readability, the researchers should present extensive findings in tables. If the findings were not supported, the consumer should—as the researcher did—attempt to identify, without finding fault, possible methodological problems (e.g., sample too small to detect a treatment effect).

From a consumer perspective, the "Discussion" section at the end of a research report is very important for determining potential application to practice.

The "Discussion" section should interpret the study's data for future research and implications for practice, including its strength, quality, gaps, limitations, and conclusions of the study. Statements reflecting the underlying theory are necessary, whether or not the hypotheses were supported. Included in this discussion are the limitations for practice. This discussion should reflect each step of the research process and potential threats to internal validity or bias and external validity or generalizability.

Finally, a concise presentation of the study's generalizability and the implications of the findings for practice and research should be evident. The last presentation can help the research consumer begin to rethink clinical practice, provoke discussion in clinical settings (see Chapters 17 and 18), and find similar studies that may support or refute the phenomena being studied to more fully understand the problem.

One study alone does not lead to a practice change. Evidence-based practice requires the you to critically read and understand each study, that is, the quality of the study, the strength of the evidence generated by the findings and its consistency with other studies in the area, and the number of studies that were conducted in the area. This assessment along with the active use of clinical judgment and patient preference leads to evidence-based practice.

CRITIQUING CRITERIA: *Research Findings*

1. Are the results of each of the hypotheses presented?
2. Is the information regarding the results concisely and sequentially presented?
3. Are the tests that were used to analyze the data presented?
4. Are the results presented objectively?
5. If tables or figures are used, do they meet the following standards?
   a. They supplement and economize the text.
   b. They have precise titles and headings.
   c. They are not repetitious of the text.
6. Are the results interpreted in light of the hypotheses and theoretical framework and all of the other steps that preceded the results?
7. If the data are supported, does the investigator provide a discussion of how the theoretical framework was supported?
8. How does the investigator attempt to identify the study's weaknesses, that is, threats to internal and external validity, and strengths, as well as suggest possible solutions for the research area?
9. Does the researcher discuss the study's clinical relevance?
10. Are any generalizations made, and if so, are they within the scope of the findings or beyond the findings?
11. Are any recommendations for future research stated or implied?
12. What is the study's strength of evidence?

CRITICAL THINKING CHALLENGES

- Do you agree or disagree with the statement that "a good study is one that raises more questions than it answers"? Support your perspective with examples.
- As the number of resources such as the Cochrane Library, meta-analysis, systematic reviews, and evidence-based reports in journals grow, why is it necessary to be able to critically read and appraise the studies within the reports yourself? Justify your answer.
- Defend or refute the following statement: All results should be reported and interpreted whether or not they support the hypothesis." If all findings are not reported, would this affect the applicability to the patient population and practice setting?
- How does a clear understanding of a study's discussion of the findings and implications for practice help you to rethink your practice?

KEY POINTS

- The analysis of the findings is the final step of a research investigation. It is in this section that the consumer will find the results printed in a straightforward manner.
- All results should be reported whether or not they support the hypothesis. Tables and figures may be used to illustrate and condense data for presentation.
- Once the results are reported, the researcher interprets the results. In this presentation, usually titled "Discussion," the consumer should be able to identify the key topics being discussed. The key topics, which include an interpretation of the results, are the limitations, generalizations, implications, and recommendations for future research.

- The researcher draws together the theoretical framework and makes interpretations based on the findings and theory in the section on the interpretation of the results. Both statistically supported and unsupported results should be interpreted. If the results are not supported, the researcher should discuss the results, reflecting on the theory, as well as possible problems with the methods, procedures, design, and analysis.
- The researcher should present the limitations or weaknesses of the study. This presentation is important because it affects the study's generalizability. The generalizations or inferences about similar findings in other samples also are presented in light of the findings.
- The research consumer should be alert for sweeping claims or overgeneralizations that a researcher may state. An overextension of the data can alert the consumer to possible researcher bias.
- The recommendations provide the consumer with suggestions regarding the study's application to practice, theory, and future research. These recommendations furnish the critiquer with a final perspective from the researcher on the utility of the investigation.
- The strength, quality, and consistency of the evidence provided by the findings are related to the study's limitations, generalizability, and applicability to practice.

REFERENCES

Bennett JA, Lyons KS, Winters-Stone K, et al: Motivational interviewing to increase activity in long-term cancer survivors, *Nurs Res* 56:18-27, 2007.

Gardner MJ, Altman DG: Confidence intervals rather than p values: estimation rather than hypothesis testing, *Brit Med J Clin Res* 292:746-750, 1986.

Gardner MJ, Altman DG, eds: Statistics with confidence, *BMJ* 255:659, 1989.

Gold M, Taylor EF: Moving research into practice: lessons from the US Agency for Healthcare Research and Quality's IDSRN program, *Implementation Science* 2:9, 2007.

Gregory KE: Clinical predictors of necrotizing enterocolitis in premature infants, *Nurs Res* 57:260-270, 2008.

Horgas AL, Yoon S, Nichols AL, et al: The relationship between pain and functional disability in black and white older adults, *Res Nurs Health* 31(4):341-354, 2008.

Jones EG, Renger R, Kang Y: Self-efficacy for health related behaviors among deaf adults, *Res Nurs Health* 30:185-192, 2007.

Meneses KD, McNees P, Loerzel VW, et al: Transition from treatment to survivorship: Effects of a psychoeducational intervention on quality of life in breast cancer survivors, *Oncol Nurs Forum* 34(5):1007-1016, 2007.

Titler MG: The evidence for evidence-based practice implementation. In Hughes R, ed: *Patient safety and quality—an evidence-based handbook for nurses*, Rockville, MD, 2008, Agency for Healthcare Research and Quality.

Wielgus KK, Berger AM, Hertzog M: Predictors of fatigue 30 days after completing anthracycline plus taxane adjuvant chemotherapy for breast cancer, *Oncol Nurs Forum* 36:38-47, 2009.

Wright DB: *Understanding statistics: an introduction for the social sciences*, London, 1997, Sage.

FOR FURTHER STUDY

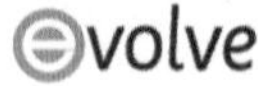

Go to Evolve at http://evolve.elsevier.com/LoBiondo/ for review questions, critiquing exercises, and additional research articles for practice in reviewing and critiquing.

16

Appraising Quantitative Research

Nancy E. Kline

LEARNING OUTCOMES

After reading this chapter, you should be able to do the following:

- Identify the purpose of the critical appraisal process.
- Describe the criteria for each step of the critical appraisal process.
- Describe the strengths and weaknesses of a research report.
- Assess the strength, quality, and consistency of evidence provided by a quantitative research report.
- Discuss applicability of the findings of a research report for evidence-based nursing practice.
- Conduct a critique of a research report.

STUDY RESOURCES

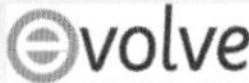

Go to Evolve at http://evolve.elsevier.com/LoBiondo/ for review questions, critiquing exercises, and additional research articles for practice in reviewing and critiquing.

Critical appraisal and interpretation of a published research report is an acquired skill that is important for nurses to master as they become consumers of the research literature. As we strive to make recommendations to change or support nursing practice, it is important for you to be able to assess the strengths and weaknesses of a research report to determine the strength, quality, and consistency of evidence provided by the design and findings of a research study.

Critical appraisal of a study is an evaluation of the strength and quality, as well as the weaknesses, of the study, not a "criticism" of the work, per se. It provides a structure for reviewing the sections of a research study. This chapter presents critiques of two quantitative studies, a randomized controlled trial (RCT) and a descriptive study, according to the critiquing criteria provided in Table 16-1. These studies provide Level II and Level IV evidence.

As reinforced throughout each chapter of this book, it is not only important to conduct and read research but to use research actively for evidence-based practice. As nurse researchers increase the depth (quality) and breadth (quantity) of studies, from RCTs to descriptive designs, the data to support evidence-informed decision making about applicability of clinical interventions that contribute to quality outcomes are more readily available. This chapter presents critiques of two studies, each of which tests research questions reflecting different quantitative designs. Criteria used to help you in judging the relative merit of a research study are found in previous chapters. An abbreviated set of critical appraisal questions presented in Table 16-1 summarize detailed criteria found at the end of each chapter and are used as a critical appraisal guide for the two sample research critiques in this chapter. These critiques are included to exemplify the critical appraisal process and the potential applicability of research findings to clinical practice, thereby enhancing the evidence base for nursing practice.

For clarification, you are encouraged to return to earlier chapters for the detailed presentation of each step of the research process, key terms, and the critiquing criteria associated with each step of the research process. The criteria and examples in this chapter apply to quantitative studies using experimental and nonexperimental designs that provided Levels II and IV evidence.

STYLISTIC CONSIDERATIONS

When you are reading research it is important to consider the type of journal in which the article is published. Some journals publish articles regarding the conduct, methodology, or results of research studies (e.g., *Nursing Research*). Other journals (e.g., *The Journal of Obstetric, Gynecologic, and Neonatal Research*) publish clinical, educational, and research articles. The author decides where to submit the manuscript based on the focus of the particular journal. Guidelines for publication, also known as "Information for Authors," are journal specific and provide information regarding style, citations, and formatting. Typically, research articles include the following:

- Abstract
- Introduction
- Background and significance
- Literature Review (sometimes includes theoretical framework)

- Methodology
- Results
- Discussion
- Conclusions

If the article is *scientifically rigorous* there is a decreased likelihood that the results occurred by chance alone, or due to extraneous conditions. Critical appraisal is the process of identifying the methodological flaws or omissions that may lead the reader to question the outcome(s) of the study or, conversely, to document the strengths and limitations and objectively judging that the work is sound and provides consistent, quality evidence that supports applicability to practice. Such judgments are the hallmark of promoting a sound evidence base for quality nursing practice.

TABLE 16-1 Summary of Major Content Sections of a Research Report and Related Critical Appraisal Guidelines

Section	Critical Appraisal Questions to Guide Evaluation
Background and Significance (see Chapters 2 and 3)	1. Is the background and significance of the research question or hypothesis appropriately presented in the introduction to the study report?
Research Question and Hypothesis (see Chapter 2)	1. What hypotheses or research questions are stated and are they appropriate to express a relationship between an independent and a dependent variable? 2. Has the research question or hypothesis been placed in the context of an appropriate theoretical framework? 3. Has the research question or hypothesis been substantiated by adequate experiential and scientific background material? 4. How have the purpose, aims, or goals of the study been substantiated? 5. Is each hypothesis or research question specific to one relationship so that each hypothesis or research question can be either supported or not supported? 6. Given the level of evidence suggested by the research question, hypothesis, and design, what is the potential applicability to practice?
Review of the Literature (see Chapter 3)	1. Does the search strategy include an appropriate and adequate number of databases and other resources to identify key published and unpublished research and theoretical resources? 2. Is there an appropriate theoretical/conceptual framework that guides development of the research study? 3. Are both primary source theoretical and research literature used? 4. What gaps or inconsistencies in knowledge or research does the literature uncover so that it builds on earlier studies? 5. Does the review include a summary/critique of each study that includes the strengths and weakness or limitations of the study? 6. Is the literature review presented in an organized format that flows logically? 7. Is there a synthesis summary that presents the overall strengths and weaknesses and arrives at a logical conclusion that generates hypotheses or research questions?

Continued

TABLE 16-1 Summary of Major Content Sections of a Research Report and Related Critical Appraisal Guidelines—cont'd

Section	Critical Appraisal Questions to Guide Evaluation
METHODS	
Internal and External Validity (see Chapter 7)	1. What are the controls for the threats to internal validity? Are they appropriate? 2. What are the controls for the threats to external validity? Are they appropriate? 3. What are the sources of bias and are they dealt with appropriately? 4. How do the threats to internal and external validity contribute to the strength and quality of evidence provided by the design and findings? 5. How was the fidelity of the study maintained?
Research Design (see Chapters 8 and 9)	1. What type of design is used in the study? 2. Is the rationale for the design appropriate? 3. Does the design used seem to flow from the proposed research question(s) or hypothesis(es), theoretical framework, and literature review? 4. What types of controls are provided by the design that increase or decrease bias?
Sampling (see Chapter 10)	1. What type of sampling strategy is used? Is it appropriate for the design? 2. How was the sample selected? Was the strategy used appropriate for the design? 3. Does the sample reflect the population as identified in the research question or hypothesis? 4. Is the sample size appropriate? How is it substantiated? 5. To what population may the findings be generalized? What are the limitations in generalizability?
Legal-Ethical Issues (see Chapter 11)	1. How have the rights of subjects been protected? 2. What indications are given that institutional review board (IRB) approval has been obtained? 3. What evidence is given that informed consent of the subjects has been ensured?
Data-Collection Methods and Procedures (see Chapter 12)	1. Physiological measurement: a. Is a rationale given for why a particular instrument or method was selected? If so, what is it? b. What provision is made for maintaining accuracy of the instrument and its use, if any? 2. Observation: a. Who did the observing? b. How were the observers trained and supervised to minimize bias? c. Was there an observation guide? d. Was interrater reliability calculated? e. Is there any reason to believe that the presence of observers affected the behavior of the subjects? 3. Interviews: a. Who were the interviewers? How were they trained and supervised to minimize bias? b. Is there any evidence of interview bias, and if so, what is it? How does it affect the strength and quality of evidence? 4. Questionnaires: a. What is the type and/or format of the questionnaires (e.g., Likert, open ended)? Are the operational definitions provided by the instruments consistent with the conceptual definition(s)? b. Is the format appropriate for use with this population? c. What type of bias is possible with this questionnaire format? 5. Available data and records: a. Are the records or data sets used appropriate for the research question(s) or hypothesis(es)? b. What sources of bias are possible with use of records or existing data sets?

TABLE 16-1 Summary of Major Content Sections of a Research Report and Related Critical Appraisal Guidelines—cont'd

Section	Critical Appraisal Questions to Guide Evaluation
Reliability and Validity (see Chapter 13)	1. Was an appropriate method used to test the reliability of the instrument(s)? 2. Was the reliability of the instrument(s) adequate? 3. Was the appropriate method(s) used to test the validity of the instrument(s)? 4. Have the strengths and weaknesses related to reliability and validity of each instrument been presented? 5. What kinds of threats to internal and external validity are presented as weaknesses in reliability and/ or validity? 6. How do the reliability and/or validity affect the strength and quality of evidence provided by the study findings?
Data Analysis (see Chapter 14)	1. Were the descriptive or inferential statistics appropriate to the level of measurement for each variable? 2. Are the inferential statistics appropriate for the type of design, hypothesis(es), or research question(s)? 3. If tables or figures are used, do they meet the following standards? a. They supplement and economize the text. b. They have precise titles and headings. c. They do not repeat the text. 4. Did testing of the hypothesis(es) or research question(s) clearly support or not support each hypothesis or research question?
Conclusions, Implications, and Recommendations (see Chapter 15)	1. Are the results of each hypothesis or research question presented objectively? 2. Is the information regarding the results concisely and sequentially presented? 3. If the data are supportive of the hypothesis or research question, does the investigator provide a discussion of how the theoretical framework was supported? 4. How does the investigator attempt to identify the study's weaknesses (e.g., threats to internal and external validity) and strengths and suggest possible research solutions in future studies in light of the limitations of this study? 5. Does the researcher discuss the study's relevance? 6. Are any generalizations made and, if so, are they made within the scope of the findings? 7. Are any recommendations for future research stated or implied?
Applicability to Nursing Practice (see Chapter 15)	1. What are the risks/benefits involved for patients if the findings are applied in practice? 2. What are the costs/benefits of applying the findings of the study? 3. Do the strengths of the study outweigh the weaknesses? 4. What is the strength, quality, and consistency of evidence provided by the study findings? 5. Are the study findings applicable in terms of feasibility? 6. Would it be possible to replicate this study in another clinical setting?

Critique of a Quantitative Research Study

The Research Study

The study "A Randomized Trial of Rocking-Chair Motion on the Effect of Postoperative Ileus Duration in Patients with Cancer Recovering from Abdominal Surgery," by Robert L. Massey, published in *Applied Nursing Research,* is critiqued. The article is presented in its entirety and followed by the critique on p. 361.

A Randomized Trial of Rocking-Chair Motion on the Effect of Postoperative Ileus Duration in Patients with Cancer Recovering from Abdominal Surgery

*Robert L. Massey, PhD, RN, NEA–BC**

Abstract

Patients who undergo abdominal surgery experience a phenomenon commonly called postoperative ileus (POI). Standard of care requires patients to get out of bed, sit in a chair, and begin ambulating the first postoperative day. No evidence supports standard care activities reduce POI duration. Rocking-chair motion has shown promise in reducing POI duration. Sixty-six participants were randomized into 2 groups. The experimental group ($n = 34$) received standard care plus the rocking-chair intervention; the control group ($n = 32$) received standard care. Participants in the experimental group had shorter duration of POI, no effect on medication use, and time to discharge.

1. INTRODUCTION

Postoperative ileus (POI) is a form of gastrointestinal dysfunction that commonly occurs after abdominal surgery and results in absent or delayed gastrointestinal motility. POI is hypothesized to be the body's sympathetic-induced response to overstimulation and stress imposed by large abdominal incisions, extensive manipulation of the bowel, and dissection of abdominal lesions (Holte & Kehlet, 2002; Le Blanc-Louvry, Costaglioli, Boulon, Leroi, & Ducrotte, 2002; Luckey, Livingston, & Tache, 2003, Miedema & Johnson, 2003; Schuster & Montie, 2002). POI presents as absent, abnormal, or disorganized motor function of the stomach, small bowel, and colon resulting in the accumulation of gas that cannot be dissipated causing abdominal distention, nausea, vomiting, and severe pain that can last for up to 7 days after surgery, complicating the full and timely recovery. Patients often describe the period immediately after surgery, prior to the resolution of POI, as the most uncomfortable part of their post abdominal surgery recovery experience. Both patients and clinicians eagerly anticipate the passage of flatus, commonly known as "surgeon's music," a sign that POI is resolving (Prasad & Matthews, 1999).

Recognized since 1899, minimal progress has been made toward the prevention and treatment of POI (Bayliss & Starling, 1899). Studies suggest there are multiple contributing causes of POI. Multiple factors have been reported to contribute to its onset and persistence

Division of Nursing, The University of Texas MD Anderson Cancer Center Houston, Texas
Received 2 November 2007; revised 27 May 2008; accepted 5 June 2008.
*Corresponding author. Tel.: +1 281 538 1949 (Home), +1 713 792 3704 (Work): fax: +1 713 794 4917. E-mail address: rlmassey@mdanderson.org.

and include activation of inflammatory mediators, secretion of gastrointestinal hormones, various forms of anesthesia during surgery, opiates given for pain control, previous abdominal surgery, surgery time, anesthesia time and American Society of Anesthesia (ASA) physical status classification have all been implicated. To date no specific interventions that prevent and successfully resolve POI have been discovered (Luckey et al., 2003; Miedema & Johnson, 2003). Physicians and nurses have had little to offer their patients other than reassurance that POI will resolve over time and bowel function will return (Matros et al., 2006).

One noninvasive postoperative standard-of-care intervention that is believed to resolve POI is having the patient get out of bed, sit in a chair, and walk beginning the first day after surgery, increasing the duration of each daily until passage of flatus or stool occurs (Waldhausen & Schirmer, 1990; Waldhausen, Shaffrey, Skenderis, Jones, & Schirmer, 1990). Evidence that these activities effectively treat POI remains unconvincing. However, there is consensus other positive benefits occur for the postoperative patient to thrombosis, and other negative physiological changes that occur with prolonged bed rest. A need exists for controlled studies of this and other interventions using randomized comparison treatment groups set into motion the design and conduct of this study.

A relatively new noninvasive clinical intervention that is believed to potentially reduce the duration and effects of POI is a rocking motion delivered using a rocking chair. The back and forth motion of rocking was previously found to reduce intestinal gas accumulation, abdominal distention, and pain associated with POI in abdominal surgery patients (Moore, Shannon, Richard, & Vacca, 1995; Thomas, Ptak, Giddings, Moore, & Opperman, 1990). Thomas et al. (1990) found that mothers who rocked after a cesarean birth used less pain medication, passed flatus earlier, and had a reduced length of hospital stay compared with those who did not rock in a rocking chair. Moore et al. (1995) reported similar findings among postoperative abdominal hysterectomy patients. Concomitant clinical observations and data analysis revealed that rocking in 10- to 20-minute increments for at least 60 minutes per day reported reduced gas pain scores, promoted earlier ambulation and expulsion of gas, and facilitated patient's discharge from the hospital earlier than patients in the nonrocking group.

1.1. Theoretical Basis for Intervention

A key physiologic factor in the development of POI is the body's response to the stress of surgery (Desborough, 2000). This surgical stress response is not limited to patients who undergo abdominal surgeries. Other surgical procedures such as hip replacement and thoracic surgeries also are implicated as stimuli for the surgical stress response and POI that is associated with abdominal dysfunction, dysmotility, and disorganization of neural stimuli that normally are responsible to coordinate propulsion within the gastrointestinal tract (Behm & Stollman, 2003). Although the exact physiological mechanisms that are influenced by rocking motions are not well known, theorists and researchers hypothesize that the gentle, rhythmic, repetitive motion of rocking stimulates the vestibular nerves to send signals of pleasure and alertness to the reticular activating system, which is the body's "flight or fight" response center (De Marco-Sinatra, 2004; Moore et al., 1995). The gentle rhythmic, repetitive motion of rocking is hypothesized to have a modulating effect on the stress response, thereby mediating the symptoms of POI, and is an important theoretical foundation for this study. No recent studies have further explained or tested the rocking intervention in both genders or in patients with cancer recovering from abdominal surgery.

1.2. Purpose

The purpose of this study was to test the effect of a nurse-derived intervention, rocking-chair motion on POI duration, total pain medication received, and time to discharge in patients with cancer recovering from abdominal surgery. This article reports the results of the effectiveness of the rocking-chair intervention in both genders of patients with cancer recovering from abdominal surgery.

1.3. Research Questions

Three research questions were evaluated. Does the rocking intervention reduce the mean time in days to passage of first flatus compared to standard care? Does the rocking intervention reduce the total mean pain Morphine Equivalent Dose (MED) medication in milligrams received compared to standard care? Does the rocking intervention reduce the mean time in days to hospital discharge compared to standard postoperative care compared to standard care?

2. METHODS

2.1. Design

This study was conducted between July 2005 and February 2007 at The University of Texas M. D. Anderson Cancer Center. A posttest-only randomized control trial design was chosen with measurement taken each day after abdominal surgery until passage of first flatus. A pretest randomized trial was not plausible owing to the subjects having to undergo surgery prior to measurement of the dependent variables: time to first flatus, postoperative pain medication received, and time to discharge. The study was approved by the institutional review board, and informed consent was obtained from each patient prior to enrollment.

2.2. Inclusion Criteria

Patients who were 21 years and older, scheduled to undergo abdominal surgery for gastrointestinal cancers, scheduled to receive postoperative patient-controlled epidural or intravenous analgesia, cognitively intact, able to read and speak English, able to tolerate rocking or sitting in a chair, and able to ambulate were eligible to participate in the study.

2.3. Setting and Sample

The study was conducted on a 32-bed surgical oncology unit composed of two separate 16-bed pods. Power calculation was based on the primary end point of time to first passage of flatus used by Disbrow, Bennett, and Owings (1993) in their study of the effects of specific instructions on POI duration, pain medication used, and time to discharge. Given the similarities in aims and research questions between the Disbrow et al. (1993) study and this study, SPSS Sample Power 2.0 (Borenstein, Rothstein, Cohen, Schoenfeld, & Berlin, 2000) software was used to perform the sample size calculations by setting the criterion for significance at .05, two-tailed tests (an effect in either direction was accepted), and power at 0.80. A total sample size of 54 participants was determined necessary to yield statistically significant results (27 in the intervention group and 27 in the control group).

2.4. Procedures

Patients scheduled to undergo abdominal surgery for gastrointestinal cancer were screened by the primary investigator during preoperative evaluation clinic visits. After completing written consent, eligible patients were randomly assigned to the intervention (rocking) or control (nonrocking) group. Study participants, nurses, and surgeons were blinded to group assignment until the first day after surgery. To reduce interaction bias, we placed intervention and control patients on separate 16-bed pods, and each pod could care for a control or intervention patient.

The control group received standard care that included walking and sitting up out of bed in a nonrocking chair beginning the first day after surgery. The experimental group received care that included walking and rocking in a rocking chair beginning the first day after surgery. The rocking intervention group had their nonrocking chair removed and replaced with a rocking chair upon arrival to the inpatient room. Only nonrocking chairs were available in the nonrocking group rooms. Intervention and control subjects were instructed to sit in the rocking and nonrocking chairs and begin to ambulate around the triangle-shaped pod beginning the first day after surgery and increase the frequency and duration of each activity each day. Nurses and surgeons were instructed and reminded of the activities for each group, and a sign was placed in the patient's chart as to group assignment. Time in rocking and nonrocking chairs and number of laps ambulated were recorded by participants, and the nurses on a datasheet for each 24-hour period.

2.5. Data Collection

The principal investigator collected all data. Demographic data and surgical characteristics collected included age, gender, ethnic group, marital status, and diagnosis, type of surgical procedure, anesthesia time, surgical time, and history of previous abdominal surgery. Each day the investigator met with each subject in each of the groups until passage of first flatus. Participants were provided a pen and pad and instructed to record the date and time they passed first flatus from the rectum after surgery.

This self-estimate assessment method was chosen because a previous study found high correlation between carbon dioxide levels expelled from the rectum and self-report of date and time of first flatus passage in abdominal surgery patients (Yukiokab, Bogod, & Rosen, 1987). Total opioid pain medication (milligrams) received was obtained every 24 hours from each patient's patient-controlled analgesia (PCA) or epidural infusion pump. Nonmorphine opioids (Fentanyl and Dilaudid) were converted to MEDs in milligrams. PCA intravenous opioids were Morphine Sulfate, Fentanyl, or Dilaudid. Epidural opioids were Fentanyl and Dilaudid. Date and time of the end of surgery were obtained from the operative record and used as a starting point for measurements of time to first flatus and time to discharge. Times of discharge were obtained from the institutional discharge system.

2.6. Data Analysis

Data were analyzed using SPSS 12.0 statistical software. Statistical analysis of demographic and clinical characteristics was summarized using descriptive statistics. The two intervention groups were compared with respect to various demographic and clinical characteristics using the appropriate statistical *t* tests for interval data and chi-square analyses for ordinal data. To examine group differences in the duration of POI (time to first passage of flatus), pain medication use (total doses in milligrams used per 24 hours), and postoperative patient recovery time (time to discharge), we used the two-sample *t* test if assumptions of normality (Levene's test) and homogeneity of variance on the dependent variable were upheld (Field, 2005). Descriptive statistics were used to summarize each outcome (time to first flatus, total pain medication used, and time to discharge). If assumptions underlying the two-sample t test were violated, appropriate nonparametric tests were run for the involved variables (Mann-Whitney *U*). A significance level of .05 was used.

TABLE 1 Demographics of Patients (N = 66)

Characteristics	Rocking, *n* (%)	Nonrocking, *n* (%)	*p*
Total patients	34 (51.5)	32 (48.5)	
	$\bar{X} \pm SD$	$\bar{X} \pm SD$	
Median age ± standard deviation	56.2 ± 10.1 years	54.8 ± 11.4 years	.600
Gender			
Male	14 (41.0)	19 (59.0)	.218
Female	20 (59.0)	13 (41.0)	
Ethnic group			
White non-Hispanic	26 (76.0)	27 (85.0)	.875
African American	2 (6.0)	1 (3.0)	
Hispanic	3 (9.0)	2 (6.0)	
Asian	3 (9.0)	2 (6.0)	
Marital status			
Single	5 (15.0)	3 (10.0)	.757
Married	27 (79.0)	25 (78.0)	
Divorced	1 (3.0)	2 (6.0)	
Widowed	1 (3.0)	2 (6.0)	
Diagnosis			
Colon cancer	20 (59.0)	22 (69.0)	.752
Liver cancer	4 (12.0)	4 (12.0)	
Sarcoma	5 (14.0)	3 (10.0)	
Gastric cancer	2 (6.0)	2 (6.0)	
Pancreatic cancer	3 (9.0)	1 (3.0)	

3. RESULTS

3.1. Sample

A total of 66 patients (n = 32 nonrocking and n = 34 rocking) completed the study. Attrition consisted of 2 rocking patients who could not continue rocking due to dizziness and returned to surgery due to internal bleeding. Both were included in the analysis based on intent-to-treat guidelines and the fact that both passed flatus after rocking during the 24 hours prior to removal from the study.

3.2. Subjects' characteristics

Demographic characteristics of the study participants are shown in Table 1. There were no significant differences between groups in age, gender, ethnicity, marital status, and diagnosis. Overall, male participants in this study were significantly older (mean age = 59.09, SD = 9.85) than female participants (mean age = 52.03, SD = 10.38; $t(64) = 2.832$, $p < .006$), but this demonstrated only a small effect size (d = 0.33).

3.3. Surgical Characteristics

Surgical attributes of the study participants are presented in Table 2. There were no significant differences between the study groups in surgical procedure types or ASA status categories. Participants in both arms of this study, overall, had high incidence of previous abdominal surgeries; however, there were no significant differences between the groups.

TABLE 2 Surgical Characteristics

Characteristic	Rocking, *n* (%)	Nonrocking, *n* (%)	*p*
Total patients	34 (51.5)	32 (48.5)	
Procedure			
Colectomy	13 (38.0)	10 (31.0)	.668
Liver resection	8 (24.0)	12 (38.0)	
Small bowel resection	1 (3.0)	1 (3.0)	
Exploratory laparotomy	12 (35.0)	9 (28.0)	
ASA status			
ASA 1	0 (0.0)	1 (3.0)	.533
ASA 2	19 (56.0)	17 (53.0)	
ASA 3	15 (44.0)	14 (41.0)	
ASA 4	0 (0.0)	1 (3.0)	
Previous abdominal surgery			
Yes	30 (88.0)	25 (78.0)	.333
No	4 (12.0)	7 (22.0)	

Note. ASA = Anesthesia Society of Anesthesia.

TABLE 3 Anesthesia and Surgery Time

Characteristic	Rocking ($n = 34$)	Nonrocking ($n = 32$)	*p*
Anesthesia time hours			
$M \pm SD$	4.77 ± 2.50	4.03 ± 2.13	.204
Surgery time hours	3.61 ± 2.35	3.01 ± 2.08	.280
$M \pm SD$	3.03	2.05	

TABLE 4 Times to First Flatus (Days)

	Rocking ($n = 34$)	Nonrocking ($n = 32$)	*p*
$M \pm SD$	3.16 ± 0.86	3.88 ± 0.80	.001*

Note. Significant $p < .05$.

3.4. Surgery and Anesthesia Duration

Durations of surgery and anesthesia in hours for each group are summarized in Table 3. The rocking group participants experienced slightly lengthier anesthesia times than nonrocking participants, and the difference was not significant ($t(64) = -1.284$, $p = .204$, $d = 0.15$). The rocking participants also experienced slightly lengthier surgical times than nonrocking participants. Again, this difference was not significant ($t(64) = -1.089$, $p = .280$, $d = 0.13$).

3.5. Time to First Flatus

The time-to-first-flatus data are presented in Table 4. The rocking group passed flatus an average 0.7 days (16.8 hours) earlier than the nonrocking group. The nonrocking group, on

TABLE 5 Total Pain Medication Received (mg)			
	Rocking ($n = 34$)	Nonrocking ($n = 32$)	p
$M \pm SD$	29.35 ± 58.99	36.48 ± 51.66	.604

TABLE 6 Surgical Characteristics			
Characteristics	Rocking ($n = 34$)	Nonrocking ($n = 32$)	p
$M \pm SD$	7.69 ± 4.57	7.89 ± 3.20	.837

average, experienced significantly longer time to passage of first flatus as compared with the rocking group ($t(64) = -3.542$, 95% confidence interval [CI] = 0.3174–1.1383, $p = .001$, $d = 0.40$). Therefore, a significant difference and effect size between means of the rocking and nonrocking group time to first flatus were identified.

3.6. Total Pain Medication Received

Data for both the rocking and nonrocking groups are presented in Table 5. Analysis of total pain medication received revealed nonnormality for both groups (nonrocking, $D(32) = .298$, $p < .001$; rocking $D(34) = .335$, $p < .001$). However, Levene's test for homogeneity was not violated (F (1, 64) = .243, $p = .624$), and therefore, the variances were assumed to be equal. The total pain medication received was, on average, greater for the nonrocking group as compared with the rocking group, and this difference was not statistically significant.

3.7. Time to Discharge

Time-to-discharge data are presented in Table 6. The time-to-discharge data with the outliers included indicated that the nonrocking group experienced essentially the same time in the hospital as compared with the rocking arm. Therefore, there was no significant difference between the means of the rocking and nonrocking groups in time to discharge from the hospital ($t(64) = .206$, $p = .837$, $d = 0.02$).

3.8. Time in Rocking/Nonrocking Chairs

Time (hours) spent in rocking and nonrocking chairs is presented in Table 7. There were no significant differences in time in chair for either group except for Day 3 when the nonrocking group spent more time in the chair ($t(64) = 2.108$, $p = .039$, CI = 0.0673–2.4996).

3.9. Laps Ambulated

Laps ambulated by the rocking and nonrocking groups are presented in Table 8. Number of laps ambulated around the triangular shaped pods were not significantly different for either the rocking or nonrocking participants.

4. DISCUSSION

4.1. Conclusions

The goal of this randomized trial was to explore the effects of rocking-chair motion on POI duration, total pain medications received, and time to discharge among patients with cancer recovering from abdominal surgery. There were no differences in age, marital status, and

TABLE 7 Laps Ambulated				
		RANDOMIZED ARM		
Time in Chair		***M***	***SD***	**Sig.**
Day 1	Nonrocking	1.13	±1.31	.307
	Rocking	1.57	±2.03	
Day 2	Nonrocking	2.28	±1.65	.567
	Rocking	2.55	±1.65	
Day 3	Nonrocking	3.25	±2.21	.039*
	Rocking	1.97	±2.23	
Day 4	Nonrocking	1.70	±2.52	.650
	Rocking	1.39	±3.02	
Day 5	Nonrocking	0.978	±2.50	.462
	Rocking	0.529	±2.41	

*Significant $p < .50$.

TABLE 8 Time in Chairs (Hours)				
		RANDOMIZED ARM		
Time in Chair		***M***	***SD***	**Sig.**
Lap Day 1	Nonrocking	4.60	±9.10	.802
	Rocking	5.01	±7.03	
Lap Day 2	Nonrocking	11.07	±19.88	.909
	Rocking	10.62	±12.07	
Lap Day 3	Nonrocking	13.93	±16.47	.759
	Rocking	15.95	±33.35	
Lap Day 4	Nonrocking	7.07	±10.92	.498
	Rocking	10.22	±23.85	
Lap Day 5	Nonrocking	3.80	±10.17	.527
	Rocking	2.14	±10.88	

ethnicity between the two groups. Surgical characteristic data revealed the rocking group experienced longer surgical and anesthesia times. However, the differences were not significant and demonstrate that these characteristics may not actually contribute to the prolonged POI duration. Both the groups had high percentages (rocking 88% and nonrocking 78%) having had previous abdominal surgery. However, this did not affect the duration of POI.

A significant difference between group means for time to first flatus provides support that the rocking-chair motion reduced the duration of POI in this group of study participants. The nonrocking group in this study, on average, used more pain medication than the rocking group. However, a lack of significance did not support rocking motion reduced pain medication use compared to previous research. Time-to-discharge data were nonsignificant and indicated the nonrocking and rocking groups experienced essentially an equal number of postoperative days in the hospital. Again, the data from this study were contrary to previous research reporting reduced time to discharge of at least 1 day.

Participants in both groups spent the same amount of time in the rocking and nonrocking chairs except on Day 3 for the nonrocking group. This can be explained due to the rocking group passing flatus an average of 0.7 days earlier than the nonrocking and were no longer participating in the study. Both groups also ambulated, on average, the same number of laps implying that both groups received similar interventions except for the rocking-chair motion in the rocking group. Therefore, this study contributes new evidence to support the use of rocking-chair motion as a modulator of POI duration in patients with cancer who have abdominal surgery.

4.2. Limitations

Limitations of this study include the small sample size, wide variation in diagnoses, surgical procedures, variation in types of pain medications used, and routes of administration. Therefore, the results of this study must be interpreted with caution.

4.3. Implications for Nursing

The standard of care that was challenged in this study has rarely been evaluated in a randomized clinical trial. This study does makes a contribution to evidence-based practice due to its statistically and clinically significant findings, as well as the limitations discussed herein may be used as guides for the design and conduct of future, more rigorous investigations. Generalization beyond this patient population is limited to patients with cancer recovering from abdominal surgery. Rocking in a rocking chair after surgery was readily accepted by the intervention group. A key factor identified is that the rocking motion had no effect on surgical incision site pain. Participants consistently voiced the rocking motion relaxed them, although relaxation was not measured.

4.4. Implications for Future Research

The results of this study indicate the feasibility of a nursing-derived intervention, rocking-chair motion, as a therapy to reduce duration of POI in patients with cancer recovering from abdominal surgery. Future research to further explore the use of rocking-chair motion on POI duration is warranted. Rocking-chair motion may provide abdominal surgery patients earlier relief from POI, the most difficult part of the postoperative recovery process, and improve short-term postoperative quality of life.

REFERENCES

Bayliss, W. M., & Starling, E. H. (1899). The movements and innervation of the small intestine. *Journal of Physiology, 24*, 99-100.

Behm, B., & Stollman, N. (2003). Postoperative ileus: etiologies and interventions. *Clinical Gastroenterology and Hepatology, 1*(2), 71-80.

Borenstein, M., Rothstein, H., Cohen, J., Schoenfeld, D., & Berlin, J. (2000). SamplePower® 2.0. Chicago, IL: SPSS, Inc.

Desborough, J. P. (2000). The stress response to trauma and surgery. *British Journal of Anesthesia, 85*, 109-117.

Disbrow, E. A., Bennett, H. L., & Owings, J. T. (1993). Effect of preoperative suggestion on postoperative gastrointestinal motility. *Western Journal of Medicine, 158*, 488-492.

De Marco-Sinatra, J. (2004). Relaxation training as a holistic nursing intervention. *Holistic Nursing Practice, 14*(3), 30-39.

Field, A. (2005). Discovering statistics using SPSS. (2nd Ed.). London: Sage Publications.

Holte, K., & Kehlet, H. (2002). Postoperative ileus: Progress towards effective management. *Drugs, 62*(18), 2603-2615.

Le Blanc-Louvry, I., Costaglioli, B., Boulon, C., Leroi, A. M., & Ducrotte, P. (2002). Does mechanical massage of the abdominal wall after colectomy reduce postoperative pain and shorten the duration of ileus? Results of a randomized study. *Journal of Gastrointestinal Surgery, 6*(1), 43-49.

Luckey, A., Livingston, E., & Tache (2003). Mechanisms and treatment of postoperative ileus. *Archives of Surgery, 138*, 206-214.

Matros, E., Rocha, F., Zinner, M., Wang, J., Ashley, S., & Breen, E., et al. (2006). Does gum chewing ameliorate postoperative ileus? Results of a prospective randomized trial. *Journal of the American College of Surgeons, 202*(5), 773-778.

Miedema, B. W., & Johnson, J. O. (2003). Methods for decreasing postoperative gut dysmotility. *Lancet Oncology, 4*(6), 365-372.

Moore, L., Shannon, M. L., Richard, P., & Vacca, G. R. (1995). Investigation of rocking as a postoperative intervention to promote gastrointestinal motility. *Gastrointestinal Nursing, 18*(3), 86-91.

Prasad, M., & Matthews, J. B. (1999). Deflating postoperative ileus. *Gastroenterology, 117*(2), 489-491.

Schuster, T. G., & Montie, J. E. (2002). Postoperative ileus after abdominal surgery. *Urology, 59*, 465-471.

Thomas, L., Ptak, H., Giddings, L. S., Moore, L., & Opperman, C. (1990). The effects of rocking, diet modifications, and antiflatulent medication of postcesarean section gas pain. *Journal of Perinatal & Neonatal Nursing, 4*(3), 12-24.

Waldhausen, J. H. T., & Schirmer, B. D. (1990). The effect of ambulation on recovery from postoperative ileus. *Annals of Surgery, 212*(6), 671-677.

Waldhausen, J. H. T., Shaffrey, M. E., Skenderis II, B. S., Jones, R. S., & Schirmer, B. D. (1990). Gastrointestinal myoelectric and clinical patterns of recovery after laparotomy. *Annals of Surgery, 211*(6), 777-785.

Yukiokab, H., Bogod, D. G., & Rosen, M. (1987). Recovery of bowel motility after surgery: Detection of time to first flatus from carbon dioxide concentration and patient estimate after nalbuphine and placebo. *British Journal of Anesthesiology, 59*, 581-584.

The Critique

This is a critical appraisal of the article, "A Randomized Trial of Rocking-Chair Motion on the Effect of Postoperative Ileus (POI) Duration in Patients with Cancer Recovering from Abdominal Surgery" (Massey, 2007) to determine its usefulness for nursing practice.

PROBLEM AND PURPOSE

The purpose of this study, "to test the effect of a nurse-derived intervention, rocking-chair motion on POI duration, medication received and time to discharge in patients with cancer recovering from abdominal surgery," is concise and clearly stated. The independent variable is the rocking-chair intervention and the dependent variables are POI duration, total pain medications, and time to discharge. The population under study is clearly defined, and the importance to nursing is evident as this is described as a "nurse-derived" intervention.

REVIEW OF THE LITERATURE

Significant physical discomfort is associated with POI, and this is well documented in the literature review. There is no prior convincing evidence that other interventions to minimize POI are useful. These measures have included the following:

- Getting the patient out of bed as soon as possible postoperatively
- Sitting in a chair
- Walking the first postoperative day
- Increasing the duration of ambulation until passage of flatus or stool occurs.

This intervention has been tested in prior abdominal surgery patients and a significant decrease in intestinal gas accumulation, abdominal distention, and pain was observed. The majority of the references in the literature review appear to be primary sources. The articles by Moore and colleagues (1995) and Thomas and colleagues (1990) are both RCTs and provide much of the rationale for the rocking-chair intervention. The identified gap in the literature is appropriately addressed by testing the intervention in patients with cancer recovering from abdominal surgery.

DEFINITIONS

The rocking-chair intervention and control group (standard care) are well defined in the "Procedures" section. The patient environment was manipulated so that nonrocking chairs were not available in rooms where patients were assigned to the intervention group so that every time the patient was up in a chair, it was a rocking chair. Passage of first flatus was recorded by the patient, and although the article does not specifically state this, it is implied that duration of POI is measured from the date and time of the end of surgery to passage of first flatus. Total opioid pain medications are operationally defined in milligrams and nonmorphine opioids were converted to milligrams and summed. Time to discharge was defined as the duration of time between the date and time of the end of surgery and hospital discharge.

RESEARCH QUESTIONS

Three research questions clearly guided this study:

1. Does the rocking intervention reduce the mean time in days to passage of first flatus compared to standard care?
2. Does the rocking intervention reduce the total mean pain Morphine Equivalent Dose (MED) medication in milligrams received compared to standard care?
3. Does the rocking intervention reduce the mean time in days to hospital discharge compared to standard postoperative care compared to standard care?

Research questions versus hypotheses are appropriate for this study because the relationships between the variables have not been previously tested.

SAMPLE

The convenience sample consisted of 66 patients with cancer who were undergoing abdominal surgery. Sample size was appropriately calculated using SPSS Sample Power 2.0, with significance set at .05 and using a two-tailed test and power of .80. A total sample of 54 subjects was determined to yield statistically significant results. Appropriately, the sample size was adjusted to account for dropouts. The final sample included 32 patients in the standard treatment group and 34 patients in the rocking intervention group. Participant attrition was minimal and included two patients who could not continue in the rocking group because of dizziness and internal bleeding, requiring return to the operating room. Although the sample was not randomly selected, there were no demographic differences between the intervention and control groups in terms of age (p = .600), gender (p = .218), ethnicity (p = .875), marital status (p = .757), and cancer diagnosis (p = .752), indicating that the groups were equivalent at baseline.

RESEARCH DESIGN

The three required elements of an RCT are present in this study, which provides Level II evidence. Participants were randomly assigned to a comparison group (standard treatment) or an intervention group (rocking-chair intervention), the control group consisted of standard treatment, and the investigator manipulated the independent variable (rocking intervention) to determine the effect on the dependent variables: POI duration, total pain medication, and time to discharge. The author draws the parallels between the physiological theory that the "gentle rhythmic repetitive motion of rocking is hypothesized to have a modulating effect on the stress response, thereby mediating the symptoms of POI," thus providing strong theoretical underpinning for this study.

THREATS TO INTERNAL VALIDITY

A strength of the study was that participants, surgeons, and nurses were blinded to the study group until the first day after surgery to reduce placebo effect and observer bias, and intervention and control patients were placed on separated 16-bed pods to reduce interaction bias. Potential subjects were screened by the investigator, and if they met inclusion criteria they were asked to participate. Selection bias may be an issue in studies that use convenience sampling. However, consenting participants were then randomized to the control or experimental group and the groups were equivalent at baseline in terms of important categorical variables, demonstrating homogeneity. Data were collected by patient report (time to passage of first flatus) and by the principal investigator. Total pain medications and time to discharge were obtained directly from the medical record and hospital discharge system so that no investigator bias was introduced.

THREATS TO EXTERNAL VALIDITY

The investigator minimized threats to external validity by maximizing control of extraneous variables. As mentioned previously, the groups were homogeneous, there was consistency in data collection with only one data collector and patient self-report at one time point, and there was manipulation of the independent variable. All of these factors minimize threats to external validity and maximize generalizability.

RESEARCH METHODOLOGY

Data collection was by patient self-report and review of medical records and hospital discharge data. Only one investigator collected data, eliminating the risk for inconsistent data collection between individuals. The patient recorded time to first passage of data at one time point, minimizing multiple measurements and variable reporting.

LEGAL-ETHICAL ISSUES

The study was reviewed and approved by the institutional review board, and informed consent was obtained from all participants before study initiation.

INSTRUMENTS

The patients were given a pen and paper and instructed to record the date and time they passed first flatus from time of surgery. The principal investigator collected all of the other data. Total medication dose was found in the patient medical record and determined by adding the total opioid pain medication in milligrams to the MED of the nonmorphine opioids. Time to discharge was determined from operating room (OR) data that indicated when the patient left the OR and then hospital discharge data that indicated when the patient went home. All data from medical records and OR and hospital databases were objective measures, not allowing for investigator bias.

DATA ANALYSIS

Gender, ethnic group, marital status, and surgical characteristics were appropriately summarized using descriptive statistics, which is the appropriate analysis of categorical variables. The mean age of patients was calculated and standard deviations were determined. The demographic variables were then compared with the use of *t* test (interval level data) and chi-square (ordinal level variables). Group differences in regard to time of passage of first flatus, total pain medications, and time to discharge were analyzed by the two-sample *t* test (*t* test for independent groups). Eight tables are used to visually display the data.

CONCLUSIONS, IMPLICATIONS, AND RECOMMENDATIONS

The author reported a significantly shorter duration of POI in the rocking-chair intervention group when compared with the standard care group (3.16 days + 0.86 days vs. 3.88 days + 0.80 days; $p = .001$). There was no significant effect on the total pain medication doses or on time to hospital discharge. The Level II RCT design, when including all required elements (e.g., randomization, intervention and control groups, and manipulation of the independent variable), is what allows the investigator to determine cause-and-effect relationships. Minimizing threats to internal validity, in this case blinding and separating patients to minimize interaction bias, strengthens the study. By ensuring a homogenous sample, maintaining consistency in data collection, manipulating the independent variable, and randomly assigning patients to groups, the threat to external validity is minimized.

Participants in both groups spent the same amount of time sitting in the designated chair except on day 3, when the non–rocking-chair group was up in the chair for a significantly longer period of time. This was not surprising, given that time to first flatus was shorter in the rocking-chair group. Time spent ambulating was not significantly different. The investigator concludes that this study "contributes new evidence to support the use of rocking-chair motion as a modulator of POI duration in patients with cancer who have abdominal surgery."

Limitations of the study, as clearly described by the investigator, included small sample size, variation in diagnoses, surgical procedures, variation in types of pain medications (opioid vs. nonopioid), and routes of administration. However, power analysis was done to justify sample size and the groups were homogeneous at baseline.

IMPLICATIONS FOR NURSING PRACTICE

This is a well-designed and well-conducted RCT that provides Level II evidence. The strengths in the study design, data-collection methods, and measures to minimize threats to internal and external validity make this strong Level II evidence that supports a nursing intervention to decrease the duration of POI. Potential risks include intolerance of the rocking motion and the potential for frail patients to exit the rocking chair safely, but the benefit of decreasing POI and the associated discomfort outweigh the risks, especially if the patient is assisted when standing. Cost may be an issue in certain institutions because of the need for purchasing rocking chairs, but in planning for replacement of existing patient furnishings, rocking chairs could be purchased instead of regular chairs for patients undergoing abdominal surgery. This study should be repeated with a larger sample, but certainly provides evidence that supports the use of this intervention to reduce duration of POI in cancer patients undergoing abdominal surgery.

Critique of a Quantitative Research Study

The Research Study

The study "The Relationships among Anxiety, Anger, and Blood Pressure in Children" by Carol C. Howell, Marti H. Rice, Myra Carmon, and Roxanne Pickett Hauber, published in *Applied Nursing Research* (2007), is critiqued. The article is presented in its entirety and followed by the critique on p. 375.

The Relationships Among Anxiety, Anger, and Blood Pressure in Children

Carol C. Howell, Marti H. Rice, Myra Carmon, Roxanne Pickett Hauber*

Abstract

Relationships between anger and anxiety have been examined in adults but less frequently in children. This investigation explored relationships among trait anxiety, trait anger, anger expression patterns, and blood pressure in children. The participants were 264 third- through sixth-grade children from five elementary schools who completed Jacob's Pediatric Anger and Anxiety Scale and Jacob's Pediatric Anger Expression Scale and had their blood pressure measured. Data were analyzed using descriptive and correlational statistics and hierarchical regression. Results have implications for the way in which anxiety and anger are perceived in children and the importance of teaching children to deal with emotions.

1. INTRODUCTION

Hypertension affects over 50 million Americans aged 6 and over and is a recognized risk factor for the development of cardiovascular disease (American Heart Association, 2004). Although few children have hypertension or cardiovascular disease, biological and psychosocial risk factors for the development of hypertension in adulthood are estimated to be present in children by the age of 8 (Solomon & Matthews, 1999). With the large number of individuals with hypertension and the progressive nature of cardiovascular disease, it is important to identify and modify risk factors early in life. Although some risk factors are not modifiable, others, such as anger and anxiety, are more amenable to change. The identification and modification of risk factors at an early age might reduce the incidence of hypertension in adulthood (Ewart & Kolodner 1994; Hauber, Rice, Howell, & Carmon, 1998; Meinginger, Liehr, Chan, Smith, & Mueller, 2004).

2. REVIEW OF THE LITERATURE

Trait anger (Johnson, 1989, 1990; Siegel, 1984), patterns of anger expression (Johnson, 1989; Muller, Grunbaum, & Labarthe, 2001; Seigel, 1984), and trait anxiety (Ewert & Kolodner, 1994; Johnson, 1989; Meinginger et al., 2004) are psychological factors that have been associated with high blood pressure in adolescents. Biological factors such as sex, height, and weight

---

Carol C. Howell, PhD, APRN-BC at Byrdine F. Lewis School of Nursing, Georgia State University, PO Box 4019, Atlanta, Georgia 30302-4019; Marti H. Rice, PhD, RN at School of Nursing, University of Alabama at Birmingham, Birmingham, Alabama 35294-1210; Myra Carmon, EdD, RN, CPNP at Byrdine F. Lewis School of Nursing, Georgia State University, PO Box 4019, Atlanta, Georgia 30302-4019; Roxanne Pickett Hauber, PhD, CNRN at Department of Nursing, University of Tampa, Tampa, FL 33615. *E-mail addresses:* chowell@gsu.edu (C.C. Howell), schauf@uab.edu (M.H. Rice), mcarmon@gsu.edu (M. Carmon), rhauber@ut.edu (R.P. Hauber).

*Corresponding author. Tel.: +1 404 651 3645 (home); +1 404 255 5453; fax: +1 404 255 1086.

have also been significantly associated with high blood pressure (Johnson, 1984, 1989; Meinginger et al., 2004; Muller et al., 2001). Although the contribution of these factors to the development of hypertension has been investigated in adults and adolescents (Ewart & Kolodner, 1994; Harburg, Gkeuberman, Russell, & Cooper, 1991; Meinginger et al., 2004), much less research has been done with children (Hauber et al., 1998). It is the intent of this study to investigate relationships among psychosocial factors, biological factors, and blood pressure in children.

2.1. Psychosocial Factors

2.1.1. Trait Anger. Trait anger is defined as an emotion that can vary from mild displeasure to rage and reflects amore permanent characteristic than state anger (Speilberger et al., 1985). Anger is thought to lead to an increase in blood pressure through its effect on the sympathetic nervous system (Meinginger et al., 2004; Muller et al., 2001; Taylor, Repetti, & Seeman, 1997; Williams & Williams, 1993). Repeated episodes of anger arousal may lead to a chronic state of elevated blood pressure or hypertension (Muller et al., 2001; Williams &Williams, 1993). Researchers have noted an association between anger scores and blood pressure (Hauber et al., 1998; Johnson, 1989, 1990; Siegel, 1984; Siegel & Leitch, 1981).

2.1.2. Anger Expression Patterns. Anger expression patterns include anger out, which implies that anger is openly expressed. Anger suppression or anger in implies that the anger is denied and held in. Anger reflection control involves a cognitive approach to resolving anger (Speilberger et al., 1985). Siegel (1984) found that subjects who had higher scores on the Frequent Anger Directed Outward factor also had higher systolic (SBP) and diastolic blood pressure (DBP). In contrast, Johnson (1984, 1989) found significant positive correlations between anger suppression and high blood pressures in male and female adolescents. In one of the few studies with children, Hauber et al. (1998), in a study of 230 third-grade children, found significant inverse relationships between anger suppression and DBP and anger reflection/control for both SBP and DBP. Muller et al. (2001) found that anger expression predicted blood pressure in 167 14-year-olds after controlling ethnicity, height, weight, percent body fat, and maturity. However, the instrument used in this study did not differentiate between anger in and anger out.

2.1.3. Trait Anxiety. Trait anxiety is defined as a subjective feeling of apprehension, tension, and worry, which is thought to be a relatively stable personality characteristic (Speilberger, Edwards, Lushene, Montuori, & Platzek, 1973). Jonas, Franks, and Ingram (1997) suggested that anxiety contributes to the development of hypertension in two ways. Anxiety has been shown to directly stimulate acute autonomic arousal (Russek, King, Russek, & Russek, 1990) and blood pressure reactivity (Krantz & Manuck, 1984; Suls & Wan, 1993; Waked & Jutai, 1990). Responding to stress- or anxiety-provoking experiences with anger has been shown to contribute to cardiovascular disease (Chang, Ford, Meoni, Wang & Klag, 2002; Wascher, 2002). The presence of anxiety has been associated with high-risk health behaviors such as smoking, drinking, low levels of physical activity, and noncompliance with prescribed medical treatments, which in turn have been associated with elevations in blood pressure (Jonas et al., 1997). In addition, Heker, Whalen, Jamner, and Delfino (2002) found that high-anxiety teenagers expressed higher levels of anger when compared with low-anxiety teenagers.

2.2. Biological Factors

2.2.1. Gender. Research with children and adolescents has shown a differential association between anger, anger expression, and blood pressure when gender is considered (Hauber et al., 1998; Johnson, 1984, 1989; Muller et al., 2001; Weinrich et al., 2000). In a study with third graders, Hauber et al. (1998) identified a positive correlation between anger reflection/control and SBP in female third graders. In male third graders, however, there was a positive correlation between anger reflection/control and DBP. Starner and Peters (2004) found a significant correlation between anger in and SBP and between anger out and SBP.

2.2.2. Height and Weight. Among the factors known to influence blood pressure in children are height and weight. Normative tables published by the National Heart, Lung, and Blood Institute (1996) (Task Force Report of High Blood Pressure in Children and Adolescents) list blood pressure standards based on height, weight, and sex in order to include body size to more accurately classify blood pressure norms. However, a more recent report no longer used weight as a factor for calculating normal blood pressure (National High Blood Pressure Education Program Working Group on High Blood Pressure in Children and Adolescents, 2004). However, the increasing occurrence of hypertension in children has been linked to the increase in weight (Couch & Daniels, 2005; Davis et al., 2005; Wyllie, 2005). Overall, the literature supports height and weight as factors that affect blood pressure (Couch & Daniels, 2005; Markovitz, Matthews, Wing, Kuller, & Meilahn, 1991, Muller et al., 2001; Muller, Wiechmann, Helms, Wulff, & Kolenda, 2000).

3. PURPOSE

The purpose of this study was to determine the relationships between trait anxiety, trait anger, height, weight, patterns of anger expression, and blood pressure in a group of elementary school children.

4. RESEARCH QUESTIONS

Specific research questions addressed were as follows:

1. What are the bivariate relationships between SBP and DBP and height, weight, and sex, trait anger and patterns of anger expression, and trait anxiety in elementary school children?
2. What is the contribution of height, weight, trait anger, anger expression patterns, and trait anxiety to SBP and DBP in elementary school boys and girls?

5. METHOD

5.1. Design

A descriptive correlational design was used in this study.

5.2. Sample and Setting

A convenience sample of 264 children was recruited from the third through the sixth grades in five public elementary schools serving kindergarten through sixth grade in a large metropolitan city in the southeastern United States. These schools served communities of varying socioeconomic levels in urban and suburban locations.

5.3. Instruments

5.3.1. Trait Anger. Trait anger was measured by the Trait Anger subscale of the Jacobs Pediatric Anger Scale (Jacobs & Blumer, 1984) (PANG Forms PPS-1 and PPS-2). The PANG is a 10-item self-report inventory developed for use with children. Reliability coefficients for the PANG range from .77 to .84 (Jacobs & Mehlhaff, 1994). A more recent study found the reliability to be .89 (M. Rice, personal communication, November 2004). Items included in the scale are in a Likert format with responses of 1, *hardly ever;* 2, *sometimes;* and 3, *often.* Scores on the PANG range from 10 to 30 and the higher the score, the greater the trait anger.

5.3.2. Anger Expression. The 15-item Jacobs Pediatric Anger Expression Scale (PAES) (Jacobs, Phelps, & Rohrs, 1989) was used to measure patterns of anger expression. The instrument contains three scales that have five items each and measure anger-out, anger suppression, and anger reflection/control. Each item is in the form of declarative statements with choices for responses of 1 for *hardly ever,* 2 for *sometimes,* and 3 for *often.* Possible scores for each scale range from 5 to 15. Alpha coefficients for the entire PAES ranged from .57 to .79 (Jacobs et al., 1989). Coefficients for anger out ranged from .66 to .78, for anger suppression from .57 to .76, and for the anger reflection/control scale from .36 to .62 (Jacobs & Mehlhaff, 1994). A more recent study found reliability measure of internal consistency for anger out to be .85, for anger suppression to be .76, and for anger reflection/control to be .70 (M. Rice, personal communication, November 2004).

5.3.3. Trait Anxiety. Measurement of trait anxiety was accomplished through use of the Jacob's Pediatric Anxiety Scale (PANX) (Jacobs & Blumer, 1984), a 10-item self-report inventory designed for use with young children. Item to total correlations range from .37 to .53 with an alpha reliability score of .78 for the total scale. A Likert format with three responses was used with a 1 for *hardly ever,* 2 for *sometimes,* and 3 for *often.* Scale scores are calculated by summing the responses on all items so that scores can range from 10 to 30. The higher the score the greater the anxiety. Alpha coefficients on the scale range from .77 to .84 (Jacobs & Mehlhaff, 1994). A more recent study found the reliability to be .80 (M. Rice, personal communication, November 2004).

5.3.4. Blood Pressure. The Hawksley's Random Zero sphygmomanometer (W. A. Braum Company Inc., Copiagne, NY), a conventional mercury sphygmomanometer with calibrations 0 to 300 mm Hg, was used to obtain blood pressure. This sphygmomanometer is designed to eliminate error variance due to operator and technique by using a shifting zero device. This allows random halting of the mercury between 0 and 20 mm Hg so that the operator cannot automatically assume a value. Mercury values must be subtracted from both systolic and diastolic readings to obtain correct blood pressure. The researchers for the study reported here were trained to use the Hawksley. Independent blood pressures on the same participant were taken until a 100% agreement rate was achieved in order to assure interrater reliability. The suggested protocol for measurement of children, including choice of correct cuff size and use of the first reading for nondiagnostic purposes, was followed (National Heart, Lung, and Blood Institute, 1996). Because blood pressure readings were not obtained for the purpose of diagnosing hypertension but for determining the relationships of blood pressure to anger and anxiety scores, only one blood pressure reading was obtained.

5.3.5. Height and Weight. Height and weight were measured by a balanced beam scale and the height rod of the balanced beam scale, respectively.

TABLE 1 Scale Scores						
	TOTAL		BOYS		GIRLS	
Variable	***M***	***SD***	***M***	***SD***	***M***	***SD***
Trait anxiety	18.66	4.16	18.13	4.23	19.0	4.11
Trait anger	17.87	4.84	18.72	4.74	17.34	4.84
Anger out	9.00	2.61	9.50	2.62	8.69	2.57
Anger suppression	9.28	2.27	9.30	2.23	9.29	2.31
Anger reflection	9.98	2.42	9.55	2.22	10.32	2.47
Systolic BP	102.58	10.96	104.66	11.03	101.16	10.75
Diastolic BP	63.28	9.83	64.30	8.72	62.55	10.50

5.4. Procedures

The human assurance committee of the university and the research committee of the county school district approved the proposal. A letter explaining the project and requesting consent for the child to participate was sent home to each child's legally designated caregiver 1 month prior to data collection at each school. On the day of data collection, children with returned completed forms were requested to sign assent forms. The assent form was read aloud to the children before they were requested to sign the form. After assent forms were signed by the children, the PANG, PAES, and PANX instruments were administered. All instruments were administered by the same investigator. Directions were read aloud, and then the children responded. Every child read and completed the scales independently. Special effort was taken to stress to the children that this was not a test and that there were no "right" or "wrong" answers. When the scales were completed, the children walked to an adjoining room where a blood pressure reading was obtained for each child.

6. RESULTS

6.1. Sample Characteristics

Of the 264 participants enrolled in the study who indicated gender and ethnicity, 107 were boys, 155 were girls; 189 were black, 58 were white, and 17 were other ethnicities.

6.2. Scale Scores

Table 1 shows scores on the study variables for the entire group and then separately for girls and boys. Boys had higher mean anger scores but lower mean anxiety scores than the girls. The girl participants had higher SBP and DBP readings, lower anger out, lower anger suppression, and higher anger reflection/control scores than the boys.

6.3. Research Question 1: Bivariate Correlations

Pearson's product-moment correlations were done in order to address Research Question 1. Table 2 shows correlation results for the children as a group and then separately for boys and girls. For the group as a whole, significant although weak correlations were found between anger reflection/control scores and DBP. Significant and moderately strong correlations were found between height and weight and both SBP and DBP. In addition, there was a significant inverse correlation between height and anger/reflection control scores. Moderate to strong correlations between height and weight and both SBP and DBP were noted for boys and

TABLE 2 Correlation Table for the Entire Group, Boys, and Girls

Variable	Trait Anger	Anger Out	Anger Suppression	Anger Reflection	Trait Anxiety	Height	Weight
SBP							
Entire group	−.02	−.04	−.04	−.08	−.07	.30***	.46***
Boys	−.04	−.03	−.14	−.13	−.02	.45***	.57***
Girls	−.00	−.06	−.04	−.20*	−.13	.27**	.45***
DBP							
Entire group	−.06	−.07	−.04	−.12*	−.04	.21**	.34***
Boys	−.19*	.08	−.07	−.07	−.04	.20	.27**
Girls	−.04	.07	−.10	−.19	−.05	.24**	.37***

* $p \leq .05$.
** $p \leq .01$.
*** $p \leq .001$.

girls. When correlation analyses were restricted to boys and then girls, different results were obtained. Significant although weak correlations were noted in the boys between DBP and trait anger. A moderate significant correlation was noted between weight and DBP, and a significant although weak correlation was noted between height and DBP in the boys. When girls were considered, a significant although weak negative correlation was found between DBP and anger reflection/control scores.

6.4. Research Question 2: Hierarchical Multiple Regression

In order to answer Research Question 2, six separate hierarchical regression analyses were performed. Two regressions were tested with the entire group, for SBP and DBP in turn, followed by two regressions restricted to sample boys and sample girls, again for SBP then DBP. The variables of height, weight, and sex were entered first as a block as these variables were correlated with blood pressure in this study. The next block included the variables of trait anger, anger out, anger reflection control, and anger suppression because links between blood pressure and anger have been widely documented. The anxiety variable was entered last. When SBP was the dependent variable, 24% of the variance was accounted for in the entire group. Only the first block contributed significantly ($p < .001$; $F = 22.58$). When DBP was the dependent variable, sex, height, and weight together accounted for 12.4% of the variance ($F = 10.21$; $p < .001$). Only the first block contributed significantly to the model.

6.4.1. Gender. In the next two multiple regression equations, the contribution of study variables to SBP and DBP was restricted to the boys in the study group. Thirty percent of the variance in SBP was accounted for by height and weight ($F = 18.05$; $p < .001$). Height and weight also accounted for 8% of the variance in DBP in the boys ($F = 3.90$; $p < .001$). In the last two multiple regression equations, the contribution of study variables to SBP and DBP was restricted to the girls in the study group. Here, the first block, sex, height, and weight, accounted for 18% of the variance in SBP ($F = 14.53$; $p < .001$). Neither the anger variables nor the anxiety variable that was added in the next block contributed significantly to the model. Height and weight accounted for 13% of the variance in DBP ($F = 10.09$; $p < .001$). Again, neither anger nor anxiety variables made significant contributions to the model.

7. DISCUSSION

In this study, support was found for the relationships of some of the identified psychosocial and biological factors and blood pressure in children. Children in the group as a whole who indicated more use of anger reflection/control had lower DBP readings. This is consistent with earlier research reporting an association between anger reflection/control and lower blood pressures in adults and children (Harburg, Blakelock, & Roeper, 1979; Harburg et al., 1991; Hauber et al., 1998; Muller et al., 2001).

There were no significant relationships between trait anxiety and blood pressure. Much of the research linking anxiety to blood pressure has been conducted with adult samples. Anxiety is thought to contribute to hypertension through repeated autonomic arousal (Jonas et al., 1997; Russek et al., 1990), blood pressure reactivity (Suls & Wan, 1993; Waked & Jutai, 1990), or through the association of anxiety and high-risk health behaviors. The findings in the current study are consistent with the work of Johnson (1989) who found that anxiety was not a predictor of blood pressure in a group of older adolescents. Perhaps the young participants in the current study, as well as Johnson's study, had not yet experienced the long-term negative effects of anxiety on blood pressure.

In this study, height and weight were significantly correlated with SBP and DBP for the entire group. In boys, height and weight were significantly correlated with SBP but not with DBP. In girls, height and weight were significantly correlated with both SBP and DBP. As noted earlier, this relationship is widely acknowledged. Blood pressure has been found to vary with the height, weight, sex, age, and fitness of an individual (Task Force Report of High Blood Pressure in Children and Adolescents, National Heart, Lung, & Blood Institute, 1996). Although weight is no longer used as a factor for calculating normal blood pressure (National High Blood Pressure Education Program Working Group on High Blood Pressure in Children and Adolescents, 2004), the results of this research strongly suggest a relationship.

A bivariate correlation between height and anger reflection control was found in this study. This implies that the taller the individual, the less anger reflection control is used. Perhaps taller children feel less inhibited about expressing their anger in more aggressive ways because their size protects them somewhat from reprisal.

Boys had significant correlations between trait anger scores and DBP. Similar findings have been reported between trait anger and higher blood pressure in both adolescents and adults (Markovitz et al., 1991; Siegel & Leitch, 1981). Girls in the present study showed negative correlations between both SBP and DBP and anger reflection/control. Similar findings were obtained in an earlier study with children (Hauber et al., 1998) where an inverse relationship was noted between anger reflection/control and SBP in girls. These findings suggest the importance of gender-specific research in the area of hypertension and cardiovascular disease. In her study of gender and gender-role identity and expression of anger, Thomas (1997) found that gender was an important factor in anger expression. She suggested that masculine sex-role identity was associated with being more anger prone, expressing anger in an outward manner, and being less likely to control anger expression. Female sex role types were less likely to express anger outwardly or to suppress anger and more likely to attempt anger control. Fabes and Eisenberg (1992) found that female preschoolers vented their anger less than their male counterparts. Fuchs and Thelen (1988) suggested that girls were socialized to hide their anger whereas boys were taught to hide their sadness or any other feeling such as anxiety that could be interpreted as a sign of weakness. Perhaps, even at this young age, anger reflection is a less acceptable choice for males and does not translate into lower blood pressure in male children in this sample. It may be that no particular expression pattern is associated with blood pressure with boys, although the characteristic of trait anger is related.

In the regression models, neither trait anxiety nor any of the other anger expression patterns accounted for any of the variance in blood pressure. Muller et al. (2001) also found that anger variables did not account for any of the variance in blood pressure in a group of 167 adolescents. In their longitudinal study with 541 normotensive middle-aged women, Raikkonen, Matthews, and Kuller (2001) found that baseline levels of anxiety and anger did not predict subsequent hypertension. However, in the 75 women who became hypertensive during this 9-year study, increases in anger and anxiety during follow-up significantly predicted the incidence of hypertension.

When separate analyses were done for boys and girls after controlling for height and weight, no additional variance in SBP or DBP was explained by trait anger, patterns of anger expression, or trait anxiety. These findings were similar to those of Johnson (1990), who identified no overall relationship between anger variables and SBP.

Although neither the anger variables nor anxiety contributed significantly to the regression model in this study, it should be recognized that factors considered in this study are thought to influence blood pressure in adulthood and are risk factors in children for the future development of hypertension. As children with these risk factors move into adulthood, they may develop hypertension due to repeated episodes of anger and anxiety, which continually stimulate the sympathetic-adrenal-medullary system. The end result is damage to cardiovascular health (Muller et al., 2001). It is important to know that these risk factors, if identified as early as childhood, can be modified before hypertension develops (Meinginger et al., 2004; Solomon & Matthews, 1999).

8. LIMITATIONS

Blood pressure readings and anger instruments were administered only once per subject. Multiple measurements could provide a pattern of blood pressure, and tracking participants for a longer period could aid in the identification of patterns across developmental periods.

9. IMPLICATIONS AND RECOMMENDATIONS

Because anger and anxiety are associated with hypertension in adults, a longitudinal study would help identify when anger and anxiety begin to contribute to the explanation of hypertension.

Current results indicate that anger reflection/control patterns are associated with lower levels of blood pressure in girls of this age. This finding is consistent with results of an earlier study with 230 third-grade boys and girls (Hauber et al., 1998) and suggests that children may benefit from anger management interventions aimed at anger control strategies. Identification of factors that influence a child's choice of anger expression patterns, the effect on blood pressure, and the contributions of gender would be helpful when designing intervention programs. The school nurse could be involved in identifying and recommending interventions for children who have frequent anger problems in the classroom or whose parents report frequent angry outbursts in the home environment.

Future research should investigate whether these findings remain consistent across younger age-groups, different socioeconomic groups, varying regions of the country, and more varied ethnic groups (Rice & Howell, 2006).

This study supports the belief that certain modifiable risk factors for hypertension are present at an early age. It has been recommended that BP should be monitored by the age of 3 for every child during every scheduled physical examination (National High Blood Pressure Education Program Working Group on High Blood Pressure in Children and Adolescents, 2004). It is important to monitor BP across a period of time to determine any elevations or pattern of BP (Cook, Gillman, Rosner, Taylor, & Hennekens, 2000). This type of assessment is most often performed by a nurse (Hauber et al., 1998). According to Moran, Panzarino, Darden, and Reigart (2003) although the rate of BP screening during well-child checkups has increased, it does not meet current recommendations. If the BP reading is normal (less than 90th percentile for sex, age, and height) it should be rechecked at the next scheduled physical exam and the nurse should encourage adequate sleep and an active lifestyle with healthy meals. A prehypertensive reading is the 90th percentile to less than the 95th percentile. This reading should be rechecked in 6 months. In this instance the nurse should counsel the parents and the child about active lifestyle and diet changes and weight reduction if the child is overweight (National High Blood Pressure Education Program Working Group on High Blood Pressure in Children and Adolescents, 2004). If hypertensive (95th–99th percentile with the addition of 5 mm Hg) the reading should be checked again on at least two occasions, usually within a few weeks to confirm the diagnosis of hypertension (National High Blood Pressure Education Program Working Group on High Blood Pressure in Children and Adolescents, 2004).

The nurse may also be the first health care professional to recognize unhealthy patterns of anger and anger expression. The nurse may be able to teach healthier means of expressing anger, such as anger reflection control, physical activity, or cognitive behavioral interventions (Rice & Howell, 2006). It is important to intervene in unhealthy lifestyles early rather than later when the disease becomes evident (Meinginger et al., 2004; Solomon & Matthews, 1999). Lifestyle changes are more easily accomplished at early ages before behavior patterns become ingrained. If risk factors for cardiovascular disease are reduced early enough, cardiovascular disease will be delayed or avoided altogether. Early anger management training for children holds promise for preventing the translation of anger into medical and behavioral problems.

Acknowledgment

This research was supported by grants from the College of Health Sciences, Georgia State University, Atlanta, Georgia.

REFERENCES

American Heart Association. (2004). Statistical supplement. Retrieved August 10, 2004, from http://www.americanheart.org.

Chang, P., Ford, D., Meoni, L., Wang, N., & Klag, M. (2002, Apr). Anger in young men and subsequent premature cardiovascular disease. *Archives of Internal Medicine*, *162*(8), 901-906.

Cook, N., Gillman, M., Rosner, B., Taylor, J., & Hennekens, C. (2000). Combining annual blood pressure measurements in childhood to improve prediction of young adult blood pressure. *Statistics in Medicine*, *19*(19), 2625-2640.

Couch, S., & Daniels, S. (2005). Diet and blood pressure in children. *Current Opinions in Pediatrics*, *17*(5), 642-647.

Davis, C., Flickinger, B., Moore, D., Bassali, R., Domel Baxter, S., & Yin, Z. (2005, Aug). Prevalence of cardiovascular risk factors in schoolchildren in a rural Georgia community. *American Journal of Medicine and Science*, *330*(2), 53-59.

Ewart, C., & Kolodner, K. (1994). Negative affect, gender and expressive style predict elevated ambulatory blood pressure in adolescents. *Journal of Personality and Social Psychology*, *66*(3), 596-605.

Fabes, R., & Eisenberg, N. (1992). Young children's coping with interpersonal anger. *Child Development*, *63*, 116-128.

Fuchs, D., & Thelen, M. (1988). Children's expected interpersonal consequences of communicating their affective state and reported likelihood of expression. *Childhood Development, 59*, 1314-1322.

Harburg, E., Blakelock, E., & Roeper, P. (1979). Resentful and reflective coping with arbitrary authority and blood pressure: Detroit. *Psychosomatic Medicine, 41*, 189-202.

Harburg, E., Gleiberman, L., Russell, M., & Cooper, M. (1991). Anger coping styles and blood pressure in black and white males: Buffalo, New York. *Psychosomatic Medicine, 41*, 189-202.

Hauber, R., Rice, M., Howell, C., & Carmon, M. (1998). Anger and blood pressure readings in children. *Psychosomatic Medicine, 11*(1), 2-11.

Heker, B., Whalen, C., Jamner, L., & Delfino, R. (2002, June). Anxiety, affect, and activity teenagers: Monitoring daily life with electronic diaries. *Journal of American Academy of Child and Adolescent Psychiatry, 41*(6), 660-670.

Jacobs, G., & Blumer, C. (1984). *The pediatric anger scale*. Vermillion: University of South Dakota, Department of Psychology.

Jacobs, G., & Mehlhaff, C. (1994). *Children's stress and the expression and experience and experience of anger.* Unpublished manuscript, University of South Dakota, Vermillion.

Jacobs, G., Phelps, M., & Rhors, B. (1989). Assessment of anger in children: The pediatric anger scale. *Personality and Individual Differences, 10*, 59-65.

Johnson, E. (1984). *Anger and anxiety as determinants of elevated blood pressure in adolescents: The Tampa study.* Unpublished doctoral dissertation, University of South Florida, Tampa.

Johnson, E. (1989). The role of the experience and expression of anger and anxiety in elevated blood pressure among black and white adolescents. *Journal of the National Medical Association, 81*(5), 573-584.

Johnson, E. (1990). Interrelationships between psychological factors, overweight, and blood pressure in adolescents. *Journal of Adolescent Healthcare, 11*, 310-318.

Jonas, B., Franks, P., & Ingram, D. (1997). Are symptoms of anxiety and depression risk factors for hypertension? *Archives of Family Medicine, 6*, 43-49.

Krantz, D., & Manuck, S. (1984). Acute psychophysiologic reactivity and risk of cardiovascular disease: A review and methodological critique. *Psychological Bulletin, 96*, 535-564.

Markovitz, J. H., Matthews, K., Wing, R. R., Kuller, L. H., & Meilahn, E. N. (1991). Psychological, biological and health behavior predictors of blood pressure changes in middle-aged women. *Journal of Hypertension, 9*, 399-406.

Meininger, J., Liehr, P., Chan, W., Smith, G., & Muller, W. (2004). Developmental, gender, and ethic group differences in moods and ambulatory blood pressure in adolescents. *Annals of Behavioral Medicine, 28*(1), 10-19.

Moran, C., Panzarino, V., Darden, P., & Reigart, J. (2003). Preventive services: Blood pressure checks at well child visits. *Clinical Pediatrics, 42*(7), 627-634.

Muller, W., Grunbaum, J., & Labarthe, D. (2001, Jul-Aug). Anger expression, body fat, and blood pressure in adolescents: Project HeartBeat. *American Journal of Human Biology, 13*(4), 531-538.

Muller, M., Wiechmann, M., Helms, C., Wulff, C., & Kolenda, K. (2000, May). Nutrient intake with low-fat diets in rehabilitation of patients with coronary heart disease. *Zeitschrift fur Kardiologie, 89*(5), 454-464.

National Heart, Lung, and Blood Institute. National Institutes of Health. (1996). *Update on the task force report on high blood pressure in children and adolescents: A working group report from the National High Blood Pressure Education Program* (SDHSS Publication No. NIH 96-3790). Washington, DC: U.S. Government Printing Office.

National High Blood Pressure Education Program Working Group on High Blood Pressure in Children and Adolescents. (2004). The fourth report on the diagnosis, evaluation, and treatment of high blood pressure in children and adolescents. *Pediatrics, 114*(2), 555-576.

Raikkonen, K., Matthews, K., & Kuller, L. (2001). Trajectory of psychological risk and incident of hypertension in middle-aged women. *Hypertension, 38*(4), 798-802.

Rice, M., & Howell, C. (2006). Differences in trait anger among children with varying levels of anger expression patterns. *Journal of Child and Adolescent Psychiatric Nursing, 19*(2), 51-61.

Russek, L., King, S., Russek, S., & Russek, H. (1990). The Harvard Mastery of Stress Study 35-year follow-up: Prognostic significance of patterns of psychophysiological arousal and adaptation. *Psychosomatic Medicine, 52*, 271-285.

Siegel, J. (1984). Anger and cardiovascular risk in adolescents. *Health Psychology, 3*, 293-313.

Siegel, J., & Leitch, C. (1981). Behavioral factors and blood pressure in adolescence: The Tacoma study. *American Journal of Epidemiology, 113*, 171-181.

Solomon, K., Matthews, K. (1999, March). *Paper presented at the American Psychosomatic Society Annual Meeting.* Vancouver, British Columbia, Canada.

Speilberger, C., Edwards, C., Lushene, R., Montuori, J., & Platzek, D. (1973). *State-trait anxiety inventory for children.* Palo Alto, CA: Consulting Psychologists Press.

Speilberger, C., Johnson, E., Russell, S., Crane, R., Jacobs, G., &Worden, T. (1985). The experience and expression of anger: Construction and validation of an anger expression scale. In M. Chesney, R. Rosenman, (Eds.), *Anger and hostility in cardiovascular and behavioral disorders* (pp. 5-30).Washington, DC: Hemisphere.

Starner, T., & Peters, R. (2004). Anger expression and blood pressure in adolescents. *Journal of School Nursing, 20*(6), 335-342.

Suls, J., & Wan, C. (1993). The relationship between trait hostility and cardiovascular reactivity: A quantitative review and analysis. *Psychophysiology, 30*, 615-626. http://www.nhlbi.nih.gov/meetings/ish/stamler.htm.

Taylor, S., Repetti, R., & Seeman, T. (1997). Health psychology: What is an unhealthy environment and how does it get under the skin? *Annual Review of Psychology, 48*, 411-447.

Thomas, S. (1997). Women's anger: Relationship of suppression to blood pressure. *Nursing Research, 46*(6), 324-330.

Waked, E., & Jutai, J. (1990). Baseline and reactivity measures of blood pressure and negative affect in borderline hypertension. *Physiological Behavior, 47*, 266-271.

Wascher, R. (2002, April). Stay at home dads and risk of cardiovascular disease. *Jewish World Review* 2002, April.

Weinrich, S., Weinrich, M., Hardin, S., Gleaton, J., Pesut, D., & Garrison, C. (2000). Effects of psychological distress on blood pressure in adolescents. *Holistic Nurse Practitioner, 5*(1), 57-65.

Williams, R., & Williams, V. (1993). *Anger kills.* New York: Harper Collins Publishers.

Wyllie, R. (2005). Obesity in childhood: An overview. *Current Opinions Pediatrics, 17*(5), 632-635.

The Critique

This critique examines a nonexperimental study that describes the relationships among anxiety, anger, and blood pressure in children (Howell et al., 2005). The objective is to critically appraise the research evidence and objectively determine applicability to nursing practice.

PROBLEM AND PURPOSE

In the introduction the authors appropriately cite information from the American Heart Association (2004) that states, "hypertension affects over 50 million Americans aged 6 and over and is a recognized risk factor for heart disease." The authors highlight the significance of this research focus by stating that although few children have hypertension or cardiovascular disease, the physical and psychosocial risk factors for development of hypertension in adulthood are present by age 8 years. It is logical for them to state that risk factors should be identified and modified early in life to decrease the incidence of hypertension in adults. The purpose of this study is clearly stated as follows: "to determine the relationship between trait anxiety, trait anger, height, weight, patterns of anger expression, and blood pressure in a group of elementary school children." The authors state that the results have implications for teaching children to deal with emotions.

REVIEW OF THE LITERATURE AND DEFINITIONS

The review of the literature clearly is divided into sections that represent psychosocial and biological factors that influence blood pressure in children. Psychosocial factors are specified to include trait anger, anger expression patterns, and trait anxiety. Biological factors appropriately include gender, height, and weight.

Trait anger is conceptually defined as "an emotion that can vary from mild displeasure to rage and reflects a more permanent characteristic than state anger." The review of the literature appropriately builds on previous research that has demonstrated a relationship between anger and hypertension. Anger expression patterns include "anger out" (the open expression of anger) and "anger in" (suppression of anger). Previous research also has demonstrated that subjects with high anger scores have higher systolic blood pressure (SBP) and diastolic blood pressure (DBP), and male and female adolescent subjects who suppress anger have higher DBP. *Trait anxiety* is conceptually defined as "a subjective feeling of apprehension, tension and worry, which is thought to be a relatively stable personality characteristic." Previous research has definitively shown that high-anxiety adolescents expressed higher levels of anger than low-anxiety adolescents.

There have been previous studies in children and adolescents that suggest associations "between anger, anger look and blood pressure when gender is considered." The increase in hypertension has also been linked to obesity in children.

The gaps in previous research are supported by the review of the literature. Although both of the independent variables (anxiety and anger) have been suggested to increase blood pressure (dependent variable) in children, this study will examine the relationships between trait anxiety, trait anger, patterns of anger expression, and the biological variables of height, weight, and blood pressure in elementary school children, which has not been done previously.

Operationalization of the variables is appropriately accomplished by the following measures: trait anger was measured by the Trait Anger subscale of the Jacobs Pediatric Anger Scale; anger expression was measured by the Jacobs Pediatric Anger Scale (PAES); trait anxiety was measured by the Jacobs Pediatric Anxiety Scale (PANX); blood pressure was measured by the Hawksley's Random Zero sphygmomanometer; and height and weight were measured by a calibrated balanced beam scale and corresponding height rod.

RESEARCH QUESTIONS

Two research questions that clearly express relationships between and among the variables guided this study: (1) "What are the bivariate relationships between SBP and DBP and height, weight, and sex, trait anger and patterns of anger expression, and trait anxiety in elementary school children?" and (2) "What is the contribution of height, weight, trait anger, anger expression patterns, and trait anxiety to SBP and DBP in elementary school boys and girls?" It would not be appropriate to use hypotheses to guide this study because of the exploratory, nonexperimental design.

SAMPLE

A convenience sample of 264 children (third through sixth grades), from five public schools in a large Southeastern city in the United States, were recruited. The authors state that these five schools served varying socioeconomic levels in suburban and urban areas, but no demographic data other than age, gender, and ethnicity were collected. One hundred seven were boys, 155 were girls, 189 were African American, 58 were white, and 17 were reported as "other" ethnicities. The sample size was not justified by power analysis, nor were inclusion and exclusion criteria defined. It is not clear if any students refused participation. Given the exploratory nature of the study, the sampling procedure is adequate but the results will need to be interpreted cautiously because of limited generalizability.

RESEARCH DESIGN

A descriptive, correlational design was used providing Level IV evidence. Data were collected at one time point (cross-sectional). This is a nonexperimental study because no randomization was done and there is no manipulation of the independent variables, nor is there a control group. The relationship of the variables can be explored, but no causality can be inferred. It is important to note that although this study provides a lower level of evidence than a randomized controlled trial, as long as the design is sound and appropriate for the research questions it may provide preliminary data to support future intervention studies. Since there is a gap in the literature, the findings of this study may provide the best available evidence.

THREATS TO INTERNAL VALIDITY

No threats from history, mortality (or attrition), or maturation affect this study. The greatest threat to internal validity is the study design and potential testing effects. Although the instruments are only administered one time, there are three individual instruments and the sample population is very young. It is impossible to know whether some of the children lost interest during the questioning process and just answered the questions to be "done." In addition, generally younger children want to please adults. There may be some social bias to answer the question in the way children perceive they "should" answer the question, versus the way they actually feel about the statement. The blood pressure readings were taken after the instruments were administered. It is also impossible to know how this might have affected the children's blood pressure measurements, although this measurement technique was consistent with all children.

THREATS TO EXTERNAL VALIDITY

There are no specific inclusion and exclusion criteria or power analysis and, because this is a convenience sample, potential bias may unknowingly be introduced, thereby limiting generalizability of the results. Although the authors mention that the schools from which the sample is recruited serve communities of varying socioeconomic levels, no demographic data are reported that describe the socioeconomic profile of the sample, another factor that limits the generalizability of the findings.

RESEARCH METHODS

All instruments were read aloud to each individual child by the same investigator. It was stressed that there were no "right" or "wrong" answers to the questions. Directions were read aloud first, and then the questions were read. The child responded aloud after each question.

It appears that data-collection methods were carried out consistently with each participant, although there was no mention of training or supervision of the data collectors to ensure systematic collection of data.

LEGAL-ETHICAL ISSUES

Both the human subjects committee of the university and the research committee of the county school district appropriately reviewed and approved the protocol. A letter was sent home to the child's legal caretaker 1 month before the data collection day. Children who returned the letter were eligible to participate. When the letter was returned the individual children were asked to sign assent, which was read aloud to them before they signed. After assent was obtained data collection proceeded.

INSTRUMENTS

The three instruments (PANG, PAES, and PANX) were read aloud by the investigator who recorded the responses. After the instruments were completed, the child went to a separate room where the child's blood pressure was taken. It is not clear from the procedures section where and when the child's weight and height were obtained. The authors do not address the possibility of social desirability bias when instruments are read aloud to subjects. This most likely was done to improve the child's understanding of the question as it was intended, but it is not addressed.

RELIABILITY AND VALIDITY

The PANG, PAES, and PANX have reported satisfactory reliability coefficients, but validity data are not reported for any of the three. Published reliability coefficients for the PANG range from .77 to .84, which suggests moderate reliability. The PAES has three subscales and a total alpha coefficient. The anger suppression subscale was reported as .57 to .76, the anger out subscale was reported as .66 to .78, the anger reflection/control scale as .36 to .62, and the total reliability score as .57 to .79. There is a more recent study cited by personal communication that shows the anger out subscale to be .85, anger suppression to be .76, and anger reflection/control to be .70. These more recent results suggest moderate reliability. The PANX has reported item to total correlations from .37 to .53 with a total reliability score of .78 to .80, again suggesting moderate reliability. The fact that validity data are not reported for any of the three instruments is a weakness and leads to questions about the accuracy with which the tools measure the variables.

DATA ANALYSIS

Scale scores reported study variables for the entire group and then separated for girls and boys (means and SD). Bivariate correlations were used to answer research question 1. Correlation analysis involves numerically assessing the strength of the relationship between two variables. Six separate hierarchical multiple regression analyses were performed to answer research question 2. Hierarchical regression is used to evaluate the relationship between a set of independent variables and a dependent variable while controlling for the impact of the independent variables on the dependent variable. Although not specifically stated, it appears that significance was set at .05. Two tables appropriately were used to visually display the data.

CONCLUSIONS, IMPLICATIONS, AND RECOMMENDATIONS

The results are discussed in terms of the relationships between some of the psychosocial and biological factors and blood pressure in children. In general, children who showed more use of anger reflection/control had lower DBP readings, a statistically significant but weak relationship. There were no significant relationships between trait anxiety and blood pressure. In terms of biological variables, height and weight showed significant correlation with blood pressure. In boys, height and weight were significantly correlated with SBP ($p < .001$), but not DBP. In girls, height and weight were significantly correlated with both (height $p < .001$; weight $p < .01$). Boys had significant correlations between trait anger and DBP ($p < .05$). Girls showed a negative correlation between anger reflection/control and SBP ($p < .05$). The regression models did not account for any of the variance in blood pressure in either group.

APPLICATION TO NURSING PRACTICE

This nonexperimental, correlational study provides data that may eventually lead to an intervention study. The findings support the association between weight and blood pressure, and suggest that anger reflection and control are associated with lower blood pressure values in girls this age. The strengths outweigh the weaknesses, although the results must be interpreted with caution because of limited generalizability. The risks are minimal, and there are no potential benefits to the individual subjects, but there may be a benefit to the greater society by the dissemination of findings in the literature and applicability to future studies.

This study should be replicated with larger and more diverse samples of young children. If the findings are replicated, gender-specific research that explores anger reflection/control interventions may be supported. The results also support previous studies that weight may be associated with increased blood pressure in children. Further longitudinal studies would be useful to confirm this. As nurses are often the first health care provider to measure weight and blood pressure, patient and family education should be provided if the child is overweight. If the blood pressure is elevated, it should be checked at routine intervals to determine if this is an ongoing finding or a spurious result limited to one clinic visit. If risk factors for hypertension are reduced in childhood, it may be possible to reduce the number of hypertensive older adults and possibly the incidence of cardiovascular disease.

CRITICAL THINKING CHALLENGES

- Discuss how the stylistic considerations of a journal impact on the researcher's ability to present the research findings of a quantitative report.
- Discuss how the limitations of a research study affect generalizability of the findings.
- Discuss how you differentiate the "critical appraisal" process from being "critical" about a research report.
- Analyze how threats to internal and external validity impact the strength and quality of evidence provided the findings of a research study.
- How would a staff nurse who has just critically appraised the study by Howell and colleagues decide if the findings of this study were applicable to practice?

REFERENCES

Howell CC, Rice MH, Carmon M, et al: The relationships among anxiety, anger, and blood pressure in children, *Appl Nurs Res* 20(2007):17-23, 2005.

Massey RL: A randomized trial of rocking-chair motion on the effect of postoperative ileus duration in patients with cancer recovering from abdominal surgery, *Appl Nurs Res (In press)*

FOR FURTHER STUDY

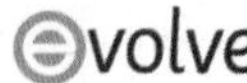

Go to Evolve at http://evolve.elsevier.com/LoBiondo/ for review questions, critiquing exercises, and additional research articles for practice in reviewing and critiquing.

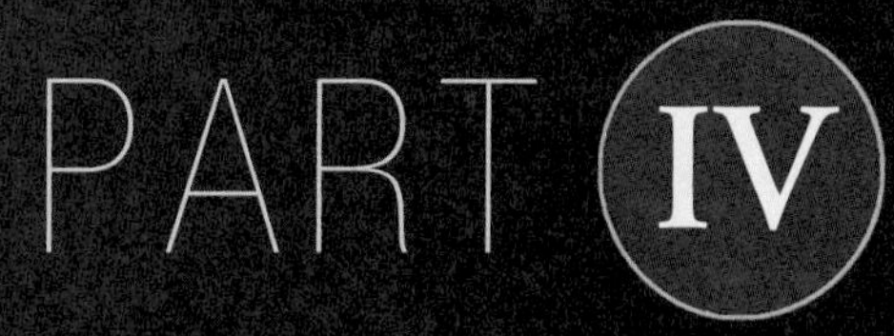

APPLICATION OF RESEARCH AND EVIDENCE-BASED PRACTICE

RESEARCH VIGNETTE

Program of Research on Substance Use Disorders

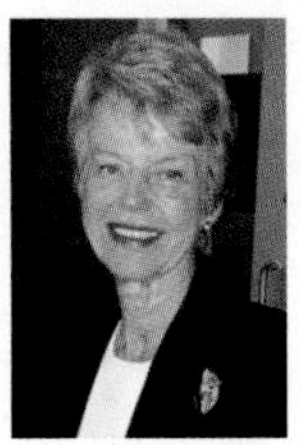

Marianne T. Marcus, EdD, RN, FAAN
John P. McGovern Professor of Addictions Nursing
University of Texas–Houston Health Science Center School of Nursing, Houston, Texas

My career trajectory illustrates the evolution of nursing education, practice, and research, as well as the impact of a chance encounter with a group in a drug treatment facility. Our school was asked to provide a voluntary primary care clinic in a long-term residential drug treatment program, a therapeutic community (TC). I was eager to have a site for students to learn physical assessment skills and primary care. That was the beginning of my focus on substance use disorders. I quickly realized that, although comfortable with my role as a clinician and educator, I knew little about addictive disorders. I questioned, "What causes addiction and how does it affect health?" "What is and how does a therapeutic community work?" And perhaps most important, "What do nurses know about substance use disorders and how do they learn it?" During this time I was completing my dissertation, a study of nurses' work in a surgical intensive care unit. I observed nurses as they worked and interviewed them. I found myself intrigued by their accounts of patients who were in the unit because of encounters with "the Clydesdales" or the "Marlboro Man," references to beer and tobacco commercials of that time period. When I asked the nurses how they had learned about alcohol and drug abuse they indicated that it was through "on-the-job training." One prevailing theme was that these patients had "done it to themselves" and would very likely "go out and do it again." I was troubled by this fatalistic attitude and my own lack of knowledge. I resolved to focus my teaching and research on substance abuse disorders.

I first explored ways to develop the necessary skills for teaching the conduct of research. This coincided with a federal initiative to increase health professional competence in meeting the challenge of substance use and abuse. Beginning in 1990 we obtained three successive faculty development grants from the Substance Abuse Mental Health Services Administration (SAMHSA), Center for Substance Abuse Prevention. Nursing and other health professions faculty acquired knowledge and skills to enhance the curriculum and begin research in substance use disorders (Marcus, 1997, 2000). We also received funding to create an addiction focus graduate program, which would develop nurse scholars in the field (Marcus & Stafford, 2002).

My experience led to my participation in Project MAINSTREAM, an initiative to prepare interdisciplinary health professional faculty to include substance abuse content in their discipline's curricula. This SAMHSA/HRSA-funded project offered opportunities to engage in educational methods research. We investigated mentoring, service-learning, interdisciplinary collaboration, and strategies to increase faculty and student competencies (Brown & Marcus, 2005; Brown, Marcus, Straussner, et al., 2006; Marcus & Brown, 2005; Marcus, Brown, Straussner, et al., 2005).

At the same time, I was pursuing my research related to TCs. I began conducting a qualitative study, using grounded theory to explore the lived experience of recovery in a therapeutic community. Residents of therapeutic communities for recovery from substance abuse participated in interviews. Therapeutic communities provide a highly structured hierarchical environment in which the community itself is the key agent for behavior change. Study participants likened the TC experience to making a career change, an arduous process that takes determination, commitment, readiness, and time. They indicated that the experience is one of translation rather than transformation, a redirection of skills to more constructive activities. The theory that emerged from this study defines the progressive steps, or stages, of recovery in TC treatment and the properties common to each stage (Marcus, 1998).

For individuals whose lives were characterized by impulsivity and lack of self-control, the rigor of a TC is restrictive and inherently stressful and the dropout rate is high. Recognizing that successful outcomes are correlated with time in treatment led me to hypothesize that stress-reduction strategies might enhance progression and retention. Mindfulness-based stress reduction (MBSR) is a meditation program to help individuals bring nonreactive, nonjudgmental attention to their present moment experiences. MBSR is congruent with the goals of the TC to encourage self-regulation, awareness insight, problem solving, and sense of well-being. Next, two feasibility studies of MBSR in the TC were conducted. The first was a quasi-experimental study, where subjects received the intervention in one facility and another group received treatment as usual in a second facility. The study investigated MBSR's effectiveness in reducing psychological problems and symptoms of psychopathology, and increasing positive coping styles (Marcus, Fine, & Kouzekanani, 2001). The second study, a pretest and post test design of MBSR in a TC, focused on physiological and psychological measures of stress. There was a decrease in self-reported stress between baseline and postmeasurement, but the change was not statistically significant. However, awakening salivary cortisol measurements were significantly lower after the intervention, suggesting the possible influence of MBSR on physiological stress (Marcus, Fine, Moeller, et al., 2003).

These findings positioned us for a larger study, a behavioral therapies trial of MBSR as an adjunct to the TC. Behavior change, in this case from harmful substance use to sobriety, is important to the prevention and treatment of many conditions caused by deleterious lifestyles. The model for behavior therapy development permits the researcher to achieve rigor for therapies commensurate with that of a pharmacological trial of a promising medication. We are currently conducting a Stage I trial of MBSR. The process includes developing a manual of MBSR adapted for TC, training the MBSR teachers, monitoring treatment integrity, and conducting a pilot study. The study's aims are to describe the stress response to TC treatment and its effect on various dimensions of behavior change associated with recovery in this setting. The Stage I trial lays the groundwork for future research. For example, if this study finds that MBSR is effective, we will be ready for a Stage II trial, a large-scale trial efficacy trial in multiple sites. A Stage III trial might investigate the effectiveness of training TC staff to include MBSR as a regular part of the curriculum. This model is useful to study therapies of potential interest to nurse researchers (Marcus, Liehr, Schmitz, et al., 2007).

As I learn more about substance use disorders, I realize there is an important role for nurses in prevention. My prevention approach is through the challenging and rewarding process of community-based participatory research (CBPR), a method that involves community stakeholders in all aspects of a study with the ultimate goal of building capacity to improve the community's health. Another chance encounter, with a youth minister who was attending a seminar where I presented on substance use, led to a fruitful collaboration. The minister and

I responded to a call for studies of human immunodeficiency virus/acquired immunodeficiency syndrome (HIV/AIDS) and substance abuse prevention in minorities. We were funded to design and implement an intervention to prevent these problems for African-American adolescents in a faith-based setting (Marcus, Walker, Swint, et al., 2004). We continue to work together to find answers to prevent substance use in vulnerable populations.

Substance use and abuse continue to compromise health in our nation. We still have much to learn about this complex problem, and nursing research can contribute a great deal to finding answers. I enjoy the daily challenge of research and I am pleased that I took this unexpected turn. My research came about because of a need to respond to a major public health problem. I have focused on the best ways to educate health professionals to meet this challenge and the development of prevention and treatment interventions.

REFERENCES

Brown RL, Marcus MT: Bearing witness: the political agenda of community-based service learning, *Substance Abuse* 26(3-4):3-4, 2005.

Brown RL, Marcus MT, Straussner SLA, et al: Project MAINSTREAM's first fellowship cohort: pilot test of a national dissemination model to enhance substance abuse curriculum at health professions schools, *Health Educ J* 65:252-266, 2006.

Marcus MT: Faculty development and curricular change: a process and outcomes model for substance abuse education, *J Prof Nurs* 13(3):168-177, 1997.

Marcus MT: Changing careers: becoming clean and sober in a therapeutic community, *Qual Health Res* 8(4):466-480, 1998. Abstracted and reviewed in *Evidence-Based Nursing* 2(1):28, 1999.

Marcus MT: An interdisciplinary team model for substance abuse prevention in communities, *J Prof Nurs* 16(3):158-168, 2000.

Marcus, MT, Brown RL: Bringing basic substance use prevention services to mainstream healthcare, *J Addictions Nurs* 16(3):93-95, 2005.

Marcus MT, Brown RL, Straussner SLA, et al: Creating change agents: a national substance abuse education project, *Substance Abuse* 26(3-4):5-15, 2005.

Marcus MT, Fine J, Kouzekanani K: Mindfulness-based meditation in a therapeutic community, *J Substance Use* 5 (5):305-311, 2001.

Marcus MT, Fine M, Moeller FG, et al: Change in stress levels following mindfulness-based stress reduction in a therapeutic community, *Addictive Disorders and Their Treatment* 2(3):63-68, 2003.

Marcus MT, Liehr P, Schmitz J, et al: Behavioral therapies trials: a case example, *Nurs Res* 56(3):210-216, 2007.

Marcus MT, Stafford L: A model for preparing nurses for the challenge of substance use disorders, *Drug and Alcohol Professional* 2(3):23-30, 2002.

Marcus MT, Walker T, Swint JM, et al: Community-based participatory research to prevent substance abuse and HIV/AIDS in African American adolescents, *J Interprofessional Care* 18(4):347-359, 2004.

17

Developing an Evidence-Based Practice

Marita Titler and Susan Adams

KEY TERMS

conduct of research
dissemination
evaluation
evidence-based practice
evidence-based practice guidelines
knowledge-focused triggers
opinion leaders
problem-focused triggers
research utilization
tailored interventions
translation science

LEARNING OUTCOMES

After reading this chapter, you should be able to do the following:

- Differentiate among conduct of nursing research, research utilization, and evidence-based practice.
- Describe the steps of evidence-based practice.
- Identify three barriers to evidence-based practice and strategies to address each.
- List three sources for finding evidence.
- Describe strategies for implementing evidence-based practice changes.
- Identify steps for evaluating an evidence-based change in practice.
- Use research findings and other forms of evidence to improve the quality of care.

STUDY RESOURCES

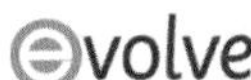

Go to Evolve at http://evolve.elsevier.com/LoBiondo/ for review questions, critiquing exercises, and additional research articles for practice in reviewing and critiquing.

The authors would like to acknowledge Kim Jordan for her superb assistance in preparing this manuscript for publication.

Evidence-based health care practices are available for a number of conditions such as asthma, smoking cessation, heart failure, management of diabetes, and others. However, these practices are not always implemented in care delivery, and variation in practices abound (Centers for Medicare and Medicaid Services [CMS], 2008; Institute of Medicine, 2001; McGlynn et al., 2003; Ward et al., 2006). Availability of high-quality research does not ensure that the findings will be used to affect patient outcomes (Institute of Medicine, 2001; McGlynn et al., 2003). Recent findings in the United States and Netherlands suggest that 30% to 40% of patients are not receiving evidence-based care, and 20% to 25% of patients are receiving unneeded or potentially harmful care (Graham et al., 2006). The use of evidence-based practices is now an expected standard as demonstrated by recent regulations from the Centers for Medicare and Medicaid Services (CMS) regarding not paying for nosocomial events such as injury from falls, Foley catheter–associated urinary tract infections, and stage 3 and 4 pressure ulcers. These practices all have a strong evidence base and when enacted, can prevent these nosocomial events. However, implementing such evidence-based safety practices is a challenge and requires use of strategies that address the complexity and systems of care, individual practitioners, senior leadership, and ultimately changing health care cultures to be evidence-based practice environments (Leape, 2005).

Conduct of research is only the first step in improving practice through the use of research (Titler & Everett, 2001). Because of the gap between discovery and use of knowledge in practice (Bootsmiller et al., 2004; Davey et al., 2005; Dopson, FitzGerald, Ferlie, et al., 2002; Titler, 2008), concentrated efforts must focus on methods to speed translation of research findings into practice. Development and dissemination of evidence-based practice guidelines are essential steps, but alone, do little to promote knowledge uptake by direct care providers (Clancy, Slutsky, & Patton, 2004a; Dopson et al., 2002; Farquhar, Stryer, & Slutsky, 2002; Institute of Medicine, 2001; Lavis et al., 2003; McGlynn et al., 2003).

Promoting use of evidence in practice is an active process that is facilitated, in part, by modeling and imitation of others who have successfully adopted the innovation, an organizational culture that values and supports use of evidence, and localization of the evidence for use in a specific health care setting (Berwick, 2003; Gillbody et al., 2003; Greenhalgh et al., 2005; Rogers, 2003a).

Translation of research into practice (TRIP) is a multifaceted, systemic process of promoting adoption of evidence-based practices in delivery of health care services that goes beyond dissemination of evidence-based guidelines (Berwick, 2003; Farquhar et al., 2002; Rogers, 2003a; Silagy, 2001; Titler & Everett, 2001). **Dissemination** activities take many forms, including publications, conferences, consultations, and training programs (Adams & Titler, in press), but promoting knowledge uptake and changing practitioner behavior requires active interchange with those in direct care (Scott et al., 2008; Titler, Herr, Brooks, et al., 2008). Although the science of translation is young, the effectiveness of interventions for promoting adoption of evidence-based practices is being studied, and federal funding is supporting research in this area (www.ahrq.gov; www.nih.gov) (Bootsmiller et al., 2004; Demakis et al., 2000; Farquhar et al., 2002; Smith et al., 2008; Stetler et al., 2008). Additionally, more evidence is available to guide selection of strategies for translating research into practice than was available several years ago (Brooks et al., 2008; Davey et al., 2005; Doebbeling et al., 2002; Feldman et al., 2005; Gravel, Légaré, & Graham, 2006; Greenhalgh et al., 2005; Katz, Muehlenbruch, Brown, et al., 2002; Murtaugh et al., 2005; Titler, 2008; Titler & Everett, 2001; Wensing, Wollersheim, & Grol, 2006). This chapter presents an overview of evidence-based practice, the process of implementing evidence in practice to improve patient outcomes, and a description of translation science.

OVERVIEW OF EVIDENCE-BASED PRACTICE

The relationships among conduct, dissemination, and use of research are illustrated in Figure 17-1. **Conduct of research** is the analysis of data collected from a homogeneous group of subjects who meet study inclusion and exclusion criteria for the purpose of answering specific research questions or testing specified hypotheses. Research design, methods, and statistical analyses are guided by the state-of-the-science in the area of investigation. Traditionally, conduct of research has included dissemination of findings via research reports in journals and at scientific conferences. In comparison, **research utilization** is the process of using research findings to improve patient care. It encompasses dissemination of scientific knowledge; critique of studies; synthesis of research findings; determining applicability of findings for practice; developing an evidence-based standard or guideline; implementing the standard; and evaluating the practice change with respect to staff, patients, and cost/resource utilization (Titler, Kleiber, Steelman, Rakel, et al., 2001).

Evidence-based practice is the conscientious and judicious use of current best evidence in conjunction with clinical expertise and patient values to guide health care decisions (Cook, 1998; Jennings & Loan, 2001; Sackett, Straus, Richardson, et al., 2000; Titler, 2006a). Best

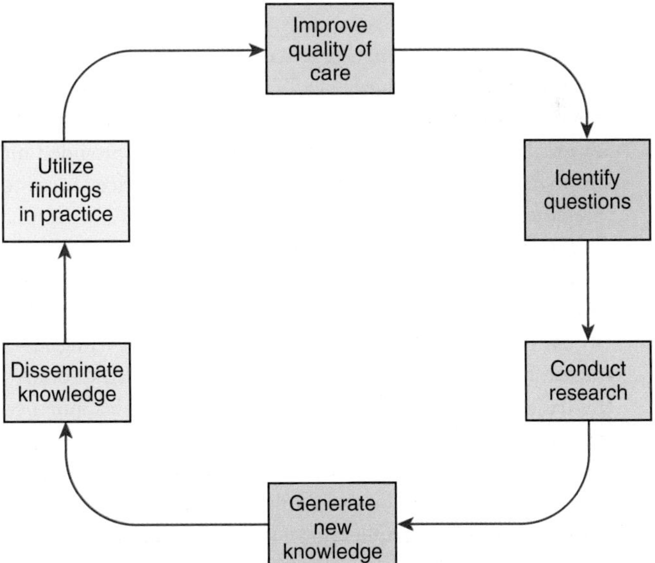

Figure 17-1 The model of the relationship among conduct, dissemination, and use of research. (Redrawn from Weiler K, Buckwalter K, Titler M: Debate: is nursing research used in practice? In McCloskey J, Grace H, eds: *Current issues in nursing,* ed 4, St Louis, 1994, Mosby.)

evidence includes empirical evidence from systematic reviews, randomized controlled trials, and evidence from other scientific methods such as descriptive and qualitative research, as well as use of information from case reports, scientific principles, and expert opinion. When enough research evidence is available, the practice should be guided by research evidence, in conjunction with clinical expertise and patient values. In some cases, however, a sufficient research base may not be available, and health care decision making is derived principally from nonresearch evidence sources such as expert opinion, and scientific principles (Titler et al., 2001). As more research is completed in a specific area, the research evidence must be incorporated into evidence-based practice (Titler, 2006a). As illustrated in the knowledge generation and use cycle (see Figure 17-1), application of research findings in practice may not only improve quality care but create new and exciting questions to be addressed via conduct of research.

The terms *research utilization* and *evidence-based practice* are sometimes used interchangeably (Jennings & Loan, 2001; Titler, Mentes, Rakel, et al., 1999). Although these two terms are related, they are not "one and the same" (Titler et al., 1999). Adopting the definition of evidence-based practice as the conscious and judicious use of the current "best" evidence in the care of patients and delivery of health care services, research utilization is a subset of evidence-based practice that focuses on the application of research findings. Evidence-based practice is a broader term that not only encompasses research utilization but also includes use of case reports and expert opinion in deciding the practices to be used in health care.

Use of Evidence in Practice

Nursing has a rich history of using research in practice, pioneered by Florence Nightingale, who used data to change practices that contributed to high mortality rates in hospitals and communities (Nightingale, 1858, 1859, 1863a, 1863b). Although during the early and mid-1900s, few nurses built on the solid foundation of research utilization exemplified by Nightingale (Titler, 1993), the nursing profession has provided major leadership for improving care through application of research findings in practice (Kirchhoff, 2004). Today nurses are being prepared as scientists in nursing, leading the way in translation science, and, as a result, the scientific body of nursing knowledge is growing (Estabrooks, Derksen, Winther, et al., 2008; Titler, 2008; Titler, Herr, Brooks, et al., 2008). It is now every nurse's responsibility to facilitate the use of nursing knowledge in practice.

Cronenwett and others describe two forms of using research evidence in practice: conceptual and decision driven (Cronenwett, 1995; Estabrooks, 2004). Conceptual-driven forms influence the thinking of the health care provider, not necessarily action. Exposure to new scientific knowledge occurs, but the new knowledge may not be used to change or guide practice. An integrative review of the literature, formulation of a new theory, or generating new hypotheses may be the result. Use of knowledge in this way is referred to as knowledge creep or cognitive application. It is often used by individuals who read and incorporate research into their critical thinking (Weiss, 1980). Decision-driven forms of using evidence in practice encompass application of scientific knowledge as part of a new practice, policy, procedure, or intervention. In this type of application of research findings, a critical decision is reached to endorse current practice or change it based on review and critique of studies applicable to that practice. Examples of decision-driven models of using research in practice are the Iowa Model of Evidence-Based Practice to Promote Quality Care (Titler et al., 2001), the Promoting Action on Research Implementation in Health Services (PARIHS) model

(Rycroft-Malone et al., 2002), and the Conduct and Utilization of Research in Nursing (CURN) model (Haller et al., 1979; Horsley et al., 1983).

Multifaceted active dissemination strategies are needed to promote use of research evidence in clinical and administrative health care decision making, and need to address both the individual practitioner and organizational perspective (Squires, Moralejo, & LeFort, 2007; Titler, 2008). When nurses decide individually what evidence to use in practice, considerable variability in practice patterns result, potentially resulting in adverse patient outcomes. For example, a solely "individual" perspective of evidence-based practice would leave the decision about use of evidence-based pressure ulcer prevention practices to each nurse. Some nurses may be familiar with the research findings for pressure ulcer prevention whereas others may not. This is likely to result in different and conflicting practices being used as nurses change shifts every 8 to 12 hours. From an organizational perspective, policies and procedures are written that are based on research, and then adoption of these practices by nurses is systematically promoted in the organization (Squires et al., 2007).

Models of Evidence-Based Practice

Multiple models of evidence-based practice and translation science are available (Barnsteiner et al., 1995; Berwick, 2003; Dufault, 2001, 2004; Goode & Piedalue, 1999; Logan et al., 1999; Olade, 2004; Rycroft-Malone et al., 2002; Soukup, 2000; Stetler, 2003; Titler & Everett, 2001; Titler et al., 2001; Wagner et al., 2001). Common elements of these models are syntheses of evidence, implementation, evaluation of the impact on patient care, and consideration of the context/setting in which the evidence is implemented. For a summary of models, the review by Grol and colleagues (2007) is recommended. Included in their recent review of models relevant to quality improvement and implementation of change in health care are cognitive, educational, motivational, social interactive, social learning, social network, and social influence theories, and also models related to team effectiveness, professional development, and leadership (Grol et al., 2007). Additional work by the Improved Clinical Effectiveness through Behavioural Research Group (ICEBeRG) has resulted in the development of a database consisting of planned action models, frameworks, and theories that explicitly describe both the concepts and action steps to be considered or taken. This database was developed from a search of social science, education, and health literature that focused on practitioner or organizational change (www.iceberg-grebeci.ohri.ca/research/kt_theories_db.html).

Although review of these models is beyond the scope of this chapter, implementing evidence in practice must be guided by a conceptual model to organize the strategies being used, and to clarify extraneous variables (e.g., behaviors and facilitators) that may influence adoption of evidence-based practices (e.g., organizational size, characteristics of users) (ICEBeRG, 2006). Conceptual models used in the TRIP I and TRIP II studies, funded by the Agency for Healthcare Research and Quality (AHRQ), were adult learning, health education, social influence, marketing, organizational, and behavior theories (Farquhar et al., 2002). Investigators (Doebbeling et al., 2002; Estabrooks et al., 2008; Jones, 2000; Titler & Everett, 2001; Titler, Herr, Schilling, et al., 2003) have used E. Rogers' Diffusion of Innovations model (Rogers, 1995), the Promoting Action on Research Implementation in Health Services (PARIHS) model (Rycroft-Malone et al., 2002), the "push/pull framework" (Lavis et al., 2003; Nutley & Davies, 2000; Nutley, Davies, & Walter, 2003), the decision-making framework (Lomas et al., 1991), and the IHI model (Berwick, 2003) in translation science and evidence-based practice.

Problem-Focused Triggers
1. Risk management data
2. Process improvement data
3. Internal/external benchmarking data
4. Financial data
5. Identification of clinical problem

Knowledge-Focused Triggers
1. New research or other literature
2. National agencies or organizational standards and guidelines
3. Philosophies of care
4. Questions from institutional standards committee

Is this topic a priority for the organization?

No → Consider other triggers

Yes → Form a team

Assemble relevant research and related literature

Critique and synthesize research for use in practice

Is there a sufficient research base?

Yes →

Pilot the Change in Practice
1. Select outcomes to be achieved
2. Collect baseline data
3. Design evidence-based practice (EBP) guideline(s)
4. Implement EBP on pilot units
5. Evaluate process and outcomes
6. Modify the practice guideline

No →

Base Practice on Other Types of Evidence
1. Case reports
2. Expert opinion
3. Scientific principles
4. Theory

Conduct research

Is change appropriate for adoption in practice?

No → Continue to evaluate quality of care and new knowledge

Yes → Institute the change in practice

Monitor and Analyze Structure, Process, and Outcome Data
- Environment
- Staff
- Cost
- Patient and family

Disseminate results

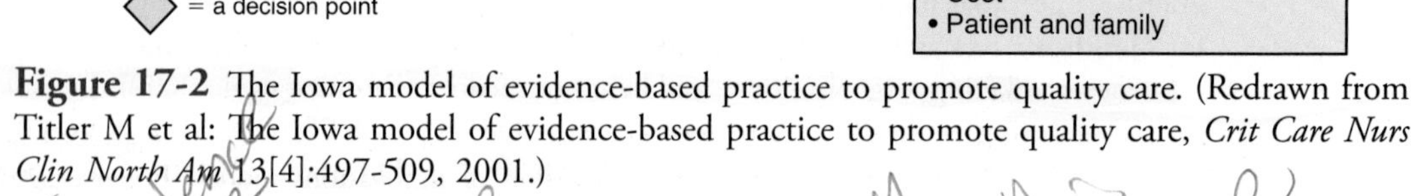

◇ = a decision point

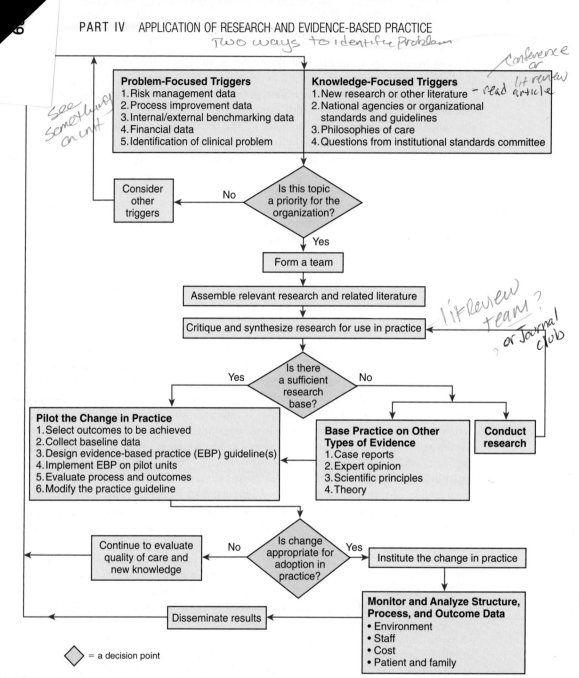

Figure 17-2 The Iowa model of evidence-based practice to promote quality care. (Redrawn from Titler M et al: The Iowa model of evidence-based practice to promote quality care, *Crit Care Nurs Clin North Am* 13[4]:497-509, 2001.)

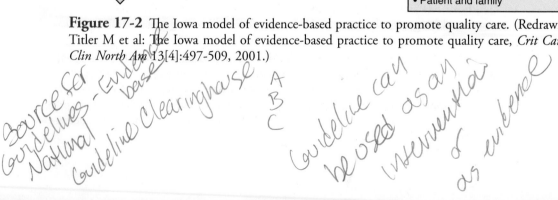

The Iowa Model of Evidence-Based Practice

An overview of the Iowa Model of Evidence-Based Practice as an example of an evidence-based practice model is illustrated in Figure 17-2. This model has been widely disseminated and adopted in academic and clinical settings (Titler et al., 2001). Since the original publication of this model in 1994 (Titler, Kleiber, Steelman, Goode, et al., 1994), the authors have received 303 written requests to use the model for publications, presentations, graduate and undergraduate research courses, and clinical research programs. It has been cited 95 times in nursing journal articles (Social Science Citation Index, 2008). It is an organizational, collaborative model that incorporates conduct of research, use of research evidence, and other types of evidence (Titler et al., 2001). Authors of the Iowa model adopted the definition of evidence-based practice as the conscientious and judicious use of current best evidence to guide health care decisions (Sackett, Rosenberg, Gray, et al., 1996). Levels of evidence range from randomized controlled trials to case reports and expert opinion.

In this model, knowledge- and problem-focused "triggers" lead staff members to question current nursing practice and whether patient care can be improved through the use of research findings. If, through the process of literature review and critique of studies, it is found that there is not a sufficient number of scientifically sound studies to use as a base for practice, consideration is given to conducting a study. Nurses in practice collaborate with scientists in nursing and other disciplines to conduct clinical research that addresses practice problems encountered in the care of patients. Findings from such studies are then combined with findings from existing scientific knowledge to develop and implement these practices. If there is insufficient research to guide practice, and conducting a study is not feasible, other types of evidence (e.g., case reports, expert opinion, scientific principles, theory) are used and/or combined with available research evidence to guide practice. Priority is given to projects in which a high proportion of practice is guided by research evidence. Practice guidelines usually reflect research and nonresearch evidence and therefore are called evidence-based practice guidelines.

An evidence-based practice guideline is developed from the available evidence. The recommended practices, based on the relevant evidence, are compared to current practice, and a decision is made about the necessity for a practice change. If a practice change is warranted, changes are implemented using a process of planned change. The practice is first implemented with a small group of patients, and an evaluation is carried out. The evidence-based practice is then refined based on evaluation data, and the change is implemented with additional patient populations for which it is appropriate. Patient/family, staff, and fiscal outcomes are monitored. Organizational and administrative support are important factors for success in using evidence in care delivery.

STEPS OF EVIDENCE-BASED PRACTICE

The Iowa Model of Evidence-Based Practice to Promote Quality Care (Titler et al., 2001) (see Figure 17-2), in conjunction with Rogers' diffusion of innovations model (Rogers, 1995, 2003a; Titler & Everett, 2001) provide guiding steps in actualizing evidence-based practice. A team approach is most helpful in fostering a specific evidence-based practice, with one person in the group providing leadership for the project.

BOX 17-1 Selection Criteria for an Evidence-Based Practice Project

1. The priority of this topic for nursing and for the organization
2. The magnitude of the problem (small, medium, large)
3. Applicability to several or few clinical areas
4. Likelihood of the change to improve quality of care, decrease length of stay, contain costs, or improve patient satisfaction
5. Potential "landmines" associated with the topic and capability to diffuse them
6. Availability of baseline quality improvement or risk data that will be helpful during evaluation
7. Multidisciplinary nature of the topic and ability to create collaborative relationships to effect the needed changes
8. Interest and commitment of staff to the potential topic
9. Availability of a sound body of evidence, preferably research evidence

Selection of a Topic

The first step in carrying out an evidence-based practice project is to select a topic. Ideas for evidence-based practice come from several sources categorized as problem- and knowledge-focused triggers. **Problem-focused triggers** are those identified by staff through quality improvement, risk surveillance, benchmarking data, financial data, or recurrent clinical problems. An example of a problem-focused trigger is increased incidence of deep venous thrombosis and pulmonary emboli in trauma and neurosurgical patients (Blondin & Titler, 1996; Stenger, 1994).

Knowledge-focused triggers are ideas generated when staff read research, listen to scientific papers at research conferences, or encounter evidence-based practice guidelines published by federal agencies or specialty organizations. This includes those evidence-based practices that CMS expects are implemented in practice and have now based reimbursement of care on adherence to indicators of the evidence-based practices. Examples include treatment of heart failure, community-acquired pneumonia, and prevention of nosocomial pressure ulcers. Each of these topics includes a nursing component such as discharge teaching and instructions for individuals with heart failure. Other examples initiated from knowledge-focused triggers include pain management, assessing placement of nasogastric and nasointestinal tubes, and use of saline to maintain patency of arterial lines. Sometimes topics arise from a combination of problem- and knowledge-focused triggers, such as the length of bed rest time after femoral artery catheterization. In selecting a topic, it is essential that nurses consider how the topic fits with organization, department, and unit priorities to garner support from leaders within the organization and the necessary resources to successfully complete the project.

Individuals should work collectively to achieve consensus in topic selection. Working in groups to review performance improvement data, brainstorm about ideas, and achieve consensus about the final selection is helpful. For example, a unit staff meeting may be used to discuss ideas for evidence-based practice; quality improvement committees may identify three to four practice areas in need of attention (e.g., urinary tract infections in elderly, reducing pressure ulcers); an evidence-based practice task force may be appointed to select and address a clinical practice issue (e.g., pain management); or a Delphi survey technique may be used to prioritize areas for evidence-based practice. Criteria to consider when selecting a topic are outlined in Box 17-1. Table 17-1 shows a helpful chart for selecting a topic.

HELPFUL HINT

Regardless of which method is used to select an evidence-based practice topic, it is critical that the staff members who will implement the potential practice changes are involved in selecting the topic and view it as contributing significantly to the quality of care.

TABLE 17-1 Tool to Use in Selecting a Topic for Evidence-Based Practice

	Topic A	**Topic B**	**Topic C**
Priority for nursing (1 = low; 5 = high)			
Priority for organization (1 = low; 5 = high)			
Magnitude of the problem (small = 1; large = 5)			
Applicability (narrow = 1; broad = 5)			
Likelihood to improve quality of care (1 = low; 5 = high)			
Likelihood to decrease length of stay/contain costs (1 = low; 5 = high)			
Likelihood to improve satisfaction (1 = low; 5 = high)			
Body of science (1 = little; 5 = multiple studies)			
TOTAL			

Modified from Titler MG: *Toolkit for promoting evidence-based practice,* Iowa City, 2002, Department of Nursing Services and Patient Care, University of Iowa Hospitals and Clinics.
Each topic should be rated by using the scoring criteria and a 1-to-5 scale.
The topic(s) receiving the higher score(s) should be considered for selection.

Forming a Team

A team is responsible for development, implementation, and evaluation of the evidence-based practice. The team or group may be an existing committee such as the quality improvement committee, the practice council, or the research committee. A task force approach also may be used, in which a group is appointed to address a specific practice issue and use research findings or other evidence to improve practice. The composition of the team is directed by the topic selected and should include interested stakeholders in the delivery of care. For example, a team working on evidence-based pain management should be interdisciplinary and include pharmacists, nurses, physicians, and psychologists. In contrast, a team working on the evidence-based practice of bathing might include a nurse expert in skin care, assistive nursing personnel, and staff nurses.

In addition to forming a team, key stakeholders who can facilitate the evidence-based practice project or put up barriers against successful implementation should be identified. A stakeholder is a key individual or group of individuals who will be directly or indirectly affected by the implementation of the evidence-based practice. Some of these stakeholders are likely to be members of your team. Others may not be team members but are key individuals within the organization or unit who can adversely or positively influence the adoption of the evidence-based practice. Examples of key stakeholders are chief nursing officers, nursing directors of clinical services or divisions, medical directors, quality improvement chairpersons, nurse managers, nurse educators, researchers, nursing supervisors, chairs of committees or councils that must approve system changes (e.g., policy/procedure revisions; changes in docu-

STAKEHOLDER INFLUENCE

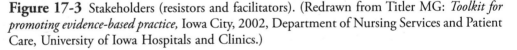

STAKEHOLDER SUPPORT	High (influence)	Low (influence)
High	• Can positively affect dissemination and adoption • Need information to gain their buy-in *Strategies:* • Collaborate • Involve and/or provide opportunities where they can be supportive • Encourage feedback • Empower High support High influence	• Can positively affect dissemination and adoption if given attention • Need attention to maintain buy-in and prevent development of ambivalence *Strategies:* • Collaborate • Encourage feedback • Elicit support via their professional status • Encourage participation, prn • Involve at some level High support Low influence
Low	Low support High influence • Can negatively affect dissemination and adoption • Need great amount of attention and information to obtain and maintain neutrality and work towards buy-in *Strategies:* • Consensus • Build relationships • Detail benefits for them • Involve some (1 or 2) of these individuals on team • Monitor their support	Low support Low influence • Least able to influence dissemination and adoption • May have some negative impact • Some attention to obtain neutrality and to work towards buy-in *Strategies:* • Consensus • Build relationships • Involve at some level — team member

Figure 17-3 Stakeholders (resistors and facilitators). (Redrawn from Titler MG: *Toolkit for promoting evidence-based practice,* Iowa City, 2002, Department of Nursing Services and Patient Care, University of Iowa Hospitals and Clinics.)

mentation forms), and patients/families. Questions to consider in identification of key stakeholders include the following:

- How are decisions made in the practice areas where the evidence-based practice will be implemented?
- What types of system changes will be needed?
- Who is involved in decision making?
- Who is likely to lead and champion implementation of the evidence-based practice?
- Who can influence the decision to proceed with implementation of an evidence-based practice?
- What type of cooperation do you need from which stakeholders to be successful?

TABLE 17-2 Using PICO to Formulate the Evidence-Based Practice Question

	Patient/Population/ Problem	Intervention/Treatment	Comparison Intervention	Outcome(s)
Tips for Building the Question	How would we describe a group of patients similar to ours?	Which main intervention are we considering?	What is the main alternative to compare with the intervention?	What can we hope to accomplish?
Example 1	Pain management for elders admitted to a hospital with a hip fracture	Pain assessment—pain tool Patient-controlled analgesia	Standard of care Nurse-administered analgesic	Regular (e.g., q4hr) pain assessment Less pain intensity Earlier mobility Decreased length of stay
Example 2	Pain assessment of cognitively impaired elders	Pain assessment tool designed for assessing pain in cognitively impaired elders in long-term care setting	Not assess pain Yes/no question	Regular pain assessment with treatment of pain Fewer residents in pain

Modified from University of Illinois at Chicago, P.I.C.O. Model for Clinical Questions, www.uic.edu/depts/lib/lhsp/resources/pico.shtml.

Failure to involve or keep supportive stakeholders informed may place the success of the evidence-based practice project at risk because they are unable to anticipate and/or defend the rationale for changing practice, particularly with resistors (nonsupportive stakeholders) who have a great deal of influence among their peer group. Use Figure 17-3 to think about the status of key stakeholders, and to strategize about interventions to engage various types of stakeholders for your evidence-based practice project.

An important early task for the evidence-based practice team is to formulate the evidence-based practice question. This helps set boundaries around the project and assists in retrieval of the evidence. A clearly defined question should specify the types of people/patients, interventions or exposures, outcomes, and relevant study designs (Alderson, Green, & Higgins, 2003). For types of people, one should specify the diseases or conditions of interest, the patient population (e.g., age, gender, educational status), and the setting. For example, if the topic for the evidence-based practice project is pain, the group needs to specify the type of pain (e.g., acute, persistent, cancer), the age of the population (e.g., children, neonates, adults, older adults), and the setting (e.g., inpatient, outpatient, ambulatory care, home care, primary care). For intervention, specify the types of interventions of interest to the project, and the comparison interventions (e.g., standard care, alternative treatments). For the pain example, the interventions of interest might include pharmacological treatment, analgesic administration methods (e.g., patient-controlled analgesia [PCA], epidural, intravenous [IV]), pain assessment, nonpharmacological treatment, and/or patient/family education regarding self-care pain management. For outcomes, select those outcomes of primary importance, and consider the type of outcome data that will be needed for decision making (e.g., benefits, harm, cost). Avoid including outcomes that may be interesting but of little importance to the project. Finally, consider the types of study designs that are likely to provide reliable data to answer the question, and search for the highest level of evidence available. A similar type of approach to formulating the practice question is PICO: Patient, Population, or Problem; Intervention/Treatment; Comparison Intervention/Treatment; and Outcome(s) (University of Illinois at Chicago, 2003). This approach is illustrated in Table 17-2 (see Chapters 1, 2, 3, and 18).

BOX 17-2 Agency for Health Care Research and Quality Evidence-Based Practice Centers

1. Blue Cross and Blue Shield (BC/BS) Association, Technology Evaluation Center (TEC), Chicago, IL
2. Duke University, Durham, NC*
3. ECRI Institute, Plymouth Meeting, PA*
4. Johns Hopkins University, Baltimore, MD
5. McMaster University, Hamilton, Ontario, Canada
6. Minnesota Evidence-Based Practice Center, Minneapolis, MN
7. Oregon Evidence-Based Practice Center, Portland, OR†
8. RTI International—University of North Carolina (UNC) at Chapel Hill, NC
9. Southern California Evidence-Based Practice Center—RAND Corporation, Santa Monica, CA
10. Tufts Medical Center, Boston, MA*
11. University of Alberta, Edmonton, Alberta, Canada*
12. University of Connecticut, Hartford, CT
13. University of Ottawa, Ottawa, Canada
14. Vanderbilt University, Nashville, TN

For contacts and additional information about the current participating evidence-based practice centers, go to www.ahrq.gov/clinic/epc/epcenters.htm.
*Evidence-based practice centers that focus on technology assessments for CMS.
†Evidence-based practice centers that focuses on evidence reports for the USPSTF.

Evidence Retrieval

Once a topic is selected, relevant research and related literature need to be retrieved and should include clinical studies, meta-analyses, integrative literature reviews, and existing evidence-based practice guidelines. As more evidence is available to guide practice, professional organizations and federal agencies are developing and making available evidence-based practice guidelines (Institute of Medicine, 2008). It is important that these guidelines are accessed as part of the literature retrieval process. In October 2007, AHRQ announced the third award of 5-year contracts for evidence-based practice centers (EPC-III) (Box 17-2) to 14 evidence-based practice centers to continue and expand the work performed by the previous group of evidence-based practice centers. Most of the third group of evidence-based practice centers were part of the initial set. However, EPC-III brings in two new institutions to the program—the University of Connecticut and Vanderbilt University—while Stanford has concluded its contract as one of the original evidence-based practice centers. Five of the evidence-based practice centers specialize in conducting technology assessments for CMS. See www.ahrq.gov/clinic/techix.htm for more information. One evidence-based practice center concentrates on supporting the work of the U.S. Preventive Services Task Force (USPSTF) (www.ahrq.gov/clinic/uspstfix.htm).

AHRQ also sponsors a National Guideline Clearinghouse where abstracts of evidence-based practice guidelines are set forth on a Web site (www.guideline.gov). Other professional organizations that have evidence-based practice guidelines available are the American Pain Society (www.ampainsoc.org); Oncology Nursing Society (www.ons.org); American Association of Critical-Care Nurses (www.aacn.org); Registered Nurses Association of Ontario (www.rnao.org); National Institute for Health and Clinical Excellence (www.nice.org.uk); Association for Women's Health, Obstetrics, and Neonatal Nursing (www.awhonn.org); Gerontological Nursing Interventions Research Center (www.nursing.uiowa.edu/excellence/nursing_interventions/index.htm); and American Thoracic Society (www.thoracic.org). Current best evidence from specific studies of clinical problems can be found in an increasing number of electronic databases such as the Cochrane Library (www3.interscience.wiley.com/cgi-bin/mrwhome/106568753/HOME?CRETRY=1&SRETRY=0), the Centers for Health

Evidence (www.cche.net), and Best Evidence (www.acponline.org) (Straus et al., 2005). Another electronic database, Evidence-Based Medicine Reviews (EBMR) from Ovid Technologies (www.ovid.com), combines several electronic databases, including the Cochrane Database of Systematic Reviews, Best Evidence, Evidence-Based Mental Health, Evidence-Based Nursing, Cancerlit, Healthstar, Aidsline, Bioethicsline, and MEDLINE, plus links to over 200 full-text journals. EBMR links these databases to one another; if a study on a topic of interest is found on MEDLINE and also has been included in a systematic review in the Cochrane Library, the review also can be readily and easily accessed (Straus et al., 2005). In using these sources, it is important to identify key search terms and to use the expertise of health science librarians in locating publications relevant to the project. Additional information about locating the evidence is in Chapter 3.

Once the literature is located, it is helpful to classify the articles as clinical (nonresearch), integrative research reviews, theory articles, research articles, synthesis reports, meta-analyses, and evidence-based practice guidelines. Before reading and critiquing the research, it is useful to read theoretical and clinical articles to have a broad view of the nature of the topic and related concepts, and to then review existing evidence-based practice guidelines. It is helpful to read articles in the following order:

1. Clinical articles to understand the state of the practice
2. Theory articles to understand the various theoretical perspectives and concepts that may be encountered in critiquing studies
3. Systematic review articles and synthesis reports to understand the state of the science
4. Evidence-based practice guidelines and evidence reports
5. Research articles, including meta-analyses

Schemas for Grading the Evidence

There is no consensus among professional organizations or across health care disciplines regarding the best system to use for denoting the type and quality of evidence, or the grading schemas to denote the strength of the body of evidence (Atkins et al., 2005; Guyatt, Oxman, Vist, et al., 2008; West et al., 2002) For example, the Scottish Intercollegiate Guidelines Network has an extensive method detailed on their Web site for appraising research and setting forth guideline recommendations (www.sign.ac.uk). The Grading of Recommendations Assessment, Development, and Evaluation (GRADE) working group, initiated in 2000, is an informal collaboration of individuals interested in addressing grading schema in health care (www.gradeworkinggroup.org). The GRADE system first rates the quality of the evidence as high, moderate, low, or very low and then grades the strength of the evidence as strong or weak in setting forth practice recommendations (GRADE working group, 2004; Guyatt, Oxman, Kunz, Jaeschke, et al., 2008; Guyatt, Oxman, Kunz, Vist, et al., 2008) (Table 17-3). Their methods are available on their Web site with grading software (GRADEpro) available. The National Guidelines Clearinghouse classifies submitted guidelines according to methods used by developers to (1) assess the quality and strength of the evidence: expert consensus; expert consensus (committee), expert consensus (Delphi method), subjective review, weighting according to a rating scheme provided by the developers; or a weighting according to a rating scheme not provided by the developers; and (2) formulate recommendations: various types of expert consensus (e.g., Delphi method; nominal group technique, consensus development conference) and balance sheets.

TABLE 17-3 Examples of Evidence-Based Practice Rating Systems

GRADE Working Group (GRADE Working Group, 2004; Guyatt, Oxman, Kunz, Vist, et al., 2008)	U.S. Preventive Services Task Force before May 2007 (Harris et al., 2001)	U.S. Preventative Services Task Force after May 2007 (Harris et al., 2001; U.S. Preventive Services Task Force, 2008)
Strength of Evidence Quality of the Evidence High: Further research is very unlikely to change our confidence in the estimate of effect. Scientific evidence provided by well-designed, well-conducted, controlled trials (randomized and nonrandomized) with statistically significant results that consistently support the guideline recommendation. Moderate: Further research is likely to have an important impact on our confidence in the estimate of effect and may change the estimate. Low: Further research is very likely to have an important impact on our confidence in the estimate of effect and is likely to change the estimate Very Low: Any estimate of effect is very uncertain. Note: The type of evidence is first ranked as follows: Randomized trial = high. Observational study = low. Any other evidence = very low. Limitations in study quality, important inconsistency of results, uncertainty about the directness of the evidence, imprecise or sparse data, and high probability of reporting bias can lower the grade of evidence. Expert opinion that supports the guideline recommendation because the available scientific evidence did not present consistent results or because controlled trials were lacking. Grade of evidence can be increased if there is (1) strong evidence of association—significant relative risk of >2 (<0.5) based on consistent evidence from two or more observational studies, with no plausible confounders (1); (2) very strong evidence of association—significant relative risk of >5 (< 0.2) based on direct evidence with no major threats to validity (2); (3) evidence of a dose response gradient (1); and (4) all plausible confounders would have reduced the effect (1).	**Quality of Evidence** I. Evidence obtained from at least one properly randomized controlled trial. II-1. Evidence obtained from well-designed controlled trials without randomization. II-2. Evidence obtained from well-designed cohort or case-control analytic studies preferably from more than one center or research group. II-3. Evidence obtained from multiple time series with or without the intervention. Dramatic results in uncontrolled experiments (such as the results of the introduction of penicillin treatment in the 1940s) also could be regarded as this type of evidence. III. Opinions of respected authorities, based on clinical experience; descriptive studies and case reports; or reports of expert committees. **Category Rating Validity of Each Study** Good = Meets all criteria for that study design. Fair = Does not meet all criteria for this study design, but has no fatal flaws that invalidates the results. Poor = Study contains a fatal flaw.	**Levels of Certainty Regarding Net Benefit** High: The available evidence usually includes consistent results from well-designed, well-conducted studies in representative primary care populations. These studies assess the effects of the preventive service on health outcomes. This conclusion is therefore unlikely to be strongly affected by the results of future studies. Moderate: The available evidence is sufficient to determine the effects of the preventive service on health outcomes, but confidence in the estimate is constrained by such factors as the following: The number, size, or quality of individual studies. Inconsistency of findings across individual studies. Limited generalizability of findings to routine primary care practice. Lack of coherence in the chain of evidence. As more information becomes available, the magnitude or direction of the observed effect could change, and this change may be large enough to alter the conclusion. Low: The available evidence is insufficient to assess effects on health outcomes. Evidence is insufficient because of one or more of the following: The limited number or size of studies. Important flaws in study design or methods. Inconsistency of findings across individual studies. Gaps in the chain of evidence. Findings not generalizable to routine primary care practice. Lack of information on important health outcomes. More information may allow estimation of effects on health outcomes.

TABLE 17-3 Examples of Evidence-Based Practice Rating Systems—cont'd

GRADE Working Group (GRADE Working Group, 2004; Guyatt, Oxman, Kunz, Vist, et al., 2008)	U.S. Preventive Services Task Force before May 2007 (Harris et al., 2001)	U.S. Preventative Services Task Force after May 2007 (Harris et al., 2001; U.S. Preventive Services Task Force, 2008)
Strength of Recommendations Strong: confident that the desirable effects of adherence to a recommendation outweigh the undesirable effects. Weak: the desirable effects of adherence to a recommendation probably outweigh the undesirable effects, but the developers are less confident. Note: Strength of recommendation is determined by the balance between desirable and undesirable consequences of alternative management strategies, quality of evidence, variability in values and preferences, and resource use.	**Recommendation Grades** A. Strongly recommends that clinicians routinely provide [the service] to eligible patients. (Found good evidence that [the service] improves important health outcomes and concludes that benefits substantially outweigh harms.) B. Recommends that clinicians routinely provide [the service] to eligible patients. (Found at least fair evidence that [the service] improves important health outcomes and concludes that benefits outweigh harms.) C. Makes no recommendation for or against routine provision of [the service]. (Found at least fair evidence that [the service] can improve health outcomes but concludes that the balance of the benefits and harms is too close to justify a general recommendation.) D. Recommends against routinely providing [the service] to asymptomatic patients. (Found at least fair evidence that [the service] is ineffective or that harms outweigh benefits.) I. Concludes that the evidence is insufficient to recommend for or against routinely providing [the service]. (Evidence that [the service] is effective is lacking, of poor quality, or conflicted and the balance of benefits and harms cannot be determined.)	**Recommendation Grades** A. The USPSTF recommends the service. There is high certainty that the net benefit is substantial. Practice: Offer or provide this service. B. The USPSTF recommends the service. There is high certainty that the net benefit is moderate or there is moderate certainty that the net benefit is moderate to substantial. Practice: Offer or provide this service. C. The USPSTF recommends against routinely providing the service. There may be considerations that support providing the service in an individual patient. There is at least moderate certainty that the net benefit is small. Practice: Offer or provide this service only if other considerations support the offering or providing the service in an individual patient. D. The USPSTF recommends against the service. There is moderate or high certainty that the service has no net benefit or that the harms outweigh the benefits. Practice: Discourage the use of this service. I. The USPSTF concludes that the current evidence is insufficient to assess the balance of benefits and harms of the service. Evidence is lacking, of poor quality, or conflicting, and the balance of benefits and harms cannot be determined. Practice: Read the clinical considerations section of USPSTF Recommendation Statement. If the service is offered, patients should understand the uncertainty about the balance of benefits and harms.

TABLE 17-4 Important Domains and Elements for Systems to Rate Quality of Individual Articles

Systematic Reviews	Randomized Clinical Trials	Observational Studies	Diagnostic Test Studies
Study question	Study question	Study question	*Study population*
Search strategy	*Study population*	Study population	*Adequate description of test*
Inclusion and exclusion criteria	*Randomization*	*Comparability of subjects*	*Appropriate reference standard*
Interventions	*Blinding*	*Exposure or intervention*	*Blinded comparison of test and reference*
Outcomes	*Interventions*	*Outcome measurement*	*Avoidance of verification bias*
Data extraction	*Outcomes*	*Statistical analysis*	
Study quality and validity	*Statistical analysis*	Results	
Data synthesis and analysis	Results	Discussion	
Results	Discussion	*Funding or sponsorship*	
Discussion	*Funding or sponsorship*		
Funding or sponsorship			

Modified from Agency for Healthcare Research and Quality: *Systems to rate the strength of scientific evidence. Evidence report/technology assessment number 47,* AHRQ pub no 02-E016, Rockville, MD, 2002, Agency for Healthcare Research and Quality, U.S. Department of Health and Human Services.
Key domains are in *italics.*

The U.S. Preventative Services Task Force (USPSTF), before May 2007, classified the hierarchy of research design, graded the quality of each study on a three-point scale (good, fair, poor), and then graded recommendations using one of five classifications (A, B, C, D, I) reflecting the strength of the evidence and magnitude of net benefit (Harris et al., 2001). After May 2007, the USPSTF made modifications in its schema and now rates the quality of evidence on a three-point scale (high, moderate, and low) based on levels of certainty regarding the net benefit, and modified the recommendations for practice to include suggestions for practice associated with each grade (A, B, C, D, I) (www.ahrq.gov/clinic/uspstf/grades.htm) (see Table 17-3).

In "grading the evidence," two important areas are essential to address: (1) the quality of the individual research; and (2) the strength of the body of evidence (West et al., 2002). Important domains and elements of any system used to rate quality of individual studies are in Table 17-4 by type of study. The important domains and elements to include in grading the strength of the evidence are defined in Table 17-5. The AHRQ technology report is necessary reading for those undertaking synthesis of evidence for practice and public policy; the scholars reviewed 121 systems (checklists, scales, guidance documents) for grading evidence as the basis of this report (West et al., 2002). From this set, 19 systems fully addressed the key domains for assessing study quality and seven systems fully addressed all three domains for grading the strength of the evidence. The information posted on the GRADE Web site (www.gradeworkinggroup.org) is also important information for readers to understand the challenges and approaches for assessing the quality of evidence and strength of recommendations. In Chapter 1, page 16 of this book, Figure 1-1 provides an evidence hierarchy used for grading the evidence that is an adaptation similar to the evidence hierarchies that appear in Table 17-3.

Before critiquing research articles, reading relevant literature, and reviewing evidence-based practice guidelines, it is imperative that an organization or group responsible for the review agree on methods for noting the type of research, rating the quality of individual articles, and grading the strength of the body of evidence (West et al., 2002). Users will have to evaluate which systems are most appropriate for the task being undertaken, the length of time to

TABLE 17-5 Important Domains and Elements for Systems to Grade the Strength of Evidence

Quality	The aggregate of quality ratings for individual studies, predicated on the extent to which bias was minimized.
Quantity	Magnitude of effect, numbers of studies, and sample size or power.
Consistency	For any given topic, the extent to which similar findings are reported using similar and different study designs.

Modified from Agency for Healthcare Research and Quality: *Systems to rate the strength of scientific evidence. Evidence report/technology assessment number 47,* AHRQ pub no 02-E016, Rockville, MD, 2002, Agency for Healthcare Research and Quality, U.S. Department of Health and Human Services.

complete each instrument, and its ease of use (West et al., 2002). It is also important to decide how the strength of the evidence will be reflected in the guideline. For example, in a guideline for acute pain management in the elderly (Herr et al., 2000), the practice recommendation is followed by the reference citations in American Psychological Association (APA) format and the evidence grade that reflects the strength of the body of evidence for the recommendation.

Critique of Evidence-Based Practice Guidelines

As the number of evidence-based practice guidelines proliferate, it becomes increasingly important that nurses critique these guidelines with regard to the methods used for formulating them and consider how they might be used in their practice. Critical areas that should be assessed when critiquing evidence-based practice guidelines include (1) date of publication or release; (2) authors of the guideline; (3) endorsement of the guideline; (4) a clear purpose of what the guideline covers and patient groups for which it was designed; (5) types of evidence (research, nonresearch) used in formulating the guideline; (6) types of research included in formulating the guideline (e.g., "we considered only randomized and other prospective controlled trials in determining efficacy of therapeutic interventions . . ."); (7) a description of the methods used in grading the evidence; (8) search terms and retrieval methods used to acquire research and nonresearch evidence used in the guideline; (9) well-referenced statements regarding practice; (10) comprehensive reference list; (11) review of the guideline by experts; and (12) whether the guideline has been used or tested in practice, and if so, with what types of patients and in what types of settings. **Evidence-based practice guidelines** that are formulated using rigorous methods provide a useful starting point for nurses to understand the evidence base of certain practices. However, more research may be available since the publication of the guideline and refinements may be needed. Although information in well-developed, national, evidence-based practice guidelines is a helpful reference, it is usually necessary to localize the guideline using institution-specific evidence-based policies, procedures, or standards before application within a specific setting. A useful tool for critiquing clinical practice guidelines is the AGREE tool available at www.agreecollaboration.org.

Critique of Research

Critique of each study should use the same methodology, and the critique process should be a shared responsibility. It is helpful, however, to have one individual provide leadership for the project and design strategies for completing critiques. A group approach to critiques is recommended because it distributes the workload, helps those responsible for implementing the changes to understand the scientific base for the change in practice, arms nurses with citations and research-based sound bites to use in effecting practice changes with peers and other disciplines, and provides novices an environment to learn critique and application of research findings. Methods to make the critique process fun and interesting include the following:

- Using a journal club to discuss critiques done by each member of the group
- Pairing a novice and expert to do critiques
- Eliciting assistance from students who may be interested in the topic and want experience doing critiques
- Assigning the critique process to graduate students interested in the topic
- Making a class project of critique and synthesis of research for a given topic

Several resources are available to assist with the critique process, including the following:

- *Evidence-Based Medicine* and accompanying compact disc (Straus et al., 2005)
- *Evidence-Based Nursing: A Guide to Clinical Practice* (DiCenso et al., 2004)
- Critiquing criteria at the end of each chapter and the critiquing criteria summary tables in Chapters 6 and 16

HELPFUL HINT

Keep critique processes simple, and encourage participation by staff members who are providing direct patient care.

Synthesis of the Research

Once studies are critiqued, a decision is made regarding use of each study in the synthesis of the evidence for application in clinical practice. Factors that should be considered for inclusion of studies in the synthesis of findings are overall scientific merit of the study; type (e.g., age, gender, pathology) of subjects enrolled in the study and the similarity to the patient population to which the findings will be applied; and relevance of the study to the topic of question. For example, if the practice area is prevention of deep venous thrombosis in postoperative patients, a descriptive study using a heterogeneous population of medical patients is not appropriate for inclusion in the synthesis of findings.

To synthesize the findings from research critiques, it is helpful to use a summary table (see Chapters 3, 6, 16, and 18) in which critical information from studies can be documented. Essential information to include in such summary is the following:

- Study purpose
- Research questions/hypotheses
- The variables studied
- A description of the study sample and setting
- The type of research design
- The methods used to measure each variable
- Detailed description of the independent variable/intervention tested
- The study findings

An example of a summary form is illustrated in Table 17-6.

TABLE 17-6 Example of a Summary Table for Research Critiques

Citation	Purpose and Research Question	Research Design	Sample	Independent Variables and Measures	Dependent Variables and Measures	Statistical Tests	Results	Implications	General Strengths	General Weaknesses	Overall Quality of Study*	Summary Statements for Practice

*Use a consistent rating system (e.g., good, fair, poor).

BOX 17-3 Consistency of Evidence from Critiqued Research, Appraisals of Evidence-Based Practice Guidelines, Critiqued Systematic Reviews, and Nonresearch Literature

1. Are there replication of studies with consistent results?
2. Are the studies well designed?
3. Are recommendations consistent among systematic reviews, evidence-based practice guidelines, and critiqued research?
4. Are there identified risks to the patient by applying evidence-based practice recommendations?
5. Are there identified benefits to the patient?
6. Have cost analysis studies been conducted on the recommended action, intervention, or treatment?
7. Summary recommendations about assessments, actions, interventions/treatments from the research, systematic reviews, evidence-based guidelines with an assigned evidence grade.
8. One example of grading the evidence:
   a. Evidence from well-designed meta-analysis or other systematic reviews.
   b. Evidence from well-designed controlled trials, both randomized and nonrandomized, with results that consistently support a specific action (e.g., assessment), intervention, or treatment.
   c. Evidence from observational studies (e.g., correlational descriptive studies) or controlled trials with inconsistent results.
   d. Evidence from expert opinion or multiple cases.

Modified from Titler MG: *Toolkit for promoting evidence-based practice,* Iowa City, 2002, Department of Nursing Services and Patient Care, University of Iowa Hospitals and Clinics.

Setting Forth Evidence-Based Practice Recommendations

Based on the critique of evidence-based practice guidelines and synthesis of research, recommendations for practice are set forth. The type and strength of evidence used to support the practice needs to be clearly delineated. Box 17-3 is a useful tool to assist with this activity. The following are examples of practice recommendation statements:

- Older people who have recurrent falls should be offered long-term exercise and balance training (Strength of recommendation = B) (American Geriatrics Society, British Geriatrics Society, American Academy of Orthopaedic Surgeons, & Panel on Falls Prevention, 2001).
- Apply dressings that maintain a moist wound environment. Examples of moist dressings include, but are not limited to, hydrogels, hydrocolloids, saline moistened gauze, and transparent film dressings. The ulcer bed should be kept continuously moist (Evidence Grade = B) (Alm et al., 1989; Colwell, Foreman, & Trotter, 1992; Folkedahl, Frantz, & Goode, 2002; Fowler & Goupil, 1984; Gorse & Messner, 1987; Kurzuk-Howard, Simpson, & Palmieri, 1985; Neill et al., 1989; Oleske et al., 1986; Saydak, 1990; Sebern, 1986; Xakellis & Chrischilles, 1992).

HELPFUL HINT

Use of a summary form helps identify commonalities across several studies with regard to study findings and the types of patients to which study findings can be applied. It also helps in synthesizing the overall strengths and weakness of the studies as a group.

Decision to Change Practice

After studies are critiqued and synthesized and evidence-based practices are set forth, the next step is to decide if findings are appropriate for use in practice. Criteria to consider in making these decisions include the following:

- Relevance of evidence for practice
- Consistency in findings across studies and/or guidelines
- A significant number of studies and/or evidence-based practice guidelines with sample characteristics similar to those to which the findings will be used
- Consistency among evidence from research and other nonresearch evidence
- Feasibility for use in practice
- The risk/benefit ratio (risk of harm; potential benefit for the patient)

It is recommended that practice changes be based on knowledge/evidence derived from several sources (e.g., several research studies) that demonstrate consistent findings.

Synthesis of study findings and other evidence may result in supporting current practice, making minor practice modifications, undertaking major practice changes, or developing a new area of practice. For example, a project on gauze versus transparent dressings did not result in a practice change because the studies reviewed substantiated current practice (Pettit & Kraus, 1995). In comparison, a guideline for assessing return of bowel motility after abdominal surgery used a combination of research findings and expert consultation and resulted in a change in practice for assessing bowel motility in this adult inpatient population (Madsen et al., 2005). This project resulted in (1) deleting bowel sound assessment as a marker of return of gastrointestinal motility; and using (2) return of flatus, first bowel movement, and absence of abdominal distention as primary indicators of return of bowel motility following abdominal surgery in adults.

HELPFUL HINT

Use a consistent approach to writing evidence-based practice standards and referencing the research and related literature.

Development of Evidence-Based Practice

The next step is to put in writing the evidence base of the practice (Haber et al., 1994) using the grading schema that has been agreed on. When results of the critique and synthesis of evidence support current practice or suggest a change in practice, a written evidence-based practice standard (e.g., policy, procedure, guideline) is warranted. This is necessary so that individuals in the setting know (1) that the practices are based on evidence, and (2) the type of evidence (e.g., randomized controlled trial, expert opinion) used in developing the evidence-based standard. Several different formats can be used to document evidence-based practice changes. The format chosen is influenced by what and how the document will be used. Written evidence-based practices should be part of the organizational policy and procedure manual and should include linkages to the references for the parts of the policy and procedure that are based on research and other types of evidence.

Clinicians (e.g., nurses, physicians, pharmacists) who adopt evidence-based practices are influenced by the perceived participation they have had in developing and reviewing the

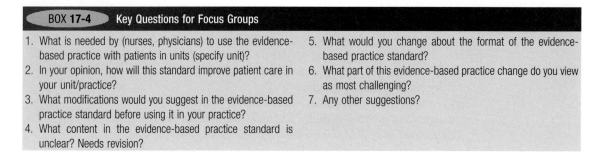

BOX 17-4 Key Questions for Focus Groups

1. What is needed by (nurses, physicians) to use the evidence-based practice with patients in units (specify unit)?
2. In your opinion, how will this standard improve patient care in your unit/practice?
3. What modifications would you suggest in the evidence-based practice standard before using it in your practice?
4. What content in the evidence-based practice standard is unclear? Needs revision?
5. What would you change about the format of the evidence-based practice standard?
6. What part of this evidence-based practice change do you view as most challenging?
7. Any other suggestions?

protocol (Greenhalgh et al., 2005; Titler, 2008). It is imperative that once the evidence-based practice standard is written, key stakeholders have an opportunity to review it and provide feedback to the individual(s) responsible for writing it. Use of focus groups is a useful way to provide discussion about the evidence-based standard and to identify key areas that may be potentially troublesome during the implementation phase. Key questions that can be used in the focus groups are in Box 17-4.

Implementing the Practice Change

If a practice change is warranted, the next steps are to make the evidence-based changes in practice. This goes beyond writing a policy or procedure that is evidence based; it requires interaction among direct care providers to champion and foster evidence adoption, leadership support, and system changes. Rogers' seminal work on diffusion of innovations (Rogers, 2003a) is extremely useful in selecting strategies for promoting adoption of evidence-based practices. Other investigators describing barriers to and strategies for adoption of evidence-based practices have used Rogers' (2003a) model (Funk et al., 1995; Gravel et al., 2006; Rutledge et al., 1996; Scott et al., 2008; Shively et al., 1997; Thompson et al., 2007; Wells & Baggs, 1994). According to this model, adoption of innovations, such as evidence-based practices, is influenced by the nature of the innovation (e.g., the type and strength of evidence; the clinical topic) and the manner in which it is communicated (disseminated) to members (nurses) of a social system (organization, nursing profession) (Rogers, 2003a; Titler & Everett, 2001). Strategies for promoting adoption of evidence-based practices must address these areas within a context of participative, planned change (Figure 17-4).

Nature of the Innovation/Evidence-Based Practice

Characteristics of an innovation or evidence-based practice topic that affect adoption include the relative advantage of the evidence-based practice (e.g., effectiveness, relevance to the task, social prestige); the compatibility with values, norms, work, and perceived needs of users; and complexity of the evidence-based practice topic (Rogers, 2003a). For example, evidence-based practice topics that are perceived by users as relatively simple (e.g., influenza vaccines for older adults) are more easily adopted in less time than those that are more complex (e.g., acute pain management for hospitalized older adults).

Strategies to promote adoption of evidence-based practices related to characteristics of the topic include practitioner review and "reinvention" of the evidence-based practice guideline to fit the local context, use of quick reference guides and decision aids, and use of clinical

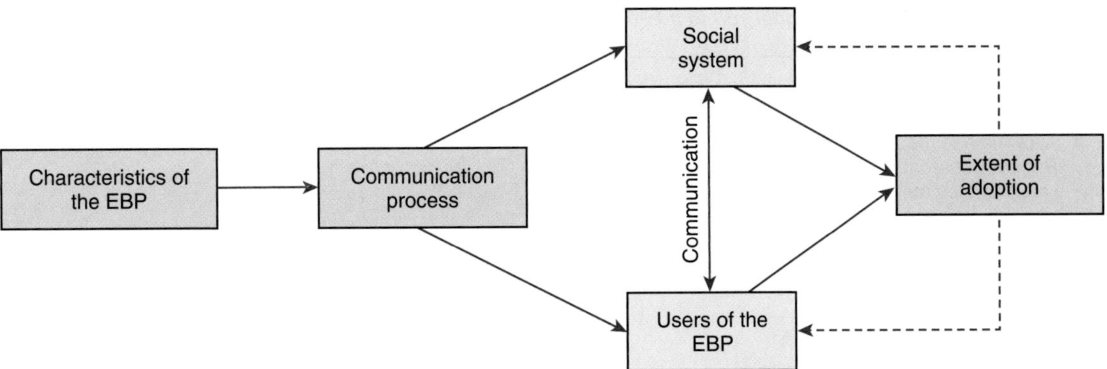

Figure 17-4 Implementation model. (Redrawn from Rogers EM: *Diffusion of innovations,* New York, 1995, Free Press; Titler MG, Everett LQ: Translating research into practice: considerations for critical care investigators, *Crit Care Nurs Clin North Am* 13(4):587-604, 2001.)

reminders (Balas et al., 2004; Berwick, 2003; Bootsmiller et al., 2004; Bradley, Schlesinger, Webster, et al., 2004; Doebbeling, Chou, & Tierney, 2006; Doebbeling et al., 2002; Fung et al., 2004; Grimshaw, Eccles, Thomas, et al., 2006; Guihan, Bosshart, & Nelson, 2004; Hunt et al., 1998; Loeb et al., 2004; Wensing et al., 2006).

An important principle to remember when planning implementation of an evidence-based practice is that the attributes of the evidence-based practice topic as perceived by users and stakeholders (e.g., ease of use, valued part of practice, etc.) are neither stable features nor sure determinants of their adoption. Rather, it is the interaction among the characteristics of the evidence-based practice topic, the intended users, and a particular context of practice that determines the rate and extent of adoption (Greenhalgh et al., 2005; Rogers, 2003a; Titler & Everett, 2001).

Studies suggest that clinical systems, computerized decision support, and prompts/quick reference guides that support practice (e.g., decision-making algorithms; paper reminders) have a positive effect on aligning practices with the evidence-base (Balas et al., 2004; Cook et al., 1997; Doebbeling et al., 2006; Farquhar et al., 2002; Grimshaw, Eccles, Thomas, et al., 2006; Hunt et al., 1998; Loeb et al., 2004; Oxman et al., 1995; Schmidt, Alpen, & Rakel, 1996; Shojania & Grimshaw, 2005; Titler, 2006a; Wensing et al., 2006).

Computerized knowledge management has consistently demonstrated significant improvements in provider performance and patient outcomes (Wensing et al., 2006). Feldman and colleagues, using a just-in-time e-mail reminder in home health care, have demonstrated (1) improvements in evidence-based care and outcomes for patients with heart failure (Feldman et al., 2005; Murtaugh et al., 2005), and (2) reduced pain intensity for cancer patients (McDonald et al., 2005). Clinical information systems should deploy the evidence base to the point of care, and incorporate computer decision support system (CDSS) software that integrates evidence for use in clinical decision making about individual patients (Bates et al., 2003; Clancy & Cronin, 2005; Doebbeling et al., 2006; James, 2003; Thompson, Dowding, & Guyatt, 2005; Titler, 2006b). There is still much to learn about the "best" manner of deploying evidence-based information through electronic clinical information systems to support evidence-based care (Jha et al., 2006). An example of a quick reference guide is shown in Figure 17-5.

Use this quick reference guide to help in the assessment of pain:

- Before patients undergo medical procedures or surgeries that can cause pain
- When patients are experiencing pain from recent surgeries, medical procedures, trauma, or other acute illness

Words that appear in color signal you to additional information on the back of this reference guide.

General principles for assessing pain in older adults:

- Verify sensory ability (Can the person see you? Hear you?).
- Allow time to respond.
- Repeat questions/instructions as necessary.
- Use printed materials with large type and dark lines.

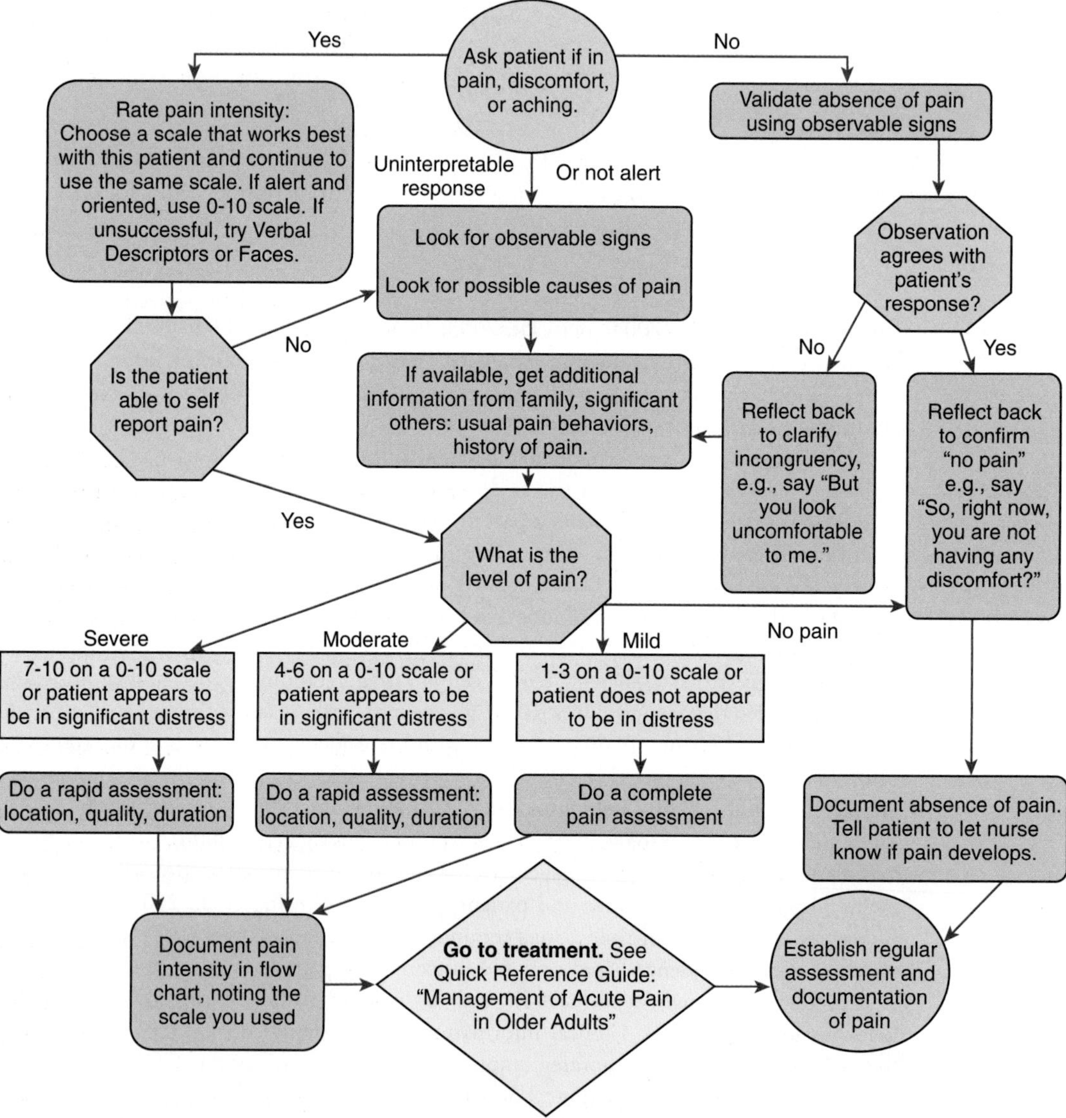

Figure 17-5 Quick reference guide: assessment of acute pain in older adults. (Redrawn from Harris RP, Helfan M, Woolf SH, et al: Current methods of the U.S. Preventive Services Task Force: a review of the process, *Am J Prev Med* 20(3S):21-35, 2001; Herr K, Titler M, Sorofman B, et al: *Evidence-based guideline: acute pain management in the elderly,* Iowa City, 2000, University of Iowa. From Book To Bedside: Acute Pain Management in the Elderly, 1 R01, HS10482-01.)

Methods of Communication

Interpersonnel communication channels, methods of communication, and influence among social networks of users affect adoption of evidence-based practices (Rogers, 2003a). Use of mass media, opinion leaders, change champions, and consultation by experts along with education are among strategies tested to promote use of evidence-based practices. Education is necessary but not sufficient to change practice, and didactic continuing education alone does little to change practice behavior (Carter et al., 2005; O'Brien, Oxman, Haynes, et al., 1999). There is little evidence that interprofessional education as compared with discipline-specific education improves evidence-based practice (Zwarenstein et al., 2000). Interactive education, used in combination with other practice-reinforcing strategies, has more positive effects on improving evidence-based practice than didactic education alone (Horbar et al., 2004; Irwin & Ozer, 2004; Jones, Fink, Vojir, et al., 2004; Loeb et al., 2004; O'Brien, Freemantle, Oxman, et al., 2001; O'Brien, Oxman, Davis, et al., 1997).

There is evidence that mass media (e.g., television, radio, newspapers, leaflets, posters, and pamphlets), targeted at the population level, has some effect on use of health services for the targeted behavior (e.g., colorectal cancer screening), although little empirical evidence is available to guide framing of messages communicated through planned mass media campaigns in order to achieve the intended change (Grilli, Ramsay, & Minozzi, 2002).

It is important that staff know the scientific basis for the changes in practice, and improvements in quality of care anticipated by the change. Disseminating this information to staff needs to be done creatively using various educational strategies. A staff in-service may not be the most effective method nor reach the majority of the staff. Although it is unrealistic for all staff to have participated in the critique process or to have read all studies used to develop the evidence-based practice, it is important that they know the myths and realities of the practice. Education of staff also must include ensuring that they are competent in the skills necessary to carry out the new practice. For example, if a pain assessment tool is being implemented to assess pain in cognitively impaired elders in the long-term care setting, it is essential that caregivers have the knowledge and skill to use the tool in their practice setting.

One method of communicating information to staff is through use of colorful posters that identify myths and realities or describe the essence of the change in practice (Titler et al., 1994; Titler et al., 2001). Visibly identifying those who have learned the information and are using the evidence-based practice (e.g., buttons, ribbons, pins) stimulates interest in others who may not have internalized the change. As a result, the "new" learner may begin asking questions about the practice and be more open to learning. Other educational strategies such as train-the-trainer programs, computer-assisted instruction, and competency testing are helpful in education of staff.

Several studies have demonstrated that opinion leaders are effective in changing behaviors of health care practitioners (Berner et al., 2003; Cullen, 2005; Dopson et al., 2001; Greenhalgh et al., 2005; Irwin & Ozer, 2004; Locock et al., 2001; O'Brien et al., 1999; Redfern & Christian, 2003), especially in combination with educational outreach or performance feedback.

Opinion leaders are from the local peer group, viewed as a respected source of influence, considered by associates as technically competent, and trusted to judge the fit between the innovation and the local situation (Berner et al., 2003; Grimshaw, Eccles, Greener, et al., 2006; Harvey et al., 2002; Heitkemper & Bond, 2004; O'Brien et al., 1999; Soumerai et al., 1998). They have a wide sphere of influence across several microsystems/units and use the innovation, influence peers, and alter group norms (Rogers, 2003a). The key characteristic of

BOX 17-5 Role Expectations of an Opinion Leader

1. Be/become an expert in the evidence-based practice.
2. Provide organizational/unit leadership for adopting the evidence-based practice.
3. Implement various strategies to educate peers about the evidence-based practice.
4. Work with peers, other disciplines, and leadership staff to incorporate key information about the evidence-based practice into organizational/unit standards, policies, procedures, and documentation systems.
5. Promote initial and ongoing use of the evidence-based practice by peers.

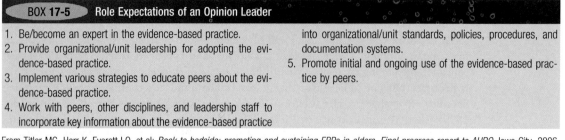

From Titler MG, Herr K, Everett LQ, et al: *Book to bedside: promoting and sustaining EBPs in elders. Final progress report to AHRQ,* Iowa City, 2006, University of Iowa College of Nursing. 2R01 HS010482-04.

an opinion leader is that he or she is trusted to evaluate new information in the context of group norms. To do this, an opinion leader must be considered by associates as technically competent and a full and dedicated member of the local group (Rogers, 2003a; Soumerai et al., 1998).

Opinion leadership is multifaceted and complex, with role functions varying by the circumstances, but few successful projects to implement innovations in organizations have managed without the input of identifiable opinion leaders (Greenhalgh et al., 2005; Rogers, 2003a; Titler & Everett, 2001; Titler, Herr, Everett, et al., 2006; Watson, 2004). Social interactions such as "hallway chats," one-on-one discussions, and addressing questions are important yet often overlooked components of translation (Berwick, 2003; Rogers, 2003a). Thus having local opinion leaders discuss the evidence-based practices with members of their peer group is necessary to translate research into practice. If the evidence-based practice that is being implemented is interdisciplinary in nature, discipline-specific opinion leaders should be used to promote the change in practice (Rogers, 2003a). Role expectations of an opinion leader are in Box 17-5.

Change champions are also helpful for implementing innovations (Rogers, 2003a, 2003b; Shively et al., 1997; Titler, 2004a; Titler et al., 2006; Titler & Mentes, 1999). They are practitioners within the local group setting (e.g., clinic; patient care unit) who are expert clinicians, are passionate about the innovation, are committed to improving quality of care, and have a positive working relationship with other health professionals (Harvey et al., 2002; Rogers, 2003a; Titler, 1998; Titler & Mentes, 1999). They circulate information, encourage peers to adopt the innovation, arrange demonstrations, and orient staff to the innovation (Shively et al., 1997; Titler, 2004a). The change champion believes in an idea; will not take "no" for an answer; is undaunted by insults and rebuffs; and above all, persists (Greer, 1988).

Because nurses prefer interpersonal contact and communication with colleagues rather than Internet or traditional sources of practice knowledge (Estabrooks, Chong, Brigidear, et al., 2005; Estabrooks, O'Leary, Ricker, et al., 2003; Estabrooks, Rutakumwa, O'Leary, et al., 2005; Thompson, 2001), it is imperative that one or two "change champions" be identified for each patient care unit or clinic where the change is being made for evidence-based practices to be enacted by direct care providers (Titler, 2003; Titler et al., 2006). Staff nurses are some of the best change champions for evidence-based practice. Conferencing with opinion leaders and change champions periodically during implementation is helpful to address questions and provide guidance as needed (Guihan et al., 2004; Horbar et al., 2004; Titler & Everett, 2001; Titler et al., 2006).

Because nurses' preferred information source is through peers and social interactions (Estabrooks, 2003; Estabrooks, Chong, Brigidear, et al., 2005; Estabrooks, O'Leary, Ricker, et al., 2003; Estabrooks, Rutakumwa, O'Leary, et al., 2005; Gerrish & Clayton, 2004; Thompson, 2001), using a "core group" in conjunction with change champions is also helpful for implementing the practice change (Barnason et al., 1998; Schmidt et al., 1996; Titler et al., 2001). A core group is a select group of practitioners with the mutual goal of disseminating information regarding a practice change and facilitating the change in practice by other staff in their unit/microsystem (Nelson et al., 2002). Core group members represent various shifts and days of the week, and become knowledgeable about the scientific basis for the practice; the change champion educates and assists them in using practices that are aligned with the evidence. Each member of the core group, in turn, takes the responsibility for imparting evidence-based information and effecting practice change with several (e.g., two to three) of their peers. They assist the change champion and opinion leader with disseminating the evidence-based information to other staff, reinforce the practice change on a daily basis, and provide positive feedback to those who align their practice with the evidence base (Titler, 2006a). Using a core group approach in conjunction with a change champion results in a critical mass of practitioners promoting adoption of the evidence-based practice (Rogers, 2003a).

Educational outreach, also known as academic detailing, promotes positive changes in practice behaviors of nurses and physicians (Feldman et al., 2005; Greenhalgh et al., 2005; Hendryx et al., 1998; Horbar et al., 2004; Jones, Fink, Vojir, et al., 2004; Loeb et al., 2004; McDonald et al., 2005; Murtaugh et al., 2005; O'Brien et al., 1997; Titler et al., 2006).

Academic detailing is done by a topic expert, knowledgeable of the research base (e.g., cancer pain management), who may be external to the practice setting and who meets one-on-one with practitioners in their setting to provide information about the evidence-based practice topic. These individuals are able to explain the research base for the evidence-based practices to others and are able to respond convincingly to challenges and debates (Greenhalgh et al., 2005). This strategy may include providing feedback on provider or team performance with respect to selected evidence-based practice indicators (e.g., frequency of pain assessment) (Horbar et al., 2004; O'Brien et al., 1997; Titler et al., 2006).

Advanced practice nurses (APNs) can provide one-on-one consultation to staff regarding use of the evidence-based practice with specific patients, assist staff in troubleshooting issues in application of the practice, and provide feedback on provider performance regarding use of the evidence-based practices. Studies have demonstrated that use of APNs as facilitators of change promote adherence to the evidence-based practice (Stetler, Legro, Rycroft-Malone, et al., 2006; Titler, 2003; Titler et al., 2008).

Users of the Innovation/Evidence-Based Practice

Members of a social system (e.g., nurses, physicians, clerical staff) influence how quickly and widely evidence-based practices are adopted (Rogers, 2003a). Audit and feedback, performance gap assessment (PGA), and trying the evidence-based practice are strategies that have been tested (Greenhalgh et al., 2005; Grimshaw, Eccles, Thomas, et al., 2006; Grimshaw, Eccles, Greener, et al., 2006; Grimshaw, Thomas, MacLennan, et al., 2004; Horbar et al., 2004; Jamtvedt et al., 2006; Jones, Fink, Vojir, et al., 2004; Katz, Brown, Muehlenbruch, et al., 2004; Katz, Muehlenbruch, Brown, et al., 2004; Titler, 2006a; Titler et al., 2006). PGA and audit and feedback have consistently shown a positive effect on changing practice behavior of providers (Duncan & Pozehl, 2000; Grimshaw, Eccles, Thomas, et al., 2006; Grimshaw, Eccles, Greener, et al., 2006; Grimshaw et al., 2004; Horbar et al., 2004; Jamtvedt et al.,

2006; Katz, Brown, Muehlenbruch, et al., 2004; Katz, Muehlenbruch, Brown, et al., 2004; Titler et al., 2006). PGA (baseline practice performance) informs members, at the beginning of change, about a practice performance and opportunities for improvement. Specific practice indicators selected for performance gap assessment are related to the practices that are the focus of evidence-based practice change such as every-4-hour pain assessment for acute pain management (Horbar et al., 2004; Titler, 2006a; Titler et al., 2006).

Audit and feedback is ongoing auditing of performance indicators (e.g., every-4-hour pain assessment), aggregating data into reports, and discussing the findings with practitioners during the practice change (Duncan & Pozehl, 2000; Greenhalgh et al., 2005; Horbar et al., 2004; Jamtvedt et al., 2006; Katz, Brown, Muehlenbruch, et al., 2004; Katz, Muehlenbruch, Brown, et al., 2004; Titler, 2004a; Titler et al., 2006). This strategy helps staff know and see how their efforts to improve care and patient outcomes are progressing throughout the implementation process. There is not clear empirical evidence for how to provide audit and feedback (Jamtvedt et al., 2006; Kiefe & Sales, 2006), although effects may be larger when clinicians are active participants in implementing change and discuss the data rather than being passive recipients of feedback reports (Hysong, Best, & Pugh, 2006; Jamtvedt et al., 2006). Examples of audit and feedback data are illustrated in Figure 17-6.

Qualitative studies provide some insight into use of audit and feedback (Bradley, Schlesinger, Webster, et al., 2004; Hysong et al., 2006). One study on use of data feedback for improving treatment of acute myocardial infarction found that (1) feedback data must be perceived as important and valid, (2) the data source and timeliness of data feedback are critical to perceived validity, (3) it takes time to establish credibility of data within a hospital, (4) benchmarking improves the validity of the data feedback, and (5) clinician leaders can enhance the effectiveness of data feedback. Data feedback that profiles an individual clinician's practices can be effective but may be perceived as punitive, data feedback must persist to sustain improved performance, and effectiveness of data feedback is intertwined with the organizational context, including physician leadership and organizational culture (Bradley, Schlesinger, Webster, et al., 2004). Hysong and colleagues (2006) found that high-performing institutions provided timely, individualized, nonpunitive feedback to providers whereas low performers were more variable in their timeliness and nonpunitiveness and relied more on standardized, facility-level reports. The concept of actionable feedback emerged as the core concept around which timeliness, individualization, nonpunitiveness, and customizability are important.

Users of an innovation usually try it for a period of time before adopting it in their practice (Greenhalgh et al., 2005; Meyer & Goes, 1988; Rogers, 2003a). When "trying an evidence-based practice" (piloting the change) is incorporated as part of the implementation process, users have an opportunity to use it for a period of time, provide feedback to those in charge of implementation, and modify the practice if necessary (Stetler, Legro, Wallace, et al., 2006). Piloting the evidence-based practice as part of implementation has a positive influence on the extent of adoption of the new practice (Greenhalgh et al., 2005; Rogers, 2003a; Stetler, Legro, Wallace, et al., 2006).

Characteristics of users such as educational preparation, practice specialty, and views on innovation may influence adoption of an evidence-based practice, although findings are equivocal (Estabrooks, Floyd, Scott-Findlay, et al., 2003; Olade, 2004; Retchin, 1997; Rogers, 2003a; Rutledge et al., 1996; Salem-Schatz et al., 1997; Schneider & Eisenberg, 1998; Shively et al., 1997). Nurses' disposition to critical thinking is, however, positively correlated with research use (Profetto-McGrath et al., 2003), and those in clinical educator roles are more likely to use research than staff nurses or nurse managers (Milner, Estabrooks, & Humphrey, 2005).

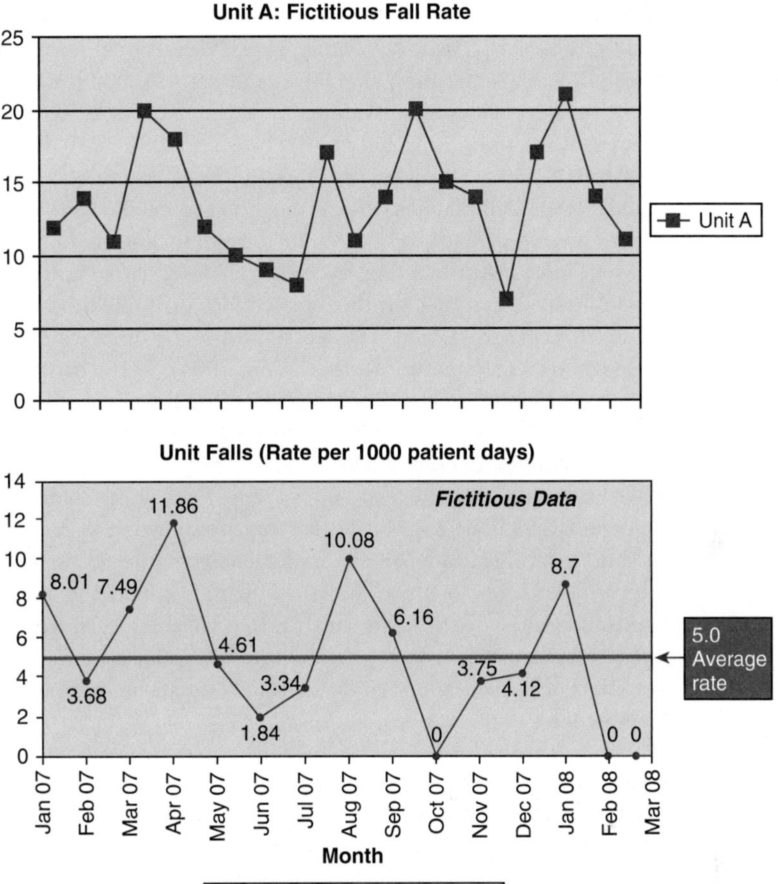

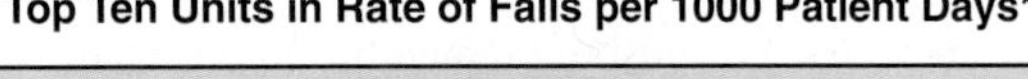

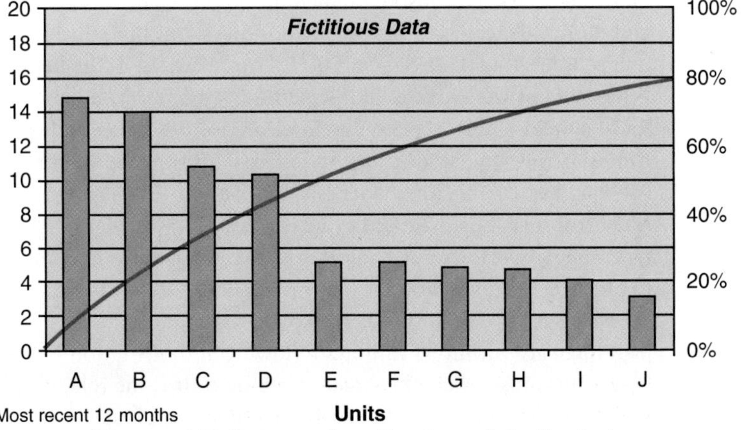

Figure 17-6 Examples of audit and feedback data.

Social System

Clearly, the social system or context of care delivery matters when implementing evidence-based practices (Anderson et al., 2004; Anderson et al., 2005; Anderson 2003; Batalden et al., 2003; Bradley, Schlesinger, Webster, et al., 2004; Ciliska et al., 1999; Denis et al., 2002; Fleuren, Wiefferink, & Paulussen, 2004; Fraser, 2004a, 2004b; Institute of Medicine, 2001; Kochevar & Yano, 2006; Litaker et al., 2006; Morin et al., 1999; Rogers, 2003a; Rycroft-Malone et al., 2004; Stetler, 2003; Vaughn et al., 2002). For example, investigators demonstrated the effectiveness of a prompted voiding intervention for urinary incontinence in nursing homes, but sustaining the intervention in day-to-day practice was limited when the responsibility of carrying out the intervention was shifted to nursing home staff (rather than the investigative team) and required staffing levels in excess of a majority of nursing home settings (Engberg, Kincade, & Thompson, 2004). This illustrates the importance of embedding interventions into ongoing processes of care.

Several organizational factors affect adoption of evidence-based practices (Cullen et al., 2005; Estabrooks, O'Leary, Ricker, et al., 2003; Greenhalgh et al., 2005; Redfern & Christian, 2003; Redman, 2004; Rogers, 2003a; Scott-Findlay & Golden-Biddle, 2005). Vaughn and colleagues (2002) demonstrated that organizational resources, physician FTEs per 1,000 patient visits, organizational size, and urbanicity affected use of evidence in the VA health care system. Large, mature, functionally differentiated organizations (e.g., divided into semiautonomous departments and units) that are specialized, with a foci of professional knowledge, extra resources to channel into new projects, decentralized decision making, and low levels of formalization will more readily adopt innovations such as new practices based on evidence.

Larger organizations are generally more innovative because size increases the likelihood that other predictors of innovation adoption will be present, such as financial and human resources (slack) and differentiation. However, these organizational determinants only account for about 15% of the variation in innovation adoption between comparable organizations (Greenhalgh et al., 2005). Adler and colleagues (2003) hypothesize that whereas more structurally complex organizations may be more innovative and hence adopt evidence-based practices relatively early, less structurally complex organizations may be able to diffuse evidence-based practices more effectively. Establishing semiautonomous teams is associated with successful implementation of evidence-based practices, and thus should be considered in managing organizational units (Adler, Kwon, & Singer, 2003; Grumbach & Bodenheimer, 2004; Shortell, 2004).

As part of the work of implementing evidence-based practices, it is important that the social system—unit, service line, and/or clinic—ensure that policies, procedures, standards, clinical pathways, and documentation systems support the use of the evidence-based practices (Bootsmiller et al., 2004; Gerrish & Clayton, 2004; Irwin & Ozer, 2004; Katz, Brown, Muehlenbruch, et al., 2004; Levine et al., 2004; Rutledge & Donaldson, 1995; Titler, 2004a). Documentation forms or clinical information systems may need revision to support changes in practice; documentation systems that fail to readily support the new practice thwart change (Wensing et al., 2006). For example, if staff members are expected to reassess and document pain intensity within 30 minutes following administration of an analgesic agent, documentation forms must reflect this practice standard. It is the role of upper- and middle-level leadership to ensure that organizational documents and systems are flexible and supportive of the evidence-based practices.

Absorptive capacity for new knowledge is another social system factor that affects adoption of evidence-based practices. Absorptive capacity is the knowledge and skills to enact the evidence-based practices, remembering that the strength of evidence alone will not promote adoption. An organization that is able to systematically identify, capture, interpret, share, reframe, and recodify new knowledge and put it to appropriate use will be better able to assimilate evidence-based practices (Barnsley, Lemieux-Charles, & McKinney, 1998; Bootsmiller et al., 2004; Ferlie et al., 2001; Wensing et al., 2006). A learning organizational culture and proactive leadership that promotes knowledge sharing are important components of building absorptive capacity for new knowledge (Estabrooks, 2003; Horbar et al., 2004; Lozano et al., 2004; Nelson et al., 2002). Components of a receptive context for evidence-based practice include the following:

- Strong leadership
- Clear strategic vision
- Good managerial relations
- Visionary staff in key positions
- A climate conducive to experimentation and risk taking
- Effective data-capture systems

Leadership is critical in encouraging organizational members to break out of the convergent thinking and routines that are the norm in large, well-established organizations (Cullen, 2005; Greenhalgh et al., 2005; Hagedorn et al., 2006; Litaker et al., 2006; Rogers, 2003a; Stetler, Legro, Wallace, et al., 2006; Ward et al., 2006).

An organization may be generally amenable to innovations but not ready or willing to assimilate a particular evidence-based practice. Elements of system readiness include the following:

- Tension for change
- Evidence-based practice–system fit
- Assessment of implications
- Support and advocacy for the evidence-based practice
- Dedicated time and resources
- Capacity to evaluate the impact of the evidence-based practice during and following implementation

If there is tension around specific work or clinical issues, and staff perceive that the situation is intolerable, a potential evidence-based practice is likely to be assimilated if it can successfully address the issues, and thereby reduce the tension (Greenhalgh et al., 2005; Hagedorn et al., 2006).

Assessing and structuring workflow to fit with a potential evidence-based practice is an important component of fostering adoption. If implications of the evidence-based practice are fully assessed, anticipated, and planned for, the practice is more likely to be adopted (Buonocore, 2004; Kochevar & Yano, 2006; Stetler, Legro, Wallace, et al., 2006). If supporters for a specific evidence-based practice outnumber and are more strategically placed within the organizational power base than opponents, the evidence-based practice is more likely to be adopted by the organization (Bradley, Schlesinger, Webster, et al., 2004; Hagedorn et al., 2006). Organizations that have the capacity to evaluate the impact of the evidence-based practice change are more likely to assimilate it. Effective implementation needs both a receptive climate and a good fit between the evidence-based practice and intended adopters' needs and values (Bradley, Holmboe, Mattera, et al., 2004; Bradley, Schlesinger, Webster, et al., 2004; Gerrish & Clayton, 2004; Greenhalgh et al., 2005; Hagedorn et al., 2006).

Leadership support is critical for promoting use of evidence-based practices (Antrobus & Kitson, 1999; Baggs & Mick, 2000; Berwick, 2003; Carr & Schott, 2002; Cullen, 2005; Katz, Brown, Muehlenbruch, et al., 2004; Katz, Muehlenbruch, Brown, et al., 2004; Morin et al., 1999; Nagy et al., 2001; Stetler, 2003), and is expressed verbally, and by providing necessary resources, materials, and time to fulfill assigned responsibilities (Omery & Williams, 1999; Rutledge & Donaldson, 1995; Stetler, Legro, Wallace, et al., 2006; Titler, Cullen, & Ardery, 2002).

Senior leadership need to create an organizational mission, vision, and strategic plan that incorporates evidence-based practice, implement performance expectations for staff that include evidence-based practice work, integrate the work of evidence-based practice into the governance structure of the health care system, demonstrate the value of evidence-based practices through administrative behaviors, and establish explicit expectations that nurse leaders will create microystems that value and support clinical inquiry (Cullen, 2005; Titler, 2002; Titler, Cullen, & Ardery, 2002). The role of the nurse manager is critical in making evidence-based practice changes a reality for staff at the bedside. Nurse managers must expect that staff will participate in evidence-based practice activities, role model the change in their practice, and provide written and verbal support for the practice change. When selecting a potential topic, it is important that the nurse manager values the idea and supports the potential changes.

APNs are critical to helping staff retrieve and critique the studies and other evidence on the selected topic. Although staff nurses are often willing to participate, the APN provides significant leadership in the process by facilitating synthesis of the research and other evidence, critically analyzing what practices should be changed, assisting staff to communicate these changes to their peers, and role modeling changes in practice.

A recent review of organizational interventions to implement evidence-based practices for improving patient care examined five major categories, and suggests the following:

- Revision of professional roles (changing responsibilities and work of health professionals such as expanding roles of nurses and pharmacists)
- Improved processes of care, but was less clear about the effect on improving patient outcomes and,
- Multidisciplinary teams (collaborative practice teams of physicians, nurses, and allied health professionals)

The review resulted in improved patient outcomes with most being tested in prevalent chronic diseases. Integrated care services (e.g., disease management and case management) resulted in improved patient outcomes and cost savings. Interventions aimed at knowledge management (i.e., optimal organization of knowledge within an organization principally via use of technology to support patient care) resulted in improved adherence to evidence-based practices and patient outcomes. The last category, quality management, had the fewest reviews available with the results uncertain. A number of organizational interventions were not included in this review (e.g., leadership, process redesign, organizational learning), and the authors note that the lack of a widely accepted taxonomy of organizational interventions is a problem in examining effectiveness across studies (Wensing et al., 2006).

An organizational intervention that is receiving increasing attention is **tailored interventions** to overcome barriers to change (Hagedorn et al., 2006; Kochevar & Yano, 2006; Shaw et al., 2005). This type of intervention focuses on first assessing needs in terms of what is causing the gap between current practice and evidence-based practice for a specified topic, what behaviors and/or mechanism need to change, what organizational units and persons should be involved, and identification of ways to facilitate the changes. This information is then used in tailoring an intervention for the setting that will promote use of the specified evidence-based practice. Based on a recent systematic review, effectiveness of tailored implementation interventions remains uncertain (Shaw et al., 2005).

BOX 17-6 Steps of Evaluation for Evidence-Based Projects

1. Identify process and outcome variables of interest.
   Example: Process variable—Patients > 65 years of age will have a Braden scale completed on admission
   Outcome variable—Presence/absence of nosocomial pressure ulcer; if present—determine stage as I, II, III, IV
2. Determine methods and frequency of data collection.
   Example: Process variable—Chart audit of all patients > 65 years old, 1 day a month
   Outcome variable—Patient assessment of all patients > 65 years old, 1 day a month
3. Determine baseline and follow-up sample sizes.
4. Design data collection forms.
   Example: Process chart audit abstraction form
   Outcome variable—pressure ulcer assessment form
5. Establish content validity of data collection forms.
6. Train data collectors.
7. Assess interrater reliability of data collectors.
8. Collect data at specified intervals.
9. Provide "on-site" feedback to staff regarding the progress in achieving the practice change.
10. Provide feedback of analyzed data to staff.
11. Use data to assist staff in modifying or integrating the evidence-based practice change.

In summary, making an evidence-based change in practice involves a series of action steps and a complex, nonlinear process. Implementing the change will take several weeks to months, depending on the nature of the practice change. Increasing staff knowledge about a specific evidence-based practice and passive dissemination strategies are not likely to work, particularly in complex health care settings. Strategies that seem to have a positive effect on promoting use of evidence-based practices include audit and feedback, use of clinical reminders and practice prompts, opinion leaders, change champions, interactive education, mass media, educational outreach/academic detailing, and the context of care delivery (e.g., leadership, learning, questioning). It is important that senior leadership and those leading evidence-based practice improvements are aware of change as a process and continue to encourage and teach peers about the change in practice. The new practice must be continually reinforced and sustained or the practice change will be intermittent and soon fade, allowing more traditional methods of care to return (Titler, 2006a).

Evaluation

Evaluation provides an opportunity to collect and analyze data with regard to use of a new evidence-based practice and then to modify the practice as necessary. It is important that the evidence-based change is evaluated, both on the pilot area and when the practice is changed in additional patient care areas. The importance of the evaluation cannot be overemphasized; it provides information for performance gap assessment, audit, and feedback, and provides information necessary to determine if the evidence-based practice should be retained, modified, or eliminated.

A desired outcome achieved in a more controlled environment, when a researcher is implementing a study protocol for a homogeneous group of patients (conduct of research), may not result in the same outcome when the practice is implemented in the natural clinical setting, by several caregivers, to a more heterogeneous patient population. Steps of the evaluation process are summarized in Box 17-6.

Evaluation should include both process and outcome measures. The process component focuses on how the evidence-based practice change is being implemented. It is important to

TABLE 17-7 Examples of Evaluation Measures

	NURSES' SELF-RATING				
Example Process Questions	**SD**	**D**	**NA/D**	**A**	**SA**
1. I feel well prepared to use the Braden Scale with older patients.	1	2	3	4	5
2. Malnutrition increases patient risk for pressure ulcer development.	1	2	3	4	5
EXAMPLE OUTCOME QUESTION					
Patient					
1. On a scale of 0 (no pain) to 10 (worst possible pain), how much pain have you experienced over the past 24 hours?	______ (Pain intensity)				

SD, strongly disagree; *D*, disagree; *NA/D*, neither agree nor disagree; *A*, agree; *SA*, strongly agree.

know if staff are using the practice in care delivery and if they are implementing the practice as noted in the written evidence-based practice standard. Evaluation of the process also should note (1) barriers that staff encounter in carrying out the practice (e.g., lack of information, skills, or necessary equipment), (2) differences in opinions among health care providers, and (3) difficulty in carrying out the steps of the practice as originally designed (e.g., shutting off tube feedings 1 hour before aspirating contents for checking placement of nasointestinal tubes). Process data can be collected from staff and/or patient self-reports, medical record audits, or observation of clinical practice. Examples of process and outcome questions are shown in Table 17-7.

Outcome data are an equally important part of evaluation. The purpose of outcome evaluation is to assess whether the patient, staff, and/or fiscal outcomes expected are achieved. Therefore it is important that baseline data be used for a preintervention/postintervention comparison (Cullen, 2005; Titler et al., 2001). The outcome variables measured should be those that are projected to change as a result of changing practice (Soukup, 2000). For example, research demonstrates that less restricted family visiting practices in critical care units result in improved satisfaction with care. Thus patient and family member satisfaction should be an outcome measure that is evaluated as part of changing visiting practices in adult critical care units. Outcome measures should be measured before the change in practice is implemented, after implementation, and every 6 to 12 months thereafter. Findings must be provided to clinicians to reinforce the impact of the change in practice and to ensure that they are incorporated into quality improvement programs. For example, an organizational task force to institute evidence-based practices for pain management included members from the Department of Nursing Quality Improvement Committee. Data collection focused on adequacy of pain control and patient satisfaction with pain management. Representatives from divisional quality improvement committees were responsible for collecting data from at least 20 patients per unit or clinical area. Results of the quality improvement monitor were distributed to each nursing unit, and staff were encouraged to use this information in identifying ways to improve pain management practices (Rakel & Titler, 2001).

When collecting process and outcome data for evaluation of evidence-based practice change, it is important that the data-collection tools are user-friendly, short, concise, and easy to complete, and have content validity. Focus must be on collecting the most essential data. Those responsible for collecting evaluative data must be trained on the methods of data collection and be assessed for interrater reliability (see Chapters 12 and 13). It is our experience that those individuals who have participated in implementing the protocol can be very helpful in evaluation by collecting data, providing timely feedback to staff, and assisting staff to overcome barriers encountered when implementing the changes in practice.

One question that often arises is how much data are needed to evaluate this change. The preferred number of patients *(N)* is somewhat dependent on the size of the patient population affected by the practice change. For example, if the practice change is for families of critically ill adult patients and the organization has 1,000 adult critical care patients annually, 50 to 100 satisfaction responses preimplementation, and 25 to 50 responses postimplementation, at 3 and 6 months should be adequate to look for trends in satisfaction and possible areas that need to be addressed in continuing this practice (e.g., more bedside chairs in patient rooms). The rule of thumb is to keep the evaluation simple, because data often are collected by busy clinicians who may lose interest if the data collection, analysis, and feedback are too long and tedious.

The evaluation process includes planned feedback to staff who are making the change. The feedback includes verbal and/or written appreciation for the work and visual demonstration of progress in implementation and improvement in patient outcomes. The key to effective evaluation is to ensure that the evidence-based change in practice is warranted (e.g., will improve quality of care) and that the intervention does not bring harm to patients. For example, when instituting a change in practice for assessing return of bowel motility following abdominal surgery in adults, it was important to inform staff that using other markers for return of bowel motility, rather than bowel sound assessment, did not result in increased paralytic ileus or bowel obstruction (Madsen et al., 2005).

HELPFUL HINT

Include patient outcome measures (e.g., pressure ulcer prevalence) and cost (e.g., cost savings, cost avoidance) in evaluation.

CREATING A CULTURE OF EVIDENCE-BASED PRACTICE

Use of research evidence to guide clinical and operational decisions is a necessity in health care delivery (Cullen & Titler, 2004). Chief nurse executives and their leadership staff set the stage and culture for evidence-based practice in their settings. How this is done varies, but essential components are necessary for evidence-based practices (both the process and product) to be an integral part of the organization.

Providing this leadership is a continuous process that involves four major building blocks (Figure 17-7):

- Incorporating evidence-based practice terminology into the mission, vision, strategic plan, and philosophy of care delivery
- Establishing explicit performance expectations about evidence-based practice for staff at all levels of the organization
- Integrating the work of evidence-based practice into the governance structure of nursing departments and the health care system
- Recognition for and rewarding of evidence-based practice behaviors

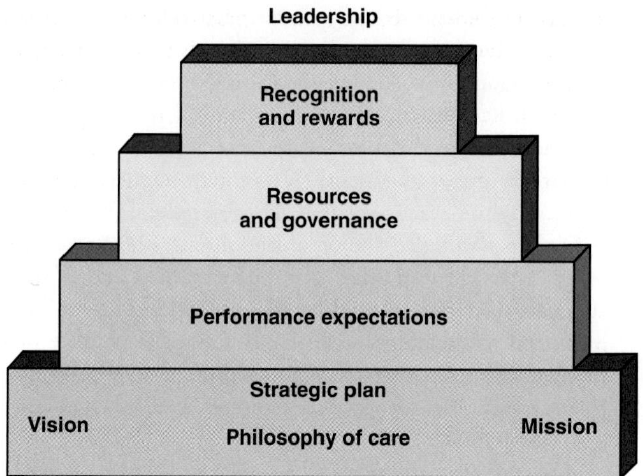

Figure 17-7 Four major building blocks.

The first building block is to ensure that the mission and vision statements of the health care system and nursing services reflect a commitment to the provision of evidence-based health care. Examples of statements that codify this commitment include the following: "The mission of the UI healthcare system is to provide evidence-based healthcare to consumers across settings and sites of care delivery." "The vision of the department of nursing services and patient care is to be an international exemplar of using evidence to guide clinical and operational decision-making." "Our mission is to provide high-quality patient care based on our strong commitments to practice, education, research, innovation, and collaboration" (UIHC Department of Nursing, 2008).

These lay the foundation for the integration of evidence-based practices throughout the organization. For evidence-based practices to be manifested in everyday work, it is necessary to incorporate into the organization's or department's strategic plan specific action statements that promote and foster evidence-based practices. Such actions might include offering an annual evidence-based practice staff nurse internship program; integrating educational content about evidence-based practice into orientation of new staff; monitoring and acting on the results of key indicators for selected evidence-based practices (e.g., acute pain management, prevention of pressure ulcers, fall prevention); and initiating two or three new evidence-based practices per year that are triggered by operational and/or quality improvement data. For example, if quality improvement data suggest that fall rates are particularly high in selected sites of care delivery, using an evidence-based process to understand the nature of the problem as well as possible solutions might be among the action statements of a strategic initiative regarding patient safety. Equally important to a mission and vision that embraces evidence-based practice is clarity about (1) the definition and meaning of evidence-based practice (some departments actually adopt a definition), (2) the organizational process or model of evidence-based practice, and (3) a philosophy of care that embraces clinical inquiry and questioning of the status quo.

The second building block is developing and using performance expectations regarding evidence-based practices. For example, evidence-based practice performance expectations for staff nurses should include critical thinking, continual questioning of practice, participating in making evidence-based practice practice changes, serving as leaders of change in their site of care delivery, and participating in evaluating evidence-based changes in practice.

The chief nurse executive sets the tone for evidence-based practice and explicates role expectations of other nurse leaders within the organization regarding the knowledge, skills, and behaviors necessary to promote adoption of evidence-based practices. Performance expectations for nurse managers include creating a culture that fosters interdisciplinary quality improvement based on evidence. Advanced practice nurses' performance expectations include leading a team, finding the evidence, and synthesis of evidence for practice. Advanced practice nurses assist staff with focusing their clinical question about improving practice, finding and evaluating the research evidence, and maneuvering through the committee structures to implement and sustain the changes in practice. The ability of APNs to meet these performance criteria is an essential part of their annual performance appraisals. Similarly, nurse managers set the tone, value, and work culture for the microsystems they lead.

Staff migrate to microsystems that foster professional growth, professional nursing practice, data-based decision making, and innovative practices; all characteristics of cultures that promote adoption of evidence-based nursing practices. Nurse managers also foster evidence-based practices in their units by allocation of resources, an important element for staff nurse participation in new evidence-based practice projects. Consequently, associate directors of nursing who hire, retain, and value, via performance appraisals, nurse managers and APNs skilled in evidence-based practice are more likely to observe development of clinical innovations, and adoption of evidence-based practices in the multiple units and sites of care delivery for which they are responsible.

Enactment of evidence-based practice behaviors by the chief nurse executive includes providing resources for evidence-based practice such as easy access to evidence-based practice Web sites, retaining personnel with expertise in evidence-based practice, supporting programs that develop a critical mass of staff nurses with expertise in evidence-based practice (e.g., an evidence-based practice staff nurse internship program) (Cullen & Titler, 2004), and providing access to assistance with analysis of data and transforming data into information. Chief nurse executives also enact the value of evidence-based practice by using information from evaluations of existing and new clinical programs in operational decisions, and by rewarding and recognizing direct care providers who make evidence-based practice a reality in their daily work. Using evidence in administrative decisions is another behavior modeled by chief nurse executives who value evidence-based practice.

Assessing the work culture of nurses that contribute to job satisfaction and retention, and then using this information, along with research evidence, to create administrative interventions that decrease turnover, is one example of an evidence-based administrative practice. As it is difficult to support multiple evidence-based practice changes simultaneously, chief nurse executives committed to evidence-based practice lead discussion and decision making regarding priority setting for areas of evidence-based practice (e.g., skin care, pain). Last, but most important, it is the chief nurse executive's responsibility to ensure that the mission, vision, philosophy of care, strategic plan, and performance criteria incorporate language about the value and commitment of the organization to evidence-based practice. Box 17-7 lists examples of performance expectations regarding evidence-based practice.

The third building block is integrating evidence-based practice into the governance of the health care system, and ensuring that resources are available to assist staff with this work. I am frequently asked, "Where should the work of evidence-based practice reside?" The short answer is "everywhere," because evidence-based practice saves health care dollars and improves

BOX 17-7 Sample Evidence-Based Practice Performance Criteria for Nursing Roles

STAFF NURSE (REGISTERED NURSE [RN])
- Questions current practices
- Participates in implementing changes in practice based on evidence
- Participates as a member of an evidence-based practice project team
- Reads evidence related to one's practice
- Participates in quality improvement (QI) initiatives
- Suggest resolutions for clinical issues based on evidence

ADVANCED PRACTICE NURSE (APN)
- Serves as coach and mentor in evidence-based practice
- Facilitates locating evidence
- Synthesizes evidence for practice
- Users evidence to write/modify practice standards
- Role models use of evidence in practice
- Facilitates system changes to support use of evidence-based practices

NURSE MANAGER (NM)
- Creates a microsystem that fosters critical thinking
- Challenges staff to seek out evidence to resolve clinical issues and improve care
- Role models evidence-based practice
- Uses evidence to guide operations and management decisions
- Uses performance criteria about evidence-based practice in evaluation of staff

ASSOCIATE DIRECTOR FOR CLINICAL SERVICES
- Hires and retains NMs and APNs with knowledge and skills in evidence-based practice
- Provides learning environment for evidence-based practice
- Uses evidence in leadership decisions
- Sets strategic directions for evidence-based practice
- Provides resources for evidence-based practice
- Integrates evidence-based practice processes into division/service line governance

CHIEF NURSE EXECUTIVE
- Ensures the governance reflects evidence-based practice if initiated in the councils and committees
- Assign accountabilty for evidence-based practice
- Ensures explicit articulation of organizational and department commitment to evidence-based practice
- Modifies mission and vision to include evidence-based practice language
- Provides resources to support evidence-based practices by direct care providers
- Articulates value of evidence-based practice to CEO and governing board
- Role models evidence-based practice in administrative decision making

patient outcomes (Brooks et al., 2008; Farquhar et al., 2002; Guyatt & Rennie, 2002; Titler et al., 2008). More explicitly, to sustain a vision of providing evidence-based health care, the work and accountability for evidence-based practice must be integrated into the governance structure. This includes interdisciplinary collaboration across departments and services, as well as coordination within discipline-specific areas of practice.

For example, in nursing, the process and evaluation of evidence-based changes in practice should be coordinated with professional nursing practice, quality improvement, research, policy and procedure, and staff education committees. An evidence-based project may be "born" out of a quality improvement committee when process or outcome indicators illustrate an opportunity to improve practice. Similarly, a professional nursing practice committee may initiate an evidence-based practice change in response to information published in research journals, by AHRQ evidence-based practice centers, or professional organizations. Evidence-based changes in practice must be coordinated with professional policy and procedure committees in order for the evidence to be reflected in practice standards. Documentation systems, be they electronic or manual, must support the evidence-based practices through reminder systems, decision-support algorithms, and easy-to-use documentation forms. Too often, we expect those in direct care to change practices without full modification of the documentation

BOX 17-8 Examples of Evidence-Based Practice Functions of Governance Committees

NURSING QUALITY MANAGEMENT COMMITTEE

- Develop mechanisms for using evidence-based practice to improve quality care.
- Assist nursing staff to interpret and use data from internal and external sources to improve care or resolve identified problems.
- Coordinate or conduct interdisciplinary performance improvement and use results of evidence-based practice projects that affect patient care delivery from multiple services.
- Promote a scientific approach to problem solving in management and delivery of patient care services.
- Promote discussion and exchange of information regarding status of evidence-based practice and process improvement projects.

PROFESSIONAL NURSING PRACTICE COMMITTEE

- Develop, evaluate, review, and revise policies and procedures related to professional nursing practice. Policies and procedures are evidence based, incorporate research findings, and reflect interdisciplinary collaboration as appropriate.

NURSING RESEARCH COMMITTEE

- Encourage and support the conduct and dissemination of nursing research regionally, nationally, and internationally.
- Develop mechanisms for using evidence-based practice to improve quality of care.
- Provide leadership for use of research findings and other evidence as an integral component of clinical practice and management decision making.
- Promote discussion and exchange of information regarding status of evidence-based practice and process improvement projects.
- Provide education and consultation to staff regarding the process and product of evidence-based practice projects.
- Maintain committee liaison and communication with the College of Nursing to encourage collaborative research and joint evidence-based practice projects between staff, faculty, and students.
- Consult with process improvement and evidence-based practice project teams about the critique of research and funding opportunities.
- Develop selected areas of interdisciplinary research and/or evidence-based practice that are strategically aligned with department and institutional goals.

RETENTION COMMITTEE

- Review the results of the National Database of Nursing Quality Indicators (NDNQI) nurse survey and identify opportunities to improve the work environment.
- Make evidence-based practice recommendations to improve nurse retention.
- Provide consultation for the use of research findings and other evidence as an integral component of management decision making regarding nurse retention.

systems that capture and reinforce the desired changes. Although the primary responsibility for tracking and promoting evidence-based practice may reside in a specific department or program (e.g., research, education, quality improvement), evidence-based practice must be viewed and valued as essential work at all levels of the organization, and within the committees/councils that govern the health care system. Examples of language reflecting evidence-based practice work in functions of committees and councils are in Box 17-8.

The fourth building block is recognition for and rewarding of evidence-based practice behaviors. Such recognition can range from submitting staff projects and names to national and international professional organizations that have recognition programs for excellence in evidence-based practice (e.g., STTI), to recognizing specific staff members in their unit at the shift change for the care they provide based on evidence. Other recognition activities include an annual recognition day with a display of posters of the evidence-based practice work occurring in each unit; recognition in a weekly or monthly internal communication; postings on Web sites; and broadcasting the stellar accomplishments in the local, regional, and national media. Some organizations integrate evidence-based practice expectations into the clinical ladder system, and others provide staff release time from direct patient care to do the work of evidence-based practice. Recognition by peers, as well as senior administrators, is important.

BOX 17-9 Outcomes of Integrating Evidence-Based Practice into Organizational Culture

SCIENTIFIC CRITERIA

1. The number of evidence-based practice projects
2. The number of evidence-based practice publications
3. The number of grants submitted and funded in which staff are investigators

ORGANIZATIONAL CLIMATE CRITERIA

1. Number of evidence-based practice standards used by staff
2. Number of staff participating in evidence-based practice activities
3. Climate of inquiry whereby staff question their practice
4. Increased number of professional nurses recruited and retained
5. Return of nurses to school for baccalaureate or higher degrees
6. National reputation, external consultations, and visits to the organization

COST AND QUALITY OF CARE

1. Decreased length of stay
2. Cost avoidance
3. Cost savings
4. Improved quality of care (e.g., decreased nosocomial urinary tract infections, improved pain management, decrease in nosocomial pressure ulcer development, increased satisfaction of families of critically ill patients)

Criteria for evaluating the success of integrating evidence-based practices into an organization's includes a combination of traditional scientific criteria, effect on the organizational climate, and improvements in providing cost-effective quality care. These criteria are summarized in Box 17-9.

TRANSLATION SCIENCE

Translation science, as discussed in this chapter, is the investigation of strategies to increase the rate and extent of adoption and sustainability of evidence-based practice by individuals and organizations to improve clinical and operational decision making (Eccles & Mittman, 2006; Titler, Everett, & Adams, 2007). It includes research to (1) understand context variables that influence adoption of evidence-based practices and (2) test the effectiveness of interventions to promote and sustain use of evidence-based health care practices. Translation science denotes both the systematic investigation of methods, interventions, and variables that influence adoption of evidence-based health care practices, as well as the organized body of knowledge gained through such research (Eccles & Mittman, 2006; Rubenstein & Pugh, 2006; Sussman et al., 2006; Titler, Everett, & Adams, 2007; Titler & Everett, 2001).

Because translation research is a young science, there are no standardized definitions of commonly used terms (Graham et al., 2006). This is evidenced by differing definitions and the interchanging of terms that, in fact, may represent different concepts to different people. Adding to the confusion, terminology may vary depending on the country in which the research was conducted (Adams & Titler, in press). A recent study done by Graham and colleagues (2006) reported identifying 29 terms in nine countries that refer to some aspect of translating research findings into practice. For example, researchers in Canada may use the terms *research utilization, knowledge-to-action, knowledge transfer,* or *knowledge translation* interchangeably, whereas researchers in the United States, the United Kingdom, and Europe may be more likely to use the terms *implementation* or *research translation* to express similar concepts (Graham et al., 2006; Graham & Logan, 2004; Titler & Everett, 2001).

The National Institutes of Health (NIH) has increased emphasis on translation research and has divided the concept into Type I and Type II. Type I translation focuses on the movement of research from basic science or bench research to efficacy trials. Type II translation is the movement from efficacy trials to effectiveness trials, dissemination trials, and implementation trials. Building a common taxonomy of terms in implementation science is of primary importance to this field and must involve input from a variety of stakeholders and researchers from various disciplines (e.g., health care, organizational science, psychology, and health services research) (Adams & Titler, in press; Institute of Medicine, 2007b).

Studies in a diversity of health care settings are beginning to build an empirical foundation of translation science (Titler, 2008). Federal agencies such as NIH, the Agency for Healthcare Research and Quality (AHRQ), and the VA have funded descriptive and intervention studies on research translation and dissemination (Brooks et al., 2008; Demakis et al., 2000; Dufault, 2004; Farquhar et al., 2002; Feldman & Kane, 2003; Hysong et al., 2006; Jones, Fink, Pepper, et al., 2004; Jones, Fink, Vojir, et al., 2004; Pineros et al., 2004; Smith et al., 2008; Stetler et al., 2006; Stetler et al., 2008; Titler, 2008; Titler et al., 2008).

These investigations and others (Estabrooks et al., 2008; Gifford et al., 2008; Godin et al., 2008; Gold & Taylor, 2007; Gravel et al., 2006; Litaker et al., 2008; Scott et al., 2008; Squires et al., 2007; Thompson et al., 2007; Wensing et al., 2006) provide a beginning scientific knowledge for promoting use of evidence in practice. The Institute of Medicine Forum on the Science of Quality Improvement and Implementation Research has sponsored several workshops on implementation science in which researchers have addressed various perspectives in conducting studies in this field (www.nap.edu). Methods used in implementation studies range from qualitative, phenomenological studies to randomized controlled trials. Links between generalizable scientific evidence for a given health care topic and the particular contexts create opportunities for experiential learning in implementation science (Institute of Medicine, 2007a).

Building this body of research knowledge demands development in many areas; theoretical developments are needed to provide frameworks and predictive theories for creating generalizable research such as how to change individual and organizational behavior. Methodological developments are also required, as well as exploratory studies aimed at understanding the experiential and organizational learning that accompanies implementation. Rigorous evaluations are needed to evaluate the effectiveness and efficiency of implementation interventions (Adams & Titler, in press). Partnerships are needed to encourage communication among researchers, theorists, and implementers and to understand what types of knowledge are needed and how that knowledge can best be developed (Adams & Titler, in press; Dawson, 2004; Gold & Taylor, 2007; Titler, 2004a; Tripp-Reimer & Doebbeling, 2004).

Nurse scientists are leaders in translation science and provide exemplars for others interested in this specialized area of research (Dawson, 2004; Donaldson, Rutledge, & Ashley, 2004; Dufault, 2004; Estabrooks et al., 2008; Feldman & McDonald, 2004; Fraser, 2004a, 2004b; Kirchhoff, 2004; Pineros et al., 2004; Rycroft-Malone et al., 2004; Stetler et al., 2008; Titler, 2004a, 2004b, 2008; Titler, Everett, & Adams, 2007; Tripp-Reimer & Doebbeling, 2004; U.S. Invitational Conference, 2004; Watson, 2004; Williams, 2004).

FUTURE DIRECTIONS

For organizations to take advantage of evidence-based practice projects from various sites throughout the country, a National Center for Evidence-Based Practice and Translation Science is needed. Such a center would encompass a computerized database of evidence-based practices that includes the relevant policy and procedure or practice standard, the population to which it applies, the quality improvement indicators and data-collection forms used in evaluation, a list of references, suggested strategies for change, the type of institutions where the evidence-based practice has been implemented, contact people at each agency, and the evidence-based practice topic content expert. This information should be available online through electronic communications such as a dedicated Listserv, or some other form of electronic media. Such a center could facilitate networking among health care professionals working on similar evidence-based topics and provide helpful consultants and educational materials (Adams & Titler, in review; Titler, 1997). This center also would provide data regarding the interventions/strategies that have been tested to translate research into practice and provide a "tool kit" of these interventions for use by all types of health care agencies (QUERI, 2004; Registered Nurses Association of Ontario, 2004; Titler, 2002). Last, such a center would also conduct translation research and provide consultation regarding research methods and design specifically for translation science (Adams & Titler, in review; Titler, 2004a).

Education of nurses must include knowledge and skills in the use of research evidence in practice. Nurses are increasingly being held accountable for practices based on scientific evidence. Thus we must communicate and integrate into our profession the expectation that it is the professional responsibility of all nurses to read and use research in their practice and to communicate with nurse scientists the many and varied clinical problems for which we do not yet have a scientific base.

CRITICAL THINKING CHALLENGES

- Discuss the differences among nursing research, research utilization, and evidence-based practice. Support your discussion with examples.
- Why would it be important to use an evidence-based practice model, such as the Iowa Model of Evidence-Based Practice, to guide a practice project focused on justifying and implementing a change in clinical practice?
- You are a staff nurse working on a cardiac step-down unit. Many of your colleagues do not understand evidence-based practice. How would you help them to understand the relevance of evidence-based practice to providing optimal care to this patient population?
- What barriers do you see to applying evidence-based practice in your clinical setting? Discuss strategies to use in overcoming these barriers.

KEY POINTS

- The terms *research utilization* and *evidence-based practice* are sometimes used interchangeably. These terms, though related, are not one and the same. Research utilization is the process of using research findings to improve practice. Evidence-based practice is a broad term that not only encompasses use of research findings but also use of other types of evidence such as case reports and expert opinion in deciding the evidence base for practice.
- There are two forms of evidence use: conceptual and decision driven.
- There are several models of evidence-based practice. A key feature of all models is the judicious review and synthesis of research and other types of evidence to develop an evidence-based practice standard.

- The steps of evidence-based practice using the Iowa Model of Evidence-Based Practice are as follows: selection of a topic, forming a team, retrieval of the evidence, grading the evidence, developing an evidence-based practice standard, implementing the evidence-based practice, and evaluating the effect on staff, patient, and fiscal outcomes.
- Adoption of evidence-based practice standards requires education and dissemination to staff and use of change strategies such as opinion leaders, change champions, use of a core group, and use of consultants.
- It is important to evaluate the change. Evaluation provides data for performance gap assessment, audit, and feedback, and provides information necessary to determine if the practice should be retained.
- Evaluation includes both process and outcome measures.
- It is important for organizations to create a culture of evidence-based practice. To create this culture requires an interactive process. To provide this culture, organizations need to provide access to information, access to individuals who have skills necessary for evidence-based practice, and a written and verbal commitment to evidence-based practice in the organization's operations.

REFERENCES

Adams S, Titler MG: Implementation science. In Mateo MA, Kirchhoff KT, eds: *Using and conducting nursing research in the clinical settings*, Philadelphia, 1999, WB Saunders.

Adams SL, Titler MG: Building a learning collaborative (unpublished). *Worldviews on Evidence-Based Nursing.*

Adler PS, Kwon SW, Singer JMK: The "Six-West" problem: professional and the intraorganizational diffusion of innovations, with particular reference to the case of hospitals. Working paper 3-15. Los Angeles, 2003, Marshall School of Business, University of Southern California. Available at www.marshall.usc.edu/web/MOR.cfm?doc_id=5561.

Alderson P, Green S, Higgins JPT: *Cochrane reviewers' handbook 4.2.1*, 2003. Retrieved March 30, 2004, from www.cochrane.org/resources/handbook/handbook.pdf.

Alm A, Hornmark AM, Fall PA, et al: Care of pressure sores: a controlled study of the use of a hydrocolloid dressing compared with wet saline gauze compresses, *Acta Derm Venereol* 149:S1-S10, 1989.

American Geriatrics Society, British Geriatrics Society, American Academy of Orthopaedic Surgeons, Panel on Falls Prevention: Guideline for the prevention of falls in older persons, *J Am Geriatr Soc* 49(5):664-672, 2001.

Anderson RA, Ammarell N, Bailey DE, et al: The power of relationship for high-quality long-term care, *J Nurs Care Qual* 20(2):103-106, 2004.

Anderson RA, Crabtree BF, Steele DJ, et al: Case study research: the view from complexity science, *Qual Health Res* 15(5):669-685, 2005.

Anderson RA, Issel LM, McDaniel RR: Nursing homes as complex adaptive systems: relationship between management practice and resident outcomes, *Nurs Res* 52(1):12-21, 2003.

Antrobus S, Kitson A: Nursing leadership: influencing and shaping health policy and nursing practice, *J Adv Nurs* 29(3):746-753, 1999.

Atkins D, Briss PA, Eccles M, et al: Systems for grading the quality of evidence and the strength of recommendations II: pilot study of a new system, *BMC Health Serv Res* 5(1):25, 2005.

Baggs JG, Mick DJ: Collaboration: a tool addressing ethical issues for elderly patients near the end of life in intensive care units, *J Gerontol Nurs* 26(9):41-47, 2000.

Balas EA, Krishna S, Kretschmer RA, et al: Computerized knowledge management in diabetes care, *Med Care* 42(6):610-621, 2004.

Barnason S, Merboth M, Pozehl B, et al: Utilizing an outcomes approach to improve pain management by nurses: a pilot study, *Clin Nurse Spec* 12(1):28-36, 1998.

Barnsley J, Lemieux-Charles L, McKinney MM: Integrating learning into integrated delivery systems, *Health Care Manage Rev* 18-28, 1998.

Barnsteiner JH, Ford N, Howe C: Research utilization in a metropolitan children's hospital, *Nurs Clin North Am* 30(3):447-455, 1995.

Batalden PB, Nelson EC, Edwards WH, et al: Microsystems in health care: part 9. Developing small clinical units to attain peak performance, *Joint Commission Journal on Quality and Safety* 29(11):575-585, 2003.

Bates DW, Kuperman GJ, Wang S, et al: Ten commandments for effective clinical decision support: making the practice of evidence-based medicine a reality, *J Am Med Informatics Assoc* 10(6):523-530, 2003.

Berner ES, Baker CS, Funkhouser E, et al: Do local opinion leaders augment hospital quality improvement efforts? A randomized trial to promote adherence to unstable angina guideline, *Med Care* 41(3):420-431, 2003.

Berwick DM: Disseminating innovations in health care, *JAMA* 289(15):1969-1975, 2003.

Blondin MM, Titler MG: Deep vein thrombosis and pulmonary embolism prevention: What role do nurses play? *Medsurg Nurs* 5(3):205-208, 1996.

Bootsmiller BJ, Yankey JW, Flach SD, et al: Classifying the effectiveness of Veterans Affairs guideline implementation approaches, *Am J Med Qual* 19(6):248-254, 2004.

Bradley EH, Holmboe ES, Mattera JA, et al: Data feedback efforts in quality improvement: lessons learned from US hospitals, *Qual Saf Health Care* 13:26-31, 2004.

Bradley EH, Schlesinger M, Webster TR, et al: Translating research into clinical practice: making change happen, *J Am Geriatr Soc* 52(11):1875-1882, 2004.

Brooks JM, Titler MG, Ardery G, et al: Effect of evidence-based acute pain management practices on inpatient costs, *Health Serv Res* 2008. Retrieved from www3.interscience.wiley.com/journal/120120473/issue.

Buonocore D: Leadership and action: creating a change in practice, *AACN Clin Issues* 15(2):170-181, 2004.

Carr CA, Schott A: Differences in evidence-based care in midwifery practice and education, *J Nurs Sch* 34(2):153-158, 2002.

Carter BL, Doucette WR, Bergus G, et al: Relationship between physician knowledge of hypertension and blood pressure control, *Am J Hypertens* 18(5, pt 2):A218, 2005.

Centers for Medicare and Medicaid Services: 2008. Retrieved December 2008 from www.cms.hhs.gov/.

Ciliska D, Hayward S, Dobbins M, et al: Transferring public-health nursing research to health-system planning: assessing the relevance and accessibility of systematic reviews, *Can J Nurs Res* 31(1):23-36, 1999.

Clancy CM, Cronin, K: Evidence-based decision making: global evidence, local decisions, *Health Aff* 24(1):151-162, 2005.

Clancy CM, Slutsky JR, Patton LT: AHRQ moves research to translation and implementation, *Health Serv Res* 39(5):xv-xxiii, 2004a.

Collins BA, Hawks JW, Davis R: From theory to practice: identifying authentic opinion leaders to improve care, *Manag Care* 9(7):56-58, 61-62, 2000.

Colwell JC, Foreman MD, Trotter JP: A comparison of the efficacy and cost-effectiveness of two methods of managing pressure ulcers, *Decubitus* 6(4):28-36, 1992.

Cook D: Evidence-based critical care medicine: a potential tool for change, *New Horizons* 6(1):20-25, 1998.

Cook DJ, Greengold NL, Ellrodt AG, et al: The relation between systematic reviews and practice guidelines, *Ann Intern Med* 127(3):210-216, 1997.

Cronenwett LR: Effective methods for disseminating research findings to nurses in practice, *Nurs Clin North Am* 30:429-438, 1995.

Cullen L: Evidence-based practice: strategies for nursing leaders. In Huber D, ed: *Leadership and nursing care management*, ed 3, Philadelphia, 2005, Elsevier.

Cullen L, Greiner J, Greiner J, et al: Excellence in evidence-based practice: an organizational and MICU exemplar, *Crit Care Nurs Clin North Am* 17(2):127-142, 2005.

Cullen L, Titler MG: Promoting evidence-based practice: an internship for staff nurses, *Worldviews on Evidence-Based Practice* 1(4):215-223, 2004.

Davey P, Brown E, Fenelon L, et al: Interventions to improve antibiotic prescribing practices for hospital inpatients, *Cochrane Database of Systematic Reviews,* 4, 2005. Art. No.: CD003543. DOI: 003510.001002/14651858.CD14003543.pub14651852.

Dawson JD: Quantitative analytical methods in translation research, *Worldviews on Evidence-Based Nursing* 1(S1):S60-S64, 2004.

Demakis JG, McQueen L, Kizer KW, et al: Quality Enhancement Research Initiative (QUERI): a collaboration between research and clinical practice, *Med Care* 38(6 suppl 1):I17-I25, 2000.

Denis JL, Hebert Y, Langley A, et al: Explaining diffusion patterns for complex health care innovations, *Health Care Manage Rev* 27(3):60-73, 2002.

DiCenso A, Ciliska D, Cullum N, et al: *Evidence-based nursing: a guide to clinical practice*, St Louis, 2004, Mosby.

Doebbeling BN, Chou AF, Tierney WM: Priorities and strategies for the implementation of integrated informatics and communications technology to improve evidence-based practice, *J Gen Intern Med* 21(S2):S50-57, 2006.

Doebbeling BN, Vaughn TE, Woolson RF, et al: Benchmarking Veterans Affairs Medical Centers in the delivery of preventive health services: comparison of methods, *Med Care* 40(6):540-554, 2002.

Donaldson NE, Rutledge DN, Ashley J: Outcomes of adoption: measuring evidence uptake by individuals and organizations, *Worldviews on Evidence-Based Nursing* 1(S1):S41-S51, 2004.

Dopson S, FitzGerald L, Ferlie E, et al: No magic targets! Changing clinical practice to become more evidence based, *Health Care Manage Rev* 27(3):35-47, 2002.

Dopson S, Locock L, Chambers D, et al: Implementation of evidence-based medicine: evaluation of the Promoting Action on Clinical Effectiveness programme, *J Health Serv Res Policy* 6(1):23-31, 2001.

Dufault MA: A program of research evaluating the effects of collaborative research utilization model, *Online Journal of Knowledge Synthesis for Nursing* 8(3):7, 2001.

Dufault MA: Testing a collaborative research utilization model to translate best practices in pain management, *Worldviews on Evidence-Based Nursing* 1(S1):S26-S32, 2004.

Duncan K, Pozehl B: Effects of performance feedback on patient pain outcomes, *Clin Nurs Res* 9(4):379-397, 2000.

Eccles MP, Mittman BS: Welcome to implementation science, *Implementation Science* 1:1, 2006.

Engberg S, Kincade J, Thompson D: Future directions for incontinence research with frail elders, *Nurs Res* 53(6S):S22-S29, 2004.

Estabrooks CA: Translating research into practice: implications for organizations and administrators, *Can J Nurs Res* 35(3):53-68, 2003.

Estabrooks CA: Thoughts on evidence-based nursing and its science: a Canadian perspective, *Worldviews on Evidence-Based Nursing* 1(2):88-91, 2004.

Estabrooks CA, Chong H, Brigidear K, et al: Profiling Canadian nurses' preferred knowledge sources for clinical practice, *Can J Nurs Res* 37(2):119-140, 2005.

Estabrooks CA, Derksen L, Winther C, et al: The intellectual structure and substance of the knowledge utilization field: a longitudinal author co-citation analysis, 1945-2004, *Implementation Science* 3:49, 2008.

Estabrooks CA, Floyd JA, Scott-Findlay S, et al: Individual determinants of research utilization: a systematic review, *J Adv Nurs* 43(5):506-520, 2003.

Estabrooks CA, O'Leary KA, Ricker KL, et al: The Internet and access to evidence: how are nurses positioned? *J Adv Nurs* 42(1):73-81, 2003.

Estabrooks CA, Rutakumwa W, O'Leary KA, et al: Sources of practice knowledge among nurses, *Qual Health Res* 15(4):460-476, 2005.

Farquhar CM, Stryer D, Slutsky J: Translating research into practice: the future ahead, *Int J Qual Health Care* 14(3):233-249, 2002.

Feldman PH, Kane RL: Strengthening research to improve the practice and management of long-term care, *Milbank Q* 81(2):179-220, 2003.

Feldman PH, McDonald MV: Conducting translation research in the home care setting: lessons from a just-in-time reminder study, *Worldviews on Evidence-Based Nursing* 1:49-59, 2004.

Feldman PH, Murtaugh CM, Pezzin LE, et al: Just-in-time evidence-based e-mail "reminders" in home health care: impact on patient outcomes, *Health Serv Res* 40(3):865-885, 2005.

Ferlie E, Gabbay J, Fitzgerald L, et al: Evidence-based medicine and organisational change: an overview of some recent qualitative research. In Ashburner L, ed: *Organisational behavior and organisational studies in health care: reflections on the future*, Basingstoke, 2001, Palgrave.

Fleuren M, Wiefferink K, Paulussen T: Determinants of innovation within health care organizations: literature review and Delphi study, *Int J Qual Health Care* 16(2):107-123, 2004.

Folkedahl B, Frantz R, Goode C: *Evidence-based protocol: treatment of pressure ulcers* (series editor: Titler MG), Iowa City, 2002, Research Dissemination Core, Gerontological Nursing Interventions Research Center, University of Iowa College of Nursing (P30 NR03979; PI: T. Tripp-Reimer).

Fowler E, Goupil DL: Comparison of the wet-to-dry dressing and a copolymer starch in the management of debrided pressure sores, *J Enterostomal Ther* 11(1):22-25, 1984.

Fraser I: Organizational research with impact: working backwards, *Worldviews on Evidence-Based Nursing* 1(S1):S52-S59, 2004a.

Fraser I: Translation research: where do we go from here? *Worldviews on Evidence-Based Nursing* 1(S1):S78-S83, 2004b.

Fung CH, Woods JN, Asch SM, et al: Variation in implementation and use of computerized clinical reminders in an integrated healthcare system, *Am J Managed Care* 10(pt 2):878-885, 2004.

Funk SG, Champagne MT, Tornquist EM, et al: Administrators' views on barriers to research utilization, *Appl Nurs Res* 8(1):44-49, 1995.

Gerrish K, Clayton J: Promoting evidence-based practice: an organizational approach, *J Nurs Manage* 12:114-123, 2004.

Gifford WA, Davies B, Graham ID, et al: A mixed methods pilot study with a cluster randomized control trial to evaluate the impact of a leadership intervention on guideline implementation in home care nursing, *Implementation Science* 3:51, 2008.

Gillbody S, Whitty P, Grimshaw J, et al: Educational and organizational interventions to improve the management of depression in primary care (a systematic review), *JAMA* 289(23):3145-3151, 2003.

Godin G, Bélanger-Gravel A, Eccles M, et al: Healthcare professionals' intentions and behaviours: a systematic review of studies based on social cognitive theories, *Implementation Science* 3:36, 2008.

Gold M, Taylor EF: Moving research into practice: lessons from the US Agency for Healthcare Research and Quality's IDSRN program, *Implementation Science* 2:9, 2007.

Goode CJ, Piedalue F: Evidence-based clinical practice, *J Nurs Admin* 29(6):15-21, 1999.

Gorse GJ, Messner RL: Improved pressure sore healing with hydrocolloid dressings, *Arch Dermatol* 123(6):766-771, 1987.

GRADE Working Group: Grading quality of evidence and strength of recommendations, *BMJ* 328:1490-1494, 2004.

Graham ID, Logan J, Harrison MB, et al: Lost in knowledge translation: time for a map? *J Contin Educ Health Prof* 26(1):13-24, 2006.

Graham K, Logan J: Using the Ottawa model of research use to implement a skin care program, *J Nurs Care Qual* 19(1):18-24, 2004.

Gravel K, Légaré F, Graham ID: Barriers and facilitators to implementing shared decision-making in clinical practice: a systematic review of health professionals' perceptions, *Implementation Science* 1:16, 2006.

Greenhalgh T, Robert G, Bate P, et al: *Diffusion of innovations in health service organisations: a systematic literature review*, Malden, MA, 2005, Blackwell.

Greer AL: The state of the art versus the state of the science, *Int J Technol AssessHealth Care* 4:5-26, 1988.

Grilli R, Ramsay C, Minozzi S: Mass media interventions: effects on health services utilisation, *Cochrane Database of Systematic Reviews*, 1, 2002. Art. No.: CD000389. DOI: 000310.001002/14651858. CD14000389.

Grimshaw J, Eccles M, Thomas R, et al: Toward evidence-based quality improvement: evidence (and its limitations) of the effectiveness of guideline dissemination and implementation strategies 1966-1998, *J Gen Intern Med* 21(suppl 2), S14-20, 2006.

Grimshaw JM, Eccles MP, Greener J, et al: Is the involvement of opinion leaders in the implementation of research findings a feasible strategy? *Implementation Science* 1(3), 2006.

Grimshaw JM, Thomas RE, MacLennan G, et al: Effectiveness and efficiency of guide dissemination and implementation strategies, *Health Technol Assess* 8(6):i-xi, 1-72, 2004.

Grol RP, Bosch MC, Hulscher ME, et al: Planning and studying improvement in patient care: the use of theoretical perspectives, *Milbank Q* 85(1):93-138, 2007.

Grumbach K, Bodenheimer T: Can healthcare teams improve primary care practice? *JAMA* 291(10):1246-1251, 2004.

Guihan M, Bosshart HT, Nelson A: Lessons learned in implementing SCI clinical practice guidelines, *SCINursing* 21(3):136-142, 2004.

Guyatt GH, Oxman AD, Kunz R, Jaeschke R, et al: Rating quality of evidence and strength of recommendations: incorporating considerations of resources use into grading recommendations, *BMJ* 336(7654):1170-1173, 2008.

Guyatt GH, Oxman AD, Kunz R, Vist GE, et al: Rating quality of evidence and strength of recommendations: what is "quality of evidence" and why is it important to clinicians? *BMJ* 336(7651):995-998, 2008.

Guyatt GH, Oxman AD, Vist G, et al: Rating quality of evidence and strength of recommendations GRADE: an emerging consensus on rating quality of evidence and strength of recommendations, *BMJ* 336:924-926, 2008.

Guyatt GH, Rennie D: *Users' guide to the medical literature: essentials of evidence-based clinical practice*, Chicago, 2002, American Medical Association.

Haber J, Feldman HR, Penney N, et al: Shaping nursing practice through research-based protocols, *J NY State Nurses Assoc* 25(3):4-12, 1994.

Hagedorn H, Hogan M, Smith JL, et al: Lessons learned about implementing research evidence into clinical practice: experiences from VA QUERI, *J Gen Intern Med* 21:S21-24, 2006.

Haller KB, Reynolds MA, Horsley JA: Developing research-based innovation protocols: process, criteria, and issues, *Res Nurs Health* 2:45-51, 1979.

Harris RP, Helfan M, Woolf SH, et al: Current methods of the U.S. Preventive Services Task Force: a review of the process, *Am J Prev Med* 20(3S):21-35, 2001.

Harvey G, Loftus-Hills A, Rycroft-Malone J, et al: Getting evidence into practice: the role and function of facilitation, *J Adv Nurs* 37(6):577-588, 2002.

Heitkemper MM, Bond EF: Clinical nurse specialist: state of the profession and challenges ahead, *Clin Nurse Spec* 18(3):135-140, 2004.

Hendryx MS, Fieselmann JF, Bock MJ, et al: Outreach education to improve quality of rural ICU care. Results of a randomized trial, *Am J Respir Crit Care Med* 158(2):418-423, 1998.

Herr K, Titler M, Sorofman B, et al: *Evidence-based guideline: acute pain management in the elderly*, Iowa City, 2000, University of Iowa. From Book To Bedside: Acute Pain Management in the Elderly, 1 R01, HS10482-01.

Horbar JD, Soll RF, Suresh G, et al: *Evidence-based surfactant therapy for preterm infants. Final progress report to AHRQ*, Burlington, VT, 2004, University of Vermont. R01 HS1052803.

Horsley JA, Crane J, Crabtree MK, et al: *Using research to improve nursing practice: a guide*, New York, 1983, Grune & Stratton.

Hunt DL, Haynes RB, Hanna SE, et al: Effects of computer-based clinical decision support systems on physician performance and patient outcomes: a systematic review, *JAMA* 280(15):1339-1346, 1998.

Hysong SJ, Best RG, Pugh JA: Audit and feedback and clinical practice guideline adherence: making feedback actionable, *Implementation Science* 1:9, 2006.

ICEBeRG: Designing theoretically-informed implementation interventions: the Improved Clinical Effectiveness through Behavioural Research Group, *Implementation Science* 1:4, 2006.

Institute of Medicine: *Crossing the quality chasm: a new health system for the 21st century*, Washington, DC, 2001, National Academies Press.

Institute of Medicine: *Advancing quality improvement research: challenges and opportunities.* Workshop summary, Washington, DC, 2007a, National Academies Press.

Institute of Medicine: *The state of quality improvement and implementation research: expert reviews.* Workshop summary, Washington, DC, 2007b, National Academies Press.

Institute of Medicine: *Knowing what works in health care: a roadmap for the nation. Committee on Reviewing Evidence to Identify Highly Effective Clinical Services*, Washington, DC, 2008, National Academies Press.

Irwin C, Ozer EM: *Implementing adolescent preventive guidelines. Final progress report to AHRQ*, San Francisco, 2004, University of California, San Francisco, Division of Adolescent Medicine U18HS11095.

James B: Information system concepts for quality measurement, *Med Care* 41(1 suppl):I71-I79, 2003.

Jamtvedt G, Young JM, Kristoffersen DT, et al: Audit and feedback: effects on professional practice and health care outcomes, *Cochrane Database of Systematic Reviews,* 2, 2006. Art. No.: CD000259. pub000252. DOI: 000210.001002/14651858.CD14000259.pub14651852.

Jennings BM, Loan LA: Misconceptions among nurses about evidence-based practice, *J Nurs Sch* 33(2):121-127, 2001.

Jha AK, Ferris TG, Donelan K, et al: How common are electronic health records in the United States? A summary of the evidence, *Health Aff* 25(6):W496-W507, 2006.

Jones J: Performance improvement through clinical research utilization: the linkage model, *J Nurs Care Qual* 15(1):49-54, 2000.

Jones KR, Fink R, Pepper G, et al: Improving nursing home staff knowledge and attitudes about pain, *Gerontologist* 44(4):469-478, 2004.

Jones KR, Fink R, Vojir C, et al: Translation research in long-term care: improving pain management in nursing homes, *Worldviews on Evidence-Based Nursing* 1(S1):S13-S20, 2004.

Katz DA, Brown RB, Muehlenbruch DR, et al: Implementing guidelines for smoking cessation: comparing the effects of nurses and medical assistants, *Am J Prev Med* 27(5):411-416, 2004.

Katz DA, Muehlenbruch DR, Brown RB, et al: Effectiveness of a clinic-based strategy for implementing the AHRQ Smoking Cessation Guideline in primary care, *Prev Med* 35:293-302, 2002.

Katz DA, Muehlenbruch DR, Brown RL, et al: Effectiveness of implementing the Agency for Healthcare Research and Quality Smoking Cessation Clinical Practice Guideline: a randomized, controlled trial, *J Natl Cancer Inst* 96(8):594-603, 2004.

Kiefe CI, Sales AE: A state-of-the-art conference on implementing evidence in health care: reasons and recommendations, *J Gen Intern Med* 21:S67-S70, 2006.

Kirchhoff KT: State of the science of translational research: from demonstration projects to intervention testing, *Worldviews on Evidence-Based Nursing* 1(S1):S6-S12, 2004.

Kochevar LK, Yano EM: Understanding health care organization needs and context: beyond performance gaps, *J Gen Intern Med* 21:S25-S29, 2006.

Kurzuk-Howard G, Simpson L, Palmieri A: Decubitus ulcer care: a comparative study, *West J Nurs Res* 7(1):58-79, 1985.

Lavis JN, Robertson D, Woodside JM, et al: How can research organizations more effectively transfer research knowledge to decision makers? *Milbank Q* 81(2):221-248, 2003.

Leape LL: *Advances in patient safety: from research to implementation, vol 3, Implementation issues*, AHRQ pub no 05-0021-3, Rockville, MD, 2005, Agency for Healthcare Research and Quality.

Levine RS, Husaini BA, Briggs N, et al: *Translating prevention research into practice. Final progress report to AHRQ,* Nashville, TN, 2004, Meharry Medical College/Tennessee State University. 5U 18HS011131.

Litaker D, Ruhe M, Weyer S, et al: Association of intervention outcomes with practice capacity for change: subgroup analysis from a group randomized trial, *Implementation Science* 3:25, 2008.

Litaker D, Tomolo A, Liberatore V, et al: Using complexity theory to build interventions that improve health care delivery in primary care, *J Gen Intern Med* 21:S30-S34, 2006.

Locock L, Dopson S, Chambers D, et al: Understanding the role of opinion leaders in improving clinical effectiveness, *Soc Sci Med* 53:745-757, 2001.

Loeb M, Brazil K, McGeer A, et al: *Optimizing antibiotic use in long term care. Final progress report to AHRQ,* Hamilton, Ontario, 2004, McMaster University. 2R18HS011113-03.

Logan J, Harrison MB, Graham ID, et al: Evidence-based pressure-ulcer practice: the Ottawa Model of Research Use, *Can J Nurs Res* 31(1):37-52, 1999.

Lomas J, Enkin M, Anderson GM, et al: Opinion leaders vs. audit and feedback to implement practice guidelines: delivery after previous cesarean section, *JAMA* 265:2202-2207, 1991.

Lozano P, Finkelstein JA, Carey VJ, et al: A multisite randomized trial of the effects of physician education and organizational change in chronic-asthma care, *Arch Pediatr Adolesc Med* 158:875-883, 2004.

Madsen D, Sebolt T, Cullen L, et al: Listening to bowel sounds: an evidence-based practice project, *Am J Nurs* 105(12):40-49, quiz 49-50, 2005.

McDonald MV, Pezzin LE, Feldman PH, et al: Can just-in-time, evidence-based "reminders" improve pain management among home health care nurses and their patients? *J Pain Symptom Manage* 29(5):474-488, 2005.

McGlynn EA, Asch SM, Adams J, et al: The quality of health care delivered to adults in the United States, *N Engl J Med* 348(26):2635-2645, 2003.

Meyer AD, Goes JB: Organizational assimilation of innovations: a multilevel contextual analysis, *Academy of Management Journal* 31:897-923, 1988.

Milner FM, Estabrooks CA, Humphrey C: Clinical nurse educators as agents for change: increasing research utilization, *Int J Nurs Stud* 42(8):899-914, 2005.

Morin KH, Bucher L, Plowfield L, et al: Using research to establish protocols for practice: a statewide study of acute care agencies, *Clin Nurse Spec* 13(2):77-84, 1999.

Murtaugh CM, Pezzin LE, McDonald MV, et al: Just-in-time evidence-based e-mail "reminders" in home health care: impact on nurse practices, *Health Serv Res* 40(3):843-858, 2005.

Nagy S, Lumby J, McKinley S, et al: Nurses' beliefs about the conditions that hinder or support evidence-based nursing, *Int J Nurs Pract* 7(5):314-321, 2001.

Neill KM, Conforti C, Kedas A, et al: Pressure sore response to a new hydrocolloid dressing, *Wounds* 1(3):173-185, 1989.

Nelson EC, Batalden PB, Huber TP, et al: Microsystems in health care: earning from high performing front-line clinical units, *J Qual Improv* 28(9):472-493, 2002.

Nightingale F: *Notes on matters affecting the health, efficiency, and hospital administration of the British Army,* London, 1858, Harrison & Sons.

Nightingale F: *A contribution to the sanitary history of the British Army during the late war with Russia,* London, 1859, John W. Parker & Sons.

Nightingale F: *Notes on hospitals,* London, 1863a, Longman, Green, Roberts, & Green.

Nightingale F: *Observation on the evidence contained in the statistical reports submitted by her to the Royal Commission on the Sanitary State of the Army in India,* London, 1863b, Edward Stanford.

Nutley S, Davies H, Walter I: *Evidence based policy and practice: cross sector lessons from the UK.* Keynote paper for the Social Policy Research and Evaluation Conference, Wellington, NZ, 2003.

Nutley S, Davies HTO: Making a reality of evidence-based practice: some lessons from the diffusion of innovations, *Public Money and Management,* October-December:35-42, 2000.

O'Brien MA, Freemantle N, Oxman AD, et al: Continuing education meetings and workshops: effects on professional practice and health care outcomes, *Cochrane Database of Systematic Reviews,* 1, 2001. Art. No.: CD003030. DOI: 003010.001002/14651858.CD14003030.

O'Brien MA, Oxman AD, Davis DA, et al: Educational outreach visits: effects on professional practice and health care outcomes, *Cochrane Database of Systematic Reviews,* 4, 1997. Art. No.: CD000409. DOI: 000410.001002/14651858.CD14000409.

O'Brien MA, Oxman AD, Haynes RB, et al: Local opinion leaders: effects on professional practice and health care outcomes, *Cochrane Database of Systematic Reviews,* 1, 1999. Art. No.: CD000125. DOI: 000110.001002/14651858.CD14000125.

Olade RA: Evidence-based practice and research utilization activities among rural nurses, *J Nurs Sch* 36(3):220-225, 2004.

Oleske DM, Smith XP, White P, et al: A randomized clinical trial of two dressing methods for the treatment of low-grade pressure ulcers, *J Enterostomal Ther* 13(3):90-98, 1986.

Omery A, Williams RP: An appraisal of research utilization across the United States, *J Nurs Admin* 29(12):50-56, 1999.

Oxman AD, Thomson MA, Davis DA, et al: No magic bullets: a systematic review of 102 trials of interventions to improve professional practice, *Can Med Assoc J* 153(10):1423-1431, 1995.

Pettit DM, Kraus V: The use of gauze versus transparent dressings for peripheral intravenous catheter sites. In Titler MG, Goode CJ, eds: *Nursing clinics of North America*, Philadelphia, 1995, WB Saunders.

Pineros SL, Sales AE, Yu-Fang L, et al: Improving care to patients with ischemic heart disease: experiences in a single network of the Veterans Health Administration, *Worldviews on Evidence-Based Nursing* 1(S1):S33-S40, 2004.

Profetto-McGrath J, Hesketh KL, Lang S, et al: A study of critical thinking and research utilization among nurses, *West J Nurs Res* 25(3):322-337, 2003.

QUERI: Retrieved November 30, 2004, from www.hsrd.research.va.gov/queri/implementation/section_2/default.cfm.

Rakel BA, Titler MG, eds: *Critical Care Nursing Clinics of North America: Pain Management in Critical Care* 13(2), 2001.

Redfern S, Christian S: Achieving change in health care practice, *J Evaluation Clin Pract* 9(2):225-238, 2003.

Redman RW: Improving the practice environment for evidence-based practice, *Res Theory Nurs Pract* 18(2-3):127-129, 2004.

Registered Nurses Association of Ontario: Implementation of clinical practice guidelines, 2004. Retrieved November 30, 2004, from www.rnao.org/bestpractices/completed_guidelines/BPG_Guide_C1_Toolkit.asp.

Retchin SM: The modification of physician practice patterns, *Clin Perform Qual Health Care* 5:202-207, 1997.

Rogers EM: *Diffusion of innovations*, New York, 1995, Free Press.

Rogers EM: *Diffusion of innovations*, ed 5, New York, 2003a, Free Press.

Rogers EM: Innovation in organizations. In Rogers EM, ed: *Diffusion of innovations,* ed 5, New York, 2003b, Free Press.

Rubenstein LV, Pugh JA: Strategies for promoting organizational and practice change by advancing implementation research, *J Gen Intern Med* 21:S58-S64, 2006.

Rutledge DN, Donaldson NE: Building organizational capacity to engage in research utilization, *J Nurs Admin* 25(10):12-16, 1995.

Rutledge DN, Greene P, Mooney K, et al: Use of research-based practices by oncology staff nurses, *Oncol Nurs Forum* 23(8):1235-1244, 1996.

Rycroft-Malone J, Kitson A, Harvey G, et al: Ingredients for change: revisiting a conceptual framework, *Qual Saf Health Care* 11:174-180, 2002.

Rycroft-Malone J, Seers K, Titchen A, et al: What counts as evidence in evidence-based practice? *J Adv Nurs* 47(1):81-90, 2004.

Sackett D, Rosenberg W, Gray J, et al: Evidence based medicine: what it is and what it isn't, *BMJ* 312:71-72, 1996.

Sackett DL, Straus SE, Richardson WS, et al: *Evidence-based medicine: how to practice and teach EBM*, London, 2000, Churchill Livingstone.

Salem-Schatz SR, Gottlieb LK, Karp MA, et al: Attitudes about clinical practice guidelines in a mixed model HMO: the influence of physician and organizational characteristics, *HMO Pract* 11(3):111-117, 1997.

Saydak SJ: A pilot test of two methods for the treatment of pressure ulcers, *J Enterostomal Ther* 17(3):139-142, 1990.

Schmidt KL, Alpen MA, Rakel BA: Implementation of the Agency for Health Care Policy and Research pain guidelines, *AACN Clin Issues* 7(3):425-435, 1996.

Schneider EC, Eisenberg JM: Strategies and methods for aligning current and best medical practices: the role of information technologies, *West J Med* 168(5):311-318, 1998.

Scott SD, Plotnikoff RC, Karunamuni N, et al: Factors influencing the adoption of an innovation: an examination of the uptake of the Canadian Heart Health Kit (HHK), *Implementation Science* 3:41, 2008.

Scott-Findlay S, Golden-Biddle K: Understanding how organizational culture shapes research use, *J Nurs Admin* 35(7/8):359-365, 2005.

Sebern MD: Pressure ulcer management in home health care: efficacy and cost effectiveness and moisture vapor permeable dressing, *Arch Phys Med Rehabil* 67(10):726-729, 1986.

Shaw B, Cheater F, Gillies C, et al: Tailored interventions to overcome identified barriers to change: effects on professional practice and health care outcomes, *Cochrane Database of Systematic Reviews,* 3, 2005. Art. No.: CD005470. DOI: 005410.001002/14651858.CD14005470.

Shively M, Riegel B, Waterhouse D, et al: Testing a community level research utilization intervention, *Appl Nurs Res* 10(3):121-127, 1997.

Shojania KG, Grimshaw JM: Evidence-based quality improvement: the state of the science, *Health Aff* 24(1):138-150, 2005.

Shortell SM: Increasing value: a research agenda for addressing the managerial and organizational challenges facing health care delivery in the United States, *Med Care Res Rev* 61(3):12s-30s, 2004.

Silagy CA: Evidence-based healthcare 10 years on: is the National Institute of Clinical Studies the answer? *Med J Aust* 175(3):124-125, 2001.

Smith JL, Williams JW Jr, Owen RR, et al: Developing a national dissemination plan for collaborative care for depression: QUERI series, *Implementation Science* 3:59, 2008.

Social Science Citation Index: Retrieved December 31, 2008, from www.thomsonreuters.com/products_services/scientific/Web_of_Science.

Soukup SM: The center for advanced nursing practice evidence-based practice model, *Nurs Clin North Am* 35(2):301-309, 2000.

Soumerai SB, McLaughlin TJ, Gurwitz JH, et al: Effect of local medical opinion leaders on quality of care for acute myocardial infarction: a randomized controlled trial, *JAMA* 279(17):1358-1363, 1998.

Squires JE, Moralejo D, LeFort SM: Exploring the role of organizational policies and procedures in promoting research utilization in registered nurses, *Implementation Science* 2:17, 2007.

Stenger K: Putting research to good use, *Am J Nurs* (suppl):30-38, 1994.

Stetler CA, Legro MW, Rycroft-Malone J, et al: Role of "external facilitation" in implementation of research findings: a qualitative evaluation of facilitation experiences in the Veterans Health Administration, *Implementation Science* 1:23, 2006.

Stetler CB: Role of the organization in translating research into evidence-based practice, *Outcomes Management* 7(3):97-105, 2003.

Stetler CB, Legro MW, Wallace CM, et al: The role of formative evaluation in implementation research and the QUERI experience, *J Gen Intern Med* 21:S1-S8, 2006.

Stetler CB, McQueen L, Demakis JG, et al: An organizational framework and strategic implementation for system-level change to enhance research-based practice: QUERI series, *Implementation Science* 3:30, 2008.

Straus SE, Richardson WS, Glasziou P, et al: *Evidence based medicine: how to practice and teach EBM*, ed 3, Philadelphia, 2005, Churchill Livingstone.

Sussman S, Valente TW, Rohrbach LA, et al: Translation in the health professions: converting science into action, *Eval Health Prof* 29(1):7-32, 2006.

Thompson CJ: The meaning of research utilization: a preliminary typology, *Crit Care Nurs Clin North Am* 13(4):475-485, 2001.

Thompson CJ, Dowding D, Guyatt G: Computer decision support systems. In DiCenso A, Guyatt G, Ciliska D, eds: *Evidence-based nursing: a guide to clinical practice*, St Louis, 2005, Mosby.

Thompson DS, Estabrooks CA, Scott-Findlay S, et al: Interventions aimed at increasing research use in nursing: a systematic review, *Implementation Science* 2:15, 2007.

Titler M: TRIP intervention saves healthcare dollars and improves quality of care (abstract/poster), 2003. Paper presented at Translating Research into Practice: What's Working? What's Missing? What's Next? Sponsored by the Agency for Healthcare Research and Quality, Washington, DC, July 22-24, 2003.

Titler MG: Critical analysis of research utilization (RU): an historical perspective, *Am J Crit Care* 2(3):264, 1993.

Titler MG: Research utilization: necessity or luxury? In McCloskey JC, Grace H, eds: *Current issues in nursing*, ed 5, St Louis, 1997, Mosby.

Titler MG: Use of research in practice. In LoBiondo-Wood G, Haber J, eds: *Nursing research*, ed 4, St Louis, 1998, Mosby–Year Book.

Titler MG: *Toolkit for promoting evidence-based practice*, Iowa City, 2002, Department of Nursing Services and Patient Care, University of Iowa Hospitals and Clinics.

Titler MG: Methods in translation science, *Worldviews on Evidence-Based Nursing* 1:38-48, 2004a.

Titler MG: Overview of the U.S. invitational conference "Advancing Quality Care through Translation Research," *Worldviews on Evidence-Based Nursing* 1(S1):S1-S5, 2004b.

Titler MG: Developing an evidence-based practice. In LoBiondo-Wood G, Haber J, eds: *Nursing research*, ed 6, St Louis, 2006a, Mosby–Year Book.

Titler MG: Evidence-based practice. In Weaver CA et al, eds: *Nursing and informatics for the 21st century: an international look at practice trends and the future*, Chicago, 2006b, HIMSS.

Titler MG: The evidence for evidence-based practice implementation. In Hughes R, ed: *Patient safety and quality—an evidence-based handbook for nurses*, Rockville, MD, 2008, Agency for Healthcare Research and Quality.

Titler MG, Cullen L, Ardery G: Evidence-based practice: an administrative perspective, *Reflections of Nursing Leadership* 28(2):26-27, 46, 2002.

Titler MG, Everett L, Adams S: Implications for implementation science, *Nurs Res* 56(4S):S53-S59, 2007.

Titler MG, Everett LQ: Translating research into practice: considerations for critical care investigators, *Crit Care Nurs Clin North Am* 13(4):587-604, 2001.

Titler MG, Herr K, Brooks JM, et al: A translating research into practice intervention improves management of acute pain in older hip fracture patients, *Health Serv Res* 2008. Retrieved from www3.interscience.wiley.com/journal/120120473/issue.

Titler MG, Herr K, Everett LQ, et al: *Book to bedside: promoting and sustaining EBPs in elders. Final progress report to AHRQ*, Iowa City, 2006, University of Iowa College of Nursing. 2R01 HS010482-04.

Titler MG, Herr K, Schilling ML, et al: Acute pain treatment for older adults hospitalized with hip fracture: current nursing practices and perceived barriers, *Appl Nurs Res* 16(4):211-227, 2003.

Titler MG, Kleiber C, Steelman V, Goode C, et al: Infusing research into practice to promote quality care, *Nurs Res* 43(5):307-313, 1994.

Titler MG, Kleiber C, Steelman VJ, Rakel BA, et al: The Iowa model of evidence-based practice to promote quality care, *Crit Care Nurs Clin North Am* 13(4):497-509, 2001.

Titler MG, Mentes JC: Research utilization in gerontological nursing practice, *J Gerontol Nurs* 25(6):6-9, 1999.

Titler MG, Mentes JC, Rakel BA, et al: From book to bedside: putting evidence to use in the care of the elderly, *Jt Comm J Qual Improv* 25(10):545-556, 1999.

Tripp-Reimer T, Doebbeling BN: Qualitative perspectives in translational research, *Worldviews on Evidence-Based Nursing* 1(S1):S65-S72, 2004.

UIHC Department of Nursing: Retrieved December 31, 2008, from www.uihealthcare.com/depts/nursing/about/index.html.

University of Illinois at Chicago: Evidence based medicine. Finding the best literature, 2003. Retrieved March 2004 from www.uic.edu/depts/lib/lhsp/resources/pico.shtml.

US Invitational Conference: *Advancing quality care through translation research*. Set of 2 CD-ROMs, 2004. Conference Proceedings.

US Preventive Services Task Force: US Preventive Services Task Force grade definitions, 2008. Retrieved May 2008 from www.ahrq.gov/clinic/uspstf/grades.htm.

Vaughn TE, McCoy KD, Bootsmiller BJ, et al: Organizational predictors of adherence to ambulatory care screening guidelines, *Med Care* 40(12):1172-1185, 2002.

Wagner EH, Austin BT, Davis C, et al: Improving chronic illness care: translating evidence into action, *Health Aff (Millwood)* 20:64-78, 2001.

Ward MM, Evans TC, Spies AJ, et al: National quality forum 30 safe practices: priority and progress in Iowa hospitals, *Am J Med Qual* 21(2):101-108, 2006.

Watson NM: Advancing quality of urinary incontinence evaluation and treatment in nursing homes through translation research, *Worldviews on Evidence-Based Nursing* 1(S2):S21-S25, 2004.

Weiss CH: Knowledge creep and decision accretion, *Knowledge Creation Diffusion Utilization* 1:381-404, 1980.

Wells N, Baggs JG: A survey of practicing nurses' research interests and activities, *Clin Nurse Spec* 8:145-151, 1994.

Wensing M, Wollersheim H, Grol R: Organizational interventions to implement improvements in patient care: a structured review of reviews, *Implementation Science* 1:2, 2006.

West S, King V, Carey TS, et al: *Systems to rate the strength of scientific evidence. Evidence report/technology assessment no. 47* (prepared by the Research Triangle Institute–University of North Carolina Evidence-Based Practice Center under contract no. 290-97-0011), AHRQ pub no 02-E016, Rockville, MD, 2002, Agency for Healthcare Research and Quality.

Williams CA: Preparing the next generation of scientists in translation research, *Worldviews on Evidence-Based Nursing* 1(S1):S73-S77, 2004.

Xakellis GC, Chrischilles EA: Hydrocolloid versus saline gauze dressings in treating pressure ulcers: a cost-effectiveness analysis, *Arch Phys Med Rehabil* 73(5):463-469, 1992.

Zwarenstein M, Reeves S, Barr H, et al: Interprofessional education: effects on professional practice and health care outcomes, *Cochrane Database of Systematic Reviews*, 3, 2000. Art. No.: CD002213. DOI: 002210.001002/14651858.CD14002213.

FOR FURTHER STUDY

evolve

Go to Evolve at http://evolve.elsevier.com/LoBiondo/ for review questions, critiquing exercises, and additional research articles for practice in reviewing and critiquing.

18

Tools for Applying Evidence to Practice

Carl A. Kirton

KEY TERMS

absolute benefit increase (ABI)
absolute risk increase (ARI)
absolute risk reduction (ARR)
confidence interval
control event rate (CER)
electronic index
experimental event rate (EER)
hazard ratio
information literacy
likelihood ratio
negative likelihood ratio
negative predictive value
null value
number needed to treat
odds ratio
positive likelihood ratio
positive predictive value
prefiltered evidence
relative benefit increase (RBI)
relative risk (RR)
relative risk reduction (RRR)
sensitivity
specificity
survival curve
systematic review

LEARNING OUTCOMES

After reading this chapter, you should be able to do the following:

- Identify the key elements of a focused clinical question.
- Discuss the use of databases to search the literature.
- Screen a research article for relevance and validity.
- Critically appraise study results and apply the findings to practice.
- Make clinical decisions based on evidence from the literature combined with clinical expertise and patient preferences.

STUDY RESOURCES

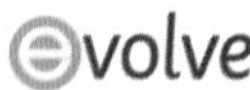

Go to Evolve at http://evolve.elsevier.com/LoBiondo/ for review questions, critiquing exercises, and additional research articles for practice in reviewing and critiquing.

In today's environment of knowledge explosion, new investigations are published at a frequency with which even seasoned practitioners have a hard time keeping pace. With so much new information, maintaining a clinical practice that is based on new evidence in the literature can be challenging. However, the development of evidence-based nursing practice is contingent on applying new and important evidence to clinical practice. A few simple techniques will help you move to a practice that is evidence oriented. This chapter will assist you in becoming a more efficient and effective reader of the professional literature. Through a few important tools and a crisp understanding of the important components of a study, you will be able to use an evidence base to determine the merits of a study for your practice and for your patients.

Consider the following case of a nurse who uses evidence from the literature to support her practice:

Nancy Sanchez is a registered nurse who works in a family practice. As part of her work in this clinic, she provides health teaching to adult and pediatric patients. Nancy is aware that many children acquire verruca plana (common warts) on their hands. She is aware that many treatments can be used to remove these warts, and in her practice it is typical that the clinic staff recommend that parents apply a small piece of duct tape to a wart for 5 to 7 days. Nancy is aware that this method of treatment is supported by evidence in the pediatric literature and has been found to be highly effective in achieving complete wart resolution (Focht et al., 2002; Gibbs & Harvey, 2006). She wonders if this method of treatment can also be recommended to her adult patients. Unaware of the answer to this question, Nancy decides to consult the literature.

EVIDENCE-BASED TOOL #1: ASKING A FOCUSED CLINICAL QUESTION

Developing a focused clinical question will help Nancy to focus on the relevant issue and prepare her for subsequent steps in the evidence-based practice process (see Chapters 1, 2, 3, and 17). A focused clinical question using the PICO format (see Chapters 1 and 2) is developed by answering the following four questions:

1. What is the *population* I am interested in?
2. What is the *intervention* I am interested in?
3. What will this intervention be *compared* to? (Note: depending on the study design, this step may or may not apply.)
4. How will I know if the intervention makes things better or worse (identify an *outcome* that is measurable)?

As you recall from Chapters 1, 2, 3, and 17, most evidence-based practitioners use the simple mnemonic **PICO** to help them recall all of the requirements for a well-designed clinical question (Table 18-1).

Because Nancy is familiar with the evidence-based practice approach for developing clinical questions, she identifies the four important components and develops the following clinical question: In adult patients with common warts, is duct tape an effective method to eradicate the common wart when compared with other methods?

TABLE 18-1 Using PICO to Formulate Clinical Questions

Patient population	What group do you want information on?	Adults with common warts
Intervention (or exposure)	What event do you want to study the effect of?	Duct tape
Comparison	Compared to what? Better or worse than no intervention at all, or than another intervention?	Physical methods (e.g., cryotherapy) or no intervention at all (i.e., placebo)
Outcomes	What is the effect of the intervention?	Wart resolution

Once a clinical question has been framed, it can be organized into one of four fundamental types of clinical categories used by clinicians:

1. **Therapy category:** When a nurse wants to answer a question about the effectiveness of a particular treatment or intervention, she or he will select studies that have the following characteristics:
   - Experimental or quasi-experimental study design (see Chapter 8)
   - Outcome known or of probable clinical importance observed over a clinically significant period of time

   When studies are in this category, the nurse uses a therapy appraisal tool to evaluate the article. A therapy tool can be accessed at www.phru.nhs.uk/Pages/PHD/resources.htm.
2. **Diagnosis category:** When a nurse wants to answer a question about the usefulness, accuracy, selection, or interpretation of a particular measurement instrument or laboratory test, he or she will select studies that have the following characteristics:
   - Cross-sectional study design (see Chapter 9) with people suspected to have the condition of interest
   - Administration to the patient of both the new instrument or diagnostic test and the accepted "gold standard" measure
   - Comparison of the results of the new instrument or test and the "gold standard"

   When studies are in this category, the nurse uses a diagnostic test appraisal tool to evaluate the article. A diagnostic tool can be accessed at www.phru.nhs.uk/Pages/PHD/resources.htm.
3. **Prognosis category:** When a nurse wants to answer a question about a patient's likely course for a particular disease state or identify factors that may alter the patient's prognosis, she or he will select studies that have the following characteristics:
   - Nonexperimental, usually longitudinal study of a particular group (cohort) for a particular outcome or disease (see Chapter 9)
   - Follow-up for a clinically relevant period of time (time is the exposure)
   - Determination of factors in those who do and do not develop a particular outcome

   When studies are in this category, the nurse uses a prognosis (sometimes called a cohort tool) appraisal tool to evaluate the article. A prognosis tool can be accessed at www.phru.nhs.uk/Pages/PHD/resources.htm.
4. **Etiology/causation/harm category:** When a nurse wants to determine whether or not one thing is related to or caused by another, he or she will select studies that have the following characteristics:

- Nonexperimental, usually longitudinal or retrospective (ex post facto or case control) study designs over a clinically relevant period of time (see Chapter 9)
- Assessment of whether or not the patient has been exposed to the independent variable

When studies are in this category, the nurse uses a harm (sometimes called a case-control tool) appraisal tool to evaluate the article. An etiology/causation/harm tool can be accessed at www.phru.nhs.uk/Pages/PHD/resources.htm.

There are two important reasons for applying clinical categories to the professional literature. First, knowing to which category a clinical question belongs helps you search the literature efficiently (see Chapter 3). Second, these structured tools, based on study research design, help the nurse to systematically appraise the strength and quality of evidence provided in research articles.

EVIDENCE-BASED TOOL #2: SEARCHING THE LITERATURE

All the skills that Nancy needs to consult the literature and answer a clinical question are conceptually defined as **information literacy** (Jacobs, Rosenfeld, & Haber, 2003). Your librarian is the best person to help you develop the necessary skills to become information literate. Part of being information literate is having the skills necessary to electronically search the literature to obtain the best evidence for answering your clinical question.

To assist nurses and other health professionals with accessing theoretical, clinical, and research articles, these publications are organized into **electronic indexes** or *databases* (see Chapter 3). Generally speaking, you can access these databases free through your health care organization or university library. Most clinical agencies recognize the importance of clinicians having immediate access to the most current health care information and thus provide access to electronic databases at the point of care.

Chapter 3 discusses the differences among databases and how to use these databases to search the literature. One or two sessions with a librarian will help you focus your search to your clinical question and structure your search to yield articles that are most likely to answer your question. You can learn how to effectively search databases through a Web-based tutorial located at www.nlm.nih.gov/bsd/disted/pubmed.html#qt.

Using the PubMed database (www.pubmed.gov), Nancy uses the search function and enters the term "duct tape." This strategy provides her with 65 articles. She does a quick scan and realizes that many of the articles do not answer her clinical question, many are not research studies, and some are not published in English-language journals. She recalls that the PubMed database has a clinical category filter option that finds citations that correspond to a specific clinical category. She reenters the search term "duct tape" and selects the therapy option (which will only yield articles that use an experimental study design). Her search yields four individual articles with a controlled study design. A careful perusal of the list of articles and a well-designed clinical question help Nancy to select the key articles.

EVIDENCE-BASED PRACTICE TIP

Prefiltered sources of evidence can be found in journal format and electronic format. Prefiltered evidence is evidence in which an editorial team has already read and summarized articles on a topic and appraised its relevance to clinical care. Prefiltered sources include *Clinical Evidence,* available online at http://clinicalevidence.com/ceweb/conditions/index.jsp and in print; *Evidence-Based Nursing* is available online at http://ebn.bmjjournals.com/ and in print.

EVIDENCE-BASED TOOL #3: SCREENING YOUR FINDINGS

Once you have searched and selected the potential articles, how do you know which articles are appropriate to answer your clinical question? This is accomplished by screening the articles for quality and relevance and credibility by answering the following three questions (D'Auria, 2007; Miser, 2000):

1. Is each article from a peer-reviewed journal? Articles published in a peer-reviewed journal have had an extensive review and editing process (see Chapter 3).
2. Are the setting and sample of each study similar to mine so that results, if valid, would apply to my practice or to my patient population (see Chapter 10)?
3. Are any of the studies sponsored by an organization that may influence the study design or results (see Chapter 11)?

Your responses to these screening questions help you decide to what extent you want to appraise an individual article. For example, if the study population is markedly different from the one to which you will apply the results, you may want to consider selecting a more appropriate study. If an article is worth evaluating, you should use the category-specific tool URLs identified in Evidence-Based Tool #1 to critically appraise the article.

Nancy reviews the abstract of the four articles retrieved from her PubMed citation lists and selects the following article: "Duct Tape for the Treatment of Common Warts in Adults: A Double-blind Randomized Controlled Trial." This study was published in Archives of Dermatology in 2007 (Wenner et al., 2007), a peer-reviewed journal. This is a clinical intervention trial that has an experimental study design and is a therapy category study. Nancy reads the abstract and finds that the objective of the study was to appraise the efficacy of duct tape occlusion therapy for the treatment of common warts in adults compared to a moleskin occlusion therapy (the placebo). The setting of the study was in a Veterans Medical Center. The study authors received funding for this investigation, and Nancy finds that there were no funding or conflict of interest issues noted. Nancy decides that this study is worth evaluating and selects the therapy category tool.

HELPFUL HINT

When appraising studies obtained in a search, consider both studies with significant findings (treatment is better) and studies with non significant findings (treatment is worse or there is no difference). Studies reporting non significant findings are more difficult to find but are equally important.

EVIDENCE-BASED TOOL #4: APPRAISE EACH ARTICLE'S FINDINGS

Applying study results to individual patients or to a specific patient population and communicating study findings to patients in a meaningful way are the hallmark of evidence-based practice. Common evidence-based practice conventions that researchers and research consumers use to appraise and report study results in clinical practice are identified by four different types of clinical categories: therapy, diagnosis (sensitivity and specificity), prognosis, and harm. The language common to meta-analysis, which is a special type of method, will also be discussed. Familiarity with these evidence-based practice clinical categories will help Nancy, as well as you, to search for, screen, select, and appraise articles appropriate for answering clinical questions.

Therapy Category

In articles that belong to the therapy category (sometimes called individual studies, experimental design studies, randomized controlled trials [RCTs], or intervention studies), investigators attempt to determine if a difference exists between two or more treatments. The evidence-based language used in a therapy article depends on whether the numerical values of the study variables are *continuous* (a variable that measures a degree of change or a difference on a range, e.g., blood pressure) or *discrete*, also known as dichotomous (measuring whether or not an event did or did not occur, e.g., the number of people diagnosed with type 2 diabetes in a community) (Table 18-2).

When investigators undertake a study to determine whether or not there is a difference between groups on a particular variable, the study author measures the variable in each of the groups and then analyzes the data to determine if there is a difference in each of the groups (this may slightly vary by study design; see Chapter 8). When researchers are interested in the differences in the variable of interest, they generally present their results as measures of central tendency (see Chapter 14). For example, in the study by Horgas and colleagues (2008) on

TABLE 18-2 Difference Between Continuous and Discrete Variables

Researcher Objective	Variable	How the Outcome Is Described in the Research Article
CONTINUOUS VARIABLES		
Researcher is interested in degree of change after exposure to an intervention	Pain score, levels of psychological distress, blood pressure, weight	Measures of central tendency (e.g., mean, median, or standard deviation)
DISCRETE VARIABLES		
Researcher is interested in whether or not an "event" occurred or did not occur	Death, diarrhea, pressure ulcer, pregnancy	Measures of event probability (e.g., relative risk, odds ratio, or number needed to treat)

TABLE 18-3 Measures of Association for Trials That Report Discrete Outcomes

Measure of Association	Definition	Comment
Control event rate (CER)	Proportion of patients in control group in which an event is observed	The CER is calculated by dividing the number of patients who experienced the outcome of interest by the total number of patients in the control group.
Experimental event rate (EER)	Proportion of patients in experimental treatment groups in which an event is observed	The EER is calculated by dividing the number of patients who experienced the outcome of interest by the total number of patients in the experimental group.
Relative risk (RR), also called risk ratio	Risk of event after experimental treatment as a percentage of original risk	The RR is calculated by dividing the EER/CER. If CER and EER are the same, the RR = 1.0 (this means there is no difference between the experimental and control group outcomes). If the risk of the event is reduced in EER compared with CER, RR < 1.0. *The further to the left of 1.0 the RR is, the greater the event, the less likely the event is to occur.* If the risk of an event is greater in EER compared with CER, RR > 1.0. *The further to the right of 1.0 the RR is, the greater the event is likely to occur.*
A NOTE REGARDING RISK: *It is important to note that the identification of a risk of an event does not imply that there is a causal relationship between the factor and the condition. However, the higher a relative risk is, the more likely it becomes that the risk of the event is causal and not due to chance.*		
When the experimental treatment *reduces* the probability of a *bad outcome* (e.g., death), the following terms are used:		
Absolute risk reduction (ARR), also called risk difference or attributable risk reduction	This value tells us the reduction of risk in absolute terms. The ARR is considered the "real" reduction because it is the difference between the risk observed in those who did and did not experience the event.	Arithmetic difference in risk of outcome between patients who have had the event and those who have not had the event, calculated as EER – CER
Relative risk reduction (RRR)	This value tells us the reduction in risk in relative terms. The relative risk reduction is an estimate of the percentage of baseline risk that is removed as a result of the therapy; it is calculated as the ARR between the treatment and control groups divided by the absolute risk among patients in the control group.	Percent reduction in risk that is removed after considering the percent of risk that would occur anyway (the control group's risk), calculated as EER – CER/CER
When the experimental treatment *increases* the probability of a *good outcome* (e.g., satisfactory hemoglobin A_{1c} levels), the following terms are used:		
Absolute benefit increase (ABI)	This is the absolute arithmetic difference in rates of good outcomes between experimental and control patients in a trial.	Calculated as EER – CER
Relative benefit increase (RBI)	This value tells us about the proportional increases in rates of good outcomes between experimental and control patients in a trial divided by the control group event rates.	Calculated as EER – CER/CER

TABLE 18-3 Measures of Association for Trials That Report Discrete Outcomes—cont'd

Measure of Association	Definition	Comment
When the experimental treatment *increases* the probability of a *bad outcome* (e.g., rash), the following terms are used:		
Absolute risk increase (ARI)	This value is the absolute arithmetic difference in rates of bad outcomes between experimental and control patients in a trial.	Arithmetic difference in risk of outcome between patients who have had the therapy and those who have not had the therapy, calculated as EER – CER
Relative risk increase (RRI)	This is the proportional increase in rates of bad outcomes between experimental and control patients in a trial.	Percent increase in risk that is added after considering the percent of risk that would occur anyway (the control group's risk), calculated as EER – CER/CER
Reporting events in terms of the probability of it occurring (good or bad):		
Odds ratio (OR)	Instead of looking at the risk of an event, we could estimate the odds of an event occurring. The OR is usually the measure of choice in the analysis of nonexperimental design studies. It is the ratio of the odds of treated or exposed patients to the odds of untreated or nonexposed patients (where the odds are the ratio of the probability of a given event occurring to the probability of the event not occurring).	If the OR = 1.0, this means there is no difference in the odds of an event occurring between the experimental and control group outcomes. If the odds of the event are reduced between groups, OR < 1.0 (i.e., the event is less likely in the treatment group than the control group). If the odds of an event are increased between groups, the OR > 1.0 (i.e., the event is more likely to occur in the treatment group than the control group).

the relationship between pain and functional disability in black and white older adults (see Appendix B), the intensity of pain was measured using a verbal descriptor scale (VDS). The researchers also measured the research subject's physical limitations using the SIP short form (SIP 68), a 21-item general physical functional disability subscale, and the subject's social functioning SIP 68 social functioning subscale. The investigators were interested in the difference in the scores between black and white adults and reported the mean score of each group by race (see Appendix C, Table 2, p. 503).

In contrast, in experimental studies with discrete variables, researchers are interested in determining the proportion of patients who either experience or do not experience an event (i.e., it either happened or did not happen). For example, An and colleagues (2006) conducted an RCT involving patients who smoked daily; they were interested in determining if telephone care by nurses increases smoking cessation compared with standard smoking cessation care. In this study, self-reported 6-month sustained abstinence was identified as the main outcome. Abstinence is a discrete outcome because at the study endpoint the researchers determined if the patient either remained abstinent or continued to smoke.

In therapy studies using discrete variables (also called outcomes), researchers generally present their results as measures of association as illustrated in Table 18-3. Understanding these measures is challenging but particularly important because they are used by nurses and other health care providers to communicate to each other and to patients the risks and benefits or lack of benefits of a treatment (or treatments). They are particularly useful to nurses because they inform decision making that validates current practice or provides evidence that supports the need for change in clinical practice.

For example, patients with heart failure (HF) generally have a poor quality of life because they often require frequent hospital admissions to manage the worsening of their disease; in fact, it is the most common diagnosis in patients older than 65 of age admitted to hospitals, and it is estimated that more than $33 billion is spent annually on the management of HF (Schocken et al., 2008). One of the HF management goals is to reduce the number of inpatient admissions to the hospital. Investigators asked the following focused clinical question: "In patients with chronic heart failure, does a telephone intervention by nurses reduce admission for worsening HF?" (GESICA Investigators, 2005).

In this RCT, participants with HF were randomized to receive usual HF care (the *control group*) or an intervention that consisted of a phone call every 2 weeks to monitor patients and make therapeutic recommendations as to medications, diet, or physical activity. The study data for the primary study endpoint is described in Table 18-4. From the calculated study data in Table 18-4, it can be concluded that a telephone intervention by nurses is effective in reducing hospitalization for worsening HF. But with so many calculated values (e.g., relative risk [RR], relative risk reduction [RRR], absolute risk reduction [ARR]), it could be difficult for you to know which one of these numerical variables is most important.

The RR and the RRR, although useful for statistical purposes, tend to overestimate treatment effects because these measures do not take into account the baseline risk for the event, in this case hospitalization, and therefore do not provide a useful measure for how the information applies to your individual patient. The ARR is a better value because it does take into account the baseline risk; however, armed with the absolute risk reduction, how does the nurse know whether or not that ARR is clinically useful? For example, in our example the ARR was 5%; it is difficult to determine if this value is impressive or not.

Two other measures can help you determine if the reported or calculated measures are clinically meaningful. They are the **number needed to treat** (NNT) and the **confidence interval** (CI). These measures allow nurses to make inferences about how realistically the results about the effectiveness of an intervention can be generalized to their individual patients and to a population of patients with similar characteristics in the research study.

The NNT is a useful measure for determining the effectiveness of the intervention and its application to individual patients. It is defined as the number of people who need to receive a treatment (or the intervention) in order for one patient to receive any benefit. The NNT may or may not be reported by the study researchers but is easily calculated from the ARR; NNT = 1/ARR. Interventions with a high NNT require considerable expense and human resources to provide any benefit or to prevent a single episode of the outcome, whereas a low NNT is desirable because it means that more individuals will benefit from the intervention. In a hypothetical situation we would be more likely to implement an intervention where the NNT = 5 versus an intervention where the NNT = 200.

Using the data from Table 18-4 we can calculate the NNT. Recall that the calculation is 1/AAR, which is 1/5 (or 100/0.05) = 20. The interpretation for the NNT is that we would have to provide 20 patients with the telephone nursing intervention for one of them to benefit from not being hospitalized. In other words, 1 in 20 patients will benefit from the nursing intervention. This gives us a very different and patient-level perspective on the intervention.

The second clinically useful measure is the confidence interval (CI). The CI is a range of values, based on a random sample of the population that often accompanies measures of central tendency and measures of association and provides you with a measure of precision or uncertainty about the sample findings. Typically, investigators record their CI results as a 95% degree of certainty; at times you may also see the degree of certainty recorded as 99%.

TABLE 18-4 Interpretation of Measures of Association

Clinical question: In patients with chronic heart failure, does a telephone intervention by nurses reduce admission for worsening heart failure (HF)?

Treatment	Total Number of Patients	Number of Patients Who Were Admitted	Number Who Were Not Admitted
Nurse intervention group	760	200	560
Usual care group	758	235	523
TOTALS	**1518**	**435**	**1083**

CALCULATIONS MADE FROM STUDY RESULTS

Experimental event rate (EER)	200/760 = 0.26 or 26% *Interpretation:* The EER is the proportion of patients in the experimental group who experienced the primary outcome, hospitalization. The interpretation is that 26% of the patients who received the nurse intervention were hospitalized.
Control event rate (CER)	235/758 = 0.31 or 31% *Interpretation:* The EER is the proportion of patients in the control group who experienced the primary outcome, hospitalization. The interpretation is that 31% of the patients who received the usual care were hospitalized.
Relative risk (RR)	EER/CER *Interpretation:* We can easily calculate the relative risk, but the study authors have already provided that information. The RR for hospital is 0.80 (if you do the calculation yourself it is not quite correct due to rounding). Recall from Table 18-3 that if the RR < 1.0, the risk of an event is reduced. In this case the intervention *reduces* the risk of hospitalization. The actual interpretation is that the risk of hospitalization is 0.80 times less than participants who did not receive the intervention.
Absolute risk reduction (ARR)	31% – 26% = 5% *Interpretation:* The RR is helpful in telling us if the risk of an event is reduced or increased. It is helpful to know by how much the event is reduced given that we now know that hospitalization occurs in those who do and do not receive the intervention. In this case 5% of the patients who received the intervention are spared hospitalization.
Relative risk reduction (RRR)	RRR = 1.0 – RR 1.0 – 0.80 = 0.20 or 20% *Interpretation:* The RRR is helpful in telling us how much of the baseline risk (the control group event rate) is removed as a result of having the intervention. In this case the nurse intervention reduced hospitalization by 20% relative to the control group.

Today, professional journals often require investigators to include CIs as one of the statistical methods used to interpret study findings. Even when CIs are not reported, they can be easily calculated from study data. The method for performing these calculations is widely available in statistical texts.

Returning to the GESICA (2005) study, it was learned that the RR for hospitalization for study participants who received the intervention was 0.80. The authors accompanied this data with a 95% CI so that the RR with CI is reported as 0.80 (0.66-.097). The CI, the number in parentheses, helps us to place the study results in context for all patients similar to those in the study (generalizability).

As a result of the calculated CI for the GESICA study, it can be stated that in adults with HF (the study population) we can be 95% certain that when a nurse provides biweekly telephone interventions the risk of hospitalization will be reduced anywhere from 0.66 times less likely to 0.97 times less likely. Although the study authors did not calculate the NNT, we now know how to do this, and when researchers report the NNT typically they also calculate the CI for the NNT. In the GESICA study, the calculated CI for the NNT of 20 is (10 to 108). With this information we now can state that the nursing intervention, when applied to our entire patient population, not just the sample, will successfully reduce hospitalization, but we would have to apply the intervention anywhere between 10 and 108 times before one patient gets any benefit. With such a large range, we might think twice about whether or not we want to implement this intervention. We would think differently about the intervention if the CI for the NNT were much narrower, say, 10 to 15 versus 10 to 108.

From a statistical standpoint such a large CI indicates that the study was not sufficiently powered; that is, the study did not enroll enough study patients to provide meaningful results (see Chapter 10). As the number of patients enrolled in a study increases, the CI narrows.

Another unique feature of the confidence interval is that it can tell us whether or not the study results are statistically significant. When an experimental value is obtained that indicates there is no difference between the treatment and control groups, we label that value "the value of no effect," or the **null value.** The value of no effect varies according to the outcome measure.

When examining a CI, if the interval does not include the null value the effect is said to be statistically significant. When the CI does contain the null value, the results are said to be nonsignificant because the null value represents the value of no difference; that is, there is no

Endpoint	Intervention (*n*=760)	Control (*n*=758)	Relative risk (95% CI)	*P* value
Primary endpoint	200 (26.3)	235 (31.0)	0.80 (0.66 to 0.97)	0.026
Heart failure admission	128 (16.8)	169 (22.3)	0.71 (0.56 to 0.91)	0.005
All cause mortality	116 (15.3)	122 (16.1)	0.95 (0.73 to 1.23)	0.690
All cause admission	261 (34.3)	296 (39.1)	0.85 (0.72 to 0.99)	0.049
Cardiovascular admission	183 (24.1)	228 (30.1)	0.76 (0.62 to 0.93)	0.006
All cause admission and/or all cause mortality	299 (39.3)	339 (44.7)	0.86 (0.73 to 1.00)	0.057
Cardiovascular admission and/or all cause mortality	239 (31.4)	288 (38.0)	0.79 (0.65 to 0.95)	0.01

The relative risk is determined by a proportion between intervention and the control group. Therefore the null value is "1." Any confidence interval that includes the null value means that the endpoint finding is not a statistically significant finding.

These confidence intervals contain the null value of "1" and as a result these endpoints are not statistically significant.

Figure 18-1 Summary of primary and secondary endpoints showing the effect of a telephone nursing intervention in patients with heart failure. Values are numbers (percentages) unless stated otherwise. (From GESICA Investigators: Randomised trial of telephone intervention in chronic heart failure: DIAL trial, *BMJ* 331:425, 2005.)

difference between the treatment and control groups. In studies of equivalence (e.g., a study to determine if two treatments are similar) this is a desired finding, but in studies of superiority or inferiority (e.g., a study to determine if one treatment is better than the other) this is not the case.

The null value varies depending on the outcome measure. For numerical values determined by proportions/ratio (e.g., relative risk, odds ratio) the null value is "1." That is, if the CI does not include the value "1," the finding is statistically significant. If the CI does include the value "1," the finding is not statistically significant. If we examine an actual table from the GESICA study we can see an excellent demonstration of this concept (Figure 18-1).

For numerical values determined by a mean difference between the score in the intervention group and the control group (usually with continuous measures), the null value is "0." In this case if the CI includes the null value of "0," the result is not statistically significant. If the CI does not include the null value of "0," the result is statistically significant as illustrated in Figure 18-2, *A* to *D*.

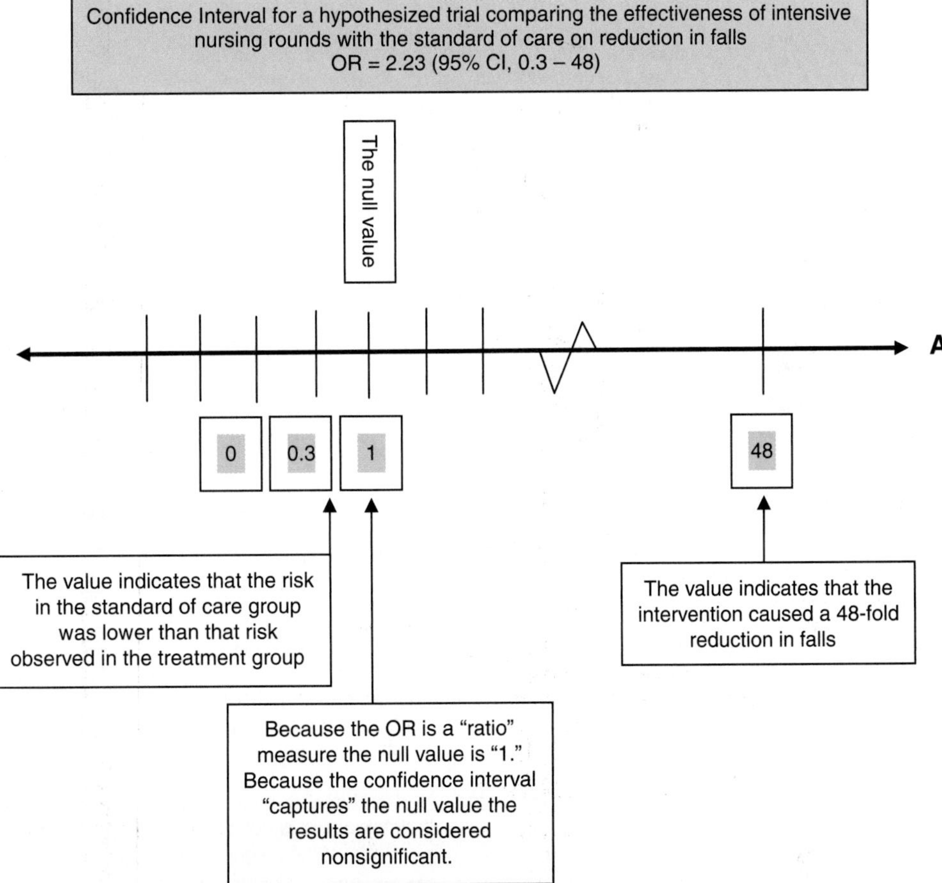

Figure 18-2 **A,** Confidence interval (nonsignificant) for a hypothesized trial comparing the ratio of events in the experimental group and control group.

Continued

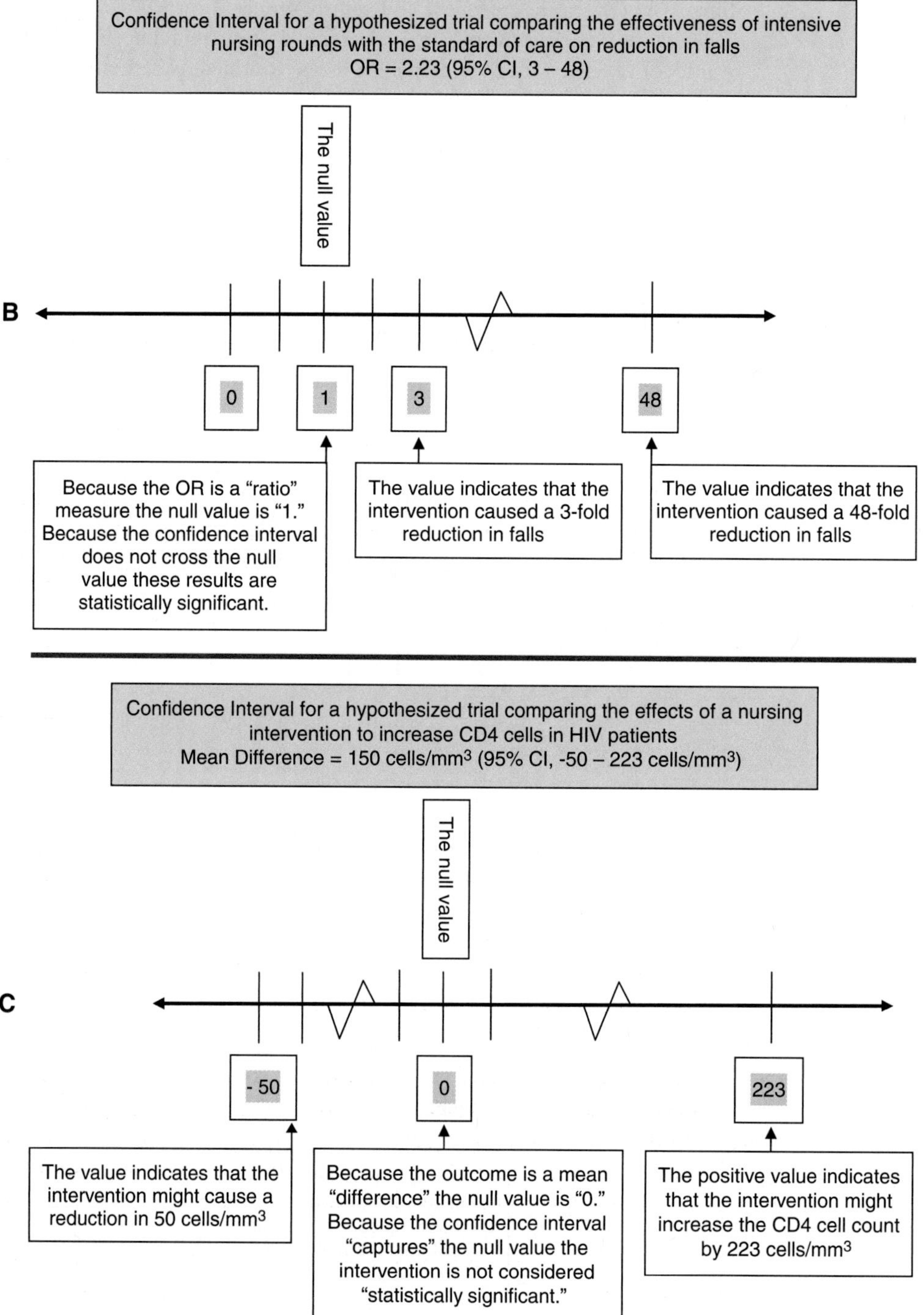

Figure 18-2, cont'd **B,** Confidence interval (significant) for a hypothesized trial comparing the ratio of events in the experimental group and control group. **C,** Confidence interval (nonsignificant) for a hypothesized control trial comparing the difference between two treatments.

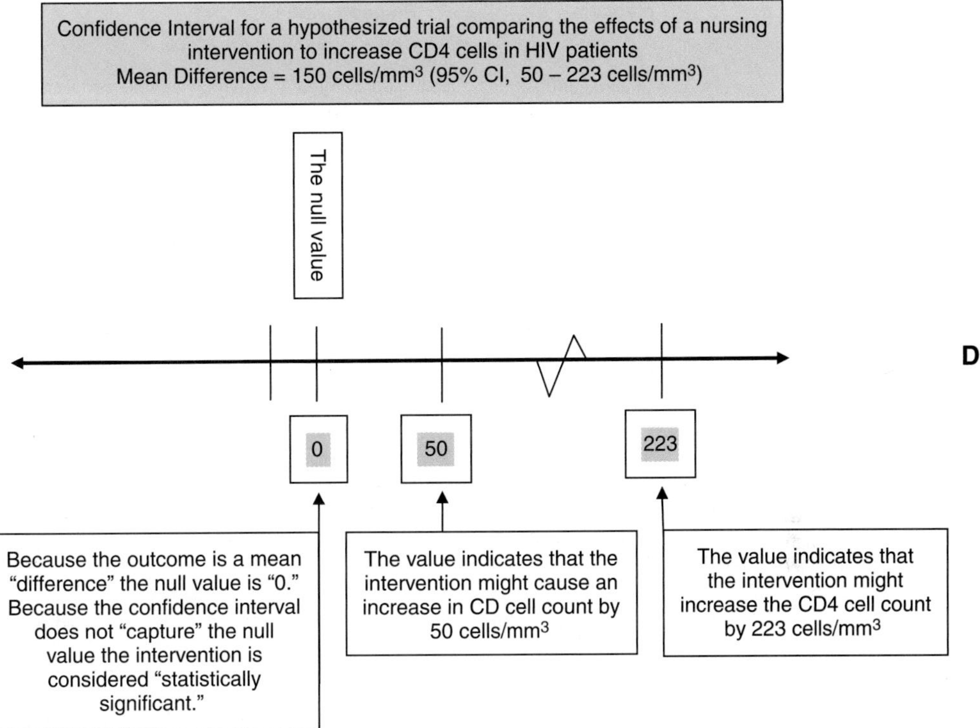

Figure 18-2, cont'd D, Confidence interval (significant) for a hypothesized control trial comparing the difference between two treatments.

Pittler and colleagues (2007) reviewed nine trials in which the use of magnets in the control of pain compared to a placebo was evaluated. Figure 18-3 summarizes the results from these nine studies. Because the difference in pain score is the outcome of analysis, the null value is "0." Looking at the table you can see that only one out of nine studies achieved statistical significance, leading this author to conclude that the evidence for use of magnets to control pain is not supported by the majority of research studies.

Diagnosis Articles

In articles that answer clinical questions of diagnosis, investigators study the ability of screening or diagnostic tests, tools, or components of the clinical examination to detect (or not detect) disease when the patient has (or does not have) the particular disease of interest. The accuracy of a test, technique, or tool is measured by its sensitivity and specificity (Table 18-5).

Sensitivity is the proportion of those with disease who test positive; that is, sensitivity is a measure of how well the test detects disease when it is really there—a highly sensitive test has few false negatives. **Specificity** is the proportion of those without disease who test negative. It measures how well the test rules out disease when it is really absent; a specific test has few false positives. Sensitivity and specificity have some deficiencies in clinical use, primarily because sensitivity and specificity are merely characteristics of the test.

Study	Magnets *n*	Magnets Pain score, mm, mean (SD)	Placebo *n*	Placebo Pain score, mm, mean (SD)	Weight, %	Weighted mean difference, random (95% CI)
Colbert et al.	13	16.0 (23.7)	12	4.0 (31.2)	2.94	12.0 (−9.8 to 33.8)
Collacott et al.	20	4.9 (16.0)	20	4.0 (18.0)	11.46	0.9 (−9.6 to 11.4)
Carter et al.	15	24.0 (27.0)	15	24.0 (26.0)	3.86	0.0 (−19.0 to 19.0)
Weintraub et al.	121	17.0 (27.6)	106	15.0 (28.2)	21.28	2.0 (−5.3 to 9.3)
Winemiller et al.	57	28.0 (25.7)	44	30.0 (27.0)	11.79	−2.0 (−12.4 to 8.4)
Harlow et al.	65	12.0 (23.4)	64	0.6 (22.4)	18.73	11.4 (3.5 to 19.3)
Mikesky et al.	20	57.6 (22.2)	20	56.3 (27.4)	5.71	1.3 (−14.2 to 16.8)
Reeser et al.	23	13.0 (18.0)	23	15.6 (18.6)	11.42	−2.6 (−13.2 to 8.0)
Winemiller et al.	36	27.0 (21.0)	47	31.0 (25.0)	12.81	−4.0 (−13.9 to 5.9)
Overall	370		351		100.00	2.0 (−1.8 to 5.8)

The statistics is the calculated mean difference in pain score between the intervention (magnets) and the control group (placebo). Therefore the null value is "0." Any confidence interval that includes the null value means that the endpoint finding is not a statistically significant finding.

This is the only study where the CI does not contain the null value of "0" and is considered statistically significant. Compare this to all of studies where the CI contains the null.

Figure 18-3 Effects of static magnets for treating pain. The outcome is the weighted mean difference in pain reduction (relative to baseline) on a 100-mm visual analogue scale with 95% confidence interval *(CI).* (From Pitter MH, Brown EM, Ernst E: Static magnets for reducing pain: systematic review and meta-analysis of randomized trials, *Can Med Assoc J* 177(7):736-742, 2007.)

Describing diagnostic tests in this way tells us how good the test is, but what is more useful is how well the test performs in a particular population with a particular prevalence of a disease. This is important because in a population in which a disease is quite prevalent, there are fewer incorrect test results (false positives), as compared with populations with low disease prevalence, for which a positive test may truly be a false positive. Predictive values are a measure of accuracy that accounts for the prevalence of a disease. As illustrated in Table 18-5, a **positive predictive value** (PPV) expresses the proportion of those with positive test results who truly have disease, and a **negative predictive value** (NPV) expresses the proportion of those with negative test results who truly do not have disease. Let us observe how these characteristics of diagnostic tests are used in nursing practice.

A study was conducted to evaluate a new method of on-site appraisal of bacteriuria in incontinent nursing home adult patients. Researchers compared a new method of pressing a urine dipstick into a wet incontinence pad and compared this method with the gold standard

TABLE 18-5 Reporting the Outcome Results of Diagnostic Trials

Measure of Accuracy	Definition	Comments
Sensitivity	A characteristic of a diagnostic test. It is the ability of the test to detect the proportion of people with the disease or disorder of interest. For a test to be useful in ruling out a disease, it must have a high sensitivity.	Formula for sensitivity: TP/(TP + FN), where TP and FN are number of true positive and false negative results, respectively
Specificity	A characteristic of a diagnostic test. It is the ability of the test to detect the proportion of people without the disease or disorder of interest. For a test to be useful at confirming a disease, it must have a high specificity.	Formula for specificity: TN/(TN + FP), where TN and FP are number of true negative and false positive results, respectively
Positive predictive value (PPV) and negative predictive value (NPV) are closely related to sensitivity and specificity (how well the test performs) but differ in that sensitivity and specificity are fixed characteristics of a diagnostic test whereas PPV and NPV consider how well the test performs in populations with difference prevalence of the disease it is testing.		
Positive predictive value	This is the proportion of people with a positive test who have the target disorder.	Formula for positive predictive value: PPV = TP/(TP + FP)
Negative predictive value	This is the proportion of people with a negative test who do not have the target disorder.	Formula for negative predictive value: NPV = TN/(TN + FN)
Likelihood ratio (LR): *A likelihood ratio is a measure that a given test result would be expected in a patient with the target disorder compared to the likelihood that the same result would be expected in a patient without the target disorder. It measures the power of a test to change the pretest into the* ***posttest probability*** *of a disease being present.*		
Positive likelihood ratio	The LR of a positive test tells us how well a positive test result does by comparing its performance when the disease is present to that when it is absent. The best test to use for ruling in a disease is the one with the largest likelihood ratio of a positive test.	Formula for positive likelihood ratio: Sensitivity/(1 – Specificity)
Negative likelihood ratio	The LR of a negative test tells us how well a negative test result does by comparing its performance when the disease is absent to that when it is present. The better test to use to rule out disease is the one with the smaller likelihood ratio of a negative test.	Formula for negative likelihood ratio: (1 – Sensitivity)/Specificity

of sending a clean-catch specimen to a laboratory for culture. The investigators compared and contrasted the new method with the gold standard using several different data combinations. The measures of accuracy using the dipstick/pad method and the result of nitrite alone are listed in Table 18-6 (Midthun et al., 2003).

The test characteristics in Table 18-6 show that the dipstick/pad method has a sensitivity of 70% and a specificity of 97%. This method compares well with the laboratory method of detecting nitrates in the urine, which has a sensitivity of 66.7% and a specificity of 98.6%. Recall that sensitivity and specificity apply to the diagnostic test alone and do not change even as the disease prevalence changes in the population. In a population in which a disease

TABLE 18-6 Nitrite Results Indicative for Bacteriuria Using the Dipstick/Pad Method

		(GOLD STANDARD) CULTURE RESULTS		
Method	**Test Result**	**Positive**	**Negative**	**Totals**
Dipstick/pad (new test)	Positive	**19** (a)	**2** (b)	21
	Negative	**8** (c)	**69** (d)	77
Totals		**27**	**71**	98

CALCULATIONS MADE FROM STUDY RESULTS

Sensitivity = a/(a + c)	19/27 = 0.70 or 70% *Interpretation:* The dipstick/pad method is 70% accurate in detecting the proportion of patients with positive tests as having bacteriuria.
Specificity = d/(b + d)	69/71 + 0.972 or 97% *Interpretation:* The dipstick/pad method is 97% accurate in detecting the proportion of patients with negative test as not having bacteriuria.
Prevalence of bacteriuria in this population (elderly, primarily female nursing home residents) = (a + c)/Total population	27/98 = 0.275 *Interpretation:* The prevalence of bacteriuria in an elderly female population is 28%.
Positive predictive value = a/(a + b)	19/21 = 0.70 or 90% *Interpretation:* 90% of primarily elderly female nursing home residents with a positive dipstick/pad method will have bacteriuria. 10% will not have bacteriuria.
Negative predictive value = d/(c + d)	69/77 = 0.896 or 90% *Interpretation:* 90% of primarily elderly female nursing home residents with a negative dipstick/pad method will not have bacteriuria. 10% will have bacteriuria.
Likelihood ratio (LR+) = Sensitivity/ (1 – Specificity)	0.70/(1 – 0.972) = 0.70/0.028 = 25 *Interpretation:* Female elderly nursing home residents with a positive dipstick/pad method test are 25 times more likely to have a urinary tract infection (UTI) than patients without bacteriuria (i.e., a positive test is very useful for ruling in UTI).
Likelihood ratio (LR–) = (1 – Sensitivity)/ Specificity	1 – 0.72/0.97 = 0.29 *Interpretation:* Female elderly nursing home residents with a negative dipstick/pad method test are 0.29 times more likely to have a UTI than patients without bacteriuria (i.e., a negative test is moderately useful for ruling out UTI; this actually is the false-negative rate. It means that we will have more false-negative tests, and this may not be so good in this population).

is very prevalent, a positive test is more meaningful compared with a positive test in a population in which the disease is very rare.

From Table 18-6 we learn that the prevalence of bacteriuria in an elderly, primarily female population is 28%. Combining this information with sensitivity and specificity, we find that the PPV is 90%; this means that 90% of primarily elderly female nursing home residents with a positive dipstick/pad method will have bacteriuria.

Combining sensitivity, specificity, PPV, NPV, and prevalence to make clinical decisions based on the results of testing is cumbersome and complex. Fortunately, all of these measures can be described by one number, the **likelihood ratio** (LR). This value tells us how many more times a positive test (or negative test) distinguished between those who have the disorder

TABLE 18-7 How Much Do Likelihood Ratio Changes Affect Probability of Disease?

Likelihood Ratio Positive	Likelihood Ratio Negative	Probability That Patient Has (+LR) or Does Not Have (–LR)
LR > 10	LR < 0.1	Large
LR 5-10	LR 0.1-0.2	Moderate
LR 2-5	LR 0.2-0.5	Small
LR < 2	LR > 0.5	Tiny
LR = 1.0		Test provides no useful information

and those who do not have the disorder. As you can see from Table 18-5, the LR is calculated from the test's sensitivity and specificity, and with more training in determining disease prevalence you could actually state the numerical probability that a patient might have a disease based on the test's LR.

As illustrated in Table 18-7, a test with a large positive likelihood ratio (e.g., greater than 10), when applied, provides the clinician with a high degree of certainty that the patient has the suspected disorder. Conversely, tests with a very low positive likelihood ratio (e.g., less than 2), when applied, provide you with little to no change in the degree of certainty that the client has the suspected disorder.

When a test has a likelihood ratio of "1," the null value, the test will not contribute to decision making in any meaningful way and should not be used. A test with a large negative likelihood ratio provides the clinician with a high degree of certainty that the patient does not have the disease. The further away from "1" the negative LR is, the better the test will be for its use in ruling out disease (i.e., there will be few false negatives). More and more journal articles require authors to provide test LRs; they may also be available in secondary sources.

HELPFUL HINT

When evaluating whether or not you should spend time reviewing an article, examine the article's tables. The information you need to answer your clinical question should be contained in one or more of the tables.

Prognosis Articles

In articles that answer clinical questions of prognosis, investigators conduct studies in which they want to determine the outcome of a particular disease or condition. Prognosis studies can often be identified by their longitudinal cohort design (see Chapter 9). At the conclusion of a longitudinal study, investigators statistically analyze data to determine which factors are strongly associated with the study outcomes. Because researchers are interested in demonstrating the occurrence of events at specific points in time, one way of presenting data is to present measures of association (see Table 18-3) for a variety of data points or several different points in time.

A more efficient manner of presenting this type of data is in survival curves. A survival curve is a graph that shows the probability that a patient "survives" in a given state for at least a specified time (or longer). Although survival curves were originally developed to study how long a patient survived symptom- or disease-free periods, almost any discrete data can be plotted on a curve (e.g., how long a patient stayed on a medication or in a nurse-managed program).

TABLE 18-8 Predictors of Institutionalization (N = 1147)

Potential Predictor	Hazard Ratio	95% Confidence Interval	*p* Value
Age*	1.06	1.03-1.10	<0.001
Sex (male vs. female)†	0.94	0.64-1.38	0.753
Education (<high school vs. >high school)†	0.84	0.61-1.12	0.843
Cognitive functioning (Mini-Mental State Examination score)*†	1.05	0.97-1.13	0.205
Living arrangement (not living alone vs. living alone)	1.15	0.70-1.87	0.588
Marital status (currently married vs. not married)†	1.08	0.65-1.79	0.774
Social support (social support score)*	1.27	1.10-1.46	0.001
Functional disability (instrumental activities of daily living score)*†	1.31	1.15-1.50	<0.001
Depression (<5 symptoms vs. >5)	0.80	0.48-1.34	0.404
History of hospitalization in past year (no vs. yes)	1.32	0.93-1.88	0.314
Number of prescription drugs*	1.21	1.11-1.32	<0.001
Dementia†	5.09	2.92-8.84	<0.001
Dementia and number of prescription drugs (interaction)†	0.81	0.70-0.95	0.001

Source: Bharucha AJ, Pandav R, Shen C, et al: Predictors of nursing facility admission: a 12-year epidemiological study in the United States, *J Am Geriatr Soc* 52:434-439, 2004.

*Continuous variable.

†All these confidence intervals contain the null value and are non-significant predictors of institutionalizations.

When analyzing survival curves, investigators often numerically report the study outcomes in terms of hazard ratios. A **hazard ratio** is essentially a weighted relative risk based on the analysis of survival curves over the whole course of the study period. The hazard is the slope of the survival curve—a measure of how rapidly subjects are dying (or some other outcome). The hazard ratio compares the slope between two groups. If the hazard ratio is 2.0, the rate of deaths (or some other outcome) in one treatment group is twice the rate in the other group. Let us see how hazard ratios are used in a longitudinal study of elderly persons.

A prospective, longitudinal study was carried out for 12 years to identify predictors of institutionalization in elderly patients based on a variety of factors measured at baseline and then every 2 years (Bharucha et al., 2004). The study outcomes after 12 years are presented in Table 18-8, with their respective CIs. In this table you will find the hazard ratios used as a measure of association.

The interpretation of hazard ratios is similar to and interpreted in the same way as the risk ratio (see Table 18-3). Also recall from our discussion that whenever we are appraising CIs (to determine statistical significance) we have to appraise the null value. Because we are evaluating a "ratio," the null value is equal to 1. Thus any hazard ratio CI interval that contains a null value of 1 is not a significant finding. This is further demonstrated by the nonsignificant *p* values that accompany all of the CI intervals in Table 18-8 that contain the null value. This table further illustrates that *p* values are not necessary to report when CI, the preferred method of reporting certainty, is given.

A review of Table 18-8 indicates that for this group, the strongest predictor of institutionalism was dementia (hazard ratio [HR] 5.09; CI 2.92 to 8.84). This means that individuals with dementia were five times more likely to be institutionalized; because the confidence interval does not include the null value, it is statistically significant. Weaker indicators for institutionalism, but nonetheless statistically significant findings, are advancing age, greater functional disability, greater number of prescription medications, and worse/less social support.

TABLE 18-9 Interpretation of Odds Ratios

	TYPE OF OUTCOME	
Odds ratio	Adverse outcome (e.g., myocardial infarction)	Beneficial outcome (e.g., adherence)
Less than 1 (e.g., 0.375)	Intervention better	Intervention worse
Equal to 1	Intervention no better/worse	Intervention no better/worse
More than 1 (e.g., 4.0)	Intervention worse	Intervention better

Using prognostic information with an evidence-based lens helps the nurse and patient focus on reducing factors that may lead to disease or disability. It also helps the nurse provide education and information to patients and their families regarding the course of the condition.

Harm Articles

In articles that answer clinical questions of harm, investigators want to determine if an individual has been harmed by being exposed to a particular event. Harm studies can be identified by their case-control design (see Chapter 9). In this type of study, investigators select the outcome they are interested in (e.g., pressure ulcers), and they examine if any one factor explains those who have and do not have the outcome of interest.

The measure of association that best describes the analyzed data in case-control studies is the odds ratio. The **odds ratio** (OR) communicates the probability of an event. An OR is calculated by dividing the odds in the treated or exposed group by the odds in the control group. Investigators typically provide the reader with the OR of factors in study tables, and thus calculation of OR is rarely necessary. The interpretation of OR is straightforward and presented in Table 18-9. Note that the null value for the OR is equal to 1.

Dubois and colleagues (2007) used a cohort of preschool children to determine risk factors associated with childhood obesity. The study authors used a large data set (n = 1,549) of preschool children and examined if preschool children who regularly consumed sugar-sweetened beverages were more obese at 5 years of age than preschool children who did not regularly consume sugar-sweetened beverages. Children who consumed sweetened beverages between meals more than four to six times per week at 2.5 to 4.5 years of age had an OR of 2.36 with a 95% CI of 1.10 to 5.05 for being obese at 5 years of age.

The interpretation of this data is relatively straightforward; children who regularly consumed sugar-sweetened beverages were 2.36 times more likely to be obese at 5 years of age than children who did not regularly consume sugar-sweetened beverages. Armed with this evidence, you can communicate to new mothers that early behaviors can affect their child later in life and work to assist them in preventing childhood obesity.

Harm data with its measure of probabilities help you to identify factors that may or may not contribute to an adverse or beneficial outcome. This information will be useful for the nursing plan of care, program planning, or patient and family education.

Meta-Analysis

Meta-analysis is not a type of study design but a research method that statistically combines the results of multiple studies (usually RCTs) to answer a focused clinical question through an objective appraisal of carefully synthesized research evidence (see Chapters 1 and 9). Meta-analysis is a systematic, analytic process used to summarize and appraise a number of studies that have researched the same question, using preestablished criteria that guide its implementation. Meta-analysis provides Level I evidence. As discussed in Chapter 9, a meta-analysis may also be called a systematic review. The strength of a meta-analysis lies in its use of statistical analysis to summarize studies. This analysis helps to remove potential bias about research findings in a particular area. A clinical question is used to guide the meta-analysis process. A team of at least two investigators search for all relevant studies, published and unpublished, on the topic or question and, again, use preestablished inclusion and exclusion criteria to determine the studies that will be used in the meta-analysis. Then at least two individuals independently assess the quality of each study, include or exclude studies based on preestablished criteria, statistically combine the results of individual studies, and present a balanced and impartial quantitative and narrative evidence summary of the findings that represents a "state-of-the-science" conclusion about the strength, quality, and consistency of evidence supporting benefits and risks of a given health care practice (Stevens, 2001).

Conducting a meta-analysis is a complex project and, as such, often is conducted by a multidisciplinary team of nurses, physicians, health scientists, clinical epidemiologists, statisticians, librarians, and informatics specialists. In the evidence-based hierarchy, the findings of a meta-analysis are considered to provide the strongest evidence (Level I) available to the clinician because they summarize large amounts of information derived from multiple experimental studies investigating the effect of the same intervention. A methodologically sound meta-analysis is more likely than an individual study to be successful in identifying the true effect of an intervention because it limits bias.

In a **systematic review** that is a meta-analysis, the data from the selected experimental studies are quantitatively combined by using their measures of association (see Table 18-3). A relative risk or, more commonly, the odds ratio is the statistic of choice for use in a meta-analysis. The same interpretation of odds ratio described in Table 18-9 applies to the odds ratios when seen in a meta-analysis.

The usual manner of displaying data from a meta-analysis is by a pictorial representation known as a *blobbogram,* accompanied by a summary measure of effect size in relative risk or odds ratio. Let us see how blobbograms and relative risk ratios are used to summarize the studies in a systematic review by practicing with the data from the Cochrane Review to determine the effectiveness of nurse-led smoking-cessation intervention. This study is located in Appendix E. On p. 555, the table "Analysis 01" lists all of the nursing studies using high-intensity nursing interventions (Analysis 01.01) and low-intensity nursing interventions (Analysis 01.02).

As you can see from the table, 24 studies are included as part of the high-intensity nursing intervention and 7 studies are included in the low-intensity nursing intervention section. In each of the next two columns there is a fraction; the numerator is the number of individuals who achieved the desired outcome (smoking cessation at longest follow-up) and the denominator represents the total number of individuals in each group. In the center of the table, you see that each trial in the analysis is represented by a horizontal line. The findings from each individual study are represented as a blob or square (the measured effect) on the vertical line. The size of the blob or square (sometimes just a small vertical line) may vary to reflect the amount of information in that individual study. The width of the horizontal line represents the 95% confidence interval. The vertical line is the line of no effect, the null value, and we know that when the statistic is the relative risk ratio, the null value is "1."

When the confidence interval of the result (horizontal line) touches or crosses the line of no effect (vertical line), we can say that the study findings did not reach statistical significance.

If the confidence interval does not cross the vertical line, we can say that the study results reached statistical significance.

In examining the blobbogram in Analysis 01.01 and Analysis 01.02, it is clear that only 5 of the 31 studies do not cross the line of no effect. Because the analysis line does not cross the line of no effect, these studies have statistically significant findings. To the far right of the blobbogram, the investigators have also provided the numerical equivalent of each blobbogram.

You will also notice other important information and additional statistical analyses that may accompany the blobbogram table, such as a test to determine how well the results of each of the individual trials are mathematically compatible (heterogeneity) and the weight the study provided to the overall analysis. The reader is referred to a book of advanced research methods for discussion of these topics.

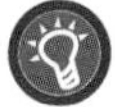

HELPFUL HINT

When appraising the different types of reviews, it is important to be able to distinguish a meta-analysis that analytically assesses studies from a systematic review that appraises the literature with or without an analytic approach to an integrative review that also appraises and synthesizes the literature but without an analytic process (see Chapter 9).

The summary ratio for all of the studies combined is represented by a diamond. There is a subtotal diamond for the high-intensity interventions and a subtotal diamond for the low-intensity interventions, and there is a total diamond that represents all of the studies combined. In this case, after statistically pooling the results of each of the controlled trials, it shows that these studies, statistically combined, overall favor the treatment (the nurse-led intervention). Because the total diamond does not touch or cross the line of no effect, the overall interpretation is that nurse-led interventions are effective for smoking cessation. Interestingly, the subtotal diamond is a statistically significant finding for high-intensity interventions but not for low-intensity interventions.

If this is a methodologically sound review (and Cochrane reviews are), it would support the clinical practice of nurse-led smoking-cessation interventions. A simple tool to help the nurse determine whether or not a systematic review is methodologically sound can be found at www.phru.nhs.uk/Pages/PHD/resources.htm.

In another example of meta-analysis, the investigators were interested in comparing the efficacy of a beta-agonist given by a metered-dose inhaler with a chamber versus a nebulizer on hospital admission in children with asthma under 5 years of age (Castro-Rodriquez and Rodrigo, 2004). The investigators searched the literature for RCTs that treated children under 5 in the emergency department (ED) with acute asthma who were randomized to receive either a metered-dose inhaler with a chamber or a nebulizer. The investigators found six trials that met this criterion (Figure 18-4). The study groups are represented by a fraction (e.g., in the trial published by Close, 4/17 children in the nebulizer group were admitted to the hospital). In the center of Figure 18-4 each trial in the analysis is represented by a horizontal line. The findings from each individual study are represented as a blob or square (the measured effect) on the vertical line. The size of the blob or square may vary to reflect the amount of information in that individual study. The width of the horizontal line represents the 95% confidence interval. A vertical line is the line of no effect (odds ratio = 1). When the confidence interval of the result (horizontal line) crosses the line of no effect (vertical line), the differences in the effect of the treatment are not statistically significant. If the confidence interval does not cross the vertical line, then the study results are statistically significant.

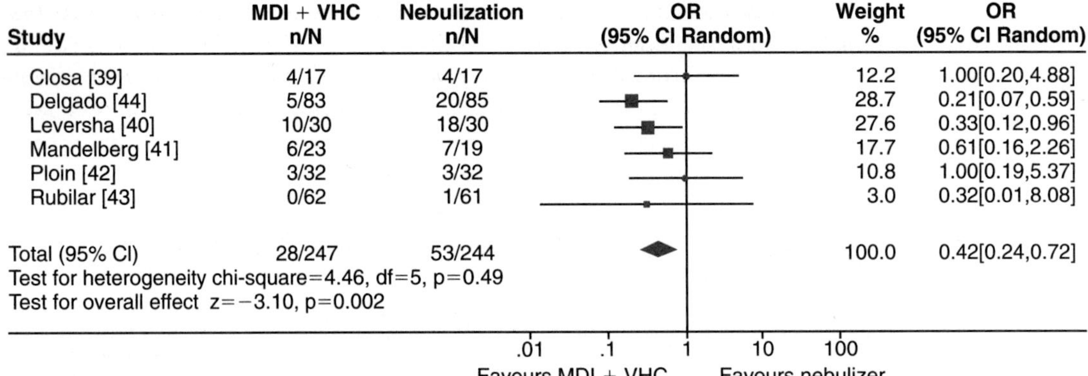

Study	MDI + VHC n/N	Nebulization n/N	Weight %	OR (95% CI Random)
Closa [39]	4/17	4/17	12.2	1.00[0.20,4.88]
Delgado [44]	5/83	20/85	28.7	0.21[0.07,0.59]
Leversha [40]	10/30	18/30	27.6	0.33[0.12,0.96]
Mandelberg [41]	6/23	7/19	17.7	0.61[0.16,2.26]
Ploin [42]	3/32	3/32	10.8	1.00[0.19,5.37]
Rubilar [43]	0/62	1/61	3.0	0.32[0.01,8.08]
Total (95% CI)	28/247	53/244	100.0	0.42[0.24,0.72]

Figure 18-4 Systematic review with meta-analysis data showing the efficacy of a beta-agonist given by metered-dose inhaler with a valved holding chamber (MDI + VHC) vs. nebulizer in children under 5 years of age with acute exacerbation of wheezing or asthma in the emergency department on hospitalization. (From Castro-Rodriquez J, Rodrigo G: Beta-agonists through metered-dose inhaler with valved holding chamber versus nebulizer for acute exacerbation of wheezing or asthma in children under 5 years of age: a systematic review with meta-analysis, *J Pediatr* 145(2):172-177, 2004.)

In the blobbogram in Figure 18-4, it is clear that only two of the six studies do not cross the line of no effect, study 2 published by Delgado and study 3 published by Leversha, and so have statistically significant findings. In columns 4 and 5 of Figure 18-4, the investigators have also provided the numerical equivalent of each blobbogram. The summary odds ratio for all of the studies combined is represented by the diamond at the bottom of Figure 18-4, which is located to the left of the vertical line, the line of no effect. In this case, after statistically pooling the results of each of the controlled trials, the pooled odds ratio, depicted by the diamond, shows that these studies, statistically combined, favor the metered-dose inhaler with chamber for preventing hospitalizations of children under 5 years of age and that this option is statistically significant.

If this were a methodologically sound meta-analysis, it would support the clinical practice of providing children under 5 years of age with asthma exacerbation with a metered-dose inhaler with a chamber to prevent hospitalization.

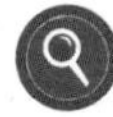

EVIDENCE-BASED PRACTICE TIP

When answering a clinical question, check to see if a Cochrane review has been performed. This will save you time searching the literature. A Cochrane review is a systematic review that primarily uses meta-analysis to investigate the effects of interventions for prevention, treatment, and rehabilitation in a health care setting or on health-related disorders. Most Cochrane reviews are based on RCTs, but other types of evidence may also be taken into account, if appropriate. If the data collected in a review are of sufficient quality and similar enough, they are summarized statistically in a meta-analysis. You should always check the Cochrane Web site, www.cochrane.org, to see if a review has been published on the nurse's topic of interest.

As Nancy evaluates the literature, she determines that the article, "Duct Tape for the Treatment of Common Warts in Adults: A Double-Blind Randomized Controlled Trial," is a clinical intervention trial that has an experimental study design and is a therapy category study. Nancy selects a therapy critical appraisal tool and answers the critical appraisal questions.

EVIDENCE-BASED TOOL #5: APPLYING THE FINDINGS

Sackett and colleagues (1996) stated that evidence-based practice is about integrating individual clinical expertise and patient preferences with the best external evidence to guide clinical decision making. With a few simple tools (see the Web links listed earlier in this chapter) and some practice, your day-to-day practice can be more evidence based. More and more studies are being conducted that demonstrate whether or not a practice that is rooted in evidence actually improves the quality of care. We know that using evidence in clinical decision making by nurses and all other health care professionals interested in matters associated with the care of individuals, communities, and health systems is increasingly important to achieving quality patient outcomes and cannot be ignored. Let us see how Nancy, our family practice nurse, uses evidence to make a clinically effective decision and perhaps make a practice change.

Nancy critically appraises the article, and she learns that for complete resolution of warts the CER = 22% and the EER = 21%. She is surprised to see that the control group (no duct tape) actually did slightly better in complete resolution of the wart at 2 months compared to the treatment group. She wants to know if this is a statistically significant finding. The study authors did not provide relative risk values or confidence intervals, but Nancy's evidence-based education allows her to perform these quick calculations (note that using rounded values will provide slightly different results). Because the researchers are investigating whether duct tape provides a benefit, we are looking at the relative benefit increase of the intervention (RBI). Nancy calculates the ABI, which is less than 1%, and she also calculates the RBI, which favors the placebo at 6.5%, and the confidence interval for the RBI is −113 to 60. Nancy notes that the confidence interval is quite wide and that it contains the null value of "1." Nancy concludes that duct tape treatment for adults patients is not more effective than plain pads without duct tape.

This finding is informative because it is in direct contrast to similar studies that found this method of treatment effective in children. The differences are not well understood but may be due to some of the limitations acknowledged by the authors of the adult study. However, without further evidence Nancy cannot recommend this method to her adult patients; she would be basing her response to the patient on the "best available evidence" for that patient population and clinical setting.

CRITICAL THINKING CHALLENGES

- How can the nurse determine if reported or calculated measures in a research study are clinically significant enough to inform evidence-based clinical decisions?
- How can a nurse in clinical practice determine whether the strength and quality of evidence provided by a diagnostic tool is sufficient to justify ordering it as a diagnostic test ? Provide an example of a diagnostic test used to diagnose a specific illness.
- Compare and contrast the use of specific statistical tests in Tables 18-3 and 18-4 for discrete and continuous variables. Provide clinical examples of discrete and continuous variables.
- Choose a meta-analysis from a peer-reviewed journal and describe how you as a nurse would use the findings of this meta-analysis in making a clinical decision about applicability of a nursing intervention for your specific patient population and clinical setting.
- How would you use the PICO format to formulate a clinical question? Provide a clinical example.

KEY POINTS

- Asking a focused clinical question using the PICO approach is an important evidence-based practice tool.
- Four types of evidence-based practice clinical categories used by nurses and other clinicians are the following: therapy, diagnosis, prognosis, and harm. These categories focus development of the clinical question, the literature search, and critical appraisal of research studies.
- An efficient and effective literature search, using information literacy skills, is critical in locating evidence to answer the clinical question.
- Sources of evidence (e.g., articles, evidence-based practice guidelines, evidence-based practice protocols) must be screened for relevance and credibility.
- Appraising the evidence generated by research studies using an accepted critiquing tool is essential in determining the strength, quality, and consistency of evidence offered by a research study.
- Articles that belong to the therapy category are designed to determine if a difference exists between two or more treatments.
- Articles that belong to the diagnosis category are designed to investigate the ability of screening or diagnostic tests, tools, or components of the clinical examination to detect whether or not the patient has a particular disease using likelihood ratios.
- Articles in the prognosis category are designed to determine the outcomes of a particular disease or condition.
- Articles in the harm category are designed to determine if an individual has been harmed by being exposed to a particular event.
- Meta-analysis is a research method that statistically combines the results of multiple studies (usually RCTs) and is designed to answer a focused clinical question through objective appraisal of synthesized evidence.

REFERENCES

An LC, Zhu S, Nelson DB, et al: Benefits of telephone care over primary care for smoking cessation: a randomized trial, *Arch Intern Med* 166:536-542, 2006.

Bharucha AJ, Pandav R, Shen C, et al: Predictors of nursing facility admission: a 12-year epidemiological study in the United States, *J Am Geriatr Soc* 52:434-439, 2004.

D'Auria JP: Using an evidence-based approach to critical appraisal, *J Pediatr Health Care* 2:343-346, 2007.

Dubois L, Farmer A, Girard M, et al: Regular sugar-sweetened beverage consumption between meals increases risk of overweight among preschool-aged children, *J Am Diet Assoc* 107(6):924-934, 2007.

Focht D, Spicer C, Fairchok M: The efficacy of duct tape vs cryotherapy in the treatment of verruca vulgaris (the common wart), *Arch Pediatr Adolesc Med* 156:971-974, 2002.

GESICA Investigators: Randomised trial of telephone intervention in chronic heart failure: DIAL trial, *BMJ* 331:425, 2005.

Gibbs S, Harvey I: Topical treatments for cutaneous warts, *Cochrane Database of Systematic Reviews*, Issue 3, 2006. Art. No.: CD001781. DOI: 10.1002/14651858.CD001781.pub2.

Horgas AL, Yoon SL, Nichols AL, et al: The relationship between pain and functional disability in black and white older adults, *Res Nurs Health* 31:1-14, 2008.

Jacobs SK, Rosenfeld P, Haber J: Information literacy as the foundation for evidence-based practice in graduate nursing education: a curriculum-integrated approach, *J Prof Nurs* 19(5):320-328, 2003.

Midthun SJ, Paur RA, Lindseth G, et al: Bacteriuria detection with a urine dipstick applied to incontinence pads of nursing home residents, *Geriatr Nurs* 24(4):206-209, 2003.

Miser WF: Critical appraisal of the literature: how to assess an article and still enjoy life. In Geyman JP, Deyo RA, Ramsey SD, eds: *Evidence based clinical practice: concepts and approaches*, Boston, 2000, Butterworth-Heinemann.

Pittler MH, Brown EM, Ernst E: Static magnets for reducing pain: systematic review and meta-analysis of randomized trials, *Can Med Assoc J* 177(7):736-742, 2007.

Sackett DL, Rosenberg WMC, Gray JAM, et al: Evidence based medicine: what it is and what it isn't, *BMJ* 312:71-72, 1996.

Schocken DD, Benjamin EJ, Fonarow GC, et al: Prevention of heart failure: a scientific statement from the American Heart Association Councils on Epidemiology and Prevention, Clinical Cardiology, Cardiovascular Nursing, and High Blood Pressure Research; Quality of Care and Outcomes Research Interdisciplinary Working Group; and Functional Genomics and Translational Biology Interdisciplinary Working Group, *Circulation* 117:2544-2565, 2008.

Stevens K: Systematic reviews: the heart of evidence-based practice, *AACN Clin Issues Adv Pract Acute Crit Care* 12(4):529-538, 2001.

Wenner R, Askari SK, Cham PMH, et al: Duct tape for the treatment of common warts in adults: a double-blind randomized controlled trial, *Arch Dermatol* 143(3):309-313, 2007.

FOR FURTHER STUDY

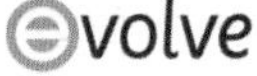

Go to Evolve at http://evolve.elsevier.com/LoBiondo/ for review questions, critiquing exercises, and additional research articles for practice in reviewing and critiquing.

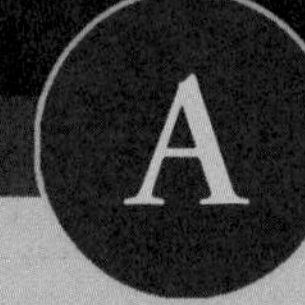

Transition from Treatment to Survivorship:

Effects of a Psychoeducational Intervention on Quality of Life in Breast Cancer Survivors

Karen Dow Meneses, PhD, RN, FAAN, Patrick McNees, PhD, FAAN, Victoria W. Loerzel, RN, MSN, AOCN®, Xiaogang Su, PhD, Ying Zhang, PhD, and Lauren A. Hassey, BSN

Purpose/Objectives: To examine the effectiveness of a psychoeducational intervention on quality of life (QOL) in breast cancer survivors in post-treatment survivorship.

Design: A randomized controlled trial.

Setting: An academic center collaborating with a regional cancer center in the southeastern United States.

Sample: 256 breast cancer survivors.

Methods: Women were randomly assigned to the experimental or wait control group. The Breast Cancer Education Intervention (BCEI) study was delivered in three face-to-face sessions and five monthly follow-up sessions (three by telephone and two in person). The control group received four monthly attention control telephone calls and the BCEI at month 6. Data were collected at baseline, three and six months after the BCEI for the experimental group, and one month after the BCEI (at month 7) for the wait control group.

Main Research Variables: Primary endpoints were overall QOL and physical, psychological, social, and spiritual well-being.

Findings: No differences in QOL were reported at baseline between groups. The experimental group reported improved QOL at three months, whereas the wait control group reported a significant decline in QOL. The experimental group reported continued maintenance of QOL at six months. Although the wait control group reported improved QOL at six months, significant differences continued to exist between the groups.

Conclusions: The BCEI was an effective intervention in improving QOL during the first year of breast cancer survivorship. Treatment effects were durable over time.

Karen Dow Meneses, PhD, RN, FAAN, is a professor and associate dean for research in the School of Nursing at the University of Alabama at Birmingham (UAB); Patrick McNees, PhD, FAAN, is a professor and the director of research, innovation, and technology in the School of Nursing and the School of Health Professions at UAB; Victoria W. Loerzel, RN, MSN, AOCN®, is an assistant professor in the School of Nursing at the University of Central Florida (UCF) in Orlando and was the project director for the Breast Cancer Education Intervention (BCEI) study at UCF; Xiaogang Su, PhD, is an associate professor in the Department of Statistics at UCF; Ying Zhang, PhD, is an associate professor in the Department of Biostatistics at the University of Iowa in Iowa City; and Lauren A. Hassey, BSN, is a research assistant for the BCEI study at UCF. (Submitted December 2006. Accepted for publication April 3, 2007.)

Implications for Nursing: Post-treatment survivorship has not been empirically studied to a large degree. The BCEI is one of the few interventions demonstrating effectiveness among survivors after primary treatment, suggesting that oncology nurses may be uniquely positioned to provide safe passage using education and support.

KEY POINTS

- Few randomized controlled trials have been conducted addressing the transition from treatment to survivorship among patients with cancer.
- Psychoeducational support interventions are demonstrated to be effective.
- The Breast Cancer Education Intervention, a psychoeducational support intervention designed for breast cancer survivors, can improve quality of life.

Quality of life (QOL) during post-treatment breast cancer survivorship is a relatively new, emerging, and promising area of investigation. Numerous multidisciplinary studies conducted since the 1980s have documented QOL in several domains, including physical function, psychological distress, social and family concerns, and spiritual issues, among breast cancer survivors. Behavioral interventions to ameliorate QOL problems include a wide variety of methods such as psychoeducational support, individual and group counseling, expressive therapy, and cognitive behavioral therapy (Institute of Medicine & National Research Council, 2004). The preponderance of behavioral interventions has been delivered primarily during active cancer treatment. A small but growing number of multidisciplinary studies have reported interventions designed for the transition from cancer treatment to cancer survivorship.

The primary purpose of this article is to report the results of the effects of the Breast Cancer Education Intervention (BCEI) Study, a QOL survivorship intervention delivered using psychoeducational support and targeting women with early-stage breast cancer in the first year of post-treatment survivorship. The aims of this article are consistent with the study aims: (a) to describe the effect of the BCEI study on overall QOL, (b) to examine whether the intervention effects were retained over time, and (c) to describe the differential effects of the BCEI study on QOL in the domains of physical, psychological, social, and spiritual well-being.

LITERATURE REVIEW

Quality of Life and Breast Cancer

The literature on QOL and breast cancer is vast and synthesizing it is outside the scope of this article. In general, however, multidisciplinary studies document the influence of breast cancer on overall QOL (Ashbury, Cameron, Mercer, Fitch, & Nielsen, 1998; Ashing-Giwa, Ganz, & Petersen, 1999; Avis, Crawford, & Manuel, 2005; Casso, Buist, & Taplin, 2004; Dirksen & Erickson, 2002; Dow, Fen-ell, Haberman, & Eaton, 1999; Dow, Fen-ell, Leigh, Ly, & Gulasekaram, 1996; Ferrans, 1994; Giedzinska, Meyerowitz, Ganz, & Rowland, 2004; Gotay & Muraoka, 1998; Heidrich, Egan, Hengudomsub, & Randolph, 2006; Holzner et al., 2001; King, Kenny, Shiell, Hall, & Boyages, 2000; Vacek, Winstead-Fry, Seeker-Walker, Hooper, & Plante, 2003; Wyatt, Kurtz, & Liken, 1993); physical functioning and treatment side effects (Armer, 2005; Armer, Fu, Wainstock, Zagar, & Jacobs, 2004; Armer & Heckathorn, 2005; Barton & Loprinzi, 2002; Barton et al., 2003; Bender et al., 2006; Berger et al., 2002, 2003; Bower et al., 2006; Carpenter & Andrykowski, 1999; Carpenter et al., 2004, 2007; Cimprich, Janz, et al., 2005; Cimprich & Ronis, 2003; Cimprich, So, Ronis, & Trask, 2005; Courneya, Blanchard, & Laing, 2001; Knobf, 2002; Loerzel, Dow, & McNees, 2006; Mock et al., 2005); psychological well-being (Bellizzi & Blank, 2006; Lewis et al., 2001); social, family, and work relationships (Bednarek & Bradley, 2005; Kinney, Rodgers, Nash, & Bray, 2003; Kurtz, Wyatt, & Kurtz, 1995; Lewis, Casey, Brandt, Shands, & Zahlis, 2006; Lewis & Deal, 1995; Mast, 1998; Northouse et al., 2002; Northouse, Kershaw, Mood, & Schafenacker, 2005; Payne, Piper, Rabinowitz, & Zimmerman, 2006; Stewart et al., 2001; Waltman et al., 2003); and spiritual concerns (Bauer-Wu & Farran, 2005; Mellon, 2002; Meraviglia, 2006; Wonghongkul, Dechaprom, Phumivichuvate, & Losawatkul, 2006). In addition, a recent comprehensive literature review evaluated the many contributions of nurse scientists that are advancing research in breast cancer (Meneses, in review).

Cancer Survivorship Intervention Research

Intervention Studies during Active Cancer Treatment:

Intervention studies historically have been developed for delivery during diagnosis and active treatment. The types of interventions used during cancer therapy include telephone counseling (Badger, Segrin, Meek, Lopez, & Bonham, 2004; Chamberlain-Wilmoth, Tulman, Coleman, Stewart, & Samarel, 2006; Coleman et al., 2005; Marcus et al., 1998; Sandgren & McCaul, 2006), cognitive-behavioral therapy (Lewis et al., 2006), face-to-face counseling and support (Braden, Mishel, & Longman, 1998), combination face-to-face and peer discussion (Helgeson, Cohen, Schulz, & Yasko, 2001; Yates et al., 2005), group intervention (Hosaka et al., 2001), education and counseling (Hoskins et al., 2001), and short-term support (Miyashita, 2005; Rawl et al., 2002). However, some longitudinal studies were initiated during active treatment and included extended follow-up in post-treatment survivorship.

Intervention Studies during Post-Treatment Survivorship:

Four breast cancer intervention studies designed for post-treatment survivorship were identified in the literature (Cimprich, Janz, et al., 2005; Mishel et al., 2005; Scheier et al., 2005; Stanton et al., 2005). The number is small because most studies conducted during post-treatment survivorship did not have interventions and, thus, were excluded from the discussion. In addition, intervention studies in advanced breast cancer were excluded from the review.

Post-treatment intervention studies used variations of psychoeducational support. The methods for intervention delivery ranged from standard National Cancer Institute (NCI) print materials, peer-modeling videotapes, or one-on-one telephone or in-person counseling (Stanton et al., 2005); four group education sessions (Scheier et al., 2005); four weekly telephone sessions (Mishel et al., 2005); to four individual sessions, two small group sessions, and two telephone contacts (Cimprich, Janz, et al., 2005). Intervention "dose" was not specifically described in the studies, but all were short-term interventions. Three studies reported intervention results (Mishel et al.; Scheier et al.; Stanton et al.), whereas one reported baseline data (Cimprich, Janz, et al.).

The literature shows the multidisciplinary interest in QOL and breast cancer. Psychoeducational support interventions have shown efficacy in QOL and breast cancer. A small but growing number of intervention studies in post-treatment survivorship have applied variations of psychoeducational and support interventions to reduce QOL-related issues.

CONCEPTUAL FRAMEWORK

QOL was the conceptual framework used to guide the identification and development of the BCEI study. QOL was defined as a multidimensional construct consisting of four domains: physical, psychological, social, and spiritual well-being (Dow et al., 1996; Ferrell, Dow, & Grant, 1995). Each domain contributes to an individual's perception of overall QOL. As individuals progress along the cancer continuum, QOL is considered dynamic. This study specifically focused on QOL in post-treatment survivorship, which is consistent with the NCI (2006) cancer survivorship research that concentrates on post-treatment concerns.

METHODS

Design

The BCEI study was a randomized trial with subjects assigned to the experimental group or the wait control group. A wait control feature was used to enhance subject retention, address ethical consideration of subjects being denied potentially helpful treatment, and allow for the evaluation of the effects of the BCEI study on all subjects. The intervention package was delivered over a six-month period. During the same six-month period, the wait control group received initial face-to-face baseline assessment, four attention control telephone calls, three face-to-face education and support sessions, and one face-to-face follow-up education and support session.

The Intervention

The BCEI study was a psychoeducational support intervention that consisted of individual face-to-face education and support sessions, telephone and face-to-face follow-up education and support sessions, and written and audiotaped reinforcement. Figure 1 shows the sequence of the various intervention components.

The three education and support sessions focused on common issues facing breast cancer survivors. Each education and support session was conducted in person and lasted about 60-90 minutes. Session 1 focused on education about physical changes after treatment, including cancer-related fatigue, lymphedema, and pain. Session 2 focused on personal and emotional changes after breast cancer (e.g., menopausal symptoms, hot flashes, sleep problems, sexual function, fertility when appropriate for premenopausal women) and ways to maintain health. Discussions about family and social relationships and work, financial, and insurance concerns also were covered, as well as ways to promote healthy lifestyle behaviors such as improving physical activity, maintaining healthy nutrition and diet, and adhering to cancer surveillance. Session 3 focused on psychological distress (e.g., mood swings, anxiety, depression, fear of recurrence) and the spiritual effects of cancer (e.g., uncertainty, meaning in illness) and its treatment.

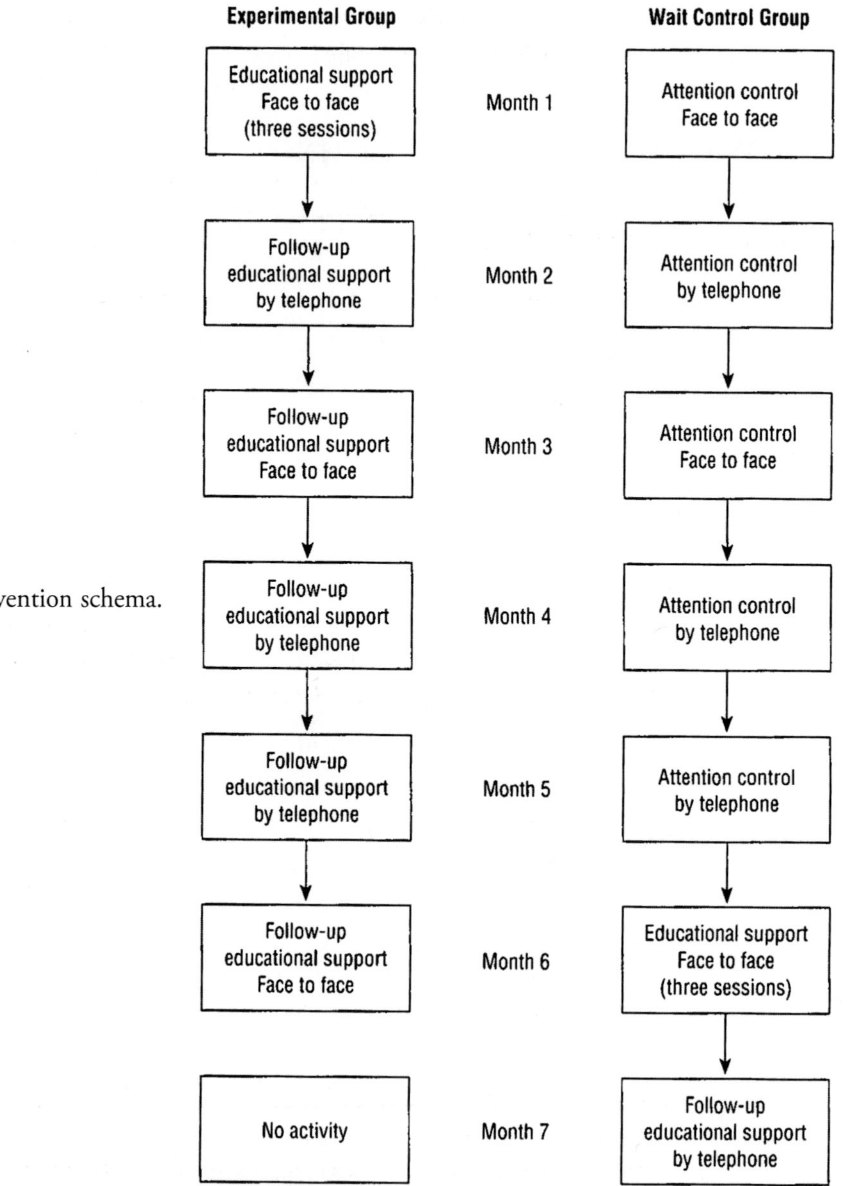

Figure 1 Intervention schema.

Face-to-face education and support sessions had a specific and unique format: In the first 30 minutes, all subjects received the same instruction, and the remaining 30 minutes were tailored to the unique problems and concerns facing each individual subject. In Session 1, subjects received information about pain, cancer-related fatigue, and lymphedema.

The intervention nurse described lymphedema, explained why subjects were at risk, and educated them about ways to prevent or manage lymphedema. The tailored component of the education and support sessions focused on unique concerns identified by each subject. For example, if a subject had specific concerns about lymphedema, the intervention nurse discussed specific ways to manage the symptom based on the subject's unique situation. The intervention nurse helped subjects to develop tailored management plans that may have included homework assignments, reading about the topic, listening to an audiotape, or trying new self-management tips.

Written and audiotaped materials supplemented the education and support sessions. Participants received the BCEI Education Binder, a 50-page notebook of materials divided into three sections that corresponded with each education and support session. Thirty-eight tip sheets ranging from one to three pages each were distributed to participants, offered management for specific concerns or problems, and used to reinforce education and support. Three audiotapes based on each of the three education and support sessions helped to reinforce learning in situations where participants preferred listening rather than reading.

Follow-up education and support sessions were conducted in person and by telephone. Each follow-up session lasted 30 minutes and was designed to evaluate subjects' symptom management, reinforce learning, and provide support. The intervention nurse also reviewed pertinent areas in the BCEI binder, tip sheets, and audiotaped materials.

Specific Aims and Hypotheses

The specific aims and hypotheses of the study were to determine the effect of the BCEI study on overall QOL and on the individual QOL domains and to examine whether the effects of the intervention were durable over time.

Subject Recruitment and Accrual

Subjects were recruited from a regional cancer center and private oncology offices in the southeastern United States. Women at least 21 years of age, with histologically confirmed stage O-II breast cancer and no evidence of local recurrence or metastatic disease, within one year of diagnosis, who had surgery at least one month before, who received radiation therapy or chemotherapy to recover from acute treatment side effects, and who were able to communicate in English were eligible to participate. Subjects may have been on hormonal therapy (i.e., aromatase inhibitor or tamoxifen) at study entry.

Procedure

Following study approval by the respective institutional review board of the university where the researchers were affiliated at the time of the study and the participating cancer centers, potential subjects were identified by the cancer center or private oncology office nursing staff using an eligibility checklist devised from consideration of the inclusion and exclusion criteria. A staff member briefly explained the study and determined eligible subjects' interest in participating.

Subjects expressing interest signed a consent form giving permission to release their name, telephone number, and address to the BCEI research office. Upon receipt of the consent form, the BCEI project director followed up with potential subjects, explained the study objectives and time commitment, and answered any questions.

Once subjects agreed to participate, they were assigned to a BCEI research nurse who obtained written informed consent consistent with university, cancer center, and federal poli-

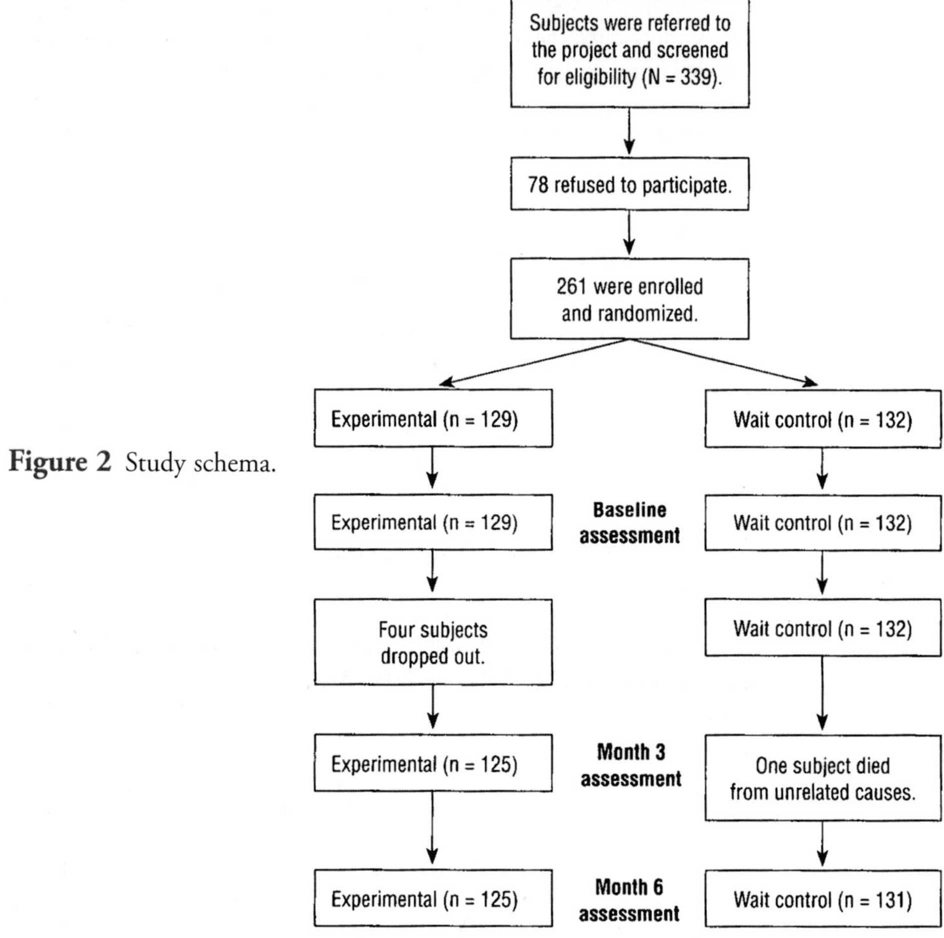

Figure 2 Study schema.

cies prior to study entry. Next, subjects completed baseline measures. They were randomly assigned to a treatment arm (i.e., experimental or wait control group) by the study biostatistician. The study eligibility and enrollment schema is depicted in Figure 2.

Instruments

The Breast Cancer Treatment and Sociodemographic Data Tool is a 32-item instrument used to capture breast cancer treatment variables (e.g., surgery, radiation therapy, chemotherapy, hormonal therapy, anti-HER2 therapy) and sociodemographic characteristics (e.g., age, race, ethnicity, education, marital status, employment status, telephone and communication patterns, family income, breast cancer history and treatment). Potential confounding variables (e.g., education, type of breast cancer therapy) were treated as covariates in data analysis.

Quality of Life–Breast Cancer Survivors is a 50-item scale that measures QOL in women with breast cancer and was adapted from the QOL–Cancer Survivors Scale (Dow et al., 1996; Ferrell et al., 1995). The items use a 10-point rating scale to describe overall QOL problems or concerns and within four identified domains—physical, psychological, social, and spiritual well-being. The tool is scored from 0-10, with lower scores indicating better QOL. Test-retest reliability of the original QOL–Cancer Survivors Scale was 0.89, and Cronbach's alpha was 0.93. Alpha coefficients for the current study were 0.93 for the total QOL score, 0.99 for the physical domain, 0.96 for the psychological domain, and 0.85 for both the social and spiritual domains.

Intervention Treatment Fidelity

Several strategies for treatment fidelity, including study design, interventionists' training, and intervention delivery and receipt, were incorporated into the BCEI study. The strategies were consistent with others reported in the literature (Bellg et al., 2004; Resnick, Bellg, et al., 2005; Resnick, Inguito, et al., 2005; Santacroce, Maccarelli, & Grey, 2004). Prior to the start of the study, an extensive BCEI procedure manual was developed; throughout the trial, the manual was reviewed regularly and updated periodically. The manual included detailed procedures for the standardized intervention protocol, ensuring consistency of data collection and management. Each member of the BCEI research team received didactic training in breast cancer survivorship, QOL, and the intervention protocol. In addition, the intervention nurses participated in three role-playing education and support sessions and follow-up sessions to standardize the intervention.

During intervention delivery, all education and support sessions were tape recorded. The study investigator reviewed a random sample of 20% of all education and support sessions using a specially designed quality assurance monitoring checklist. When any disagreement with the checklist occurred, outcomes were reviewed with the intervention nurses and adjustments made as needed. In addition, the BCEI research team discussed intervention delivery and fidelity issues at monthly team meetings. Strategies to monitor receipt of treatment were devised during follow-up education and support sessions where the intervention nurses reviewed the subjects' homework, provided feedback, and assessed ongoing behavioral changes.

After completion of the clinical trial, study subjects were asked to participate in a summative evaluation of the delivery of the BCEI intervention components (i.e., education and support, follow-up education and support, face-to-face and telephone discussions, written materials, and audiotapes).

Data Analysis

The research design is essentially a randomized, controlled longitudinal intervention study. The baseline measurements together with the longitudinal data enable comparison before and after the intervention. Simultaneously, the inclusion of the wait control group facilitated a natural history study of QOL in breast cancer survivors. By comparing the experimental group with the wait control group, the researchers were able to obtain a more genuine assessment of the BCEI. In addition, the wait control group received the BCEI at the end of the study.

To measure the efficacy of the BCEI, the endpoint variable of interest was the QOL score, which is the overall average computed from four subscale measures (physical, psychological, social, and spiritual well-being). The analysis was based on data collected at three time points—baseline, month 3 (time 2), and month 6 (time 3).

The generalized estimating equation (GEE) method for longitudinal data (Liang & Zeger, 1986) was the primary approach used to establish the efficacy of the BCEI study.

The analysis was performed with and without adjustment for baseline covariates to account for a possible imbalance in baseline characteristics between the two groups and identify potential confounding effects on the intervention treatment.

The GEE approach is flexible enough to allow for an intent-to-treat analysis by naturally integrating the few patients who dropped out after enrollment in the study. A number of two sample *t* tests and paired *t* tests were used with a Bonferroni type adjustment to make detailed comparisons, which helped to assess the sustained effect of the BCEI. Data were entered using SPSS® version 12 (SPSS Inc.). Statistical analysis was conducted using R (R Development Core Team, 2006).

RESULTS

Baseline Characteristics

A total of 261 women participated in the study. Four women in the experimental group withdrew during the first month of participation. One subject in the wait control group died from a non–cancer-related cause during the study. A total of 256 subjects remained in the study, and complete data for the subjects at all study time points were available (98% retention).

Subjects' mean age was 54.5 years (SD = 11.58); 82% were Caucasian, 9% were African American, 6% were Hispanic, and the remainder were Asian, Middle Eastern, and Native American. English was the primary language for 95%, and Spanish was the primary language for 4%. Almost 30% had a high school education but did not attend college, and 48% had a college education. Sixty-eight percent were married or living with a partner; 32% were single, divorced, or widowed. Sixty-two percent of subjects were employed full- or part-time, with 45% having annual family incomes of less than $50,000. More than 90% had not received counseling or participated in cancer support groups.

When breast cancer treatment was considered, more than 60% had breast-conserving surgery and 40% had single or bilateral mastectomy. More than 69% received primary or postoperative radiation therapy, and 54% received combination chemotherapy. More than 76% were taking tamoxifen or an aromatase inhibitor. Baseline demographic characteristics and treatment variables were compared to determine whether any significant baseline differences existed between groups, but none was found.

Effect of the Intervention on Overall Quality of Life

At baseline, no significant difference existed in overall QOL scores between groups. Figure 3 plots the mean QOL scores at the three time points for both groups. A lower value represents an improvement in QOL, whereas a higher value represents a decline in QOL. Both groups had similar mean QOL scores at baseline, which was confirmed by the associated two-sample *t* test (0.1613 with two-sided $p = 0.872$). At time 2, QOL scores in the wait control group were slightly worse, but they improved by time 3. In contrast, the experimental group showed dramatic improvement in QOL at time 2 and continued improvement at time 3. Overall QOL remained better at time 3 for those in the experimental group compared with the wait control group.

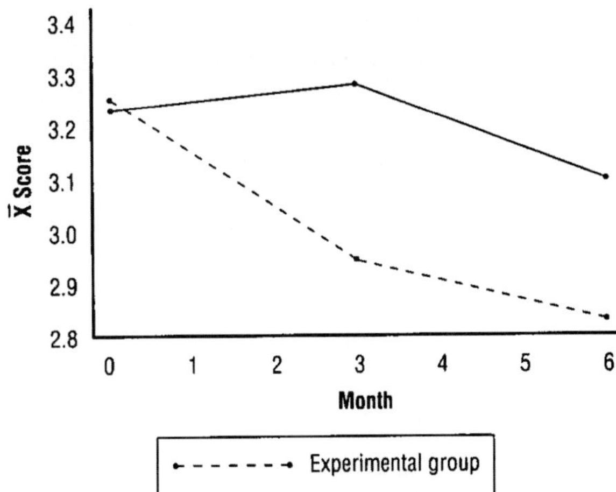

Figure 3 Plot of mean quality-of-life scores.

The GEE approach was used to draw the overall statistical conclusion about the effectiveness of the BCEI study. To proceed, two difference scores, time 2 versus baseline and time 3 versus baseline, were computed for each subject. The GEE marginal model was based on the two difference scores. A binary variable that distinguishes the two treatment groups was added into the model as a predictor. As a result, the within-group effect was filtered out so that the GEE approach could focus better on the between-group comparison while dealing with the correlation between two difference scores from the same subject. Other than the original demographic variables, a binary covariate of time, taking values at time 2 and time 3, also was included. Taken together, they were used as covariates in the GEE model and could be potential effect modifiers or confounders for the intervention effect.

Two GEE marginal models were fit: One included month as a covariant, and the other included all covariates. No significant interaction terms were found between the intervention and other covariates, including time, in both models. The slope estimates for the treatment effect (i.e., the BCEI) are −0.298 and −0.308, respectively, without and with adjustment for other covariates (both having $p < 0.001$), suggesting that the confounding effect of other covariates on the BCEI study was negligible.

Within-group differences were considered. Because the researchers made a total of six inferences, applying Bonferroni-type adjustment would lead to a joint significance level of 0.05 divided by 6 = 0.0083. Results showed that the experimental group's QOL greatly improved at both time points when compared to their baseline and to the wait control group. QOL in the wait control group declined by time 2 but did improve at time 3. Thus, the BCEI study was effective in improving QOL in the experimental group at time 2 and time 3. Furthermore, significant between-group differences in QOL were found at time 3.

Retention of Intervention Effects Over Time

The second specific aim examined whether the effects of the BCEI on QOL were retained through time 3 for the experimental group; the researchers hypothesized that the intervention effects would be durable. Table 1 presents the comparisons among three points: (a) baseline

TABLE 1 Between- and Within-Group Comparisons in Overall Quality of Life

	SCORE CHANGES			
Time Frame	**$\bar{X}$**	**SD**	**Paired *t* Test**	***p***
BASELINE TO MONTH 3				
Wait control group	0.042	0.752	0.642	0.522
Experimental group	−0.309	0.834	−4.142	<0.001
Two-sample *t* test	−28.420	—	—	<0.001
BASELINE TO MONTH 6				
Wait control group	−0.162	0.765	−2.423	<0.016
Experimental group	−0.405	0.879	−5.151	<0.001
Two-sample *t* test	−18.895	—	—	<0.001
MONTH 3 TO MONTH 6				
Wait control group	−0.199	0.784	−2.090	<0.004
Experimental group	−0.100	0.661	−1.687	<0.094
Two-sample *t* test	−1.096	—	—	<0.274

Experimental group $N = 125$
Wait control group $N = 132$
Note. The paired *t* test was used to assess changes between each pair of time points for each group, whereas the two-sample *t* test was used to compare the mean score changes between the experimental and wait conrol groups. All reported *p* values are two-sided.

and time 2, (b) baseline and time 3, and (c) time 2 and time 3. The values represent mean score changes. The paired *t* test was used to assess changes between every pair of time points for each group, and the two-sample *t* test was used to compare the mean score changes between the experimental group and the wait control group.

At time 2, the experimental group reflected significantly superior overall QOL scores compared to baseline scores ($p < 0.001$). At time 3, overall QOL in the experimental group remained significantly better compared to baseline ($p < 0.001$).

Although the primary intent of time 2 to time 3 analysis for the experimental group was to determine the durability of the BCEI study effect, the group experienced improved QOL from time 2 to time 3. Therefore, the effect of the BCEI was retained through time 3.

The intervention's Effect on the Quality-of-Life Domains

The third specific aim of this study was to determine the effects of the BCEI on the four QOL domains: physical, psychological, social, and spiritual well-being. Figure 4 plots the mean scores for each domain; the QOL pattern is similar to Figure 3. Both groups had similar mean domain QOL scores at baseline; but at times 2 and 3, the experimental group had lower mean scores (i.e., improved QOL) compared to the wait control group. The results were evident in psychological and social well-being scores between the two groups. The improvements can be attributed to the efficacy of the BCEI in enhancing QOL.

The GEE approach was used to draw a statistical conclusion (see Table 2). GEE analysis showed significant differences in overall QOL and psychological and social well-being scores between the two groups ($p < 0.001$). However, GEE analyses showed no significant differences in physical or spiritual well-being.

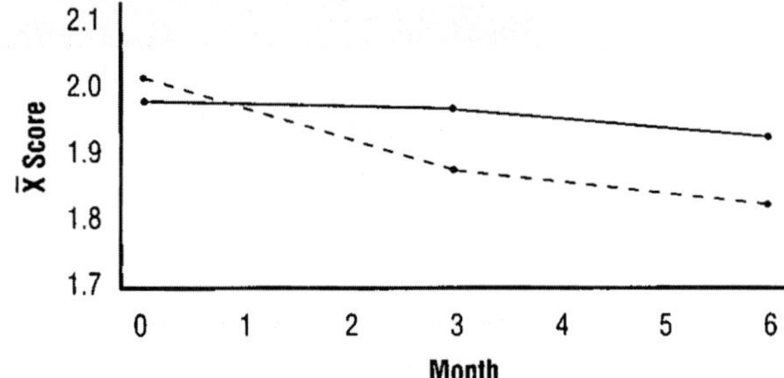

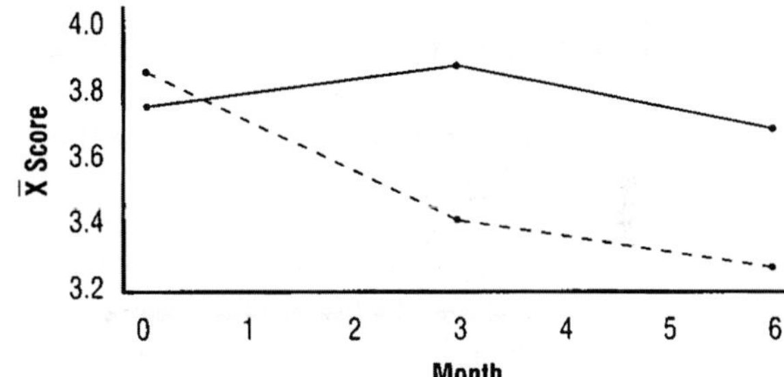

Figure 4 Plots of the mean domain scores.

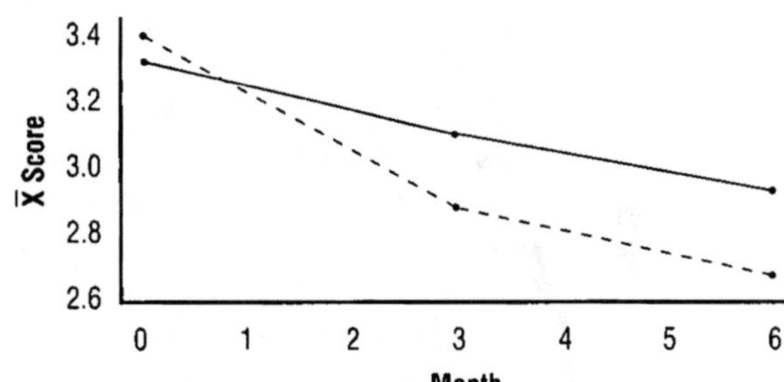

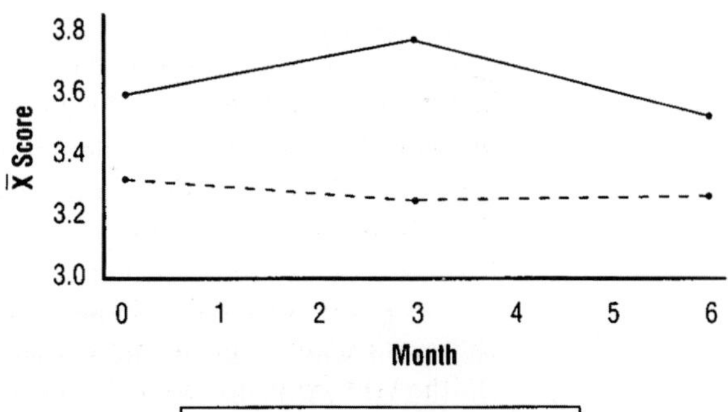

TABLE 2 Generalized Estimating Equation Comparisons Between Overall Quality of Life and Quality-of-Life Domain With and Without Covariates

Covariate Adjustment	With Covariates	*p*	Without Covariates	*p*
Overall quality of life	−4.144	<0.001	−4.356	<0.001
Physical well-being	−0.960	0.338	−1.129	0.258
Psychological well-being	−4.842	<0.001	−4.994	<0.001
Social well-being	−2.900	0.004	−2.974	0.003
Spiritual well-being	−0.652	0.514	−0.704	0.482

Note. All *p* values are two-sided.

DISCUSSION

At baseline, no differences existed in QOL scores between the two groups, thus establishing comparability. However, after the BCEI study was initiated, a significant difference in QOL emerged between the two groups. The experimental group's QOL scores showed significant improvement, whereas the wait control group's QOL scores showed decline. Thus, the efficacy of the BCEI has been established.

The researchers anticipated that the BCEI study effects would be maintained through time 3 for the experimental group, but QOL actually improved for that period. The positive effects of the BCEI for the experimental group through time 3 compared with moderate QOL improvement for the wait control group. The improvement from time 2 to time 3 in the wait control group resulted in less pronounced between-group differences. However, the experimental group continued to reflect significantly better overall QOL than did the wait control group. Thus, not only was the durability of the intervention demonstrated, but the differences between groups were maintained.

Several aspects of the results are interesting and deserve additional consideration. During what is perhaps a critical period early after treatment, the BCEI resulted in substantial improvements in QOL; however, those who did not receive the BCEI experienced a decline in QOL. That period could represent an at-risk time when patients are particularly vulnerable, in need of supporting alternatives for safe passage to later survivorship, and highly amenable to intervention.

The effects of the BCEI in the experimental group were not only maintained over the three-month period from time 2 to time 3, but QOL improved during that period. The study design does not allow for a definitive conclusion, but the QOL improvement may be because the BCEI is an ongoing, six-month intervention process in which follow-up reinforcement of education and support are critical.

QOL for the wait control group improved from time 2 to time 3, which is noteworthy. Marked between-group differences still existed at time 3, but the improvements in the wait control group are nonetheless impressive. The period immediately following treatment may be one in which patients are particularly vulnerable and has been mentioned previously (Institute of Medicine & National Research Council, 2006). Improvements in QOL for the wait control group may be a result of longer-term adaptation or resilience of breast cancer survivors that surfaces after a few months, or the improvement in QOL scores for the wait control group may be related to a reinterpretation of "normalcy" after treatment.

In examining the differential effect of the BCEI study on the physical, psychological, social, and spiritual well-being domains of QOL between the two groups, several explanations are offered. First, study results add further evidence in the literature that demonstrates enhanced psychological and social adjustment with psychoeducational interventions (Scheier et al., 2005; Stanton et al., 2005). Second, although the experimental group slightly improved and the wait control group declined in physical well-being scores at time 2, the differences were less evident at time 3. Subjects may have attributed aches, pains, and fatigue to aging or conditions preexisting cancer (e.g., arthritis, osteoporosis) or may have been in a phase of relatively good physical well-being.

Third, the differences in spiritual well-being scores showed a marked difference between the two groups at time 2, with similar improvement in the experimental group and a decline in the wait control group. However, by time 3, the wait control group showed improvement. Perceptions about the meaning of illness may have been incorporated over the six-month period with reduced certainty over the future.

IMPLICATIONS FOR RESEARCH AND PRACTICE

Several implications for practice and research become apparent. First, this randomized trial adds to a very small but growing body of psychoeducational interventions to improve QOL in post-treatment survivorship. Differential aspects of QOL contributed to overall improvement in QOL, notably psychological and social interventions. Determining what proportion of education or emotional support contributed to improved outcomes is important in future cancer survivorship research.

Second, this study contributes to a clearer articulation and description of the actual components of the intervention to help future researchers clarify their respective descriptions of delivery methods. Although this study used a combination of individual face-to-face and telephone delivery over a six-month period, additional modes or delivery systems for providing psychoeducational support interventions tailored to the target population should be examined in future studies. For example, telephone or electronic communication may be the most efficacious for at-risk, underserved populations in rural areas, whereas electronic means may be best for international breast cancer survivors (Fogel, Albert, Schnabel, Ditkoff, & Neugut, 2002; Gustafson et al., 2005; Meneses & McNees, in press). In brief, if an effective intervention or treatment is identified, the optimal delivery system for various populations remains a question of considerable interest.

Third, the intervention dose for each education and support component can be measured in future studies to further develop intervention treatment standards and adhere to treatment fidelity. Additionally, a discussion about treatment fidelity deserves attention in future behavioral intervention studies. A detailed description of the actual delivery components with treatment dose and strategies for treatment fidelity can improve the confidence in study results.

Theoretical and conceptual underpinnings currently are based on a variety of frameworks that do not fully describe the timing of interventions after treatment. The number of long-term cancer survivors is growing, so future studies that combine a theoretical or conceptual framework within a cancer survivorship context would help to illuminate the differences in post-treatment concerns. Such differences may be critically important in helping practitioners discern optimal routines, processes, and systems so that patients move from treatment to survivorship without being "lost in transition" from treatment to survivorship (Institute of Medicine & National Research Council, 2006).

From a clinical practice perspective, translation of research findings into practice can be accomplished in several venues—through established and new cancer survivorship clinics, in comprehensive breast health and breast cancer programs, and in individual practice. The study results also demonstrate that oncology nurses with their strong background in education and support are well positioned to lead the translation of research findings into practice.

If patients are to be provided safe passage from treatment to survivorship, oncology nurses will be very prominent, if not central, figures, in providing that conduit as well as the support and access to resources after treatment ends. The present study underscores the value and importance of that role.

REFERENCES

Armer, J., Fu, M.R., Wainstock, J.M., Zagar, E., & Jacobs, L.K. (2004). Lymphedema following breast cancer treatment, including sentinel lymph node biopsy. *Lymphology*, 37(2), 73-91.

Armer, J.M. (2005). The problem of post-breast cancer lymphedema: Impact and measurement issues. *Cancer Investigation*, 23, 76-83.

Armer, J.M., & Heckathorn, P.W. (2005). Post-breast cancer lymphedema in aging women: Self-management and implications for nursing. *Journal of Gerontological Nursing*, 57(5), 29-39.

Ashbury, F.D., Cameron, C, Mercer, S.L., Fitch, M., & Nielsen, E. (1998). One-on-one peer support and quality of life for breast cancer patients. *Patient Education and Counseling*, 55(2), 89-100.

Ashing-Giwa, K., Ganz, P.A., & Petersen, L. (1999). Quality of life of African-American and white long term breast carcinoma survivors. *Cancer*, 85, 418-426.

Avis, N.E., Crawford, S., & Manuel, J. (2005). Quality of life among younger women with breast cancer *Journal of Clinical Oncology*, 23, 3322-3330.

Badger, T., Segrin, C, Meek, P., Lopez, A.M., & Bonham, E. (2004). A case study of telephone interpersonal counseling for women with breast cancer and their partners. *Oncology Nursing Forum*, 31, 997-1003.

Barton, D., & Loprinzi, C. (2002). Novel approaches to preventing chemotherapy-induced cognitive dysfunction in breast cancer: The art of the possible. *Clinics in Breast Cancer*, i(Suppl. 3), S12I-S127.

Barton, D.L., Loprinzi, C.L., Novotny, P., Shanafelt, T., Sloan, J., Wahner-Roedler, D., et al. (2003). Pilot evaluation of citalopram for the relief of hot flashes. *Journal of Supportive Oncology*, 7(1), 47-51.

Bauer-Wu, S., & Farran, C.J. (2005). Meaning in life and psycho-spiritual functioning: A comparison of breast cancer survivors and healthy women. *Journal of Holistic Nursing*, 23, 172-190.

Bednarek, H.L., & Bradley, C.J. (2005). Work and retirement after cancer diagnosis. *Research in Nursing and Health*, 28, 126-135.

Bellg, A.J., Borrelli, B., Resnick, B., Hecht, J., Minicucci, D.S., Ory, M., et al. (2004). Enhancing treatment fidelity in health behavior change studies: Best practices and recommendations from the NIH Behavior Change Consortium. *Health Psychology*, 23, 443-451.

Bellizzi, K.M., & Blank, T.O. (2006). Predicting posttraumatic growth in breast cancer survivors. *Health Psychology*, 25(1), 47-56.

Bender, CM., Sereika, S.M., Berga, S.L., Vogel, V.G., Brufsky, A.M., Paraska, K.K., et al. (2006). Cognitive impairment associated with adjuvant therapy in breast cancer. *Psycho-Oncology*, 15, 422-430.

Berger, A.M., VonEssen, S., Kuhn, B.R., Piper, B.F, Agrawal, S., Lynch, J.C., et al. (2003). Adherence, sleep, and fatigue outcomes after adjuvant breast cancer chemotherapy: Results of a feasibility intervention study. *Oncology Nursing Forum*, 30, 513-522.

Berger, A.M., VonEssen, S., Kuhn, B.R., Piper, B.F, Farr, L., Agrawal, S., et al. (2002). Feasibility of a sleep intervention during adjuvant breast cancer chemotherapy. *Oncology Nursing Forum*, 29, 1431-1441.

Bower, J.E., Ganz, P.A., Desmond, K.A., Bernaards, C, Rowland, J.H., Meycrowitz, B.E., et al. (2006). Fatigue in long-term breast carcinoma survivors: A longitudinal investigation. *Cancer*, 106, 751-758.

Braden, C.J., Mishel, M.H., & Longman, A.J. (1998). Self-help intervention project: Women receiving breast cancer treatment. *Cancer Practice*, 6, 87-98.

Carpenter, J.S., & Andrykowski, M.A. (1999). Menopausal symptoms in breast cancer survivors. *Oncology Nursing Forum*, 26, 1311-1317.

Carpenter, J.S., Elam, J.L., Ridner, S.H., Carney, P.H., Cherry, G.J., & Cucullu, H.L. (2004). Sleep, fatigue, and depressive symptoms in breast cancer survivors and matched healthy women experiencing hot Flashes. *Oncology Nursing Forum*, 31, 591-598.

Carpenter, J.S., Storniolo, A.M., Johns, S., Monahan, PO., Azzouz, F, Elam, J.L., et al. (2007). Randomized, double-blind, placebo-controlled crossover trials of venlafaxine for hot flashes after breast cancer. *Oncologist*, 12, 124-135.

Casso, D., Buist, D.S., & Taplin, S. (2004). Quality of life of 5-10 year breast cancer survivors diagnosed between age 40 and 49. *Health and Quality of Life Outcomes*, 2, 25.

Chamberlain-Wilmoth, M., Tulman, L., Coleman, E.A., Stewart, C.B., & Samarel, N. (2006). Women's perceptions of the effectiveness of telephone support and education on their adjustment to breast cancer. *Oncology Nursing Forum*, 33, 138-144.

Cimprich, B., Janz, N.K., Northouse, L., Wren, P.A., Given, B., & Given, C.W. (2005). Taking CHARGE: A self-management program for women following breast cancer treatment. *Psycho-Oncology*, 14, 704-717.

Cimprich, B., & Ronis, D.L. (2003). An environmental intervention to restore attention in women with newly diagnosed breast cancer. *Cancer Nursing*, 26, 284-292.

Cimprich, B., So, H., Ronis, D.L., & Trask, C. (2005). Pre-treatment factors related to cognitive functioning in women newly diagnosed with breast cancer *Psycho-Oncology* 14, 70-78.

Coleman, E.A., Tulman, L., Samarel, N., Wilmoth, M.C, Rickel, L., Rickel, M., et al. (2005). The effect of telephone social support and education on adaptation to breast cancer during the year following diagnosis. *Oncology Nursing Forum*, 32, 822-829.

Courneya, K.S., Blanchard, CM., & Laing, D.M. (2001). Exercise adherence in breast cancer survivors training for a dragon boat race competition: A preliminary investigation. *Psycho-Oncology*, 10, 444-452.

Dirksen, S.R., & Erickson, J.R. (2002). Well-being in Hispanic and non-Hispanic white survivors of breast cancer. *Oncology Nursing Forum*, 29, 820-826.

Dow, K.H., Ferrell, B.R., Haberman, M.R., & Eaton, L. (1999). The meaning of quality of life in cancer survivorship. *Oncology Nursing Forum*, 26, 519-528.

Dow, K.H., Ferrell, B.R., Leigh, S., Ly, J., & Gulasekaram, P. (1996). An evaluation of the quality of life among long-term survivors of breast cancer. *Breast Cancer Research and Treatment*, 39, 261-273.

Ferrans, C.E. (1994). Quality of life through the eyes of survivors of breast cancer. *Oncology Nursing Forum*, 21, 1645-1651.

Ferrell, B.R., Dow, K.H., & Grant, M. (1995). Measurement of the quality of life of cancer survivors. *Quality of Life Research*. 4, 523-531.

Fogel, J., Albert, S.M., Schnabel, F., Ditkoff, B.A., & Neugut, A.I. (2002). Internet use and social support in women with breast cancer. *Health Psychology*, 21, 398-404.

Giedzinska, A.S., Meyerowitz, B.E., Ganz, P.A., & Rowland, J.H. (2004). Health-related quality of life in a multiethnic sample of breast cancer survivors. *Annals of Behavioral Medicine*, 28, 39-51.

Gotay, C.C., & Muraoka, M.Y. (1998). Quality of life in long-term survivors of adult-onset cancers. *Journal of the National Cancer Institute*, 90, 656-667.

Gustafson, D.H., McTavish, F.M., Stengle, W., Ballard, D., Hawkins, R., Shaw, B.R., et al. (2005). Use and impact of eHealth System by low income women with breast cancer. *Journal of Health Communication*, 10(Suppl. 1), 195-218.

Heidrich, S.M., Egan, J.J., Hengudomsub, P., & Randolph, S.M. (2006). Symptoms, symptom beliefs, and quality of life of older breast cancer survivors: A comparative study. *Oncology Nursing Forum*, 33, 315-322.

Helgeson, V.S., Gohen, S., Schulz, R., & Yasko, J. (2001). Long-term effects of educational and peer discussion group interventions on adjustment to breast cancer. *Health Psychology*, 20, 387-392.

Holzner, B., Kemmler, G., Kopp, M., Moschen, R., Schweigkofler, H., Dunser, M., et al. (2001). Quality of life in breast cancer patients—Not enough attention for long-term survivors? *Psychosomatics*, 42, 117-123.

Hosaka, T., Sugiyama, Y., Hirai, K., Okuyaina, T., Sugawara, Y., & Nakamura, Y., (2001). Effects of a modified group intervention with early-stage breast cancer patients. *General Hospital Psychiatry*, 23, 145-151.

Hoskins, G.N., Haber, J., Budin, W.G., Gartwright-Alcarese, F., Kowalski, M.O., Panke, J., et al. (2001). Breast cancer: Education, counseling, and adjustment—A pilot study. *Psychological Reports*, 89, 677-704.

Institute of Medicine & National Research Council. (2004). Meeting the psychosocial needs of women with breast cancer (vol. 2005). Washington, DC: National Academies Press.

Institute of Medicine & National Research Council. (2006). From cancer patient to cancer survivor: Lost in transition. Washington, DC: National Academies Press.

King, M.T., Kenny, P., Shiell, A., Hall, J., & Boyages, J. (2000). Quality of life three months and one year after first treatment for early stage breast cancer: Influence of treatment and patient characteristics. *Quality of Life Research*, 9, 789-800.

Kinney, G.K., Rodgers, D.M., Nash, K.A., & Bray, G.O. (2003). Holistic healing for women with breast cancer through a mind, body, and spirit self-empowerment program. *Journal of Holistic Nursing*, 21, 260-279.

Knobf, M.T. (2002). Carrying on: The experience of premature menopause in women with early stage breast cancer. *Nursing Research*, 51, 9-17.

Kurtz, M.E., Wyatt, G., & Kurtz, J.C. (1995). Psychological and sexual well-being, philosophical/spiritual views, and health habits of long-term cancer survivors. *Health Care for Women International*, 16, 253-262.

Lewis, F.M., Gasey, S.M., Brandt, P.A., Shands, M.E., & Zahlis, E.H. (2006). The enhancing connections program: Pilot study of a cognitive-behavioral intervention for mothers and children affected by breast cancer, *Psycho-Oncology*, 15, 486-497.

Lewis, F.M., & Deal, L.W. (1995). Balancing our lives: A study of the married couple's experience with breast cancer recurrence. *Oncology Nursing Forum*, 22, 943-953.

Lewis, J.A., Manne, S.L., DuHatnel, K.N., Vickburg, S.M., Bovbjerg, D.H., Gurrie, V., et al. (2001). Social support, intrusive thoughts, and quality of life in breast cancer survivors. *Journal of Behavioral Medicine*, 24, 231-245.

Liang, K.Y., & Zeger, S.L. (1986). Longitudinal data analysis using generalized linear models. *Biometrika*, 73, 13-22.

Loerzel, V.W., Dow, K.H., & McNees, P. (2006, February). Why women with breast cancer use or don't use lymphedema prevention and management strategies. Presented at the American Psychosocial Oncology Society Third Annual Conference, Amelia Island, FL.

Marcus, A.C., Garrett, K.M., Gella, D., Wenzel, L.B., Brady, M.J., Grane, L.A., et al. (1998). Telephone counseling of breast cancer patients after treatment: A description of a randomized clinical trial. *Psycho-Oncology*, 7, 470-482.

Mast, M.E. (1998). Survivors of breast cancer: Illness uncertainty, positive reappraisal, and emotional distress. *Oncology Nursing Forum*, 25, 555-562.

Mellon, S. (2002). Comparisons between cancer survivors and family members on meaning of the illness and family quality of life. *Oncology Nursing Forum*, 29, 1117-1125.

Meneses, K. (in review). Breast cancer research by oncology nurse scientists. In C.R. King & J. Mitchell-Phillips (Eds.), *Advancing oncology nursing science.* Pittsburgh, PA: Oncology Nursing Society.

Meneses, K., & McNees, P. (in press). Transdisciplinary integration of electronic communication technology and nursing research. *Nursing Outlook.*

Meraviglia, M. (2006). Effects of spirituality in breast cancer survivors [online exclusive]. *Oncology Nursing Forum*, 33, EI-E7. Retrieved July 26, 2007, from http://www.ons.org/publications/journals/QNF/volutne33/issuel/pdf7330137.pdf.

Mishel, M.H., Germino, B.B., Gil, K.M., Belyea, M., Laney, I.C, Stewart, J., et al. (2005). Benefits from an uncertainty management intervention for African-American and Caucasian older long-term breast cancer survivors, *Psycho-Oncology*, 14, 962-978.

Miyashita, M. (2005). A randomized intervention study for breast cancer survivors in Japan: Effects of short-term support group focused on possible breast cancer recurrence. *Cancer Nursing*, 2S, 70-78.

Mock, V., Frangakis, C., Davidson, N.E., Ropka, M.E., Pickett, M., Poniatowski, B., et al. (2005). Exercise manages fatigue during breast cancer treatment: A randomized controlled trial. *Psycho-Oncology*, 14.

National Cancer Institute. (2006). About cancer survivorship research: Survivorship definitions. Retrieved February 16, 2007, from http://dccps.nci.nih.gov/ocs/definitions.html.

Northouse, L., Kershaw, T, Mood, D., & Schafenacker, A. (2005). Effects of a family intervention on the quality of life of women with recurrent breast cancer and their family caregivers, *Psycho-Oncology*, 14, 478-491.

Northouse, L.L., Mood, D., Kershaw, T., Schafenackei, A., Mellon, S., Walker, J., et al. (2002). Quality of life of women with recurrent breast cancer and their family members. *Journal of Clinical Oncology*, 20, 4050-4064.

Payne, J., Piper, B., Rabinowitz, I., & Zitntnemian, B. (2006). Biomarkers, fatigue, sleep, and depressive symptoms in women with breast cancer: A pilot study. *Oncology Nursing Forum*, 33, 775-783.

Rawl, S.M., Given, B.A., Given, C.W., Ghatnpion, V.L., Kozachik, S.L., Kozachik, S.L., et al. (2002). Intervention to improve psychological functioning for newly diagnosed patients with cancer. *Oncology Nursing Forum*, 29, 967-975.

R Development Core Team. (2006). A language and environment for statistical computing: Reference index (version 2.3.1). Retrieved July 25, 2007, from http://cran.r-project.org/doc/manuals/fullrefman.pdf.

Resnick, B., Bellg, A.J., Borrelli, B., Defrancesco, G., Breger, R., Hecht, J., et al. (2005). Examples of implementation and evaluation of treatment fidelity in the BGG studies: Where we are and where we need to go. *Annals of Behavioral Medicine*, 29(Suppl.), 46-54.

Resnick, B., Inguito, P., Orwig, D., Yahiro, J.Y., Hawkes, W., Werner, M., et al. (2005). Treatment fidelity in behavior change research: A case example. *Nursing Research*, 54, 139-143.

Sandgren, A.K., & McGaul, K.D. (2006), Long-term telephone therapy outcomes for breast cancer patients. *Psycho-Oncology*, 16, 38-47.

Santacroce, S.J., Maccarelli, L.M., & Grey, M. (2004). Intervention fidelity. *Nursing Research*, 53, 63-66.

Scheier, M.R., Helgeson, V.S., Schulz, R., Golvin, S., Berga, S., Bridges, M.W., et al. (2005). Interventions to enhance physical and psychological functioning among younger women who are ending nonhormonal adjuvant treatment for early-stage breast cancer. *Journal of Clinical Oncology*, 23, 4298-4311.

Stanton, A.L., Ganz, P.A., Kwan, L., Meyerowitz, B.E., Bower, J.E., Krupnick, J.L., et al. (2005). Outcomes from the Moving Beyond Cancer psychoeducational, randomized, controlled trial with breast cancer patients. *Journal of Clinical Oncology*, 23, 6009-6018.

Stewart, D.E., Cheung, A.M., Duff, S., Wong, R., McQuestion, M., Cheng, T., et al. (2001). Long-term breast cancer survivors: Confidentiality, disclosure, effects on work and insurance. *Psycho-Oncology*, 10, 259-263.

Vacek, P.M., Winstead-Fry, P., Seeker-Walker, R.H., Hooper, G.J., & Plante, D.A. (2003). Factors influencing quality of life in breast cancer survivors. *Quality of Life Research*, 12, 527-537.

Waltman, N.L., Twiss, J.J., Ott, C.D., Gross, G.J., Lindsey, A.M., Moore, T.E., et al. (2003). Testing an intervention for preventing osteoporosis in postmenopausal breast cancer survivors. *Journal of Nursing Scholarship*, 35, 333-338.

Wonghongkul, T., Dechaprom, N., Phumivichuvate, L., & Losawatkul, S. (2006). Uncertainty appraisal coping and quality of life in breast cancer survivors. *Cancer Nursing*, 29, 250-257.

Wyatt, G., Kurtz, M.E., & Liken, M. (1993). Breast cancer survivors: An exploration of quality of life issues. *Cancer Nursing*, i6, 440-448.

Yates, P., Aranda, S., Hargraves, M., Mirolo, B., Clavarino, A., McLachlan, S., et al. (2005). Randomized controlled trial of an educational intervention for managing fatigue in women receiving adjuvant chemotherapy for early-stage breast cancer. *Journal of Clinical Oncology*, 23, 6027-6036.

B

Self-Efficacy for Health-Related Behaviors Among Deaf Adults

Elaine G. Jones[1]*, *Ralph Renger*[2]*, *and Youngmi Kang*[1†]

ABSTRACT

The purpose of this quasi-experimental, pre-post-test study was to test the effectiveness of the Deaf Heart Health Intervention (DHHI) in increasing self-efficacy for health-related behaviors among culturally deaf adults. The DHHI targets modifiable risk factors for cardiovascular disease. A sample of 84 participants completed time-1 and time-2 data collection. The sign language version of the Self-Rated Abilities Scale for Health Practices (SRAHP) was used to measure self-efficacy for nutrition, psychological well-being/stress management, physical activity/exercise, and responsible health practices. Total self-efficacy scores were significantly higher in the intervention group than in the comparison group at time-2, controlling for scores at baseline (F [1, 81] = 26.02, $p < .001$). Results support the development of interventions specifically tailored for culturally deaf adults to increase their self-efficacy for health behaviors. © 2007 Wiley Periodicals, Inc. *Res Nurs Health* 30:185-192, 2007.

Keywords: deaf; health; self-efficacy

The purpose of this study was to test the effectiveness of the Deaf Heart Health Intervention (DHHI) in increasing self-efficacy for health behaviors related to risk for cardiovascular disease (CVD) among culturally deaf adults. There are an estimated two million adults who are members of a deaf cultural community. Culturally deaf adults typically experience significant hearing loss at an early age, communicate primarily through sign language in adulthood, and participate in deaf community activities (Dolnick, 1993; Stebnicki & Coeling, 1999). American Sign Language (ASL) is the primary language for culturally deaf

[1]University of Arizona, College of Nursing, Tucson, AZ
[2]University of Arizona, College of Public Health, Tucson, AZ
Correspondence to Elaine G. Jones, 1305 N. Martin, Room 411, University of Arizona, College of Nursing, Tucson, AZ 85721-0203.
*Associate Professor.
†Doctoral Candidate.
Published online in Wiley InterScience (www.interscience.wiley.com) DOI: 10.1002/nur.20196

communities who are often considered a linguistic minority. Adults with hearing loss beginning in adulthood ("late-deafened" or hard-of-hearing) face communication issues different from culturally deaf adults. Late-deafened and hard-of-hearing adults typically continue to rely on spoken language. They are usually literate in their first language and rarely learn sign language.

CVD remains a leading cause of premature death and disability in the United States (Centers for Disease Control and Prevention [CDC], 2005a). There are no data specifically about health status or CVD, in particular, among culturally deaf adults. People with hearing loss are included together, with no distinction between culturally deaf, late-deafened, or hard-of-hearing people, in health statistics of people with physical disabilities. In general, people with disabilities are at greater risk for CVD than people without disabilities. For example, 19% of people with disabilities have high total blood cholesterol, compared to 17% of people without disabilities (CDC, 2005b). In addition, many culturally deaf adults are from ethnic minority groups who are known to have greater CVD risk than white non-Hispanic populations. For example, CVD mortality rates are consistently higher among black Americans than white Americans (CDC, 2005a) and many deaf persons are black (Gallaudet Research Institute, 2005).

There have been extensive efforts to promote health behaviors to decrease modifiable risks for CVD in varied populations specifically related to heart-healthy diets, physical activity, and stress management. Deaf adults may lack the prerequisite behavioral capabilities (knowledge and skills) for achieving high levels of self-efficacy for health-related behaviors to decrease their risk for CVD (Advocate Health Care [AHC] & Sinai Health System [SHS], 2004; Jones, Renger, & Firestone, 2005), yet no published reports exist of interventions specifically targeting self-efficacy for heart-health behaviors among culturally deaf adults. AHC and SHS (2004) collaborated to survey 203 culturally deaf adults in the Chicago area about their health status, health care experiences, communication styles, barriers to accessing health care and health knowledge and behaviors. Overall, about 44% of respondents said they were overweight. Participants were asked how many days per week they exercised at least 20 minutes. AHC participants averaged 3.4 days and SHS participants averaged 1 day per week. Regarding cholesterol, 31% of the total sample said they had been told that they had high cholesterol, but only 38% could correctly define the term *cholesterol* and many participants (42% at SHS and 12% at AHC) were unable to name any ways to control blood cholesterol levels. Many could not identify any risk factors for a heart attack or stroke (47% at SHS and 16% at AHC). The researchers concluded that deaf participants who were more educated, reported a higher household income, and who were non-Hispanic and white had higher levels of knowledge than their less educated, poorer, and non-white counterparts consistent with correlates of poor health in other groups. In addition, the researchers noted that the deaf adults in their study were receiving health care from deaf-friendly organizations and that the health knowledge and health status of deaf adults who have less access to health information, are likely worse than their study sample.

Jones et al. (2005) reported results of interviews (in sign language) with 111 culturally deaf adults regarding CVD risk factors. Nearly half (49%) reported diets that were moderate-high fat, and 43% were overweight (BMI > 25) or obese. The majority (54%) said they exercised less than three times each week. In response to questions about how often they had felt angry or frustrated in the last month (to assess stress), more than half said "some of the time," and 13% said "most of the time." Most (82%) thought their cholesterol was normal because no one had told them it was high. Yet, the data collectors were unsure whether the participants were familiar with the term *cholesterol.* Results of this community analysis provided the foundation for developing and pilot testing the DHHI, which is the only intervention we are aware of specifically designed to lower culturally deaf adults' CVD risk factors.

BARRIERS TO ACCESSING HEALTH INFORMATION IN DEAF ADULTS

For many culturally deaf adults, English functions as a second language, and for a variety of reasons, the average reading level of many culturally deaf adults is at the third- to fourth-grade level. The most recent study of literacy among deaf and hard-of-hearing students found that the median reading comprehension subtest scores for 17- to 18-year-old deaf/hard-of-hearing students corresponded with a fourth-grade level for hearing students (Gallaudet Research Institute, 1996; Holt, Traxler, & Allen, 1997). Many culturally deaf adults are, therefore, virtually unable to access information available to hearing adults through sound or written language. With television, radio, computers, newspapers, and health professionals relying on spoken or written English, a limited number of culturally deaf individuals can benefit from health-related information as typically provided. Closed captioning may be useful for late-deafened persons or for the minority of truly bilingual (Sign/English) deaf adults. Basic health information and skills are prerequisite to gaining the self-efficacy (confidence) necessary to enact behaviors linked to positive health (Baranowski, Perry, & Parcel, 2002). In addition to communication barriers, culturally deaf adults' lower average socioeconomic status (Olkin, Abrams, Preston, & Kirshbaum, 2006) and membership in ethnic minority groups may compound their risk for poor health outcomes (Adler & Newman, 2002).

Deaf adults are more often unemployed or underemployed and often have less education than their hearing counterparts (McCrone, 1990; Olkin et al., 2006). The ethnic composition of the culturally deaf community reflects the ethnic composition of the general public (Foster & Kinuthia, 2003); however, most deaf adults' primary language is ASL, rather than the language of their ethnic group. Despite the numerous risk factors for poor health outcomes, culturally deaf adults, like other groups with physical disabilities or language barriers, are rarely included in health promotion research.

SELF-EFFICACY FOR HEALTH-RELATED BEHAVIORS

Defined as the belief in one's ability to perform a certain task, self-efficacy is a key construct in understanding and modifying health behaviors (Bandura, 1986, 1995). Self-efficacy is a major factor in decisions to adopt healthy behaviors among people with varying health states, ages, and ethnic groups (Maase & Anderson, 2003; Resnick, 1998; Sohng, Sohng, & Yeom, 2002; Taylor, 2000). Yet self-efficacy may vary with the specific health behavior in question (Faryna & Morales, 2000; Hickey, Owen, & Froman, 1992; Horan, Kim, Gendler, Froman, & Patel, 1998). Self-efficacy in engaging in one health behavior does not guarantee self-efficacy when engaging in another. For example, the skills needed to manage stress (more psychological) are different from those needed to engage in exercise (more physical). A high degree of self-efficacy for a specific health behavior correlates strongly with actual enactment of that behavior (Yarcheski, Mahon, Yarcheski, & Cannella, 2004).

Two studies of health-related self-efficacy among adults with physical disabilities provided data relevant for comparison to culturally deaf adults' scores for health-related self-efficacy. Stuifbergen and Becker (1994) included measures of self-efficacy for specific health behaviors in a sample of 117 adults with 22 disabilities, 10 of whom were hearing-impaired. Scores of the hearing-impaired participants were not reported separately. The mean age of the sample was 44 years (range 20-74). The sample included approximately equal numbers of men and women; 85% had at least some college education. The majority (88%) were Anglo, and the ethnicity of the remaining subjects was not reported. The mean Self-Rated Abilities Scale for Health Practices (SRAHP) score was 79.87 (range 41-112, *SD* = 7.03). In addition, self-efficacy scores for specific health behaviors were highly correlated with scores for actual health behaviors. The researchers concluded that interventions designed to strengthen perceptions of self-efficacy could be successful in promoting higher rates of health behaviors in nutrition and exercise among persons with disabilities.

Tate et al. (2002) included assessment of health-related self-efficacy in their study to evaluate the effectiveness of a wellness program for men and women with spinal cord injury (*n* = 68 at baseline). Forty-four completed post-testing: 23 in the intervention group and 21 in the control group. The mean age of the sample was 47 years (range 22-80); the majority were men (68%) and white (93%). A minority (23%) had high school education, 40% had some college education, and 37% were college graduates. The intervention was a series of six 4-hour workshop sessions. The SRAHP was used as the pre- and post-test measure of health-related self-efficacy. The mean score at baseline was 88 (*SD* = 17.8) for the intervention group and 92.8 (*SD* = 12.7) for the control group. There was a significant improvement in the SRAHP scores for the intervention group (increased to a mean of 95.4; *p* = .03), while the control group scores showed no significant change (*p* = .88).

THE DEAF HEART HEALTH INTERVENTION

The DHHI was designed specifically for implementation with culturally deaf adults whose preferred communication was in sign language (Jones et al., 2005). Its health content draws heavily from recommendations from the American Heart Association (2006b) for primary prevention of CVD. The teaching-learning strategies incorporated in the DHHI were based on principles of health behavior change in social cognitive theory (Bandura, 1986, 1995) and research on preferred teaching-learning strategies among culturally deaf adults (Lang, McKee, & Conner, 1993; Lang, Stinson, Basile, Kavanagh, & Liu, 1999). Participants attended class once each week for 2 hours over 8 weeks. Classes were highly interactive and were taught entirely in sign language by a trained deaf lay heart-health teacher. The training for the deaf DHHI teacher consisted of 12 hours of didactic instruction about modifiable CVD risk factors and principles of health behavior change, followed by supervised teaching of the entire 16 hour DHHI with three deaf volunteers.

The DHHI begins with discussion of heart disease, CVD risk factors, and discussion of reasons for joining the classes and goals for participation. Activities to increase self-efficacy for heart-healthy eating include a presentation about the food pyramid (knowledge building), practice in planning heart-healthy daily menus and reading food labels (skill building), and discussing strategies for overcoming barriers to healthy eating (problem solving). Activities to strengthen self-efficacy for exercise and physical activity include information about safety during exercise and physical activity (American Heart Association, 2006a), practice counting heart-rate and discussion about overcoming barriers to exercise and physical activity. Activities related to stress and stress management include discussion of the effects of stress on health, practice with guided relaxation using a lava lamp, and discussions about different stress management strategies. The final class focuses on celebrating progress and planning strategies for maintaining health behaviors over time. The study hypothesis was that culturally deaf adults who receive the DHHI would demonstrate greater self-efficacy for targeted health-related behaviors than deaf adults who did not receive the DHHI.

METHOD

We used a quasi-experimental, pre-post-test design. Participants were recruited through networking within the deaf community and advertising on a Web site frequented by deaf individuals. sample of 105 deaf adults was recruited in Phoenix and Tucson, Arizona. The 84 participants who completed both time-1 and time-2 data collection included more women (58%) than men, and had a median education level of high school and a mean age of 51 years (range 18-85, *SD* = 18.34). There was a significant difference between the intervention and comparison groups in ethnic composition (composition (χ^2 [1, N = 84] = 8.17, p = .004), with more participants in the intervention group (37%) who were members of ethnic minorities (mainly Mexican-American) than in the comparison group (8%). American Sign Language is used throughout the deaf community, regardless of ethnic or language background. The mean SRAHP scores for deaf participants from ethnic minorities were lower (71.9, *SD* = 21.3) than the mean scores of the white/non-Hispanic (81.5, *SD* = 15.0) deaf participants, but the differences did not reach statistical significance.

The intervention group in Tucson received the 8-week (16 hours) DHHI, and the Phoenix comparison group received an alternative treatment of 16 hours of social activities, such as movies, game nights, and potluck dinners over 8 weeks. Both the DHHI and the social activities were conducted in small group meetings, in cohorts of 5-10 persons, at locations in the community.

During the study, the PI visited selected classes to ensure fidelity in conducting the DHHI. The DHHI teacher completed evaluation forms after each class, reporting time spent on each topic (dose), and any deviation from the class plans. The social activities for the comparison group were designed to enhance their interest in continued participation in the study and control for the Hawthorne effect by engaging participants in activities unlikely to affect their heart health behaviors over the course of the study.

Participants in Tucson and Phoenix were not randomly assigned to intervention versus comparison groups because the deaf community in each city is relatively small and close-knit. Cross-talk would probably occur between deaf adults assigned to different treatment groups within the same city. Tucson was selected as the site for conducting the intervention group because the intervention group required more intensive supervision than the comparison group, and the majority of the research team resided in Tucson.

Sample

Selection criteria included: (a) 18 years or older and (b) self-identified as a member of deaf culture. Persons under 18 years of age were not eligible for participation because the content and teaching strategies of the intervention were designed for adults. Persons who had a prior diagnosis of CVD were disqualified for participation because the DHHI is a primary prevention intervention. Participants in the comparison group were invited to free presentations about heart health at the conclusion of the study. The study was approved by the University of Arizona Institutional Review Board for Protection of Human Subjects prior to subject recruitment. The consent form was translated into ASL, presented to potential participants on videotape, and any questions were answered in sign language as part of the consenting procedure.

Instruments and Procedures

Self-efficacy for the targeted health behaviors was measured with the SRAHP (Becker, Stuifbergen, Oh, & Hall, 1993; Stuifbergen & Becker, 1994). The SRAHP is a 28-item self-report questionnaire designed to measure self-efficacy in the areas of nutrition, psychological well-being/stress management, physical activity/exercise, and responsible health practices. Individuals are asked to rate their ability to perform a health behavior on a five-point scale from 0 (not at all) to 4 (completely). The stem for each item is "I am able to ..." The Cronbach's alpha for the total scale was .94 in two samples, totaling 298 subjects, and 2-week test-retest reliability for a sample of 70 students was r = .70.

The Nutrition Subscale has seven items to measure beliefs about ability to perform practices in nutrition. The Psychological Well-Being (Stress Management) Subscale has seven items to measure psychological well-being. These questions correspond to stress management skills taught in many stress management classes, such as the DHHI. For example, one question on the psychological well-being scale asks how confident the individual is that he/she can "change things in my life to reduce my stress" or "figure out things I can do to help me relax," and "get help from others when I need it." The Physical Activity Subscale has seven items to measure beliefs about ability to perform physical activity/exercise. The Responsible Health Practices Subscale has seven items about the individual's confidence in interacting effectively with health providers: for example, "I am able to find a doctor or nurse who gives me good advice about how to stay healthy." Although this last subscale was not specifically relevant to the targeted modifiable CVD risk factors, it was administered along with the other items to enable us to make comparisons to total SRAHP scores from other study samples.

The SRAHP scale was previously used with a sample of 117 adults with disabilities, including 10 hearing-impaired persons. The original written English SRAHP was translated into ASL on videotape (Jones & Kay, 1992; Jones, Lee, Phillips, Zhang, & Jaciedo, 2001; Jones, Mallinson, Phillips, & Kang, 2006) and administered to 24 adults who were bilingual in English and ASL prior to use in pilot testing the DHHI. The correlation between total scores on the original written English SRAHP and the signed SRAHP was excellent (r = .92), and internal consistency was high (Cronbach's alpha of .91 and .90, respectively), supporting the comparability of the written English and signed SRAHP. We assessed the psychometric soundness of the signed SRAHP with the larger sample of deaf participants (n = 105) before proceeding to analyze scores. The internal consistency remained high (Cronbach's alpha = .92) and item-total correlations ranged from .39 to .79.

Data Analysis

Data were analyzed using SPSS 12.0. Chi-square was used to assess demographic differences between the intervention and comparison groups. *T*-tests were performed to identify differences in self-efficacy scores at baseline between the intervention and comparison groups. ANCOVA was used to control for initial difference on self-efficacy scores between the intervention and comparison groups and to test the effectiveness of the DHHI in increasing self-efficacy for targeted health-related behaviors. Statistical significance was set at a p value <.05 for a two-tailed test.

RESULTS

A sample of 105 deaf adults was recruited in southern Arizona for participation in this study: 41 in the Tucson intervention group and 64 in the Phoenix comparison group at baseline (Time 1). Eighty-four participants completed data collection at time 2 (Table 1): 32 from the intervention group and 52 from the comparison group, representing an 80% return rate at time 2 or, conversely, a 20% attrition rate for time-2 data collection. Only participants who completed both time-1 and time-2 data collection were included in data analysis to evaluate the effectiveness of the DHHI in increasing self efficacy for health-related behaviors.

The hypothesis was supported. The mean total SRAHP score for the total sample (n = 84) was 77.87 (range 38-107, SD = 17.85) at time 1. SRAHP scores of total and of each subscale at time 1 were significantly higher in the comparison group ($p < .05$) than in the intervention group. Therefore, ANCOVA was used to test the effectiveness of the DHHI controlling for self-efficacy score at time 1. Assumptions of ANCOVA were met. Total self-efficacy scores were significantly higher in the intervention group than in the comparison group after the DHHI, controlling for the total self-efficacy score at baseline (F [1, 81]) = 26.02, $p < .05$). Scores of each subscale were significantly higher in the intervention group than in the

TABLE 1 Demographic Characteristics of Participants

Variable	Intervention Group (n = 32)	Comparison Group (n = 52)
Age		
$M \pm SD$ (range)	51.3 ± 15.4 (18-83)	50.6 ± 20.1 (22-85)
Education		
$M \pm SD$ (range)	11.8 ± 2.9 (5-18)	11.9 ± 3.5 (4-20)
Sex		
Men	14 (43.8%)	21 (40.4%)
Women	18 (57.2%)	31 (59.6%)
Ethnicity		
White (NH*)	20 (62.5%)	45 (86.5%)
Hispanic (MA**)	10 (31.3%)	2 (3.8%)
African American	0 (0.0%)	2 (3.8%)
Other	2 (6.2%)	2 (3.8%)
Missing	0	1 (2.1%)
Living situation		
Married/partnered	15 (46.9%)	17 (32.7%)
Single	16 (50.0%)	34 (65.4%)
Missing	1 (3.1%)	1 (1.9%)

NH* = Non-Hispanic; MA** = Mexican American.

TABLE 2 The Self-Rated Abilities Scale for Health Practices: Intervention versus Comparison Groups	PRE-TEST		POST-TEST	
	M (SD)	Range	M* (SE)	Range
Intervention group (n = 32)				
Total	65.85 (18.06)	38-99	83.90 (2.17)	59-104
Nutrition	16.34 (5.60)	5-26	22.00 (0.58)	12-26
Psychological well-being	17.23 (5.01)	4-26	20.55 (0.69)	10-27
Physical activity	13.89 (7.13)	2-26	20.26 (0.79)	9-27
Responsible health practices	18.39 (4.76)	4-27	20.84 (0.71)	9-27
Comparison group (n = 32)				
Total	85.27 (13.20)	59-107	80.78 (1.64)	60-112
Nutrition	20.89 (3.84)	12-28	19.94 (0.44)	12-28
Psychological well-being	20.83 (3.89)	12-28	20.29 (0.53)	13-28
Physical activity	21.00 (5.53)	5-28	20.07 (4.86)	7-28
Responsible health practices	22.55 (4.07)	14-28	21.71 (0.54)	13-28

M* = Corrected Mean.

comparison group at time 2, controlling for scores of self-efficacy at baseline: the nutrition subscale (F [1, 81] = 42.51, $p < .05$), the psychological well-being/stress management subscale (F [1, 81] = 9.86, $p < .05$), the physical activity/exercise subscale (F [1, 81] = 29.06, $p < .05$), and the responsible health practices subscale (F [1, 81] = 12.90, $p < .05$). SRAHP scores in the intervention and comparison group at both time 1 and time 2 are presented in Table 2.

DISCUSSION

A comparison of self-efficacy scores of deaf participants in our study with other research suggests that deaf adults may have lower levels of self-efficacy for health behaviors than other groups. The mean SRAHP scores of the total DHHI sample were lower at baseline than mean SRAHP scores of adults with physical disabilities in two other studies (Stuifbergen & Becker, 1994; Tate et al., 2002). The mean total SRAHP score in the Stuifbergen and Becker study of adults with diverse physical disabilities (n = 117) was 79.87 (range 41-112, SD = 7.03), and the mean scores in the Tate et al. sample (n = 68) of adults with spinal cord injuries was 88 at baseline (SD = 13) and 92 (SD = 18) after an intervention. The mean score of the total sample of deaf adults (n = 84) was lower at baseline in the DHHI study (77.87, range 38-107, SD = 17.85). After receiving the DHHI, the intervention group mean total scores were increased to 83.90, while the mean total scores of the DHHI comparison group remained virtually unchanged at 80.78.

Limitations of this study include a relatively small sample of culturally deaf adults and nonrandomized assignment to groups, precluding meaningful analysis of interactions between multiple demographic characteristics (such as ethnicity and age) and SRAHP scores. Results support our hypothesis that the DHHI is effective in increasing deaf adults' self-efficacy for health behaviors to improve modifiable risk factors for CVD.

CONCLUSIONS

The DHHI was effective in increasing culturally deaf adults' self-efficacy for targeted health behaviors related to modifiable CVD risk factors. A clinical trial of the DHHI will be necessary to evaluate the theoretical correlations between self-efficacy and targeted behaviors, and the effectiveness of the DHHI in decreasing risk for CVD among culturally deaf adults. Further study also is needed to learn more about the relationships among ethnicity, socioeconomic status, health-related self-efficacy, and health behaviors in culturally deaf communities.

The DHHI represents synthesis of cultural competency and scientific evidence to create an effective theory-based intervention for an underserved population. However, the difficulty experienced by culturally deaf adults in accessing health-related information (Barnett, 2002), deficits in health knowledge (Steinberg, Wiggins, Barmada, & Sullivan, 2002), and vulnerability to poor health outcomes are apparent in many other areas: breast cancer education (Sadler et al., 2001), maternity services (Underwood, 2004), mental health services (Munro-Ludders, Simpatico, & Zvetina, 2004), prostate and testicular cancer screening (Folkins et al., 2005), and end-of-life care (Allen, Meyers, Sullivan, & Sullivan, 2002). The DHHI prototype could be used in designing interventions targeting other urgent health issues, and advancing the national health agenda.

The DHHI supports the National Institute of Nursing Strategic Plan (2006) for research (a) focusing on risk reduction (b) eliminating health disparities (c) using community-based approaches to facilitate risk reduction and (d) behavior interventions to achieve biological outcomes. However, a great deal more effort will be necessary to eliminate disparities in health care for culturally deaf Americans.

REFERENCES

Adler, N.E., & Newman, K. (2002). Socioeconomic disparities in health: Pathways and policies. *Health Affairs*, 21(2), 60-76.

Advocate Health Care & Sinai Health System. (2004, February). Improving access to health and mental health for Chicago's Deaf community: A survey of Deaf adults. Final Survey Report. [Electronic version]. Retrieved October 27, 2006 from http://healthtrust.net/inex.php?option=com_content&task=view&id=29&Itemid=61.

Allen, B., Meyers, N., Sullivan, J., & Sullivan, M. (2002). American Sign Language and end-of-life care: Research in the deaf community. *HEC Forum*, 14(3), 197-208.

American Heart Association. (2006a). Heart attack, stroke and cardiac arrest warning signs. Retrieved October 27, 2006 from http://www.americanheart.org/presenter.jhtml?identifier=10000015&q=&x=44&y=10

American Heart Association. (2006b). Healthy lifestyle. Retrieved October 27, 2006 from http://www.americanheart.org/presenter.jhtml?identifier=1200000

Bandura, A. (1986). *Social foundations of thought and action: A social cognitive theory.* Englewood Cliffs, NJ: Prentice-Hall.

Bandura, A. (1995). *Self-efficacy in changing societies.* New York: Cambridge University Press.

Baranowski, T., Perry, C.L., & Parcel, G.S. (2002). How individuals, environments, and health behavior interact. In K. Glanz, R.K. Rimer, & F.M. Lewis (Eds.), *Health behavior and health education: Theory, research, and practice* (pp. 165-184). San Francisco: Jossey-Bass.

Barnett, S. (2002). Cross-cultural communication with patients who use American Sign Language. *Family Medicine*, 34, 376-382.

Becker, H., Stuifbergen, A., Oh, H.S., & Hall, S. (1993). The self-rated abilities for health practices scale: A health self-efficacy measure. *Health Values*, 17(5), 42-50.

Centers for Disease Control and Prevention. (2005a). Division for heart disease and stroke prevention: Fact sheet and at-a-glance report. Retrieved August 23, 2005 from http://www.cdc.gov/DHDSP/library/fs_heart_disease.htm.

Centers for Disease Control and Prevention. (2005b). Disability and health in 2005: Promoting the health and well-being of people with disabilities. Retrieved August 23, 2005 from http://www.cdc.gov/ncbddd/dh.

Dolnick, E. (1993, September). Deafness as culture. *The Atlantic Monthly*, 272(3), 37-53.

Faryna, E.L., & Morales, E. (2000). Self-efficacy and HIV-related risk behaviors among multiethnic adolescents. *Cultural Diversity and Ethnic Minority Psychology*, 6, 42-56.

Folkins, A., Sadler, G.R., Ko, C., Branz, P., Marsh, S., & Bovee, M. (2005). Improving the deaf community's access to prostate and testicular cancer information: A survey study. *BioMed Central Public Health*, 5, 63-74.

Foster, S., & Kinuthia,W. (2003). Deaf persons of Asian American, Hispanic American, and African American backgrounds: A study of intra-individual diversity and identity. *Journal of Deaf Studies and Deaf Education*, 8, 271-290.

Gallaudet Research Institute. (1996). *Stanford Achievement Test, 95th Edition, Form S, Norms booklet for deaf and hard-of-hearing students.* Washington, DC: Gallaudet University.

Gallaudet Research Institute. (2005). Regional and national summary report of data from the 2004-2005 annual survey of deaf and hard of hearing children and youth. Washington, DC: GRI, Gallaudet University. Retrieved October 24, 2006 from http://gri.gallaudet.edu/Demographics/

Hickey, M.L., Owen, S.V., & Froman, R.D. (1992). Instrument development: Cardiac diet and exercise self-efficacy. *Nursing Research*, 41, 347-351.

Holt, J.A., Traxler, C.B., & Allen, T.E. (1997). *Interpreting the scores: A user's guide to 9th edition Stanford Achievement Test for educators of deaf and hard-of-hearing students.* Gallaudet Research Institute Technical Report 97-100. Washington, DC: Gallaudet University.

Horan, M.L., Kim, K.K., Gendler, P., Froman, R.D., & Patel, M.D. (1998). Development and evaluation of the Osteoporosis Self-Efficacy Scale. *Research in Nursing and Health*, 21, 395-403.

Jones, E.G., & Kay, M. (1992). Instrumentation in cross cultural research. *Nursing Research*, 41, 186-188.

Jones, E.G., Mallinson, R.K., Phillips, L., & Kang, Y. (2006). Challenges in language, culture, and modality: Translating English measures into American Sign Language. *Nursing Research*, 55, 75-81.

Jones, E.G., Renger, R., & Firestone, R. (2005). Deaf community analysis for health education priorities. *Public Health Nursing*, 22, 27-35.

Jones, P.S., Lee, J.W., Phillips, L.R., Zhang, X.E., & Jaciedo, K.B. (2001). An adaptation of Brislin's translation model for cross cultural research. *Nursing Research*, 50, 300-304.

Lang, H.G., McKee, B.G., & Conner, K.N. (1993). Characteristics of effective teachers: A descriptive study of perceptions of faculty and deaf college students. *American Annals of the Deaf*, 138, 252-259.

Lang, H.G., Stinson, M.S., Basile, M., Kavanagh, F., & Liu, Y. (1999). Learning styles of deaf college students and teaching behaviors of their instructors. *Journal of Deaf Studies and Deaf Education*, 4, 16-27.

Maase, L.C., & Anderson, C.B. (2003). Ethnic differences among correlates of physical activity in women. *American Journal of Health Promotion*, 17, 357-360.

McCrone, W.P. (1990). A summary of the Americans with Disabilities Act and its specific implications for hearing impaired people. *Journal of the American Deafness and Rehabilitation Association*, 23, 60-63.

Munro-Ludders, B., Simpatico, T., & Zvetina, D. (2004). Making public mental-health services accessible to deaf consumers: Illinois Deaf Services 2000. *American Annals of the Deaf*, 148, 396-402.

National Institute of Nursing Research. (2006). NINR strategic plan. Retrieved on October 27, 2006 from http://ninr.nih.gov/assets/Documents/NINR_StrategicPlan.pdf.

Olkin, R., Abrams, K., Preston, P., & Kirshbaum, M. (2006). Comparison of parents with and without disabilities raising teens: Information from the NHIS and two national surveys. *Rehabilitation Psychology*, 51(1), 43-49.

Resnick, B. (1998). Efficacy beliefs in geriatric rehabilitation. *Journal of Gerontological Nursing*, 24(7), 34-44.

Sadler, G.R., Gunsauls, D.C., Huang, J., Padden, C., Elion, L., Galey, T., et al. (2001). Bringing breast cancer education to deaf women. *Journal of Cancer Education*, 16, 225-228.

Sohng, K.Y., Sohng, S., & Yeom, H.A. (2002). Health promoting behaviors of elderly Korean immigrants in the United States. *Public Health Nursing*, 19, 294-300.

Stebnicki, J.A.M., & Coeling, H.V. (1999). The culture of the deaf. *Journal of Transcultural Nursing*, 10, 350-357.

Steinberg, A.G., Wiggins, E.A., Barmada, C.H., & Sullivan, V.J. (2002). Deaf women: Experiences and perceptions of healthcare system access. *Journal of Women's Health*, 11, 729-741.

Stuifbergen, A.K., & Becker, H.A. (1994). Predictors of health-promoting lifestyles in persons with disabilities. *Research in Nursing and Health*, 17, 3-13.

Tate, D.G., Chiodo, A., Nelson, V., Roller, S., Zemper, E., & Forchheimer, M. (2002). The effect of a holistic health promotion program on individuals with spinal cord injury. The National Center on Physical Activity and Disability. Retrieved October 27, 2006 from http://www.ncpad.org/programming/fact_sheet.php?sheet=116&PHPSESSID=

Taylor, M.J. (2000). The influence of self-efficacy on alcohol use among American Indians. *Cultural Diversity and Ethnic Minority Psychology*, 6, 152-167.

Underwood, C. (2004). Maternity services are failing deaf women. *Journal of Family Health Care*, 14(2), 30-31.

Yarcheski, A., Mahon, N.E., Yarcheski, T.J., & Cannella, B.L.A. (2004). Meta-analysis of predictors of positive health practices. *Journal of Nursing Scholarship*, 3, 102-108.

C

The Relationship Between Pain and Functional Disability in Black and White Older Adults

Ann L. Horgas,[1*] *Saunjoo L. Yoon,*[1†] *Austin Lee Nichols,*[2‡] *and Michael Marsiske*[3*]

ABSTRACT

In this study we examined pain and disability in 115 community-dwelling, urban, older adults (mean age = 74 years; 52% black, 48% white). Participants completed a survey of pain (pain presence, intensity, locations, and duration) and disability (Sickness Impact Profile). Sixty percent of the sample reported pain; black and white adults did not differ on any pain variable. In structural equation models controlling for socioeconomic factors and health, pain did not mediate the relationship between race and disability. Race moderated the pain-disability relationship; pain was more associated with disability among whites than blacks. This study highlights the need for greater understanding of health disparities between black and white older adults as they relate to pain and disability. © 2008 Wiley Periodicals, Inc. *Res Nurs Health.*

Keywords: pain; disability; race; aging; health disparities

[1]Department of Adult and Elderly Nursing, College of Nursing, University of Florida, HPNP Complex, P.O. Box 100197, Gainesville, FL 32610-0197

[2]Department of Psychology, College of Liberal Arts and Sciences, University of Florida, Gainesville, FL

[3]Department of Clinical and Health Psychology, College of Public Health and Health Professions, University of Florida, Gainesville, FL

Correspondence to Ann L. Horgas

*Associate Professor.

†Assistant Professor.

‡Graduate Student.

Published online in Wiley InterScience (www.interscience.wiley.com) DOI: 10.1002/nur.20270

Pain is a persistent problem in the daily lives of many older community-dwelling adults (American Geriatrics Society, 2002). Approximately 50% of community-dwelling adults have pain (Herr, 2002), which is largely due to the high prevalence of chronic health problems, such as osteoarthritis, in this population (Helme & Gibson, 2001). Acute conditions such as cancer, cardiovascular disease, and other painful medical diseases and syndromes are also prevalent in this age-group (Feldt, Warne, & Ryden, 1998). Pain, from both acute and chronic conditions, is a key indicator of physical impairment; it is associated with depression and decreased physical/social functioning and quality of life (Helme & Gibson; Herr).

Recently, researchers have studied racial and/or ethnic differences in the pain experience, finding that African Americans report more pain, have more untreated pain, and have less access to pain medications (Cintron & Morrison, 2006). Others have reported that black Americans have more activity limitations due to pain (Green, Baker, Smith, & Sato, 2003). Few of these studies, however, have been conducted in older adult populations. Thus, we sought to investigate the relationships among race, pain, and functional disability in older adults.

In the cascade model (Kahana, Kahana, Namazi, Kercher, & Stange, 1997), based on the classic biopsychosocial approach proposed by Engle (1962), pain is considered a key factor in the progression (or cascade) from chronic illness to social and physical disability among older adults. Kahana et al. posited that pain has a direct effect on disability (indicated by physical and social activity limitations) and that pain is influenced by demographic characteristics (e.g., age, sex, income, education, marital status) and chronic illness. In a different model, the biocultural model of pain, ethnocultural identity is theorized to influence the experience and expression of pain, and provides a framework for considering the role of race in the pain-disability pathway (Bates, 1987; Bates, Edwards, & Anderson, 1993). Thus, we added race to the cascade model as a predictor of pain and disability, and tested it in a sample of community-dwelling older adults (Fig. 1).

In the pain literature, the terms *race* (i.e., ancestry) and *ethnicity* (i.e., culture) are often used interchangeably, although they are conceptually distinct. For this paper, we use the term *race* because participants were asked to self-identify their race on the survey question (as opposed to ethnic identity). In our literature review, however, we employ terms used by authors to describe their research. Thus inconsistencies in language and spelling (e.g., African American hyphenated or not) reflect discrepancies in this literature. When we reference our own data, we use the terms *black,* recognizing that many blacks are not of African heritage, and *white,* to reflect racial group identity without reference to heritage, ancestry, or culture.

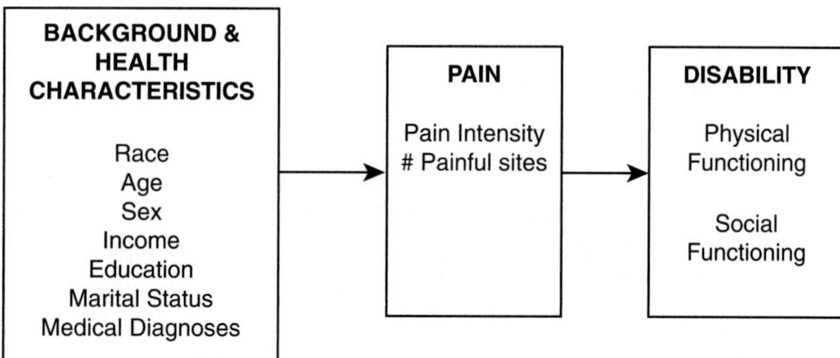

Figure 1 Conceptual model.

RELATIONSHIP BETWEEN PAIN AND FUNCTIONAL DISABILITY

There is ample literature to support the relationship between persistent pain and functional disability among older adults. In many studies, functional disability has been measured as limitations in both physical and social ability (Osborne, Jensen, Ehde, Hanley, & Kraft, 2007; Weiner, Rudy, Morrow, Slaboda, & Lieber, 2006; C. S. Williams, Tinetti, Kasl, & Peduzzi, 2006). Others measured functional disability in physical functioning only (R. R. Edwards, 2006; Reyes-Gibby, Aday, Todd, Cleeland, & Anderson, 2007; Scudds & Robertson, 2000). Physical disability typically refers to impaired performance of Instrumental Activities of Daily Living in studies of older adults (R. R. Edwards, 2006; Lichenstein, Dhanda, Cornell, Escalante, & Hazuda, 1998; Reyes-Gibby, Aday, & Cleeland, 2002). In a study of community-dwelling Canadian seniors, Scudds and Robertson (2000) reported that 73% of respondents had musculoskeletal pain in the 2 weeks prior to the study, and almost 70% had physical disability. They found that pain-related variables, including more painful body locations, higher pain intensity, greater pain frequency, and more pain medications used, were significantly associated with more physical disability. Lichtenstein et al. also reported that pain intensity was strongly associated with limitations in physical functioning among older adults. In a sample of older adults with osteoarthritis, other investigators reported that pain severity was a stronger determinant of physical disability than structural joint changes (as measured by x-ray; Creamer, Lethbridge-Cejku, & Hochberg, 2000).

A number of researchers have found a relationship between social disability and pain (Bookwala, Harralson, & Parmalee, 2003; Cano, Mayo, & Ventimiglia, 2006; McCracken & Eccleston, 2005; C.S. Williams et al., 2006). Typically, social disability was measured with a psychosocial disability subscale of the Sickness Impact Profile (SIP; Cano et al.; McCracken & Eccleston), Short Form-36 (SF-36; Dawson et al., 2005; De Filippis et al., 2004) or with the Established Populations of Epidemiologic Studies of the Elderly Interview (C.S. Williams et al.). In the study reported by Dawson and colleagues, persistent pain was related to social functioning when measured longitudinally. The authors concluded that hip or knee pain worsened over time in older adults, and pain severity was related to a decline in social functioning. Bookwala and colleagues measured 21 social and leisure activities over 1 month to examine associations with pain, and reported that people with greater osteoarthritis-related pain had more physical and social disability.

RELATIONSHIPS AMONG RACE, PAIN, AND PAIN-RELATED FUNCTIONAL DISABILITY

Over the past decade, there has been a growing interest in understanding differences in the pain experience of black Americans and Caucasians (C.L. Edwards, Fillingim, & Keefe, 2001). In several laboratory-based studies researchers have reported significant differences in experimental pain sensitivity among African Americans compared to Caucasians (R.R. Edwards, Doleys, Fillingim, & Lowery, 2001; R.R. Edwards & Fillingim, 1999). In another laboratory-based study, Rahim-Williams et al. (2007) demonstrated significant differences in pain tolerance (using cold pressor and thermal pain) between ethnic groups; African American and

Hispanic participants showed lower pain tolerance than non-Hispanic white Americans. This study was conducted in a young student volunteer sample.

In some clinical investigations, African Americans with arthritis reported more severe pain compared to Caucasians/whites (R.R. Edwards et al., 2001; Golightly & Dominick, 2005), but not in others (Ang, Ibrahim, Burant, & Kwoh, 2003; Riley et al., 2002). Based on data from a pain clinic, Green et al. (2003) found that black Americans reported significantly higher pain intensity, more suffering associated with pain, and more activity limitations due to pain than did white Americans. In a follow-up study using retrospective clinic data, Baker and Green (2005) examined within-race group differences in the pain experience, comparing young black Americans to older black Americans and young white Americans to older white Americans. They concluded that younger participants reported higher pain intensity than older participants within each racial group, but found no within-group differences in pain suffering or pain-related disability. The pattern of results was not significantly different between black and white Americans. Other researchers have indicated that health disparities between blacks and whites in America are the widest and most persistent when compared to other racial/ethnic groups (Green, Todd, Lebovits, & Francis, 2006). This highlights the importance of investigating similarities and differences between blacks and whites in the pain-disability pathway.

Using national survey data, Reyes-Gibby et al. (2007) examined differences in pain prevalence, pain severity, and pain-related activity limitations between non-Hispanic whites, non-Hispanic blacks, and Hispanics in a community-based sample of older adults (≥51 years). Significant racial/ethnic group differences were noted: Hispanics reported higher prevalence of pain than the other two groups, Hispanics and blacks reported more severe usual pain, and blacks reported more activity limitations due to pain than either Hispanics or whites. These authors noted that socioeconomic characteristics (e.g., Medicaid recipient or lower education level) were significant predictors of severe pain and helped to explain racial/ethnic differences in pain symptoms. Other researchers have concurred, reporting the importance of socioeconomic differences in the pain experience across the adult age range, particularly with regard to dental pain (Riley, Gilbert, & Heft, 2003; Vargas, Macek, & Marcus, 2000). In a telephone survey of community-residing adults with persistent pain, Portenoy, Ugarte, Fuller, and Hass (2004) found that non-Hispanic blacks and Hispanics reported more severe pain than whites. In addition, participants with low income and less than a high school education were more likely to report significant pain. Neither race nor ethnicity predicted disabling pain, but minority participants were more likely to have the socioeconomic indicators associated with functionally limiting pain.

These studies suggest that racial/ethnic characteristics are related to the pain experience. Blacks and Hispanics have reported higher levels of pain, and some evidence suggests that they experience more pain-related functional limitations than whites. Socioeconomic disadvantage appears, in some findings, to be more important than race in predicting disabling pain.

There is evidence that race does matter; people of minority races are more likely to have their pain severity under-estimated by providers, have more under-treated pain, and have less access to opioids for severe pain (Cintron & Morrison, 2006). Given that race and socioeconomic status (SES) are often confounded, these findings may be more attributable to socioeconomic disadvantage, which limits access to health care and resource-rich environments, than to race.

It should be noted that most of the studies reported were conducted with general adult populations, not with older adults. In fact, in studies reporting participants' ages, the upper cutoff was approximately age 65, generally considered the portal into old age in the aging literature (Maddox, 1995). Among blacks, chronic health conditions (including those typically associated with pain) are noted at an earlier age compared to whites (Green et al., 2003), so we elected to include adults aged 60 and over in our study.

The few published clinical studies on this topic have focused on samples of adults recruited from pain clinics, which limits generalizability. Very few researchers have examined relationships between pain and disability in black and white older adults, and even fewer have controlled for socioeconomic and sociodemographic variables (such as income and education; Reyes-Gibby et al., 2007). Given the prevalence of pain among older adults and the rapidly-aging U.S. population, relationships among race, pain experience, and pain-related disability warrant further investigation.

The purpose of the study was to examine relationships among race (black or white), pain, and functional disability (physical and social functioning) in older adults. We asked the following research questions:

(1) Do self-reported pain (pain sites and pain intensity) and disability (physical and social functional limitations) differ between black and white older adults?
(2) Consistent with the cascade model, does pain mediate the relationship between race (black or white) and disability, after controlling for other sociodemographic (age, sex, marital status, income, and education) and health (number of limiting diagnoses) variables?
(3) Does race (black or white) moderate the relationship between pain and disability, after controlling for other sociodemographic and health variables?

METHOD

Sample and Setting

A convenience sample was recruited from five senior centers and two churches in a large, racially diverse city in the Midwest in 2000. All seniors present in the facility on the day of the survey were invited to participate. Inclusion criteria were: ≥60 years old, willing to participate, and able to provide informed consent. Ability to consent was ascertained by explaining the study to potential participants, who were then asked to describe the study. Participants were excluded if they were unable to explain the study and provide consent or were unable to complete the survey. Because this was a community-based, volunteer sample, very few participants were excluded on this basis (approximately 5% of participants who expressed interest in the study were unable to consent or complete the survey).

A total of 115 community-dwelling older adults completed the survey. The sample was predominantly female, had an age range of 62-95 years, and was almost equally divided between black and white older adults (see Table 1). As shown in Table 1, blacks and whites differed significantly in several sociodemographic and health variables. black participants were generally older; more likely to be female, unmarried, and have lower levels of education and income; and more blacks suffered from functionally limiting medical conditions than whites in this sample. Thus, these variables were included as covariates in the statistical analyses.

Measures

A paper-and-pencil questionnaire was developed to assess the main study variables. The measures are described below.

TABLE 1 Sample Characteristics, Overall ($N = 115$) and by Race

Characteristic	Category	Total Sample, *n*	BY RACE Black, *n*	White, *n* (%)	*p*
Race*	Black	60 (52.2%)			
	White	55 (47.8%)			
Sex	Male	26 (22.6%)	9 (15%)	17 (30.9%)	$p < .05$
	Female	89 (77.4%)	51 (85%)	38 (69.1%)	
Marital status	Married	34 (29.6%)	7 (11.7%)	27 (49.1%)	$p < .001$
	Unmarried	80 (69.5%)	53 (88.3%)	27 (49.1%)	
	Missing	1 (0.9%)	0	1 (1.8%)	
Education	<HS Graduate	38 (33%)	34 (56.7%)	4 (7.3%)	$p < .001$
	HS Graduate	41 (35.7%)	14 (23.3%)	27 (49.1%)	
	≥College	35 (30.4%)	12 (20%)	23 (41.8%)	
	Missing	1 (0.9%)	0	1 (1.8%)	
Income	Under $10,000	40 (34.8%)	34 (56.7%)	6 (10.9%)	$p < .001$
	$10,000-$29,000	43 (37.4%)	14 (23.3%)	29 (52.7%)	
	$30,000-$49,000	10 (8.7%)	1 (1.7%)	9 (16.4%)	
	Over $50,000	3 (2.6%)	0	3 (5.5%)	
	Missing	19 (16.5%)	11 (18.3%)	8 (14.5%)	
Age	Mean (SD)	74 (7.3%)	76 (7.9)	72 (6.1)	$p < .05$
Limiting diagnoses	Mean (SD)	1.7 (0.7%)	1.9 (0.8)	1.5 (0.7)	$p < .05$

*Participants self-identified their race from eight categories: black/African American, white/Caucasian, Asian, Native Hawaiian/Pacific Islander, American Indian/Alaskan Native, Hispanic, Arabic, and other (open ended). No respondents selected any category other than black or white.

Pain

The presence, intensity, duration, and locations of pain were assessed. Pain presence was measured with the question, "Do you currently have pain?" Response choices were *yes* or *no.* The intensity of pain (in the most painful location) was assessed via a verbal descriptor scale (VDS), an instrument recommended for measuring pain in older adults (Herr, 2002). This tool measures pain intensity by asking participants to select a word that best describes their present pain ([0] *no pain* to [6] *worst pain imaginable*). This measure has been found to be a reliable and valid measure of pain intensity, and it has demonstrated concurrent validity with other pain intensity scales (Taylor & Herr, 2003). In addition, the VDS is easy to complete, rated as most preferred by older adults relative to other pain intensity measures (Herr & Mobily, 1993), and appropriate for use in African American and white American populations (Taylor & Herr). Participants were also asked to indicate how long they had experienced pain in their most painful location. Responses were coded into <1, 1-5, 6-10, 11-15 years, or more than 15 years. The pain map from the McGill Pain Questionnaire (Melzack, 1975) was used to assess pain locations. Pain locations were scored with a transparent template divided into 36 anatomical areas (Escalante, Lichtenstein, White, Rios, & Hazuda, 1995), and a sum score, indicating number of painful locations, was created. This widely used measure has been validated in several epidemiologic studies and has demonstrated high inter-rater reliability (Escalante et al., 1995; Margolis, Tait, & Krause, 1986).

Functional Disability

The SIP Short Form (SIP68), one of the most widely used generic measures of health-related functioning, was used to measure physical and social disability. The SIP, originally developed as a broad measure of health-related behavior (Bergner, Bobbit, Carter, & Gilson, 1981), was reported to be valid and reliable (de Bruin, deWitte, Stevens, & Diederiks, 1992), but it was considered to be too lengthy and burdensome for some older adults to complete. The SIP68 has 68 items with 6 subscales: somatic autonomy, mobility control, psychic autonomy, and communication (mental functioning and verbal communication), social behavior, emotional stability, and mobility range (de Bruin, de Witte, & Diedriks, 1994). Psychometric evaluation of the new instrument has been conducted in several studies of adults with chronic disease and revealed high internal consistency reliability for the total scale, as well as high test-retest reliability over periods ranging from 1 week to 3 months (de Bruin, Diederiks, de Witte, Stevens, & Philipsen, 1997; Nanda, McLendon, Andresen, & Armbrecht, 2003). The SIP has also demonstrated high reliabilities when used with blacks and whites (Cano et al., 2006). In the present study, three subscales of the SIP68 were used, as described below.

Physical functioning was evaluated based on mobility control and mobility range subscales. The mobility control subscale has 12 questions about the level of control an individual has over his or her body. Items address walking and upper extremity control. The mobility range subscale has nine questions about the range of activities a person does to sustain his or her lifestyle, such as "I stay at home most of the time." For this study, the mobility control and range subscales were combined to create a 21-item general physical functional disability subscale. Response choices for each item are (1) yes or (0) no. The SIP physical functioning score is a sum of the number of limitations reported by participants, with a possible range of 0-21; higher scores indicate more functional limitations. The Cronbach's alpha was .89 in this sample.

Social functioning was assessed via the social behavior subscale of the SIP68, which has 11 questions about a person's social functioning in relation to others and to the community. Sample questions include, "I am doing fewer social activities with groups of people." Response choices for each item are (1) *yes* or (0) *no.* The SIP social functioning score is a sum of the number of limitations reported by participants, with a possible range of 0-11; higher scores indicate more social functional limitations. The Cronbach's alpha was .82 in this sample.

Demographic Characteristics

Demographic data were collected with a survey that included items regarding age (in years), sex (coded as 0 = *male* and 1 = *female*), level of education (in years), income, and marital status. Race was measured by the question, "What race do you consider yourself?" Education was assessed with a question that ascertained the highest grade of school completed. Educational level scores were recoded into three groups: 1 = less than 12th grade, 2 = high school graduate, or 3 = some college education or more. Marital status was categorized as married or unmarried. Income was assessed as current annual household income on a 16-point categorical scale and re-categorized into the following four groups: 1 = less than $10,000, 2 = $10,000-$29,999, 3 = $30,000-49,999, and 4 = $50,000 or more. Missing data on the income variable (19 cases) were estimated using regression-based imputation analyses (Penn, 2007).

Health Conditions

To assess health conditions, participants were asked to respond to the question, "Has a doctor or nurse ever told you that you have the following conditions?" A 24-item medical conditions checklist from the Older Americans Resources and Services (OARS) Multidimensional

Assessment, a measure widely used in geriatric research, was used as an indicator of health status (George & Fillenbaum, 1985). An expert panel of four advanced practice nurses reviewed the checklist, and identified 12 medical conditions often associated with disability (including physical and social functional limitations). These were coded as functionally limiting medical conditions for subsequent analyses and included vision impairments (cataracts, diabetic retinopathy, and macular degeneration), cardiovascular conditions (angina, myocardial infarction, stroke, and congestive heart failure), arthritis, diabetes, asthma, cancer, and Alzheimer's disease. A sum score was created to reflect the total number of functionally limiting medical conditions (potential score = 0-12).

Procedure

Approvals were obtained from the two Institutional Review Boards of the two appropriate institutions, where data were collected and analyzed for this study. All printed materials were written at an eighth-grade reading level and printed in 14-point font on white paper to assist participants in reading the text. Most participants read and completed the survey independently, but a few asked for assistance due to writing difficulties.

When participants asked for help, the PI or research assistant read the question and response choices aloud verbatim, and recorded the answer verbatim. No prompts were given. If the participants stated they wanted to stop or appeared to have difficulty completing the survey due to reasons other than physical disability, they were thanked for their time and the survey was discontinued. Upon completion (approximately 30 minutes), participants were compensated with $10.00.

Statistical Analyses

Descriptive statistics were computed to describe sample characteristics. Chi-square analyses and t tests were used to examine relationships between race and pain, pain intensity, and functional disability between racial groups. Structural equation modeling (SEM) was used to examine relationships among race, pain, and functional disability.

Modeling Approach

Several guidelines in the literature indicate that the sample size of the current analyses (N = 115) was sufficient for the relatively simple measurement and structural regression models planned (Bollen, 1989; Kline, 1998; MacCullum, Browne, & Sugawara, 1996; Quintana & Maxwell, 1999). Analyses for research questions 2 (evaluation of pain as a mediator of race effects in disability) and 3 (race as a moderator of the pain-disability relationship) were conducted as structural equation models in a hierarchical model framework. Pain (indicated by measures of pain intensity and number of pain sites) and disability (indicated by scales of physical and social disability) were estimated as latent constructs. Race effects on pain and disability were estimated controlling for other sociodemographic (age, sex, income, education, and marital status) and health (number of limiting diagnoses) variables, to ensure that race effects were estimated in a way relatively unconfounded with other variables. For research question 3 (which addressed whether race moderated the pain-disability relationship, after controlling for other sociodemographic and health variables), a two-group (blacks and whites) structural equation model was conducted. A nested model was used to examine whether the pain-function relationship could be constrained to equality in the two groups.

The covariance matrices were analyzed, and maximum likelihood was used as the estimation method because it has been found to be a robust estimation procedure (Hoyle & Panter, 1995; Quintana & Maxwell, 1999). Moreover, full-information maximum likelihood estimation was used, such that each parameter was based on all available data, so no listwise deletion of missing cases was required. Overall model fit was evaluatedwith incremental fit indices (Hu & Bentler, 1995). Each fit index compares the estimated model to a null (no predictor) model and is generally expected to exceed .90 (Hoyle & Panter, 1995). Individual parameter estimates provided by the program were examined, including the nonnormed fit index (NNFI), the normed fit index (NFI), the relative fit index (RFI), the comparative fit index (CFI), and the incremental fit index (IFI; Bentler, 1989; Bentler & Bonett, 1980; Marsh, Balla, & McDonald, 1988). Chi-square statistics are also reported, with smaller values generally indicative of better reproduction of the input correlation matrix among measures; however, since Chi-square is often inflated by small departures from normality and increasing sample sizes, it was not evaluated as a primary indicator of fit (Tabachnick & Fidell, 2007). Although all models were conducted in covariance metric, results are presented as completely standardized solutions for ease of interpretation.

RESULTS

Descriptive Findings

Pain

Sixty percent of the sample reported experiencing pain. See Table 2 for description.

Functional Disability

In this sample, 66 (57.4%) participants reported having physical limitations in at least one item on the physical mobility subscale of the SIP. The most frequently reported limitations were related to walking, such as walking more slowly (n = 58, 50.4%), going up and down stairs more slowly (n = 56, 48.7%), and walking shorter distances (n = 52, 45.2%). In addition, 71 (61.7%) participants indicated they had limitations in at least one area of the social behavior subscale. The most commonly reported social limitations were going out for entertainment less often (n = 53, 46.1%) and doing hobbies and recreation for shorter periods (n = 52, 45.2%). Mean scores for both subscales are presented in Table 2.

Differences in Pain and Disability by Race

Pain

Chi-square analysis and t tests were conducted to examine the association between the presence of pain and race (black or white); no statistically significant association was found (χ^2 = 2.32, df = 1, p = .09). Blacks and whites did not differ significantly in intensity (t = −1.14, df = 44, p = .26) or duration of self-reported pain (χ^2 = 3.68, df = 3, p = .30), or in the number of pain locations reported (t = −1.12, df = 67, p = .23; see Table 2).

Disability

With regard to functional disability, significant differences between blacks and whites were noted for both physical limitations (t = −5.24, df = 113) and social limitation subscales

TABLE 2 Description of Pain and Disability, Overall Sample and by Race ($N = 115$)

	Category	Total Sample, *n*	BY RACE Black ($n = 60$), *n*	White ($n = 55$), *n*	*p*
Pain					
Pain presence	Yes	69 (60%)	40 (66.7%)	29 (52.7%)	n.s.
	No	46 (40%)	20 (33.3%)	26 (47.3%)	n.s.
Pain duration	0	46 (40%)	20 (33.3%)	26 (47.3%)	n.s.
	<1 year	22 (19.1%)	16 (26.7%)	6 (10.9%)	
	1-5 years	31 (27.0%)	17 (28.3%)	14 (25.5%)	
	6-10 years	8 (7.0%)	4 (6.7%)	4 (7.3%)	
	≥11 years	8 (7.0%)	3 (5.0%)	5 (9.1%)	
Pain intensity (range = 0-6)	Mean (SD)	2.9 (1.0)	2.8 (0.8)	3.0 (1.2)	n.s.
# of pain locations (range = 0-8)	Mean (SD)	2.0 (2.5)	1.2 (1.0)	1.0 (1.0)	n.s.
Pain regions*	Upper extremities	50 (72.5%)	32 (80.0%)	18 (62.1%)	n.s.
	Lower extremities	26 (37.7%)	16 (40%)	10 (34.5%)	n.s.
	Back	23 (33.3%)	13 (32.5%)	10 (34.5%)	n.s.
	Head	7 (10.1%)	4 (10.0%)	3 (10.3%)	n.s.
	Abdomen	9 (13.0%)	4 (10.0%)	5 (17.2%)	n.s.
	Hip	10 (14.5%)	6 (15.0%)	4 (13.8%)	n.s.
Disability					
Physical limitations (scale = 0-21)	Mean (SD)	5.8 (4.1)	7.6 (4.3)	3.9 (3.0)	$p < .001$
Social limitations (scale = 0-11)	Mean (SD)	4.1 (2.6)	5.0 (2.7)	3.1 (2.2)	$p < .001$

*Frequencies are shown for those who reported pain ($n = 69$). Note that participants could report pain in more than one region of the body.

($t = -4.03$, $df = 113$). In both domains, blacks reported significantly more functional limitations than did whites (see Table 2).

Pain as a Mediator of the Race-Disability Relationship, Controlling for Sociodemographic and Health Variables

In structural equation models, criteria for mediation can be evaluated simultaneously. Analyses for this question were conducted in three steps. In step one, a fully recursive model was estimated with seven singly-indicated exogenous variables (age, sex, education, income, marital status, number of limiting diagnoses, and race [dichotomously coded as 0 = *white* and 1 = *black*]). Each of these variables was allowed to have direct effects on both the latent constructs of pain (pain sites + pain intensity) and disability (physical + social functional limitations). In addition, a path was specified from pain to disability; such that the exogenous variables could also have indirect effects on function, mediated through pain. All possible correlations among the seven exogenous predictors were freely estimated. The fit of this first model was generally good: χ^2 (15) = 24.16, $p = .06$, NNFI = .92, NFI = .95, RFI = .82, IFI = .98, CFI = .98. Along with a non-significant chi-square statistic, the fit indices were uniformly excellent. Chi-square statistics were used to permit a nested model test with the subsequent model.

In step two, a reduced-form equation was estimated in which the path from race to pain was eliminated. Based on the previous descriptive analyses, we expected that race and pain would not be related. Thus, a statistical comparison of the two nested models would provide a test of whether any of the race effect on disability was mediated through pain. The fit of this second model was virtually identical to the preceding model: χ^2 (16) = 25.79, p = .06, NNFI = .92, NFI = .95, RFI = .82, IFI = .98, CFI = .98. A nested model test (chi-square difference between models) revealed that the elimination of the race-pain path did not significantly reduce model fit: χ^2 (1) = 1.63, p = .20. Thus, while race was a significant direct predictor of disability, pain did not mediate the relationship between race and disability.

In a third step, we noted that, after controlling for all exogenous variables, the unique relationship between race and disability was no longer statistically significant. Therefore, we eliminated the direct path from race to disability and recomputed the model. Again, the fit of this model was virtually unchanged: χ^2 (17) = 28.45, p = .04, NNFI = .92, NFI = .94, RFI = .88, IFI = .98, CFI = .97. A nested model test between the second and third models showed that elimination of the race-disability path did not significantly worsen the model fit (χ^2 [1] = 2.66, p = .10). We also compared this final reduced model to the original model (in which race had direct effects on both pain and disability), and the elimination of all direct effects of race did not significantly reduce the model fit (χ^2 [2] = 4.29, p = .12).

The final accepted model, with standardized coefficients, is shown in Figure 2. Significant coefficients are indicated in bold text. Additional findings from the model indicated that having more functionally limiting medical diagnoses was associated with increased pain; no other demographic or socioeconomic variables showed significant direct effects on pain. Males and those with lower education and more functionally limiting diagnoses had significantly more functional disability. In addition, more pain was associated with significantly more disability. The model explained 16% of the reliable variance in pain, and 61% of the reliable variance in disability.

Pain as a Moderator of the Race-Disability Relationship, Controlling for Sociodemographic and Health Variables

To examine whether race moderated the relationship between pain and disability, a two-group model was conducted. The sample was split into black and white sub-samples. Age, sex, education, income, marital status, and limiting diagnoses were treated as exogenous variables and were allowed to have direct effects on pain and disability. A path from pain to disability was again specified, so that sociodemographic and health variables could have both direct and indirect (mediated through pain) effects on disability. To facilitate group comparisons, invariant indicator loadings on the pain and disability factors wereassumed. Two model steps were estimated. In Step 1, the pain-disability path was constrained to equality in black and white groups; the fit of this model was good: χ^2 (29) = 44.08, p = .04, NNFI = .85, NFI = .89, IFI = .96, CFI = .95. In Step 2, the pain-disability path was allowed to vary between groups; the fit of this model was χ^2 (28) = 38.52, p = .09, NNFI = .88, NFI = .90, IFI = .97, CFI = .97. The difference between the two models was not significant [χ^2 (1) = 5.56, p = .01], indicating that a hypothesis of invariant pain-disability relationships in black and white participants was not supported. Race moderated the pain-disability relationship. The standardized pain-disability path was .81 in whites and .18 in blacks. To verify that these differences reflected true trends in the data and were not just disattenuated artifacts of the modeling procedure, we inspected the original bivariate correlations between the pain and disability indicators separately for the two race groups. These correlation coefficients are shown in Table 3; values in the left two columns are for blacks and in the right two columns, for whites. Even

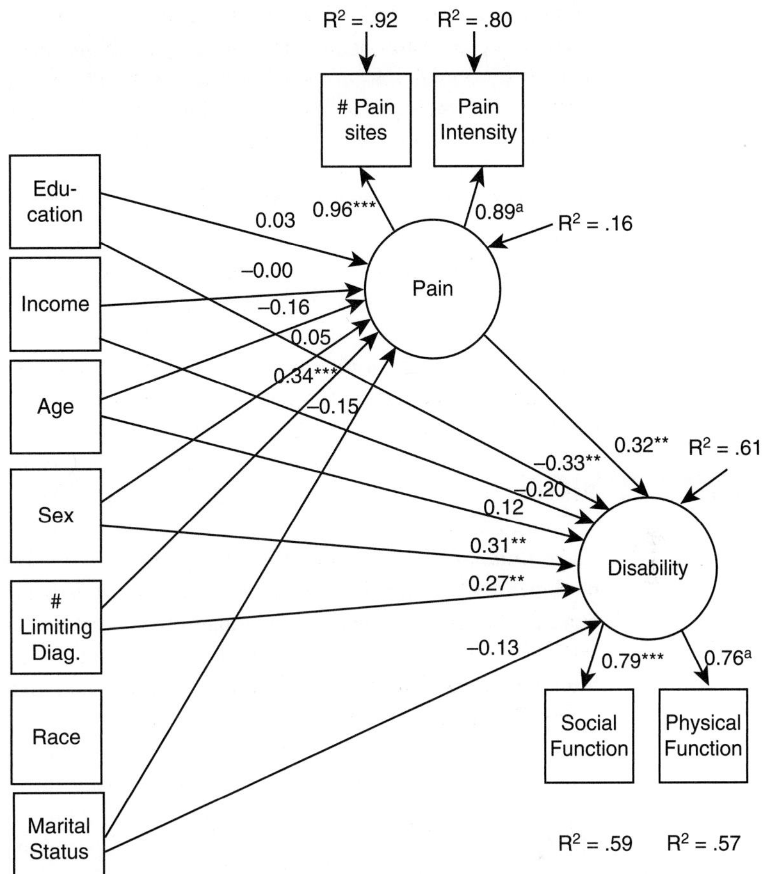

Notes: * $p < .05$, ** $p < .01$, *** $p < .001$, [a]fixed parameter for solution scaling

Correlations among exogenous predictors:

	(1) Education	(2) Income	(3) Age	(4) Sex	(5) # Limiting diagnoses	(6) Race	(7) Marital Status
(1)	1.00						
(2)	0.496***	1.00					
(3)	−0.279*	−0.314**	1.00				
(4)	−0.044	−0.246*	0.105	1.00			
(5)	−0.141	−0.160	0.149	0.247*	1.00		
(6)	−0.496***	−0.579***	0.221*	0.190*	0.245*	1.00	
(7)	0.186*	0.565***	−0.247*	−0.331**	−1.40	−0.416***	1.00

Figure 2 Final structural model.

TABLE 3 Bivariate Correlations Between Pain and Disability Indicators, by Race

	BLACK (N = 60)		WHITE (N = 55)	
	Physical Limitations	Social Limitations	Physical Limitations	Social Limitations
Pain intensity	.23	.16	.62†	.30*
Pain locations	.13	.08	.59†	.22

$^*p < .05$.
$†p < .001$.

when attenuated by measurement error and at the indicator level, pain had a much stronger relationship with disability in whites than in blacks.

DISCUSSION

These findings highlight important information about relationships among pain, race, and disability in community-dwelling older adults. Pain is a common problem, and its high prevalence (60%) in this sample of individuals over 60 years of age is consistent with epidemiological studies of pain (Reyes-Gibby et al., 2007). Pain was significantly associated with greater functional disability in both physical and social functional domains, highlighting the important real-world consequences of living with pain.

Contrary to previous research, race was not related to pain in this sample. In bivariate analyses, black and white participants were equally likely to report experiencing pain and described equivalent pain intensity, pain duration, and number of pain locations. This lack of a significant association between race and pain persisted after controlling for demographic, health, and socioeconomic indicators in structural equation models.

There are several possible explanations for these discrepant findings. First, studies supporting racial differences in pain have been primarily laboratory-based. In these investigations, blacks consistently report more pain than whites (Edwards & Fillingim, 1999; Rahim-Williams et al., 2007). Laboratory pain, however, is intrinsically different from clinical pain, because it is experimentally induced with a known stimulus type and amount, is short-term acute pain, and is scheduled to end within a relatively short time frame. This is markedly different from pain associated with a disease condition or medical procedure (e.g., post-surgical pain) in which the course of the pain is often less predictable and, especially among older adults, more persistent (e.g., arthritic pain). Second, the few published investigations of relationships between race and pain have focused on younger populations, and results have been equivocal (C. L. Edwards et al., 2001). Third, most researchers have investigated racial differences in pain clinic populations. These individuals, by definition, have persistent and/or severe pain that has not responded to usual care, and it has been documented that blacks are undertreated for pain relative to non-blacks (Cintron & Morrison, 2006; Green, Baker, & Ndao-Brumblay, 2004), a fact likely to have exacerbated their pain experience. Consequently, blacks who seek specialized treatment from a pain clinic are likely to have substantially worse pain than their white peers. Therefore, differences in pain experience between blacks and whites using pain clinics may be more pronounced than in the general population. Fourth, the finding that black or white race was not associated with pain in this study may reflect measurement differences. In this study, we examined the role of race—as measured by self-declared racial category of black or white—and not ethnicity. It may be that ethnicity or ethnic identity, as noted by Rahim-Williams et al. (2007), is a more important predictor of pain. This is a potentially important distinction that should be addressed in future research. Finally, it is possible that in non-clinical populations, differences between racial groups in the experience of pain are less important than differences within racial groups. Future researchers should examine variability in the pain experience within racial groups, as suggested by Baker and Green (2005).

While race was unrelated to pain in this study, it had an association with disability, with blacks reporting disproportionately more physical and social disability than whites. This undoubtedly reflects socioeconomic and health disparities between these two racial groups; blacks had lower education and income, were older, and had more functionally limiting diagnoses than did whites. Findings reflect the ongoing health and socioeconomic disparities between blacks and whites in the literature (Betancourt, 2006; Portenoy et al., 2004; D. R. Williams, 2005), and this is supported by results of the structural equation models. When race, socioeconomic, demographic, and health variables were considered simultaneously, race no longer had a significant direct effect on disability in this sample. This indicates that race is less important in predicting disability in older adults than the socioeconomic disparities for which black or white race is a proxy. Because race was unrelated to both the dependent variable (disability) and the mediator (pain) in these models, no evidence supported pain as a mediator in the race-disability relationship. The cascade model, used as the theoretical foundation for this study, did not explain the pathway from race or other sociodemographic variables to pain and disability outcomes. Instead, only the presence of more functionally limiting medical conditions was significantly associated with pain, a finding that is consistent with other studies (Leong, Farrell, Helme, & Gibson, 2007). More theoretical work is needed to understand and explain the mechanisms by which race and other sociodemographic indicators influence pain and disability in older adult populations.

There was a robust relationship between pain and disability in this study. This relationship persisted in both the bivariate and multivariate analyses. Even after controlling for SES and health factors, more pain was associated with greater physical and social limitations. This finding highlights the importance of pain in the daily lives of older adults and the need to effectively assess and treat pain to avoid exacerbating or causing functional or social limitations.

The relationship between pain and disability differed for blacks and whites. Race was a significant moderator of the pain-disability relationship; that is, the impact of more pain (greater severity and number of painful body locations) on physical and social limitations was worse for whites than for blacks. This may reflect racial group differences in the experience of living with pain and other health conditions throughout the life span; blacks may be more used to living with adversity, and pain may be less salient factor in their daily functioning. The health disparities literature indicates that black adults experience the onset of chronic diseases, including those associated with disability, at a younger age than whites (Geronimus, 2001). Consequently, disability may be normalized in the daily experience of blacks and less likely to be attributed to pain. In contrast, the effect of pain on functional status in whites may be more noticeable because it is a more recent phenomenon and an obvious deviation from their normal condition. These differential findings may also reflect differences in coping strategies and coping effectiveness, as well as other possible characteristics such as hardiness and resilience.

Several limitations of this study should be noted. First, we examined the role of race, measured by racial category, not ethnicity. Our convenience sample of modest size, recruited from churches and senior centers in one urban metropolitan area in the Midwest, limited to those able to participate in community-based activities, may have excluded housebound or more functionally impaired older adults. The non-randomly selected sample was not fully representative of the older adult population. Finally, several variables might have been overlooked in this cross-sectional study. Participants were not asked, for example, if they had taken pain medications prior to being interviewed about their pain, potentially altering their pain descriptions. If analgesics were used (but not assessed), the prevalence of pain reported in this study is an underestimate, and the impact of pain on disability may actually be more pronounced than we detected.

Findings from this study indicate that race, reflected by black or white identification, did not influence characteristics of pain in a general, nonclinic population of older adults. Pain had negative consequences for daily functioning of this population, a finding more apparent in whites than blacks. This emphasizes the need for better understanding of health disparities between older adults of different races as these disparities relate to pain and disability. It also highlights the need for more comprehensive assessment of ethnicity and cultural identity to fully understand the pain experiences of older adults.

REFERENCES

American Geriatrics Society Panel on Persistent Pain in Older Persons. (2002). Clinical practice guidelines: The management of persistent pain in older persons. *Journal of the American Geriatrics Society*, 50, 1-20.

Ang, D.C., Ibrahim, S.A., Burant, C.J., & Kwoh, C.K. (2003). Is there a difference in the perception of symptoms between African Americans and whites with osteoarthritis? *Journal of Rheumatology*, 30, 1305-1310.

Baker, T.A., & Green, C.R. (2005). Intrarace differences among black and white Americans presenting for chronic pain management: The influence of age, physical health, and psychosocial factors. *Pain Medicine*, 6, 29-38.

Bates, M.S. (1987). Ethnicity and pain: A biocultural model. *Social Science and Medicine*, 24, 47-50.

Bates, M.S., Edwards, W.T., & Anderson, K.O. (1993). Ethnocultural influences on variation in chronic pain perception. *Pain*, 52, 101-112.

Bentler, P.M. (1989). *EQS structural equations manual.* Los Angeles: BMDP Statistical Software.

Bentler, P.M., & Bonett, D.G. (1980). Significance tests and goodness of fit in the analysis of covariance structures. *Psychological Bulletin*, 88, 588-606.

Bergner, M., Bobbit, R.A., Carter,W.B., & Gilson, B.S. (1981). The Sickness Impact Profile: Development and final evaluation of a health status measure. *Medical Care*, 19, 787-805.

Betancourt, J.R. (2006). Eliminating racial and ethnic disparities in health care: What is the role of academic medicine? *Academic Medicine*, 81, 788-792.

Bollen, K.A. (1989). *Structural equations with latent variables.* New York: Wiley Interscience.

Bookwala, J., Harralson, T.L., & Parmelee, P.A. (2003). Effects of pain on functioning and well-being in older adults with osteoarthritis of the knee. *Psychology and Aging*, 18, 844-850.

Cano, A., Mayo, A., & Ventimiglia, M. (2006). Coping, pain severity, interference, and disability: The potential mediating and moderating roles of race and education. *The Journal of Pain*, 7, 459-468.

Cintron, A., & Morrison, R.S. (2006). Pain and ethnicity in the United States: A systematic review. *Journal of Palliative Medicine*, 9(6), 1454-1473.

Creamer, P., Lethbridge-Cejku, M., & Hochberg, M.C. (2000). Factors associated with functional impairment in symptomatic knee osteoarthritis. *Rheumatology*, 39, 490-496.

Dawson, J., Linsell, L., Zondervan, K., Rose, P., Carr, A., & Randall, T, et al. (2005). Impact of persistent hip or knee pain on overall health status in elderly people: A longitudinal population study. *Arthritis and Rheumatism*, 53, 368-374.

de Bruin, A.F., Diederiks, J.P.M., de Witte, L.P., Stevens, F.C.J., & Philipsen, H. (1997). Assessing the responsiveness of a functional status measure: The Sickness Impact Profile versus the SIP68. *Journal of Clinical Epidemiology*, 50, 529-540.

de Bruin, A.F., deWitte, L.P., & Diedriks, J.P.M. (1994). The Sickness Impact Profile: SIP68 a short generic version: First evaluation of the reliability and reproducibility. *Journal of Clinical Epidemiology*, 47, 863-871.

de Bruin, A.F., deWitte, L.P., Stevens, F., & Diedericks, J.P.M. (1992). Sickness Impact Profile: The state of the art of a generic functional status measure. *Social Science and Medicine*, 35, 1003-1014.

De Filippis, L.G., Gulli, S., Caliri, A., D'Avola, G., Lo Gullo, R., & Morgante, S, et al. (2004). Factors influencing pain, physical function and social functioning in patients with osteoarthritis in Southern Italy. *International Journal of Clinical Pharmacology and Research*, 24, 103-109.

Edwards, C.L., Fillingim, R.B., & Keefe, F. (2001). Race, ethnicity and pain. *Pain*, 94, 133-137.

Edwards, R.R. (2006). Age differences in the correlates of physical functioning in patients with chronic pain. *Journal of Aging and Health*, 16, 56-69.

Edwards, R.R., Doleys, D.M., Fillingim, R.B., & Lowery, D. (2001). Ethnic differences in pain tolerance: Clinical implications in a chronic pain population. *Psychosomatic Medicine*, 63, 316-323.

Edwards, R.R., & Fillingim, R.B. (1999). Ethnic differences in thermal pain responses. *Psychosomatic Medicine*, 61, 346-354.

Engle, G. (1962). *Psychological development in health and disease*. Philadelphia: Saunders.

Escalante, A., Lichtenstein, M.J., White, K., Rios, N., & Hazuda, H.P. (1995). Reliability and validity of a method for scoring the pain map of the McGill Pain Questionnaire for use in epidemiologic studies of the elderly. *Aging: Clinical Experimental Research*, 7, 358-366.

Feldt, K.S., Warne, M.A., & Ryden, M.B. (1998). Examining pain in aggressive cognitively impaired older adults. *Journal of Gerontological Nursing*, 24,14-22.

George, L.K., & Fillenbaum, G.G. (1985). OARS methodology: A decade of experience in geriatric assessment. *Journal of the American Geriatrics Society*, 33, 607-615.

Geronimus, A.T. (2001). Understanding and eliminating racial inequalities in women's health in the United States: The role of the weathering conceptual framework. *Journal of American Medical Women's Association*, 56, 133-136.

Golightly, Y.M., & Dominick, K.L. (2005). Racial variations in self-reported osteoarthritis symptom severity among veterans. *Aging: Clinical and Experimental Research*, 17, 264-269.

Green, C.R., Baker, T.A., & Ndao-Brumblay, S.K. (2004). Patient attitudes regarding health care utilization and referral: A descriptive comparison in African and Caucasian Americans with chronic pain. *Journal of the National Medical Association*, 96, 31-42.

Green, C.R., Baker, T.A., Smith, E.M., & Sato, Y. (2003). The effect of race in older adults presenting for chronic pain management: A comparative study of black and white Americans. *The Journal of Pain*, 4, 82-90.

Green, C.R., Todd, K.H., Lebovits, A., & Francis, M. (2006). Disparities in pain: Ethical issues. *Pain Medicine*, 7, 530-533.

Helme, R.D., & Gibson, S.J. (2001). The epidemiology of pain in elderly people. *Clinics in Geriatric Medicine*, 17, 417-431.

Herr, K. (2002). Chronic pain: Challenges and assessment strategies. *Journal of Gerontological Nursing*, 28, 20-27.

Herr, K.A., & Mobily, P.R. (1993). Comparison of selected pain assessment tools for use with the elderly. *Applied Nursing Research*, 6, 39-46.

Hoyle, R.H., & Panter, A.T. (1995). Writing about structural equation models. In R.H. Hoyle (Ed.), *Structural equation modeling: Concepts, issues, and applications* (pp. 158-176). Thousand Oaks, CA: Sage.

Hu, L., & Bentler, P.M. (1995). Evaluating model fit. In R.H. Hoyle (Ed.), *Structural equation modeling: Concepts, issues, and applications* (pp. 76-99). Thousand Oaks, CA: Sage.

Kahana, B., Kahana, E., Namazi, K., Kercher, K., & Stange, K. (1997). The role of pain in the cascade from chronic illness to social disability and psychological distress in late life. In D.C. Turk & R. Melzack (Eds.), *Handbook of pain assessment* (pp. 185-206). New York: Guilford.

Kline, R. (1998). *Principles and practice of structural equation modeling.* New York: Guilford Press.

Leong, I.Y., Farrell, M.J., Helme, R.D., & Gibson, S.J. (2007). The relationship between medical comorbidity and self-rated pain, mood disturbance, and function in older people with chronic pain. *Journal of Gerontology: Medical Sciences*, 62A, M550-M555.

Lichenstein, M.J., Dhanda, R., Cornell, J.E., Escalante, A., & Hazuda, H.P. (1998). Disaggregating pain and its effect on physical functional limitations. *Journal of Gerontology: Medical Sciences*, 53A, M361-M371.

MacCullum, R.C., Browne, M., & Sugawara, H. (1996). Power analysis and determination of sample size for covariance structure modeling. *Psychological Methods*, 1, 130-149.

Maddox, G.L. (1995). *The encyclopedia of aging* (2nd ed.). New York: Springer.

Margolis, R.B., Tait, R.C., & Krause, S.J. (1986). A rating system for use with patient pain drawings. *Pain*, 24, 57-65.

Marsh, H.W., Balla, J.R., & McDonald, R.P. (1988). Goodness-of-fit indexes in confirmatory factor analysis: The effect of sample size. *Psychological Bulletin*, 103, 391-410.

McCracken, L.M., & Eccleston, C. (2005). A prospective study of acceptance of pain and patient functioning with chronic pain. *Pain*, 118, 164-169.

Melzack, R. (1975). The McGill Pain Questionnaire: Major properties and scoring methods. *Pain*, 1, 277-299.

Nanda, U., McLendon, P.M., Andresen, E.M., & Armbrecht, E. (2003). The SIP68: An abbreviated sickness impact profile for disability outcomes research. *Quality of Life Research*, 12, 583-595.

Osborne, T.L., Jensen, M.P., Ehde, D.M., Hanley, M.A., & Kraft, G. (2007). Psychosocial factors associated with pain intensity, pain-related interference, and psychological functioning in persons with multiple sclerosis and pain. *Pain*, 127, 52-62.

Penn, D.A. (2007). Estimating missing values from the General Social Survey: An application of multiple imputation. *Social Science Quarterly*, 88, 573-584.

Portenoy, R.K., Ugarte, C., Fuller, I., & Hass, G. (2004). Population-based survey of pain in the United States: Differences among white, African American, and Hispanic subjects. *The Journal of Pain*, 5, 317-328.

Quintana, S.M., & Maxwell, S.E. (1999). Implications of recent developments in structural equation modeling for counseling psychology. *The Counseling Psychologist*, 27, 485-527.

Rahim-Williams, F.B., Riley, J.L., Herrera, D., Campbell, C.M., Hastie, B.A., & Fillingim, R.B. (2007). Ethnic identity predicts experimental pain sensitivity in African American and Hispanics. *Pain*, 129, 177-184.

Reyes-Gibby, C.C., Aday, L., Cleeland, C. (2002). Impact of pain on self-rated health in the community-dwelling older adults. *Pain*, 95, 75-82.

Reyes-Gibby, C.C., Aday, L., Todd, K.H., Cleeland, C.S., & Anderson, K.O. (2007). Pain in aging community-dwelling adults in the United States: Non-Hispanic whites, Non-Hispanic blacks, and Hispanics. *The Journal of Pain*, 8, 75-84.

Riley, J.L., Gilber, G.H., & Heft, M.W. (2003). Socioeconomic and demographic disparities in symptoms of orofacial pain. *Journal of Public Health and Dentistry*, 63, 166-173.

Riley, J.L.,Wade, J.B., Myers, C.D., Sheffeld, D., Papas, R.K., & Price, D.D. (2002). Racial/ethnic differences in the experience of chronic pain. *Pain*, 100, 291-298.

Scudds, R.J., & Robertson, J.M. (2000). Pain factors associated with physical disability in a sample of community-dwelling senior citizens. *Journal of Gerontology: Medical Sciences*, 55A, M393-M399.

Tabachnick, B.G., & Fidell, L.S. (2007). *Using multivariate statistics* (5th ed.). Boston, MA: Pearson/Allyn & Bacon.

Taylor, L.J., & Herr, K. (2003). Pain intensive assessment: A comparison of selected pain intensity scales for use in cognitively intact and cognitively impaired African American older adults. *Pain Management Nursing*, 4, 87-95.

Vargas, C.M., Macek, M.D., & Marcus, S.E. (2000). Sociodemographic correlates of tooth pain among adults: United States, 1989. *Pain*, 85, 87-92.

Weiner, D.K., Rudy, T.E., Morrow, L., Slaboda, J., & Lieber, S. (2006). The relationship between pain, neuropsychological performance, and physical function in community-dwelling older adults with chronic low back pain. *Pain Medicine*, 7, 60-70.

Williams, C.S., Tinetti, M.E., Kasl, S.V., & Peduzzi, P.N. (2006). The role of pain in the recovery of instrumental and social functioning after hip facture. *Journal of Aging and Health*, 18, 743-762.

Williams, D.R. (2005). The health of U.S. racial and ethnic populations. *Journals of Gerontology: Series B*. 60B, 53-62.

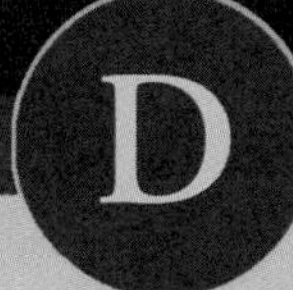

Perceptions of Adult Patients on Hemodialysis Concerning Choice Among Renal Replacement Therapies

Kandace J. Landreneau and Peggy Ward-Smith

Purpose: The aim of this study was to explore what patients on hemodialysis perceive concerning choice among three types of renal replacement therapies: transplantation, hemodialysis, and peritoneal dialysis.

Method: A qualitative phenomenological research design was employed in this exploratory, descriptive study. A convenience sample was recruited from two urban dialysis units in the southern part of the United States. The analysis was performed using Colaizzi's (1978) phenomenological technique.

Results: Two themes emerged from analysis: knowledge and choice. Participants perceived choice in their renal replacement therapies. The predominant theme reflected that most participants had knowledge about at least two of the three types of renal replacement therapies.

Conclusion: The areas of choice among renal replacement therapies, education about all renal replacement therapies, and other dynamics that impact choice, need to be studied. Inquiry needs to remain treatment specific and include all renal replacement treatments available to the patient. Future studies should continue to investigate perceptions of choice, and no assumption should be made about whether patients undergoing hemodialysis are receiving information or education on all the options for renal replacement therapy. Additional research within this area will validate needs and concerns of these patients.

Kandace J. Landreneau, PhD, RN, CCTC, is Associate Professor of Nursing, University of Texas, Tyler, TX. She is a member of ANNA's Acadiana Chapter. For more information on this article, contact the author at kandacel@msn.com.

Peggy Ward-Smith, PhD, RN, is Associate Professor of Nursing, University of Missouri, Kansas City, MO.

Note: The authors reported no actual or potential conflict of interest in relation to this continuing nursing education article.

This offering for 1.5 contact hours is being provided by the American Nephrology Nurses' Association (ANNA).

ANNA is accredited as a provider of continuing nursing education (CNE) by the American Nurses Credentialing Center's Commission on Accreditation.

ANNA is a provider approved by the California Board of Registered Nursing, provider number CEP 00910.

This CNE article meets the Nephrology Nursing Certification Commission's (NNCC's) continuing nursing education requirements for certification and recertification.

GOAL

Explore what patients on hemodialysis perceive concerning choice among three types of renal replacement therapies.

OBJECTIVES

1. State the three types of renal replacement therapies.
2. Discuss two themes which emerged from the study.
3. Formulate a statement about how a patient on hemodialysis could perceive their choice among renal replacement therapies.

Currently, the United States ESRD program is the only national catastrophic Medicare program that offers access regardless of the patient's ability to pay (CMS, 2006). Prior to the ESRD program and the improved success rate of transplantation, the decision to dialyze a patient was based on a selection process and private insurance availability (Bevan, 2000). After this legislation was passed, minorities, women, and the economically disadvantaged were given equal access (Young & Gaston, 2000).

Medicare funding alleviates this large financial burden for the patient, yet the cost of the ESRD program is burdensome for the federal government. The treatment costs to the federal government are different among the therapies. The health care dollar cost to society for a kidney transplant is considerably less than the cost for 2 years on dialysis or a lifetime of dialysis (CMS, 2006; United Network of Organ Sharing [UNOS], 2006). According to the UNOS (2006), it is estimated that the cost of a kidney transplant pays for itself 2 years after surgery and the cost of dialysis keeps increasing year after year. Since the early 1980s, research has demonstrated that renal transplants have offered the possibility and probability of a return to life "without kidney failure," therefore greatly improving quality of life (Headley & Wall, 1999; Kutner, Zhang, & McClellan, 2000; Linqvist, Carlsson, & Sjoden, 2000). Currently, more than 450,000 people have ESRD, with less than 25% listed as candidates for transplant (CMS, 2006; UNOS, 2006).

Considerable attention has been given in reviews and research studies in the nursing science literature on renal replacement therapies for people with ESRD (Bevan, 2000; Linqvist et al., 2000; Murray & Conrad, 1999; Rittman, Northsea, Hausauer, Green, & Swanson, 1993; Weil, 2000). Although there is a large amount of literature on different renal replacement therapies, most of the research has been conducted from the health care providers' perspectives (Gordon et al., 2000; Keogh et al., 1999; Starzomski et al., 2000). The literature reveals a division as to either the study of dialysis therapy or the study of transplant therapy. The perceptions of the choice of renal replacement therapy for patients on hemodialysis remain unknown.

To date, there is little or no data to allow us to better understand the question of why patients receive one renal replacement therapy versus another. No research has addressed patient perception of choice while considering all three available treatments: transplantation, peritoneal dialysis, and hemodialysis.

STUDY

Aim

The aim of this study was to explore what patients on hemodialysis perceive concerning choice among the three types of renal replacement therapies: transplantation, hemodialysis, and peritoneal dialysis.

Design

This study was an exploratory, descriptive study using a phenomenological approach (Husserl, 1913) to describe what patients on hemodialysis perceive about their choice among renal replacement therapies. Qualitative methods provided the means to "grasp and sense the lived experience" of patients on hemodialysis (Streubert & Carpenter, 1999, p. 1). Based on a review of literature and the lack of research examining perceptions about choice among all renal replacement therapies, the research question was refined to an open-ended guide.

Pilot Study

A pilot study with 2 patients on hemodialysis, 2 patients on peritoneal dialysis and 2 patients who had functioning kidney transplants was conducted to determine the feasibility and effectiveness of recruitment strategies, interview, and data analysis techniques. The strategies and methods successfully used in the pilot study were again used in the larger study. Data from the pilot study were so broad in scope that the decision was made to limit the larger study to just one of the three groups. Because the patients on hemodialysis had the richest descriptions in the pilot study, the decision was made to focus on that population in the larger study (Landreneau & Ward-Smith, 2006).

Sample and Setting

A purposive, convenience sample was recruited from the population of patients on hemodialysis who dialyzed at 2 dialysis units in the southern part of the U.S. Participants were selected based on their experience with the phenomenon of choice among renal replacement therapies, and the ability to share that knowledge. This type of sampling was used to obtain information-rich cases for in-depth analysis. Issues of central importance to the purpose of this research, such as individual patients' perceptions of their disease trajectories, were elucidated through purposive sampling.

The criteria for sample selection were: (a) diagnosis of ESRD; (b) over 18 years of age; (c) receiving hemodialysis therapy only for more than 1 week; (d) present at the study site for more than one hemodialysis treatment; and (e) able to converse and understand English. The criteria for exclusion were: (a) medical conditions that would make participation in this study a hardship on the individual; (b) absent during the usual hemodialysis treatment time; and (c) co-morbid psychiatric conditions.

Data Collection

With the approval of the university internal review board for the protection of human subjects, approval from the dialysis units' internal review board, and permission of both dialysis units, the researcher approached 190 patients on hemodialysis from the 2 dialysis units and invited them to participate in the current study. Of the 190 patients on hemodialysis, 175 (92%) verbally consented and 20 were randomly selected to begin the study. Each participant consented to provide the researcher with his or her phone number and was phoned to discuss the study. A script was used to describe the study. Phone consent was obtained and the researcher scheduled a time to meet with the participant at the dialysis unit. The demographic data sheet was completed after written informed consent was obtained, and interviews were audiotaped. The interviews ranged from 30–45 minutes each. Each participant's consent form and audio-tape was encoded with a number designation (Participant #1, Participant #2, etc. rather than their name) and contained no identifying information. Data collection was completed over a 5-day period. All tapes were transcribed within 2 weeks following the interviews. A research assistant transcribed the tapes verbatim and the researcher proofread the content while listening to the audiotapes.

Sampling continued until saturation of data was achieved. Once repetition and confirmation of previously collected data were noted, recruitment was discontinued. After the 12th interview, no new information was shared by participants.

Table 1 describes the demographics of the sample. Demographic data were obtained from 11 of the participants, with one participant declining to complete the demographic sheet. Concurrent medical conditions were also self-disclosed. Renal failure was identified by all of

TABLE 1 Demographic Data (N = 12)

Participant	Age	Gender	Marital Status	Ethnicity	Education	Income	Medical Status	Years in ESRD
#1	21	Female	Missing	Caucasian	10	Missing	Hypertension	5
#2	51	Female	Married	Caucasian	12	$10,001+	Hypertension	2
#3	50	Male	Divorced	Caucasian	12	$60,001+	Diabetes mellitus Hypertension	1
#4	40	Male	Single	African American	BA	0+	Hypertension	2
#5	32	Female	Single	African American	12	0+	Hypertension	5
#6	77	Male	Married	Caucasian	MS	$30,001+	Diabetes mellitus Hypertension	1
#7	55	Male	Single	African American	6	0+	Hypertension	2
#8	44	Female	Married	Caucasian	GED	$10,001+	Hypertension	2
#9	66	Male	Married	African American	12	0+	Diabetes mellitus Hypertension	2
#10	63	Female	Married	Caucasian	12	$10,001+	Hypertension	4
#11	Missing	Male	Missing	missing	Missing	missing	missing	Missing
#12	58	Male	Single	African American	8	missing	Diabetes mellitus Hypertension	4

Note: BA = Bachelor of Arts; MS = Master of Science; GED = General Education Development.

the participants, with 8 (66%) of them stating they had the condition for at least 2 years. Ten (83%) of the participants stated the cause of their renal failure: hypertension was identified by 11 (92%) as a comorbidity, and diabetes was identified by 4 (33%) as a comorbidity. One participant had no comorbidities stated on the demographic form.

An open-ended guide was used for the individual interview. The researcher told the participants "I am interested in knowing more about the choices that you thought about when you were deciding on which treatments were best for your kidney failure. Usually these choices are transplantation, hemodialysis, or peritoneal dialysis. Please tell me, in as much detail as possible, what perceptions you have concerning your choice among kidney failure treatments. Please share all your thoughts, feelings, and perceptions concerning your choices among kidney failure treatments." All participants were encouraged to express as many of their thoughts as possible.

Validity and Reliability

Rigor refers to establishing the trustworthiness of data and was demonstrated through attention to, and confirmation of, information discovery (Denzin & Lincoln, 2000). Lincoln and Guba (1985) have outlined the current gold standard criteria for qualitative researchers by which to establish the trustworthiness of qualitative data. These criteria include credibility, dependability, confirmability, and transferability.

Several operational techniques were used to increase the likelihood that credible findings would be produced (Streubert & Carpenter, 1999): (a) use of open-ended interviewing techniques: tape recordings and verbatim transcriptions increased the accuracy of describing each participant's experience; (b) use of peer debriefings—there were no changes in coding descriptions; (c) use of member checks in which participants were asked to comment on the data themes and the researcher's interpretations in a follow-up telephone call—no changes were suggested by any of the four validating member checks/participants; and (d) an extensive literature review.

The second criterion in assessing trustworthiness is dependability or stability of the data over time and over conditions (Denzin & Lincoln, 2000). The investigator interviewer had significant clinical background in renal replacement therapy, and, as such, had biases. Data collection over a short time frame was helpful by providing so much data in a concentrated period that these biases were largely minimized. Dependability was also established through the consistency of the data descriptions from each interview, through the reading of verbatim transcripts along with listening to the participant's audiotape, and through the validation of the 4 participants/member checks concerning what was described. There was a time lapse between the interview and the transcription of the audiotapes. There was also a time lapse between the transcription and the 4 member checks. The stability of the data was seen throughout these time settings and conditions and contributes to the dependability of this study.

The third criterion is confirmability, or objectivity of the data (Denzin & Lincoln, 2000). Confirmability of this study was objectively grounded by the researcher's use of bracketing along with the researcher's reflexive journal, available audit trail, and peer debriefings.

Transferability is the fourth criterion and reveals how the findings have meaning to others in similar situations (Denzin & Lincoln, 2000). These descriptions and findings were read by an experienced nurse researcher who was familiar with chronic illness and with patients' perceptions of choice in medical treatments. Similarities and differences between these 2 groups were evident to the experienced nurse researcher. While the results of this study may be transferable to other patients with ESRD who are being treated in settings where transplantation is accessible, it is recognized that they may not be generalizable to all patients with ESRD.

Data Analysis

Data analysis began when data collection began. Data were analyzed using Colaizzi's (1978) framework for phenomenological analysis. Beliefs and assumptions were separated from the raw data throughout the investigation by the use of bracketing and intuiting. Following this reductive phenomenology approach, the researcher wrote down any ideas, feelings, and responses that emerged during data collection (Streubert & Carpenter, 1999). The researcher's own experiences were considered data and were examined within the context of the study.

As each interview was conducted, the researcher carefully listened to each participant's words to discover meanings. This questioning and verifying was part of the analysis. This researcher became immersed in the data, and listened multiple times to the audiotapes prior to transcription. Through this immersion, the researcher committed to fully understand what was spoken by each participant. Each transcript was read, analyzed, and synthesized in order to describe their meanings about the phenomenon of choice about renal replacement therapy.

The first extraction of meaning yielded 515 significant statements from the texts of the 12 interviews. Data analysis revealed 63 statements with the word "choice" or a synonym of choice. Knowledge was identified in 263 significant statements. Formulated meanings were created from each statement, which were then validated in a collaborative method with both the researcher for this study and another nurse researcher with experience and knowledge of qualitative research and data analysis. These debriefings between the researcher and another nurse researcher were useful in validation of the themes. These statements then readily collapsed into three themes. Reflexive journal notes were maintained by the researcher throughout data collection and analysis.

FINDINGS

Two themes emerged from the significant statements: knowledge and choice. Each of the statements relates to participants' perceptions concerning choice of renal replacement therapy. The two themes, knowledge and choice, came directly from all of the participants' responses to the research question/statement.

Theme One: Knowledge

Knowledge was a theme mentioned in 263 significant statements. Each participant mentioned knowledge regarding renal replacement therapies 10 to 36 times (mean = 22). All participants discussed at least 2 of the 3 replacement therapies. An example of knowledge was described as "hemodialysis cleans my blood," "peritoneal dialysis is sterile and can't be done at my home," and "I'm going to get a kidney transplant from a relative." Knowledge regarding renal replacement therapy was obtained from a variety of sources. The most frequent source mentioned was information received from health care professionals, specifically the physician. One participant stated:

I was being treated for uh, for high blood pressure and I asked him [doctor] about did he ever sign me up for a transplant and he said he couldn't cause my kidneys has hardened and there wasn't no use to try to go in with no transplant. Now what's his name, I don't know what he had told me, I mean the doctor.

Another frequent source mentioned was the transplant surgeon. A participant noted:

[T]he day I found out that my kidneys had failed, uh, the doctors there told me that I would have to go on dialysis and uh, they asked me would you want a kidney transplant. And I said, yes I would, cause I didn't want to do this all my life. So, I told them to put me on the list.

The dialysis nurses were also mentioned as a source. One participant noted:

Some nurses told me. Just a few nurses. They just told me about the risks and it's like a 6-hour operation and it's just a risk between life and death. That's mostly what I know about it, you know, now. They were dialysis nurses.

Additional knowledge was obtained from a social worker and others with renal failure. Lastly, knowledge was obtained from family members and "street people." The knowledge acquired by patients was not always accurate. Much of the knowledge shared by participants revealed outdated and inaccurate medical information regarding renal replacement therapy. For example: *Hemodialysis is the best treatment of all, You have to have a sterile home to do peritoneal dialysis,* and *A kidney transplant is a risk of life and death.*

A final feature of the knowledge category was the timing of when renal replacement therapy choice was presented to participants. Each participant stated that they obtained knowledge regarding treatment choice, yet this knowledge was provided at inconsistent points of the illness trajectory. Some knowledge was obtained when hemodialysis treatment was initiated: *All I could do was dialysis. I am sick and cannot have a transplant and I did not want to do the peritoneal thing.*

Theme Two: Choice

The theme of choice was mentioned from 2 to 12 times (mean 5) by each participant. Choice was directly described by each participant and the word "choice" was often used. When using the word "choice," the participants described the process of deciding which treatment among various alternatives they selected. There were 63 significant statements regarding choice.

One participant described her choice of treatment by stating that:

My choice was to have hemodialysis. And I am on the list for a kidney transplant, and I've been on the list for, you know, several years.

Another participant spoke of his choice as:

I chose hemo because, I guess this is more, it's more sterile. I mean I'm more sterile, but if I was at home when you do the peritoneal you have to be real, well with this you have to be sterile too, but I don't know. This type was the best type for me. You know, come in 3 days a week and let them do it. The other way it was at home, I guess, I think you can do it when you get home. Peritoneal you do it when you want to.

Another aspect of the choice category was who made the choice:

My doctor says this is the treatment for me. I've heard of the other things but this works for me. I choose hemodialysis.

When considering choice, ethical issues must be considered. One must consider and incorporate the medically appropriate time to present the types of renal replacement therapies and the patient's option to choose among the renal replacement therapies. Several sources indicated that patients on hemodialysis are not given the knowledge necessary to make an informed treatment choice at the medically appropriate time (Alexander & Sehgal, 1998; Breckenridge, 1997; Gordon et al., 2000). Alexander and Sehgal (1998) noted that the timing of transplantation as a treatment choice was influenced by socio-demographic differences and access to the transplant waiting list rather than lack of interest in transplantation. Problems of timing the presentation of treatment options was also noted in this current study. Several participants stated they were told by the nephrologist that they must start dialysis treatment first, even though several were in chronic renal failure and had been treated for up to a year or longer before becoming end stage. It should be noted that these participants were treated by other physicians before starting dialysis with their present physician. These participants also knew about transplantation after they started dialysis and talked with their "dialysis doctor" about transplantation. This may be a factor of different physicians' opinions or philosophies concerning the promotion of different types of renal replacement therapies.

DISCUSSION

Based on the findings of this study, these patients on hemodialysis perceived that they had a choice in renal replacement therapy even when they had limited participation in choosing their treatment. The predominant theme reflects that most participants had knowledge about renal replacement therapies even though their knowledge included extensive amounts of misinformation regarding the current state-of-the-art of the treatments. The themes identified from the data support these conclusions and provided a forum for discussion. Access to all renal replacement therapies, and the ever-changing medical improvements in these therapies, has expanded the need for understanding health outcomes. In evaluating these therapies for risks and benefits, we see how the treatment affects the patient in her or his areas of choice and requires evaluation. Since this was the first study to explore perceptions concerning choice among all renal replacement therapy in patients on hemodialysis, findings should be viewed with caution. Concerns about participants' knowledge base, and participants' perceptions of choice were strengths of this research.

Knowledge was obtained from a variety of medical and nonmedical sources and at a variety of times. However, many of their statements were medically inaccurate. Published literature does not support knowledge-related statements made by the participants. At the time of this study, transplantation was considered the medically optimal and first choice therapy for ESRD and, more specifically, this population of patients on hemodialysis (CMS, 2006; UNOS, 2006). Just knowing about renal replacement therapies may not assist the patient to make the best personal choice. If the patient's knowledge is not current or accurate, then having a choice may prove to be personally satisfying, yet medically inappropriate.

The primary finding from this study was that these participants on hemodialysis perceived they did have a choice in renal replacement therapy even though they didn't discuss that they had limited participation in the choice, which was not an expected finding and not consistent with the pilot study themes.

In the pilot study, the findings were different. The pilot study themes from the 2 participants on hemodialysis, the 2 participants on peritoneal dialysis, and the 2 participants who had functioning renal transplants were consistent with "no choice among renal replacement therapies" and the "nephrologist chose" the renal replacement therapy (Landreneau & Ward-Smith, 2006). However, in this larger study, all of the participants stated they had a choice. This perception of choice was universal.

In reviewing the literature, only one study was found that addressed patients' perceptions concerning their choice, and this choice was only related to renal transplant (Gordon & Sehgal, 2000). This triangulated study explored discussions between patients and nephrologists regarding transplantation as a treatment option for ESRD. This pioneering study concluded that treatment options, and the order of the presentation of options, influenced renal transplantation as a choice. There was no mention of knowledge obtained from sources other than the nephrologists.

Making treatment choice is possible without accurate knowledge; yet, appropriate and timely information given would better prepare the patient for making a choice. Prior to choosing a treatment, the patient needs to know the potential impact of the treatment (Waitzkin, 1985). Waitzkin (1985) found that the desire for information regarding medical care and the time dedicated to providing this information was underestimated by the physician. Thus, choice may occur prior to all information being disclosed to the patient. If a treatment leads to a decrease in one's risks and an increase in benefits, the patient may be concerned about the choice to be made. Therefore, without accurate and current medical information, neither the clinician nor the patient can make a fully informed choice about therapy.

Breckenridge (1997) discussed that treatment options were selected because of clinical or practical circumstances and some of the participants had no choice in the timing of the treatment or decision. Gordon and Sehgal (2000) stated that nephrologists provided information on treatment options over several weeks to months and they generally presented the option of dialysis first and transplant later. Each type of renal replacement therapy, its risks and benefits, physical changes, and survival statistics are different. The patient's perception concerning choice may carry an impact on the patient's long-term outcomes. The timing of treatment is important for the reduction in mortality and morbidity, with selecting transplantation to eliminate ESRD altogether. Thus, the impact of choice among each therapy has distinct levels of risks and benefits that can be ranked according to medical research, with transplantation as the first choice, peritoneal dialysis as the second, and hemodialysis the least optimal (CMS, 2006; ESRD Network, 2006; Gould & Wainwright, 1997; Gudex, 1995; Starzomski & Hilton, 2000). The medically appropriate time to discuss renal replacement therapy would be during the chronic renal failure phase while most renal failure patients have time to think and decide about their future therapy. Whether patients are receiving this information at the medically appropriate time requires additional research since the available literature does not speak to this important issue.

When discussing the issues of choice and knowledge among the participants of this study, the issue of education becomes apparent. Who best provides the education is unknown. A review of the literature identified only one set of standards for education—those provided by the American Nephrology Nurses Association (ANNA). The ANNA's *Nephrology Nursing Standards of Practice and Guidelines for Care* include 2 patient outcomes in preparation for replacement therapy stating the patient will participate in the decision-making process for treatment modality selection and will have completed evaluation for a kidney transplant, if appropriate, along with a patient teaching plan for renal replacement therapies (Burrows-Hudson & Prowant, 2005). The data from this study suggest that the transference of research about education on all different types of renal replacement therapies to practice is not apparent. There was much misinformation regarding knowledge, among the participants, and standardized teaching outline. Standardized teaching outlines could be developed among the national organizations and should be a priority. Research that identifies what is being taught, and the educational knowledge of health care professionals providing the education to patients with ESRD, should be assessed as this information would provide a foundation for future studies.

Findings in this study support Waitkin's (1985) research on the impact of medical treatment and its effect on choice. Namely, risks and benefits are taken into account when making treatment choice. Data from the present study demonstrated that other treatments carry risks that participants perceived, often incorrectly, as too great and influenced their treatment choice.

Research with samples of patients choosing renal transplantation as a treatment indicated that the order of presentation impacts treatment choice (Gordon & Sehgal, 2000). When comparing the results of this study to the available research regarding treatment choice among patients with ESRD, several issues can be highlighted. The medically appropriate time to provide education, the practical circumstances that surround this timing of education, and who provides this information have all been shown to affect treatment choice (Alexander & Sehgal, 1998; Breckenridge, 1997; Gordon & Sehgal, 2000). The present study did not aim to determine the order of presentation, thus, the impact this may have on treatment choice, within the population of patients on hemodialysis, remains unknown. Findings in this study begin to develop a new body of knowledge, which certainly requires additional research.

CONCLUSIONS

Future research with this population should focus on the areas of choice, education, and other dynamics that impact choice. Data obtained in this study provide a very important first step in the investigation of perceptions concerning choice of renal replacement therapy in patients on hemodialysis. More research is needed to understand each type of renal replacement therapy, not just hemodialysis. Choice and knowledge as essential features of the decision-making process for patients on hemodialysis would necessitate inquiry that is treatment specific and include all treatments available to the patient.

Increasing numbers of people are succumbing to ESRD. This is related to the increase in obesity and diabetes among the general population (CMS, 2006). In the last few years, diabetes has replaced hypertension as the number one cause of ESRD (White & Grenyer, 1999; ESRD Network, 2006; CMS, 2006). More nursing research is needed about the provision of education concerning choice among all renal replacement therapies during their chronic renal failure phase. Many of these patients are in chronic renal failure for more than 5 years (CMS, 2006). With the best medical option, renal transplantation, these patients may find greater opportunity for a living-related or non-related donor transplant. At the end of this equation is a person, a person with health needs requiring nursing professionals to step in and provide an atmosphere in which every patient receives adequate, timely, and accurate information to make an informed choice for renal replacement therapies.

REFERENCES

Alexander, G.C., & Sehgal, A.R. (1998). Barriers to cadaver renal transplant among blacks, women, and the poor. *Journal of the American Medical Association*, 280(13), 1148-1152.

Bevan, M.T. (2000). Dialysis as "deus ex machine:" A critical analysis of haemodialysis. *Journal of Advanced Nursing*, 31(2), 437-443.

Breckenridge, D.M. (1997). Patients' perceptions of why, how, and by whom dialysis treatment modality was chosen. *ANNA Journal*, 24(3), 313-319.

Burrows-Hudson, S., & Prowant, B. (Eds.). (2005). *Nephrology nursing standards of practice and guidelines for care*. Pitman, NJ: American Nephrology Nurses' Association.

Center for Medicare and Medicaid Services (2006). *United States renal data system 2005 annual report*. Retrieved March 31, 2006 from www.cms.hhs.gov

Colaizzi, P. (1978). Psychological research as the phenomenologist views it. In K. Valle & I. King (Eds.), *Existential phenomenological alternatives for psychology*. New York: Oxford Press.

Denzin, N.K., & Lincoln, Y.S. (2000). *Handbook of qualitative research*. London: Sage Publications.

ESRD Network. (2006). Retrieved March31, 2006 from www.esrdnetworks.org.

Gordon, E.J., & Sehgal, A.R. (2000). Patient-nephrologist discussion about kidney transplantation as a treatment option. *Advances in Renal Replacement Therapy*, 7(2), 177-183.

Gould, D., & Wainwright, S.P. (1997). Stress and quality of life in the renal transplant patient: A preliminary investigation. *Journal of Advanced Nursing*, 25(1), 562-570.

Gudex, C.M. (1995). Health related quality of life in end stage renal failure. *Quality of Life Research*, 4(4), 359-366.

Headley, C.M., & Wall, B. (1999). Acquired cystic kidney disease in ESRD. *ANNA Journal*, 26(4), 381-389.

Hesse-Biber, S., Kinder, T.S., Dupuis, P.R., Dupuis, A., & Tormabene, E. (1994). *HyperRESEARCH: A content analysis tool for the qualitative research*. Randolph, MA: Researchware, Inc.

Husserl, E. (1913). *Ideas*. London: George Allen and Unwin (1962, Republished, New York: Colliers).

Keogh, A.M., & Feehally, J. (1999). A quantitative study comparing adjustment and acceptance of illness in adults on renal replacement therapy. *ANNA Journal*, 26(5), 471-477.

Kutner N.G., Zhang, R., & McClellan, W.M. (2000). Patient-reported quality of life early in dialysis treatment: effects associated with usual exercise activity. *Nephrology Nursing Journal*, 27(4), 357-367.

Landreneau, K., & Ward-Smith, P. (2006). Patients' perceptions concerning choice among renal replacement therapies: A pilot study. *Nephrology Nursing Journal*, 33(4), 397-402.

Lincoln, Y.S., & Guba, E.G. (1985). *Naturalistic inquiry*. Newbury Park, CA: Sage.

Lindqvist, R., Carlsson, M., & Sjoden, P. (2000). Coping strategies and health related quality of life among spouses of continuous ambulatory peritoneal dialysis, haemodialysis, and transplant patients. *Journal of Advanced Nursing*, 31(6), 1398-1408.

Murray, L.R., & Conrad, N.E. (1999). Perceptions of kidney transplant by persons with end stage renal disease. *ANNA Journal*, 26(5), 479-500.

Rittman, M., Northsea, C., Hausauer, N., Green, C., & Swanson, L. (1993). Living with renal failure. *ANNA Journal*, 20(3), 327-332.

Social Security Amendments of 1972. (PL 92-603, 30 Oct. 1972), 86. United States Statutes at Large, 1463-1464.

Starzomski, R., & Hilton, A. (2000). Patient and family adjustment of kidney transplant with and without an interim period of dialysis. *Nephrology Nursing Journal*, 27(1), 17-32.

Streubert, H.J., & Carpenter, D.F. (1999). *Qualitative research in nursing: Advancing the humanistic imperative* (2nd ed., pp. 1-62). Philadelphia: Lippincott Williams & Wilkins.

United Network for Organ Sharing (UNOS). (2006). *Annual report*. Retrieved March 31, 2006 from www.unos.org

Waitzkin, H. (1985) Information giving in medical care. *Journal of Health and Social Behavior*, 26, 81-101.

Weil, C.M. (2000). Exploring hope inpatients with end stage renal disease on chronic hemodialysis. *Nephrology Nursing Journal*, 27(2), 219-224.

White, Y., & Grenyer, B.F. (1999). The biopsychosocial impact of end stage renal disease: The experience of dialysis patients and their partners. *Journal of Advanced Nursing*, 30(6),1312-1320.

Young, C.J., & Gaston, R.S. (2000). Renal transplantation in black Americans. *New England Journal of Medicine*, 343(21), 1545-1552.

E

Nursing Interventions for Smoking Cessation (Review)

Rice VH and Stead LF

Contribution of author(s)	VHR extracted data andwrote the review. LS conducted searches, extracted data and assisted in drafting the review. Both authors contribute to review updates.
Issue protocol first published	1998/3
Review first published	1999/3
Date of most recent amendment	13 November 2007
Date of most recent SUBSTANTIVE amendment	21 October 2007
What's New	Updated for 2008 issue 1 with 12 new studies (identified inNotes column of Characteristics of Included Studies table). No major changes to results. The conclusions have not changed.
Date new studies sought but none found	Information not supplied by author
Date new studies found but not yet included/excluded	Information not supplied by author
Date new studies found and included/ excluded	21 October 2007
Date authors' conclusions section amended	15 September 2003
Contact address	Prof Virginia Hill Rice College of Nursing Wayne State University 5557 Cass Avenue Detroit Michigan 48202 USA E-mail: vfrice@aol.com Tel: +1 313 577 4064 Fax: +1 313 577 5777
DOI	10.1002/14651858.CD001188.pub3
Cochrane Library number	CD001188
Editorial group	Cochrane Tobacco Addiction Group
Editorial group code	HM-TOBACCO

ABSTRACT

Background Healthcare professionals, including nurses, frequently advise patients to improve their health by stopping smoking. Such advice may be brief, or part of more intensive interventions.

Objectives To determine the effectiveness of nursing-delivered smoking cessation interventions.

Search strategy We searched the Cochrane Tobacco Addiction Group specialized register and CINAHL in July 2007.

Selection criteria Randomized trials of smoking cessation interventions delivered by nurses or health visitors with follow-up of at least six months.

Data collection and analysis Two authors extracted data independently. The main outcome measure was abstinence from smoking after at least six months of follow-up. We used the most rigorous definition of abstinence for each trial, and biochemically validated rates if available. Where statistically and clinically appropriate, we pooled studies using a Mantel-Haenszel fixed effect model and reported the outcome as a risk ratio (RR) with 95% confidence interval (CI).

Main results Forty-two studies met the inclusion criteria. Thirty-one studies comparing a nursing intervention to a control or to usual care found the intervention to significantly increase the likelihood of quitting (RR 1.28, 95% CI 1.18 to 1.38). There was heterogeneity among the study results, but pooling using a random effects model did not alter the estimate of a statistically significant effect. In a subgroup analysis there was weaker evidence that lower intensity interventions were effective (RR 1.27, 95% CI 0.99 to 1.62). There was limited indirect evidence that interventions were more effective for hospital inpatients with cardiovascular disease than for inpatients with other conditions. Interventions in non-hospitalized patients also showed evidence of benefit. Nine studies comparing different nurse-delivered interventions failed to detect significant benefit from using additional components. Five studies of nurse counselling on smoking cessation during a screening health check, or as part of multifactorial secondary prevention in general practice (not included in the main meta-analysis) found nursing intervention to have less effect under these conditions.

Authors' conclusions The results indicate the potential benefits of smoking cessation advice and/or counselling given by nurses to patients, with reasonable evidence that intervention is effective. The evidence of an effect is weaker when interventions are brief and are provided by nurses whose main role is not health promotion or smoking cessation. The challenge will be to incorporate smoking behaviour monitoring and smoking cessation interventions as part of standard practice, so that all patients are given an opportunity to be asked about their tobacco use and to be given advice and/ or counselling to quit along with reinforcement and follow-up.

PLAIN LANGUAGE SUMMARY

Advice and Support from Nurses to Help People Stop Smoking, Especially When They Are in Hospital

Most smokers want to quit, and may be helped by advice and support from healthcare professionals. Nurses are the largest healthcare workforce, and are involved in virtually all levels of health care. This review of clinical trials covered 42 studies, with more than 15,000 participants included in the analyses. It found that advice and support from nursing staff could increase people's success in quitting smoking, especially in a hospital setting. Similar advice and encouragement given by nurses at health checks or prevention activities seems to be less effective, but may still have some impact.

Status: Updated

This record should be cited as: Rice VH, Stead LF. Nursing interventions for smoking cessation. Cochrane Database of Systematic Reviews 2008, Issue 1. Art. No.: CD001188. DOI: 10.1002/14651858.CD001188.pub3.

This version first published online: 23 January 2008 in Issue 1, 2008. Date of most recent substantive amendment: 21 October 2007

BACKGROUND

Tobacco-related deaths and disabilities are on the increase worldwide, because of continued use of tobacco (mainly cigarettes). Tobacco use has reached epidemic proportions in many developing countries, while steady use continues in industrialized nations (Davis 2007; West 2006; DHHS 2004).The following two factors may help to reduce the prevalence of cigarette smoking: (1) 79% to 90% (Coultas 1991) of smokers want to quit smoking (NIH 2006) and (2) 70% of smokers visit a healthcare professional each year (Cherry 2003). Nurses, with the largest number of healthcare providers worldwide, are involved in the majority of these visits and could therefore have a profound effect on the reduction of tobacco use (Percival 2003; Whyte 2003).

Systematic reviews (e.g., Lancaster 2004) have confirmed the effectiveness of advice to stop smoking from physicians. The Agency for Health Care Research and Quality Clinical Practice Guideline (AHRQ 2000) notes strong support for physicians to advise every patient who smokes to quit. The findings for advice by nonphysician clinicians have been weaker, although the guideline recommends that all clinicians provide interventions. A review of nursing's role in smoking cessation is essential if the profession is to endorse the American Nurses Association position, "patient education and preventive healthcare interventions to stop tobacco use should be part of nursing practice" (ANA 1995).

The aim of this review is to examine and summarize randomized clinical trials where nursing provided smoking cessation interventions. The review therefore focuses on the nurse as the intervention provider, rather than on a particular type of intervention. Smoking cessation [efforts] targeting pregnant women are not included here, because of the particular circumstance and motivation among these women. Interventions for pregnant smokers have been reviewed elsewhere (Lumley 2004).

OBJECTIVES

The primary objective of this review was to determine the effectiveness of nursing-delivered interventions on smoking behaviour in adults. *A priori* study hypotheses were that nursing-delivered smoking cessation interventions:

(i) are more effective than no intervention
(ii) are more effective if the intervention is more intense
(iii) differ in effectiveness with health state and setting of the participants
(iv) are more effective if they include follow-ups
(v) are more effective if they include aids that demonstrate the pathophysiological effect of smoking

This review does not address the incremental effects of providing nicotine replacement therapy (NRT) by nurses, as NRT effectiveness is addressed in a separate Cochrane review (Stead 2008). Studies in which advice about nicotine replacement was part of the nursing intervention are included.

CRITERIA FOR CONSIDERING STUDIES FOR THIS REVIEW

Types of Studies

Inclusion criteria for studies were:

(i) they had to have at least two treatment groups

(ii) allocation to treatment groups must have been stated to be "random"

Studies that used historical controls were excluded.

Types of Participants

Participants were adult smokers, 18 years and older, of either gender and recruited in any type of healthcare setting. The only exceptions were studies that had exclusively recruited pregnant women. Trials in which "recent quitters" were classified as smokers were included, but sensitivity analyses were performed to determine whether they differed from trials that excluded such individuals.

Types of Intervention

Nursing intervention was defined as the provision of advice, counselling, and/or strategies to help patients quit smoking. The review includes cessation studies that compared usual care with an intervention, brief advice with a more intensive smoking cessation intervention or different types of interventions. Studies of smoking cessation interventions as a part of multifactorial lifestyle counselling or rehabilitation were included only if it was possible to discern the specific nature and timing of the intervention, and to extract data on the outcomes for those who were smokers at baseline. Advice was defined as verbal instructions from the nurse to "stop smoking" whether or not information was provided about the harmful effects of smoking. Interventions were grouped into low and high intensity for comparison. *Low intensity* was defined as trials where advice was provided (with or without a leaflet) during a single consultation lasting 10 minutes or less with up to one follow-up visit. *High intensity* was defined as trials where the initial contact lasted more than 10 minutes, there were additional materials (e.g., manuals) and/or strategies other than simple leaflets, and usually participants had more than one follow-up contact. Studies where patients were randomized to receive advice versus advice plus some form of nicotine replacement therapy (NRT) were excluded, since these were primarily comparisons of the effectiveness of NRT rather than nursing interventions.

Types of Outcome Measures

The principal outcome was smoking cessation rather than a reduction in withdrawal symptoms, or reduction in number of cigarettes smoked. Trials had to report follow-up of at least six months for inclusion in the review. We excluded trials which did not include data on smoking cessation rates. We used the strictest available criteria to define abstinence in each study, e.g., sustained cessation rather than point prevalence. Where biochemical validation was used, only participants meeting the biochemical criteria for cessation were regarded as abstainers. Participants lost to follow-up were regarded as continuing smokers (intention-to-treat analyses).

SEARCH METHODS FOR IDENTIFICATION OF STUDIES

See: Cochrane Tobacco Addiction Group methods used in reviews. We searched the Tobacco Addiction Review Group specialized register for trials (most recent search July 2007). This register includes trials located from systematic search of MEDLINE, EMBASE and PsycINFO and hand searching of specialist journals, conference proceedings, and reference lists of previous trials and overviews. We checked all trials with "nurse" or "health visitor" in the title, abstract, or keywords for relevance. We also searched the Cumulative Index to Nursing and Allied Health Literature (CINAHL) on OVID for "nursing" and "smoking cessation" from 1983 to July 2007.

METHODS OF THE REVIEW

Data Extraction

The authors extracted data from the published reports independently. Disagreements were resolved by referral to a third person. For each trial, the following data were extracted: (i) author(s) and year; (ii) country of origin, study setting, and design; (iii) number and characteristics of participants and definition of "smoker"; (iv) description of the intervention and designation of its intensity (high or low); and (v) outcomes and biochemical validation. In trials where the details of the methodology were unclear or where the results were expressed in a form that did not allow for extraction of key data, we approached the original investigators for additional information. We treated participants lost to follow-up as continuing smokers. We excluded from totals only those participants who died before follow-up or were known to have moved to an untraceable address.

Quality Assessment

We assessed the studies in relation to the four general sources of bias described in the Cochrane Handbook.

(i) selection bias—systematic differences in the securing of the comparison groups
(ii) performance bias—systematic differences in care apart from the intervention of interest
(iii) attrition bias—systematic withdrawals from the trial
(iv) detection bias—systematic differences in outcome assessment

Only the control of selection bias at entry has been shown empirically to result in systematic differences in the assessment of effect size (Schulz 1995). We used a three-point scale, with a grading of A if the effort to control selection bias had been optimal (e.g., a randomly-generated table of assignment established before contact with potential participants); a grading of B if there was uncertainty as to how and when random assignments had been made; and a grading of C if group allocation had definitely not been adequately concealed.

Data Analysis

Following changes to the Cochrane Tobacco Addiction Group's recommended method of data analysis since this review was last updated, we have changed the way in which we summarise the effects of treatment. We now use the risk ratio rather than the odds ratio for summarising individual trial outcomes and for the estimate of the pooled effect. Treatment effects will seem larger when expressed as odds ratios than when expressed as risk ratios, unless the event rates are very low. For example, if 20 out of 100 participants have quit in the intervention group, and 10 out of 100 in the control group the risk ratio is 2.0 [(20/100)/(10/100)], whilst the odds ratio is 2.25 [(20/80)/(10/90)]. Whilst there are circumstances in which odds ratios may be preferable, there is a danger that they will be interpreted as if they are risk ratios, making the treatment effect seem larger (Deeks 2006). Where we judged a group of studies to be sufficiently clinically and statistically homogenous we used the Mantel-Haenszel fixed-effect method (Greenland 1985) to calculate a weighted average of the risk ratios of the individual trials, with 95% confidence intervals.

To assess statistical heterogeneity between trials we used the I^2 statistic (Higgins 2003). This measures the percentage of total variation across studies due to heterogeneity rather than to chance. Values of I^2 over 75% indicate a considerable level of heterogeneity. We append the Cochrane Tobacco Addiction Group's Glossary of tobacco-related terms as an additional table (Table 01).

TABLE 01 Glossary of Terms

Term	Definition
Abstinence	A period of being quit, i.e., stopping the use of cigarettes or other tobacco products. May be defined in various ways; see also: point prevalence abstinence; prolonged abstinence; continuous/sustained abstinence.
Biochemical verification	Also called "biochemical validation" or "biochemical confirmation": A procedure for checking a tobacco user's report that he or she has not smoked or used tobacco. It can be measured by testing levels of nicotine or cotinine or other chemicals in blood, urine, or saliva, or by measuring levels of carbon monoxide in exhaled breath or in blood.
Bupropion	A pharmaceutical drug originally developed as an antidepressant, but now also licensed for smoking cessation; trade names Zyban, Wellbutrin (when prescribed as an antidepressant).
Carbon monoxide (CO)	A colourless, odourless highly poisonous gas found in tobacco smoke and in the lungs of people who have recently smoked, or (in smaller amounts) in people who have been exposed to tobacco smoke. May be used for biochemical verification of abstinence.
Cessation	Also called "quitting." The goal of treatment to help people achieve abstinence from smoking or other tobacco use, also used to describe the process of changing the behaviour.
Continuous abstinence	Also called "sustained abstinence." A measure of cessation often used in clinical trials involving avoidance of all tobacco use since the quit day until the time the assessment is made. The definition occasionally allows for lapses. This is the most rigorous measure of abstinence.
"Cold turkey"	Quitting abruptly, and/or quitting without behavioural or pharmaceutical support.
Craving	A very intense urge or desire [to smoke]. See: Shiffman et al. "Recommendations for the assessment of tobacco craving and withdrawal in smoking cessation trials," *Nicotine and Tobacco Research* 2004:6(4):599-614.
Dopamine	A neurotransmitter in the brain which regulates mood, attention, pleasure, reward, motivation and movement.

TABLE 01 Glossary of Terms—cont'd

Term	Definition
Efficacy	Also called "treatment effect" or "effect size": The difference in outcome between the experimental and control groups.
Harm reduction	Strategies to reduce harm caused by continued tobacco/nicotine use, such as reducing the number of cigarettes smoked, or switching to different brands or products, e.g., potentially reduced exposure products (PREPs), smokeless tobacco.
Lapse/slip	Terms sometimes used for a return to tobacco use after a period of abstinence. A lapse or slip might be defined as a puff or two on a cigarette. This may proceed to relapse, or abstinence may be regained. Some definitions of continuous, sustained or prolonged abstinence require complete abstinence, but some allow for a limited number or duration of slips. People who lapse are very likely to relapse, but some treatments may have their effect by helping people recover from a lapse.
nAChR [neural nicotinic acetylcholine receptors]	Areas in the brain which are thought to respond to nicotine, forming the basis of nicotine addiction by stimulating the overflow of dopamine.
Nicotine	An alkaloid derived from tobacco, responsible for the psychoactive and addictive effects of smoking.
Nicotine replacement therapy (NRT)	A smoking cessation treatment in which nicotine from tobacco is replaced for a limited period by pharmaceutical nicotine. This reduces the craving and withdrawal experienced during the initial period of abstinence while users are learning to be tobacco-free. The nicotine dose can be taken through the skin, using patches, by inhaling a spray, or by mouth using gum or lozenges.
Outcome	Often used to describe the result being measured in trials that is of relevance to the review. For example, smoking cessation is the outcome used in reviews of ways to help smokers quit. The exact outcome in terms of the definition of abstinence and the length of time that has elapsed since the quit attempt was made may vary from trial to trial.
Pharmacotherapy	A treatment using pharmaceutical drugs, e.g., NRT, bupropion.
Point prevalence abstinence (PPA)	A measure of cessation based on behaviour at a particular point in time, or during a relatively brief specified period, e.g., 24 hours, 7 days. It may include a mixture of recent and long-term quitters; cf. prolonged abstinence, continuous abstinence.
Prolonged abstinence	A measure of cessation which typically allows a "grace period" following the quit date (usually of about two weeks), to allow for slips/lapses during the first few days when the effect of treatment may still be emerging. See: Hughes et al. Measures of abstinence in clinical trials: issues and recommendations, *Nicotine and Tobacco Research,* 2003:5(1);13-25.
Relapse	A return to regular smoking after a period of abstinence.
Secondhand smoke	Also called passive smoking or environmental tobacco smoke [ETS]. A mixture of smoke exhaled by smokers and smoke released from smouldering cigarettes, cigars, pipes, bidis, etc. The smoke mixture contains gases and particulates, including nicotine, carcinogens, and toxins.
Self-efficacy	The belief that one will be able to change one's behaviour, e.g., to quit smoking.
SPC [summary of product characteristics]	Advice from the manufacturers of a drug, agreed with the relevant licensing authority, to enable health professionals to prescribe and use the treatment safely and effectively.
Tapering	A gradual decrease in dose at the end of treatment, as an alternative to abruptly stopping treatment.
Tar	The toxic chemicals found in cigarettes. In solid form, it is the brown, tacky residue visible in a cigarette filter and deposited in the lungs of smokers.
Titration	A technique of dosing at low levels at the beginning of treatment, and gradually increasing to full dose over a few days, to allow the body to get used to the drug. It is designed to limit side effects.
Withdrawal	A variety of behavioural, affective, cognitive, and physiological symptoms, usually transient, which occur after use of an addictive drug is reduced or stopped. See: Shiffman et al. Recommendations for the assessment of tobacco craving and withdrawal in smoking cessation trials, *Nicotine and Tobacco Research* 2004:6(4):599-614.

DESCRIPTION OF STUDIES

Forty-two trials met the inclusion criteria. They were of nursing interventions for smoking cessation for adults who used tobacco (primarily cigarettes), published between 1987 and 2007. One trial (Sanders 1989a; Sanders 1989b) had two parts with randomization at each stage, so is treated here as two separate studies, making a total of 43 studies in the Table of Included Studies. Thirty studies contributed to the primary meta-analysis that compared a nursing intervention to a usual care or minimal intervention control. Nine studies included a comparison between two nursing interventions, involving different components or different numbers of contacts. Four studies did not contribute to a meta-analysis and their results are described separately. Sample sizes of studies contributing to a meta-analysis ranged from 25 to 2700 but were typically between 150 and 500.

Sixteen trials took place in the USA, nine in the UK, three in Canada, two each in Australia, Denmark, Japan, The Netherlands, Norway and Spain, and one trial each was reported from South Korea and from Sweden.

Seventeen trials intervened with hospitalized patients (Taylor 1990; Rigotti 1994; DeBusk 1994; Allen 1996; Carlsson 1997; Miller 1997; Lewis 1998; Feeney 2001; Bolman 2002; Hajek 2002; Quist-Paulsen 2003; Froelicher 2004; Hasuo 2004; Chouinard 2005; Hennrikus 2005; Nagle 2005; Hanssen 2007). One trial (Rice 1994) recruited hospitalized patients, but with follow-up after discharge. Nineteen studies recruited from primary care or outpatient clinics (Janz 1987; Sanders 1989a/Sanders 1989b; Risser 1990; Vetter 1990; Nebot 1992; Hollis 1993; OXCHECK 1994; Family Heart 1994; Tonnesen 1996; Campbell 1998; Lancaster 1999; Steptoe 1999; Canga 2000; Aveyard 2003; Ratner 2004; Tonnesen 2006; Kim 2005; Hilberink 2005; Sanz-Pozo 2006). In some trials, the recruitment took place during a clinic visit whilst in others the invitation to enroll was made by letter. One study (Terazawa 2001) recruited employees during a workplace health check, two enrolled community-based adults motivated to make a quit attempt (Davies 1992; Alterman 2001), one recruited mothers taking their child to a paediatric clinic (Curry 2003) and one recruited people being visited by a home healthcare nurse (Borrelli 2005).

Twelve of the studies focused on adults with diagnosed cardiovascular health problems (Taylor 1990; DeBusk 1994; Family Heart 1994; Rice 1994; Rigotti 1994; Allen 1996; Carlsson 1997; Miller 1997 (subgroup with cardiovascular disease); Campbell 1998; Feeney 2001; Bolman 2002; Hajek 2002); two studies were with patients with respiratory diseases (Tonnesen 1996; Tonnesen 2006) and one with patients with diabetes (Canga 2000). One study recruited people attending a surgical pre-admission clinic (Ratner 2004).

All studies included adults 18 years and older who used some form of tobacco. Allen 1996, Curry 2003 and Froelicher 2004 studied females only, and Terazawa 2001 males only. The definition of tobacco use varied and in some cases included recent quitters.

Five of the studies examined a smoking cessation intervention as a component of multiple risk factor reduction interventions in adults with cardiovascular disease (DeBusk 1994; Allen 1996; Carlsson 1997; Campbell 1998; Hanssen 2007). In the first three of these studies, the smoking cessation component was clearly defined, of high intensity, and independently measurable. In the fourth and fifth studies the smoking component was less clearly specified.

Thirty-one studies with a total of over 15,000 participants contributed to the main comparison of nursing intervention versus control. We classified 24 as high intensity on the basis of the planned intervention, although in some cases implementation may have been incomplete. In seven, we classified the intervention as low intensity (Janz 1987; Vetter 1990; Davies 1992; Nebot 1992; Tonnesen 1996; Aveyard 2003; Nagle 2005). All of these were conducted in outpatient, primary care or community settings. One further study (Hajek 2002) may be considered as a comparison between a low intensity intervention and usual care. Patients in the usual care control group received systematic brief advice and self-help materials from the same nurses who provided the intervention. Unlike the other trials in the low intensity subgroup, this trial was conducted amongst inpatients with cardiovascular disease. Since the control group received a form of nursing intervention, we primarily classified the trial as a comparison of two intensities of nursing intervention. But since other studies had usual care groups that may have received advice from other healthcare professionals, we also report the sensitivity of the main analysis results to including it there as a low intensity nursing intervention compared to usual care control.

Hajek 2002 and eight other studies contributed to a second group comparing two interventions involving a nursing intervention. Three of these tested additional components as part of a session; demonstration of carbon monoxide (CO) levels to increase motivation to quit (Sanders 1989b); CO and spirometry feedback (Risser 1990); CO feedback, additional materials and an offer to find a support buddy (Hajek 2002). Three involved additional counselling sessions from a nurse (Alterman 2001; Feeney 2001; Tonnesen 2006). One other study compared two interventions with a usual care control (Miller 1997). The minimal intervention condition included a counselling session and one telephone call after discharge from hospital. In the intensive condition, participants received three additional telephone calls, and those who relapsed were offered further face-to-face meetings, and nicotine replacement therapy if needed. We classified both interventions as intensive in the main meta-analysis, but compared the intensive and minimal conditions in a separate analysis of the effect of additional follow-up. Chouinard 2005 also assessed the effect of additional telephone support as an adjunct to an inpatient counselling session, so is pooled in a subgroup with Miller 1997. We included in the same subgroup a study that tested additional telephone follow-up as a relapse prevention intervention for people who had inpatient counselling (Hasuo 2004).

Four studies (Family Heart 1994; OXCHECK 1994; Campbell 1998; Steptoe 1999) were not included in any meta-analysis and do not have results displayed graphically because their designs did not allow appropriate outcome data to be extracted. The first part of a two-stage intervention study is also included here (Sanders 1989a); the second part (Sanders 1989b) is included in one of the meta-analyses. These five studies are discussed separately in the results.

We determined whether the nurses delivering the intervention were providing it alongside clinical duties that were not smoking related, were working in health promotion roles, or were employed specifically as project nurses. Of the high intensity intervention studies, seven used nurses for whom the intervention was a core component of their role (Hollis 1993; DeBusk 1994; Allen 1996; Carlsson 1997; Terazawa 2001; Quist-Paulsen 2003; Froelicher 2004). In eight studies the intervention was delivered by a nurse specifically employed by the project (Taylor 1990; Rice 1994; Rigotti 1994; Miller 1997; Lewis 1998; Canga 2000; Hennrikus 2005; Hanssen 2007). In three of these, the same nurse provided all the interventions (Rigotti 1994; Lewis 1998; Canga 2000). One study (Kim 2005) employed retired nurses who were trained to provide brief intervention using the "5 As" framework. In only four studies were intensive interventions intended to be delivered by nurses for whom it was not a core task (Lancaster 1999; Bolman 2002; Curry 2003; Sanz-Pozo 2006). Most of the low intensity interventions were delivered by primary care or outpatient clinic nurses. One low intensity inpatient intervention was delivered by a clinical nurse specialist (Nagle 2005).

A brief description of the main components of each intervention is provided in the "Characteristics of Included Studies" table. Follow-up periods for reinforcement and outcome measurements varied across studies, with a tendency for limited reinforcement and shorter follow-up periods in the older studies. All trials had some contact with participants in the first three months of follow-up for restatement of the intervention and/or point prevalence data collection. Five of the studies had less than one year final outcome data collection (Janz 1987; Vetter 1990; Davies 1992; Lewis 1998; Canga 2000). The rest had follow-up at one year or beyond. Outcome used for the meta-analysis was the longest follow-up (six months and beyond). There was no evidence from a subgroup analysis that the differences in length of follow-up explained any of the heterogeneity in study results.

Characteristics of Included Studies	
Study	**Allen 1996**
Methods	Country: USA (Maryland) Recruitment setting: hospital inpatients. Intervention: Prior to hospital discharge and 2 weeks post discharge Randomization: computer assignment with balanced allocation. Allocation concealed
Participants	116 female post CABG patients. 25 smokers amongst them. Smoker defined by use of cigs in 6 months before admission. Nurses provided intervention as part of their core role
Interventions	1. Multiple risk factor intervention, self efficacy programme: 3 sessions with nurse using AHA Active Partnership Program and a follow-up call 2. Usual care (standard discharge teaching and physical therapy instructions) Intensity: high
Outcomes	Abstinence at 12m ("current use") Validation: none
Notes	Data on number of quitters derived from percentages. Likely to include some who stopped prior to intervention.
Allocation concealment	A—Adequate
Study	**Alterman 2001**
Methods	Country: USA Recruitment setting: community volunteers, motivated to quit, cessation clinic Randomization: "urn technique", no description of concealment
Participants	160 smokers (>= 1 pack/day) in relevant arms
Interventions	All received nicotine patch 21mg 8 weeks incl weaning Medium Intensity: 4 sessions over 9 weeks, 15-20 mins, advice & education from nurse practitioner Low Intensity: single 30 min session with nurse, 3 videos
Outcomes	Abstinence at 12m, not defined Validation: CO < 9 ppm, urine cotinine <50 ng/ml
Notes	No control group so not in main analysis. High intensity intervention not included in review. Authors give 77 as ITT denominator for medium intensity group. N randomized of 80 used here.
Allocation concealment	B—Unclear

Characteristics of Included Studies—cont'd	
Study	**Aveyard 2003**
Methods	Country: UK Recruitment setting: 65 general practices, invitation by letter Randomization: questionnaire read optically, allocation by computer using minimization
Participants	831 current smokers in relevant arms, volunteers but not selected by motivation (>80% precontemplators) Intervention from practice nurses with 2 days training in Pro-Change system
Interventions	1. In addition to tailored self help in 2, asked to make appointment to see practice nurse. Single postal reminder if no response. Up to 3 visits, at time of letters. Reinforced use of manual. 2. Self-help manual based on Transtheoretical model, maximum of 3 letters generated by expert system. No face-to-face contact. Intensity: low (Standard S-H control and telephone counselling arms not used in review.)
Outcomes	Abstinence at 12m, self-reported sustained for 6m Validation: saliva cotinine <14.2 ng/ml
Notes	Low uptake of nurse component, 20% attended 1st visit, 6% 2nd and 2% 3rd, also more withdrawals (20%). Nursing arm discontinued part way through recruitment. We use only the Manual (control) group recruited during 4 arm section of trial (3/418, data from author Web site www.publichealth.bham.ac.uk/berg/pdf/Addiction2003.pdf, compared to 15/683 for Manual group across the entire trial). This increases apparent benefit of nurse intervention. A sensitivity analysis did not alter any findings from the meta-analysis.
Allocation concealment	A—Adequate
Study	**Bolman 2002**
Methods	Country: Netherlands Recruitment setting: cardiac ward patients in 11 hospitals Randomization: by hospital, 4/11 selected condition (exclusion of these did not change results)
Participants	789 smokers who had smoked in previous week. 25 deaths, 38 refusals, 64 missing baseline data excluded from analysis denominator. Nurses had 2 hours training and delivered intervention alongside normal duties
Interventions	1. Cardiologist advice on ward and 1st checkup, GP notified, Nurse provided stage of change-based counselling and provided a self-help cessation manual and a brochure on smoking and CHD. Nurse assessed smoking behaviour, addiction, motivation, addressed pros and cons, barriers and self-efficacy, encouraged a quit date. 2. Usual care (nurses on control wards intended to be blind to status) Intensity: High (but not consistently delivered)
Outcomes	Abstinence at 12 m (no smoking since hospital discharge) Validation: none ("bogus pipeline")
Notes	Process analysis indicated some implementation failure. Due to cluster randomization there were baseline differences between intervention and control participants. Raw numbers quit are misleading. Regression analyses suggest no significant effect on continuous abstinence at 12m, so numbers quit in intervention group in meta-analysis adjusted to approximate the odds ratio & confidence interval from regression analysis
Allocation concealment	C—Inadequate

Continued

Characteristics of Included Studies—cont'd	
Study	**Borrelli 2005**
Methods	Country: USA Recruitment/setting: Home healthcare nursing service Randomization: cluster randomized by nurse, method of allocation not described
Participants	278 smoking patients of home healthcare nurses, not selected by motivation 54% F, av. age 57, av. cpd 21 Home healthcare nurses trained to deliver intervention during usual visits
Interventions	1. Motivational enhancement. 3 × 20-30 min sessions during nursing visits. 5 min follow-up call. 2. Standard care control based on 5As model, single 5-15 min session with brief support at subsequent nursing visits, consistent with guidelines. Intensity: High
Outcomes	Abstinence at 12m (no smoking since 6m assessment) Validation: CO < 10 ppm obtained for 60%, informant report also used
Notes	New for 2008/1 update Nurses treated an average of 4 patients (range 1-13). Within-nurse correlation low, so multilevel models not reported. 39 deaths & 5 who quit before intervention excluded from denominators. Included in high intensity subgroup. Control intervention was more than usual care.
Allocation concealment	B—Unclear
Study	**Campbell 1998**
Methods	Country: UK (Scotland) Recruitment setting: GP (Family Practice) Intervention: within 3m of enrolment Randomization: centrally, stratified for age, sex & practice
Participants	Approx 200 smokers amongst 1343 patients with CVD diagnosis
Interventions	1. Multiple risk factor intervention, at least one 45min counselling session plus follow-up visits 2. Usual care
Outcomes	Abstinence at 12 m Validation: none
Notes	Not included in meta-analysis. Data presented as odds ratio for non-smoking
Allocation concealment	A—Adequate
Study	**Canga 2000**
Methods	Country: USA Recruitment: 15 primary care centres, 2 hospitals Intervention: After enrolment Randomization: computer-generated sequence, sealed envelope used but not specified to be numbered & opaque.
Participants	280 smokers with diabetes (incl 16 recent quitters) Intervention delivered by a single research nurse
Interventions	1. Individual counselling based on NCI physician manual: 40 min, follow-up with phone call, 2 further visits, letter. 2. Usual care Intensity: High
Outcomes	Abstinence at 6m for >5 m. Validation: urine cotinine

Characteristics of Included Studies—cont'd

Study	**Canga 2000—cont'd**
Notes	NRT offered to 105 of intervention group but only accepted by 25. No reported use in control group. Quit rate for NRT user subgroup not stated. 6 in int and 4 in control failed/refused validation
Allocation concealment	B—Unclear
Study	**Carlsson 1997**
Methods	Country: Sweden Recruitment setting: Hospital CCU. Intervention at home 4 weeks after discharge. Randomization: method not stated
Participants	168 survivors of AMI. 67 smokers amongst them defined as present smoker by questionnaire. Intervention delivered by a trained nurse rehabilitator
Interventions	1. Multiple risk factor intervention in secondary prevention unit, 1.5 hrs smoking cessation component as part of 9 hours group/individual counselling. 4 visits to nurse during 9m. 2. Usual care, follow-up by general practitioners Intensity: High
Outcomes	Abstinence at 12m Validation: none
Notes	
Allocation concealment	B—Unclear
Study	**Chouinard 2005**
Methods	Country: Canada Recruitment setting: Inpatients with cardiovascular disease (MI, angina, CHF) or PVD, unselected by motivation Randomization: In blocks of 3-6, sealed envelope
Participants	168 past-month smokers. Av. age 56 Intervention delivered by a research nurse
Interventions	1. Counselling by research nurse (1x, 10-60 mins, av. 40 min, based on Transtheoretical Model, included component to enhance social support from a significant family member), 23% used pharmacotherapy. 2. As 1, plus telephone follow-up, 6 calls over 2m post-discharge, 29% used pharmacotherapy 3. Control: cessation advice, 11% used pharmacotherapy.
Outcomes	Abstinence at 6m (sustained at 2m & 6m) Validation: Urine cotinine or CO
Notes	New for 2008/1 update Two interventions combined versus control in high intensity subgroup. 1 versus 2 used in higher versus lower comparison. Four deaths (3 in Grp 1., 1 in Grp 2.) and 3 not meeting follow-up criteria excluded from MA denominators. Other losses to follow-up included.
Allocation concealment	A—Adequate

Continued

Characteristics of Included Studies—cont'd

Study	**Curry 2003**
Methods	Country: USA Recruitment setting: mothers attending 4 paediatric clinics, unselected by motivation Randomization: selection of coloured ping-pong ball
Participants	303 women (any smoking), 23% in precontemplation av age 33, av cpd 12 Intervention delivered either by clinic nurses or a study interventionist. Nurses received 8 hours individual training in motivational interviewing
Interventions	1. Clinician advice based on 5A's (1-5mins), Self-help materials targeted for mothers. Asked to meet a nurse or health educator who provided motivational interviewing during visit. Up to 3 phone calls over 3m. 2. No intervention Intensity: High (but implementation incomplete)
Outcomes	Abstinence at 12 m (Sustained at 3m & 12 m. PP also reported) Validation: CO < 10 ppm, only for women followed up in person. Tabulated rates based on self-report
Notes	Intervention included physician advice. Not all participants received intervention. Based on counsellor records, 74% received face-to-face intervention, average length 13 mins, and 78% had at least 1 phone call. Nurses provided intervention as part of their normal duties.
Allocation concealment	C—Inadequate
Study	**Davies 1992**
Methods	Country: Canada Recruitment setting: healthy adult community-based volunteers Randomization: method not stated. Each participating nurse visited a control patient first, then received training.
Participants	307 essentially healthy adult smokers of at least 5 cpd
Interventions	1. "Time To Quit" programme delivered by a student nurse trained in programme 2. Visit by same student nurse prior to receiving training Intensity: Low
Outcomes	Abstinence at 9m Validation: Cotinine < 100 ng/ML
Notes	Effect of training and manuals on nurse intervention
Allocation concealment	B—Unclear
Study	**DeBusk 1994**
Methods	Country: USA (California) Recruitment setting: inpatients with AMI at 5 hospitals Randomization: centralized computer allocation. Both smokers and non-smokers randomized.
Participants	131/293 intervention and 121/292 control patients were smokers as defined by any use of tobacco in 6m before admission. Nurses provided intervention as part of their core role
Interventions	1. Multiple risk factor intervention case-management system with smoking cessation, nutritional counselling, lipid lowering therapy and exercise therapy. Smoking cessation: 2 min physician then nurse counselling with repeated telephone follow-ups x8. NRT offered only to highly addicted patients who relapsed post-discharge. 2. Usual care including physician counselling. Group cessation programmes available for US$50 (2% enrolled)
Outcomes	Abstinence at 1yr (PP) Validation: plasma cotinine <10 ng/mL, or 11-15 ng/mL with expired CO < 10 ppm.

Characteristics of Included Studies—cont'd

Study	**DeBusk 1994—cont'd**
Notes	Number of quitters derived from smoking cessation rates based on number of baseline smokers. Author contacted for smoker drop-out rates.
Allocation concealment	A—Adequate
Study	**Family Heart 1994**
Methods	Country: UK Recruitment setting: Male general practice (family practice) patients aged 40-59 and partners, identified by household Randomization: by practice (one of a pair in each of 14 towns), and within intervention practices by individuals to screening/ intervention or 1 year screening
Participants	7460 male and 5012 female medical practice patients who reported "smoking" on a questionnaire.
Interventions	1. Screening for cardiovascular risk factors, risk-related lifestyle intervention during a single 1.5 hr visit. 2. Delayed screening (at 1 year) for families in the same practice (internal control) and the paired practice (external control)
Outcomes	Smoking prevalence at 1yr Validation: CO
Notes	Not included in meta-analysis because outcome not directly comparable with cessation studies. Smoking prevalence was lower in the intervention subjects at 1yr than in either internal or external practice controls. But non-returners in the intervention group had a higher smoking prevalence at baseline than returners.
Allocation concealment	B—Unclear
Study	**Feeney 2001**
Methods	Country: Australia Recruitment/setting: CCU, single hospital Randomization: numbered sealed envelopes (but admin error led to more in control)
Participants	198 smokers in previous week, unselected for motivation. 9 deaths (4/5) excluded from denominator in analysis
Interventions	1. Stanford Heart Attack Staying Free programme. Review by Alcohol & Drug Assessment Unit (ADAU) physician. Self-help manual, high relapse risk patients counselled on coping strategies, audiotapes. On discharge ADAU nurse contacted weekly for 4 weeks & 2,3,12 m. 2. Verbal and written didactic advice, video, review by ADAU nurse, supportive counselling and follow-up offered at 3,6,12 m
Outcomes	Abstinence at 12m, continuous and validated at 1 m & 3 m. Validation: urine cotinine <400 ng/ml at each ADAU clinic visit
Notes	Both intervention and control included a nursing component so not in main analysis. Only participants who attended basic ADAU follow-up programme assessed, so large number of drop-outs. More drop-outs in group 2 (79%) than group 1 (51%), so treating drop-outs as smokers may overestimate treatment effect.
Allocation concealment	A—Adequate

Continued

Characteristics of Included Studies—cont'd	
Study	**Froelicher 2004**
Methods	Country: USA Recruitment/setting: Inpatients with CVD or PVD admitted to 10 hospitals Randomization: permuted blocks stratified by hospital
Participants	277 female current smokers or recent quitters (smoked in month before admission), willing to make serious quit attempt at discharge. Av. age 61, av. cpd 18-19 Intervention delivered by trained research nurses
Interventions	1. As usual care + nurse-managed cessation & relapse prevention: 30-45 min individual counselling predischarge with multimedia materials. Up to 5 phone calls (5-10 min) at 2, 7, 21, 28, 90 days. Relapsers offered additional session. 2. Usual care; brief physician counselling, Self-help pamphlet, list of resources Patch or gum offered to selected women after discharge who had relapsed and wanted to try to quit (pharmacotherapy used by 20% of intervention and 23% of control group). Intensity: High
Outcomes	Abstinence at 12m (7-day PP). (Also followed at 24m, 30m but validation not attempted) Validation: Saliva cotinine <14 ng/ml or family/friend verification
Notes	New for 2008/1 update 11 deaths at 12m, excluded from cessation denominators. 73% of participants reached at all 4 follow-ups
Allocation concealment	A—Adequate
Study	**Hajek 2002**
Methods	Country: UK Recruitment/setting: inpatients with MI or for CABG at 17 hospitals Randomization: serially numbered opaque sealed envelopes
Participants	540 smokers or recent quitters (26%) who had not smoked in hospital & motivated to quit. 26 deaths, 9 moved address excluded from denominator in analysis Intervention delivered by nurses alongside other duties
Interventions	1. As control, +CO reading, booklet on smoking & cardiac recovery, written quiz, offer to find support buddy, commitment, reminder in notes. Implemented by cardiac nurses during routine work, est time 20mins. 2. Verbal advice, Smoking and Your Heart booklet
Outcomes	Abstinence at 12m, sustained (no more than 5 cigs since enrolment & 7day PP) Validation: saliva cotinine <20 ng/ml (CO used at 6 week follow-up and for visits at 12m)
Notes	Control meets criteria for a low intensity intervention so not included in comparison 1, but included there and in inpatient CVDcategory in sensitivity analyses (Comparisons 4 & 5).
Allocation concealment	A—Adequate
Study	**Hanssen 2007**
Methods	Country: Norway Recruitment/setting: inpatients with AMI Randomization: Computer-generated list, sequence in sealed opaque envelopes but not stated to be numbered. Fewer control group participants raises possibility of selection bias so not classified as A
Participants	133 daily smokers amongst 288 participants. Not selected by motivation. Demographics not given for smoking subgroup Intervention delivered by research nurses

Characteristics of Included Studies—cont'd	
Study	**Hanssen 2007—cont'd**
Interventions	1. Structured but individualized telephone support addressing lifestyle issues including smoking, diet and exercise. Nurse-initiated calls at 1, 2, 3, 4, 6, 8, 12, 24 weeks post-discharge. Smoking not explicitly addressed at each call. Reactive phone support line available 6 hrs/week 2. Usual care; outpatient visit at 6-8 weeks and primary care follow-up Intensity: High
Outcomes	Abstinence at 6m (not defined). Primary trial outcome was health-related quality of life Validation: none
Notes	New for 2008/1 Smoking was part of a multicomponent intervention.
Allocation concealment	A—Adequate
Study	**Hasuo 2004**
Methods	Country: Japan Recruitment: Inpatients (all diagnoses) Randomization: By hospital clerk using computer programme; stratified by smoking status, FTND, and self efficacy
Participants	120 current smokers or recent quitters (smoked in past month) who intended to be quit on day of discharge Diagnoses include cancer (n = 37), cardiac (n = 57)
Interventions	1. Intervention: nurse counselling (3 × 20min sessions). Telephone follow-up with focus on relapse prevention at 7, 21, 42 days (5 min/call) 2. Control: Same inpatient counselling but no follow-up contact
Outcomes	Abstinence at 12m (not defined). Validation: urinary cotinine
Notes	New for 2008/1 Both groups included inpatient counselling so not used in main comparison; effect of telephone follow-up. Intervention was intended to prevent relapse. MA denominators exclude 6 deaths, but include 8 who were still smoking on day of discharge. This gives marginally larger relative effect.
Allocation concealment	A—Adequate
Study	**Hennrikus 2005**
Methods	Country: USA Recruitment/setting: Inpatients (all diagnoses) admitted to 4 hospitals Selected: Invited to participate. Randomization: by research assistant from a list of randomly ordered assignments, but blinding at time of enrolment not specified
Participants	2095 current smokers (smoked in past week and considered self to be regular smoker for at least a month in past year) Not selected by motivation; approx 10% in each group confident they could quit. Av. age 47 Intervention delivered by research nurses
Interventions	1. Brief advice: as control, plus labels in records to prompt advice from nurses and physicians. 2. Brief advice and counselling: As 1. plus 1 bedside (or phone) session using motivational interviewing and relapse prevention approaches and 3 to 6 calls (2-3 days, 1 wk, 2-3 wk, 1m, 6m) 3. Control: modified usual care: smoking cessation booklet in hospital (not used in meta-analysis) Intensity: High Pharmacotherapy not offered.

Continued

Characteristics of Included Studies—cont'd	
Study	**Hennrikus 2005—cont'd**
Outcomes	Abstinence at 12m (7-day PP). Validation: saliva cotinine <15 ng/ml
Notes	New for 2008/1 update Brief advice & counselling regarded as nurse intervention, compared to Brief advice. Including Usual Care in control as well would marginally increase Relative Risk but not change conclusion of no effect. High and differential levels of refusal to provide validation and of misreporting 78 deaths and ineligible for follow-up excluded from denominators
Allocation concealment	B—Unclear
Study	**Hilberink 2005**
Methods	Country: Netherlands Recruitment/setting: Patients with COPD identified by prescription & diagnosis codes in 43 general practices Randomization: cluster randomized by practice. 5/48 dropped out after randomization, leading to an imbalance of numbers of participants
Participants	392 current smokers with COPD. Not selected for motivation, ~50% willing to quit within 6m, different between groups 50% F, av. age 59 Parts of intervention delivered by practice nurses alongside other duties
Interventions	1. SMOCC intervention: booklet for COPD population & video. Stage-based intervention: Precontemplators given information on advantages of quitting. Contemplators received self-efficacy enhancing intervention, discussion of barriers, info on NRT if dependent & further visit at 2 weeks. Preparers had visit to GP to schedule quit date & max 2 follow-ups, & max 3 phone calls from practice nurse/assistant. 2. Usual care Intensity: High
Outcomes	Abstinence at 6m (PP) Validation: none (people told their reports would be validated)
Notes	New for 2008/1 update Only the telephone follow-up for people in preparation stage was explicitly provided by a nurse. Paper notes that practices differed in amount of tasks delegated to practice nurses. Paper reports use of multilevel modelling. No adjustment to crude Relative Risk need for clustering. Denominators exclude 2 deaths and those for whom follow-up not attempted
Allocation concealment	C—Inadequate
Study	**Hollis 1993**
Methods	Country: USA (Portland, OR) Recruitment: Internal medicine/family clinics Randomization: By 2 random digits in health record number. Physicians blind to assignment.
Participants	2691 internal medicine/family clinic adults who reported being a smoker on a questionnaire.
Interventions	1. Brief physician advice (30 sec and pamphlet from nurse) 2. Brief physician message plus nurse who promoted self quit attempts—advice, CO feedback, 10 min video & manual (1 of 3 types) + follow-up call & materials 3. Brief physician advice plus nurse-promoted group programme—advice, CO, + video-ask to join group with schedule, coupon, etc., follow-up calls 4. Brief physician advice, and nurse-offered choice between self-directed and group-assisted quit—shown both types of materials. Intensity: High

Characteristics of Included Studies—cont'd	
Study	**Hollis 1993—cont'd**
Outcomes	Abstinence at 1 yr (2 PP) Validation: Saliva cotinine at 12 m
Notes	All three nurse-mediated interventions compared with 1. Saliva samples only obtained for approx half of reported quitters. Compliance and confirmation rates did not differ between groups.
Allocation concealment	C—Inadequate
Study	**Janz 1987**
Methods	Country: USA (Michigan) Recruitment setting: OP Dept Med Clinic (R.A.) Randomization: Half-day clinics assigned to treatment status.
Participants	Smokers (>=5 cpd) attending clinics
Interventions	1. Physician discussed personal susceptibility, self efficacy & concern, trained nurse counselled on problems and strategies. 2. As 1, and self-help manual "Step-by-Step Quit Kit". + 1 telephone call 3. Usual Care control (from physicians not involved in study) Intensity: Low
Outcomes	Abstinence at 6m (self-report by telephone) Validation: none
Notes	1 & 2 vs 3. Interventions included both physician and nurse components. Data derived from graphs of percentages. Original data sought but not available.
Allocation concealment	C—Inadequate
Study	**Kim 2005**
Methods	Country: South Korea Recruitment/setting: Internal medicine outpatient department Randomization: 12 allocation strata. Assignments in sealed opaque envelopes.
Participants	401 daily smokers, 65% willing to quit within 1 m 92% M, av. age 52
Interventions	Test of 5As approach recommended by US AHCPR guideline. All participants Asked about smoking status & Advised to quit by physicians. Counsellors (retired nurses trained in cessation) Assessed willingness to quit, and enrolled & randomized patients. 1. Intervention: Counsellors provided Assist and Arrange components to participants willing to quit within 1m; set quit date, provided Self-help materials, supplied cigarette substitute. Culturally specific for Koreans. Other participants given 4Rs 2. Control: Counsellors told participants to quit without further assistance.
Outcomes	Abstinence at 5m Validation: CO <= 7 ppm
Notes	New for 2008/1 update Marginal to include because 5m follow-up and counsellors were retired nurses
Allocation concealment	A—Adequate

Continued

Characteristics of Included Studies—cont'd	
Study	**Lancaster 1999**
Methods	Country: UK Recruitment setting: General practice, recruitment during a visit or by letter. Smokers who completed a questionnaire about smoking habits. Randomization: computer-generated allocation in sealed envelopes
Participants	497 smokers (av. cpd 17)
Interventions	1. Physician advice (face-to-face or in a letter) and a leaflet 2. As 1, plus invitation to contact a trained practice nurse for more intensive tailored counselling. Up to 5 follow-up visits offered.
Outcomes	Abstinence at 12m (sustained at 3 m & 12 m) Validation: saliva cotinine at 3m & 12m
Notes	2 vs 1. Only 30% took up offer of extended counselling. Included in high intensity subgroup based on intended intervention but sensitivity analysis for effect of treating as low intensity
Allocation concealment	A—Adequate
Study	**Lewis 1998**
Methods	Country: USA Recruitment setting: hospital inpatients (excluding some cardiac conditions) Randomization: predetermined computer-generated code
Participants	185 hospitalized adults; self-reported "regular use" for at least one year. Counselling intervention delivered by research nurse
Interventions	1. Minimal care (MC): motivational message from physician to quit plus pamphlet 2. Counselling and nicotine patch (CAP). 3. Counselling and placebo patch (CPP). In addition groups 2 & 3 received a motivational message & instructions on patch use from physician, 4 sessions of telephone counselling by nurse based on cognitive behavioural therapy and motivational interviewing. Intensity: high
Outcomes	Abstinence at 6m (7 day PP) Validation: CO <= 10ppm
Notes	Compared 3 vs 1; Nurse counselling and placebo patch compared to minimal care to avoid confounding with effect of NRT.
Allocation concealment	A—Adequate
Study	**Miller 1997**
Methods	Country: USA (California) Recruitment setting: hospital inpatients Randomization: sealed envelopes
Participants	1942 hospitalized smokers (any tobacco use in week prior to admission) Counselling delivered by a research nurse
Interventions	1. Intensive: 30min inpatient counselling, video, workbook, relaxation tape + 4 phone calls after discharge 2. Minimal: 30min counselling etc. + 1 phone call 3. Usual care Intensity: High
Outcomes	Abstinence at 12m, (PP, sustained abstinence also reported, but not by disease subgroup) Validation: plasma cotinine or family member collaboration at 12m

Characteristics of Included Studies—cont'd	
Study	**Miller 1997—cont'd**
Notes	1 + 2 vs 3 in main analysis—classifying both interventions as high intensity. Cardiovascular and other diagnoses separated in analysis by setting. 1 vs 2 in analysis of effect of additional telephone contact (sustained abstinence).
Allocation concealment	A—Adequate
Study	**Nagle 2005**
Methods	Country: Australia Recruitment/setting: Inpatients (all diagnoses) admitted to 1 teaching hospital (excluding intensive care units), invited to participate. Randomization: stratified by smoking status in past month, blocks of 20, using handheld computer with random number programme
Participants	1422 current smokers or quitters (including 331 who had quit in past 12m). Not selected by motivation. 40% male in intervention group, 33% male in controls Main part of intervention delivered by specialist
Interventions	1. Assessment and identification of smokers with the Smoking Cessation Clinical Pathway as chart reminder for ward nurses, Clinical Nurse Specialist provided 2 brief counselling sessions, offer of NRT (3% provided), discharge letter. 2. Usual care & assessment of smoking status, no standardized clinical assessment. Intensity: Low (borderline)
Outcomes	Abstinence at 12m (7-day validated PP, continuous self-reported abstinence also given) Validation: Saliva cotinine <=15 ng/ml.
Notes	New for 2008/1 update Study includes recent quitters; no difference in intervention effect. 85% of recent smokers received at least 1 counselling session, 38% received 2. 28 deaths at 12m excluded from denominator
Allocation concealment	A—Adequate
Study	**Nebot 1992**
Methods	Country: Spain Recruitment: Primary Care Centre (patients not selected for motivation to quit) Randomization: Primary care teams randomized to perform 3 interventions in successive weeks
Participants	425 smokers (at least 1 cpd in past week)
Interventions	1. Physician advice 2. Physician advice & nicotine gum 3. Nurse counselling (up to 15 mins) Intensity: Low All received booklet and offer of follow-up visit or call.
Outcomes	Abstinence at 12m (sustained at 2m & 12m) Validation: 1/4 validated by expired CO at 2m.
Notes	3 vs 1
Allocation concealment	C—Inadequate
Study	**OXCHECK 1994**
Methods	Country: UK Recruitment: patients aged 35-64 in 5 urban general practices (family practice) who returned a baseline questionnaire Randomization: by household, to health checks in one of 4 years

Continued

Characteristics of Included Studies—cont'd	
Study	**OXCHECK 1994—cont'd**
Participants	11,090 general practice patients
Interventions	1. Health check and risk factor counselling 2. Delayed intervention
Outcomes	Smoking prevalence, and reported quitting in previous year
Notes	Not included in meta-analysis because outcome not directly comparable with cessation studies. When all intervention patients (including non-attenders) are compared to controls there was no significant difference in the proportion who had stopped smoking in previous year.
Allocation concealment	B—Unclear
Study	**Quist-Paulsen 2003**
Methods	Country: Norway Recruitment/setting: Inpatients admitted to cardiac ward of 1 general hospital, invited to participate Randomization: Serially numbered sealed envelopes
Participants	240 current smokers (smoked daily before symptoms began). Av. 15 cpd Intervention delivered by 3 cardiac nurses
Interventions	1. Intervention: Usual care plus 1-2 sessions with nurse using booklet focusing on fear arousal and relapse prevention. 5 telephone follow-ups at 2, 7, 21 days, 3m, 5m. Clinic visit to nurse at 6wks. Gum or patch encouraged for subjects with strong urges to smoke in hospital. 2. Control: usual care (advice to quit + booklet) Intensity: High
Outcomes	Abstinence at 12m (PP) Validation: urine cotinine <2.0 mmol/mol creatinine
Notes	New for 2008/1 update. Included in CVD subcategory 5 deaths and 2 people who changed address at 12m excluded from denominators.
Allocation concealment	A—Adequate
Study	**Ratner 2004**
Methods	Country: Canada Recruitment: Patients having presurgical assessment Method of randomization: sealed envelope, computer-generated assignment
Participants	237 smokers (past 7 days) awaiting elective surgery 52% female Av. 12 cpd
Interventions	1. Pre-admission clinic 15 min counselling from trained research nurse, materials, nicotine gum, quit kit, hotline number. Post-operative counselling in hospital. 9 follow-up calls over 16 wks. 2. Usual care Intensity: High
Outcomes	Abstinence at 12m (PP) Validation: urine cotinine (NicoMeter)
Notes	New for 2008/1 update 9 deaths at 12 m excluded from denominators. Included in hospitalized patient subgroup for Comparison 2 although the initial intervention delivered pre-admission
Allocation concealment	A—Adequate

Characteristics of Included Studies—cont'd

Study	**Rice 1994**
Methods	Country: USA (Michigan) Recruitment: Previously hospitalized; self-referral or by provider Randomization: table of random numbers
Participants	255 smokers (>=10 cpd) with CVD
Interventions	1. Smokeless (R) programme, individual delivery by nurse, 5 sessions 2. Same programme, 5 group sessions 3. Same programme, written self-help format 4. Usual care control Intensity: High
Outcomes	Abstinence at 12m. Validation: saliva thiocyanate measured, but self-report used as outcome.
Notes	1 + 2 + 3 vs 4
Allocation concealment	B—Unclear
Study	**Rigotti 1994**
Methods	Country: USA (Boston) Setting/Recruitment: Cardiac surgery unit Randomization: method not described
Participants	87 smokers (1+ pack of cigs in past 6 m) scheduled for CABG.
Interventions	1. 3 sessions behavioural model with video tape and face-to-face counselling by registered nurse 2. Usual care control Intensity: High
Outcomes	Sustained abstinence at 12 m Validation: saliva cotinine <20 ng/mL
Notes	Abstinence rates include some smokers who had quit prior to surgery
Allocation concealment	B—Unclear
Study	**Risser 1990**
Methods	Country: USA Setting: Nurse-staffed health promotion clinic Randomization: method not described
Participants	90 smokers attending health promotion clinic for annual visit
Interventions	1. 50min session, self-help materials, offer of training and counselling program. 2. as 1, plus 10min personalized motivational intervention with spirometry, CO measurement and discussion of symptoms.
Outcomes	Abstinence at 1yr (PP) Validation: expired CO
Notes	Not in main comparison: effect of additional components. No group without intervention. (No true control group.)
Allocation concealment	B—Unclear
Study	**Sanders 1989a**
Methods	Country: UK Setting: Primary care clinics (11) Randomization: by day of week, randomized across weeks and practices.
Participants	4210 primary care clinic attenders identified by questionnaire as smokers

Continued

Characteristics of Included Studies—cont'd	
Study	**Sanders 1989a—cont'd**
Interventions	1. Asked by doctor (following advice to quit) to make appointment with nurse for health check. Advice, discussion, leaflet and offer of follow-up by nursing 2. Usual care control Intensity: Low
Outcomes	Sustained abstinence at 12m (self-report of not smoking at 1m and 12m and gave date on which they last smoked as before the 1m follow-up) Validation: urine cotinine
Notes	Only a sample of usual care group followed up so not appropriate to use data in main meta-analysis. A significant effect of the intervention was apparent only for the sustained cessation outcome. 12m PP abstinence rates were 11.2% for intervention, 10% for control (NS).
Allocation concealment	C—Inadequate
Study	**Sanders 1989b**
Methods	Country: UK Setting: Primary care clinics (11) Randomization: method not described
Participants	751 smokers who attended a health check (having been randomly allocated to an intervention offering a health check—see Sanders 1989a)
Interventions	1. Health check from a practice nurse; advice, leaflet and offer of follow-up 2. As 1, with demonstration of expired CO levels.
Outcomes	Sustained abstinence at 1 yr (self report of not smoking at 1m and 12m and who gave date on which they last smoked as before the 1m follow-up) Validation: urine cotinine in a sample of participants indicated a relatively high deception rate.
Notes	2 vs 1 for effect of CO demonstration as an adjunct to nurse advice. This was part of same study as Sanders 1989a, and randomized a subgroup of participants in the main study
Allocation concealment	B—Unclear
Study	**Sanz-Pozo 2006**
Methods	Country: Spain Setting: Primary care clinic Randomization: method not described
Participants	125 daily smokers attending clinic, motivated to make a quit attempt but not interested in using pharmacotherapy Intervention 52% F, Control 62% F, av. age ~40, av. cpd 19
Interventions	1. Brief advice from doctor at recruitment, appointment with clinic nurse 7 days before TQD, on TQD, 1wk, 1 m, 2 m, 3 m. 2. Brief advice only. No pharmacotherapy
Outcomes	Sustained abstinence at 24 m (from 12 m) Validation: CO < 8 ppm
Notes	New for 2008/1 Control group rates also higher at 12 m follow-up. Some baseline differences but logistic regression did not alter conclusion of no effect
Allocation concealment	B—Unclear

Characteristics of Included Studies—cont'd	
Study	**Steptoe 1999**
Methods	Country: UK Setting: Primary care clinics (20) Randomization: cluster randomized by practice
Participants	404 smokers (from total of 883 patients with modifiable CVD risk factors)
Interventions	1. Behavioural counselling using stages of change approach. 2-3 20min sessions + 1-2 phone contacts. NRT used if appropriate. 2. Usual care
Outcomes	Sustained abstinence at 12 m (4 m & 12 m) Validation: saliva cotinine
Notes	Not included in meta-analysis. Used practice-based analysis. Differential drop-out rates for smokers in intervention & control groups.
Allocation concealment	B—Unclear
Study	**Taylor 1990**
Methods	Country: USA (California) Recruitment setting: Hospital (patients with AMI) Randomization: Random numbers in sealed envelopes
Participants	173 smokers following AMI. Smoker defined as any use of tobacco.
Interventions	1. Nurse counselling on self efficacy, benefits and risks, + manual coping with high risk situations. Further telephone counselling as needed up to 6 m. 2. Usual care control Intensity: High
Outcomes	Abstinence at 12m Validation: serum thiocyanate <110 nmol/L, expired CO < 10 ppm
Notes	Nurses averaged 3.5 hours/patient including phone contact Slightly higher loss to follow-up in control group. Nicotine gum was prescribed to 5 patients.
Allocation concealment	A—Adequate
Study	**Terazawa 2001**
Methods	Country: Japan Recruitment setting: Workplace annual health check Randomization: by employee ID number. Assigned prior to contact
Participants	228 male smokers, Av age 39, av cpd 23
Interventions	1. 15-20min stage-matched counselling by trained nurses. 4 follow-up calls for those willing to set a quit date. 1 wk after intervention, 3-4 days. 1m, 3m after cessation 2. Usual care
Outcomes	Sustained abstinence at 12 m (>6 m, validated at 6 m & 12 m) Validation: CO, urine
Notes	25 from intervention group set quit date. More intervention group in preparation/contemplation II subgroups at baseline; 17 vs 7.
Allocation concealment	A—Adequate
Study	**Tonnesen 1996**
Methods	Country: Denmark Recruitment setting: outpatient chest clinic Randomization: method not described

Continued

Characteristics of Included Studies—cont'd	
Study	**Tonnesen 1996—cont'd**
Participants	507 smokers of <10 cpd or of >10 cpd who had refused a trial of nicotine replacement, age 20-70 yrs Intervention delivered by clinic nurses given 8hr training and 3 problem-solving meetings
Interventions	1. Motivational approach, 5 min of benefits/risks, brochures on hazards and how to quit. 4-6 wks letter sent 2. Control—questionnaire and CO measurement. No advice to stop smoking. Intensity: Low
Outcomes	Sustained abstinence at 1yr (stopped during intervention and no reported smoking during year) Validation: CO <10 ppm
Notes	
Allocation concealment	B—Unclear
Study	**Tonnesen 2006**
Methods	Country: Denmark Recruitment setting: 7 outpatient chest clinics Randomization: by block randomization list at each centre. Double blind but allocation concealment not specifically described
Participants	370 smokers of >1 cpd with COPD 52% F, av. age 61, av. cpd 20
Interventions	Factorial trial. Nicotine sublingual tablet and placebo arms collapsed in MA 1. High support: 7 × 20-30min clinic visits (0, 2, 4, 8, 12wks, 6m, 12m) & 5 × 10min phone calls (1, 6, 10 wks. 4.5 m. 9 m), total contact time 4.5 h. 2. Low support: 4 clinic visits (0, 2 wks, 6 m, 12 m) & 6 phone calls (1, 4, 6, 9, 12 wks, 9 m), total time 2.5 hrs
Outcomes	Sustained abstinence at 12m (validated at all visits from wk 2, PP also reported) Validation: CO < 10 ppm
Notes	New for 2008/1 update Not in main comparison; compares different intensities of nurse counselling
Allocation concealment	B—Unclear
Study	**Vetter 1990**
Methods	Country: UK (Wales) Recruitment setting: general practice (family practice) Randomization: method not described
Participants	226 smokers aged 60+ in general practice who completed a health questionnaire. Unselected by motivation to quit.
Interventions	1. Letter asking patient to visit doctor who advised on importance of stopping smoking, opportunity to see practice nurse who gave advice on lifestyle factors concentrating on quitting smoking 2. No contact, completed questionnaire only Intensity: Low
Outcomes	Abstinence at 6m (PP) Validation: expired CO (cut off point not stated)
Notes	Intervention included nursing and physician advice
Allocation concealment	B—Unclear

AHCPR = Agency for Health Care Policy and Research; CABG = coronary artery bypass graft; CCU = coronary care unit; CHD = coronary heart disease; CHF = congestive heart failure; CO = carbon monoxide; COPD = chronic obstructive pulmonary disease; cpd = cigarettes per day; CVD = cardiovascular disease; FTND: Fagerstrom Test for Nicotine Dependence; ITT = intention-to-treat; m = month(s); (A)MI = (Acute) Myocardial Infarction; NRT = nicotine replacement therapy; NS: not statistically significant; PP = point prevalence; PVD = peripheral vascular disease; SMOCC = smoking cessation for patients with COPD in general practice; TQD = target quit date

Characteristics of Excluded Studies	
Study	**Reason for Exclusion**
Andrews 2007	Cluster-randomized trial with only 2 community clusters & baseline differences between participants. Nurse-led counselling confounded with NRT availability and personal contact from a community health worker for the duration of the trial.
Browning 2000	Not a randomized trial, uses historical control
Carlsson 1998	Describes 5 studies, only 1 reporting smoking cessation is included in review separately (Carlsson 1997).
Chan 2005	Follow-up less than 6m.
Fletcher 1987	Number of quitters after 6m not stated. (Total of 20 participants)
Galvin 2001	Only 3m follow-up. (Total of 42 participants)
Griebel 1998	Maximum follow-up was 6 wks post-hospital discharge.
Haddock 1997	No long-term follow-up. Randomization unclear.
Hall 2007	Follow-up less than 6m
Jelley 1995	Not RCT. Control and intervention ran sequentially.
Johnson 1999	Not RCT. No equivalent study groups, intervention allocated according to cardiac unit of admission.
Johnson 2000	Population and intervention not within scope. Recruited women who had stopped smoking during pregnancy for a relapse prevention intervention.
Kendrick 1995	Intervention in pregnant smokers. See review by Lumley et al 2004.
Lifrak 1997	Four advice sessions with a nurse practitioner compared with a more intensive intervention of 16 weekly therapy sessions. All also received nicotine patch therapy.
McHugh 2001	Multiple risk factor intervention with shared care. Cannot evaluate effect of nursing.
O'Connor 1992	Intervention in pregnant smokers. See review by Lumley et al 2004.
Pozen 1977	Intervention in post-MI patients. Only 1m follow-up, and number of smokers at baseline not described.
Reeve 2000	Follow-up less than 6m.
Reid 2003	Stepped care intervention from nurse counsellor confounded with nicotine patch therapy (no evidence of effect of the combination).
Rigotti 1997	Intervention not given by a nurse.
Stanislaw 1994	Follow-up less than 6m.
Sun 2000	Follow-up less than 6m.
Wadland 1999	Not randomized. The 2 groups were recruited by different means and given different interventions, both of which included telephone counselling by nurses or counsellors
Wadland 2001	Follow-up less than 6m (90 days). Nurses and counsellors provided telephone-based intervention.
Wewers 1994	Follow-up less than 6m.
Woollard 1995	No data presented on number of smokers or quitting.
van Elderen 1994	Multicomponent intervention, smoking cessation element not clear.

METHODOLOGICAL QUALITY

Of the 31 studies contributing to the primary meta-analysis, we graded 15 (48%) as A for reporting a randomization and allocation concealment process likely to avoid selection bias. The majority employed some form of computer-generated allocation system. Six studies (20%) were classified as potentially inadequate (graded C). In one of these studies the last two digits on the patient record was used for assignment (Hollis 1993), and in a second study participants drew a coloured ball from a bag (Curry 2003). Four studies allocated interventions by provider rather than by individual participant: by clinic session (Janz 1987); by intervention teams (Nebot 1992); by primary care clinic (Hilberink 2005) and by hospital (Bolman 2002). In Hilberink 2005 some clinics dropped out after randomization due to problems identifying and recruiting participants. This raised the possibility of selection bias, and it was noted that the distribution of participants' stage of change differed between the intervention and control groups. In Bolman 2002, four of eleven hospitals selected their condition, although seven were randomly allocated. There were also baseline differences among smokers, and although raw data suggested a benefit for the intervention, a logistic regression analysis did not detect a significant effect. In order to include this study in the meta-analysis we adjusted the number of quitters in the intervention group to match the odds ratio derived from the logistic regression. Excluding the study completely did not change the pooled effect. The remaining ten studies (40%) did not specify exactly how random assignment and allocation concealment were achieved (graded B). A sensitivity analysis including only the results of studies graded A did not alter the main conclusions. Of the five studies not used in any meta-analysis one was adequate (Campbell 1998), three were unclear (Family Heart 1994; OXCHECK 1994; Steptoe 1999), and one was inadequate (Sanders 1989a).

Definitions of abstinence ranged from single point prevalence to sustained abstinence (multiple point prevalence with self-report of no slips or relapses). In one study (Miller 1997) we used validated abstinence at one year rather than continuous self-reported abstinence because only the former outcome was reported for disease diagnosis subgroups. Validation of smoking behaviour using biochemical analysis of body fluids (e.g., cotinine or thiocyanate) was reported in 15 (47%) of the thirty-one studies in the primary meta-analysis. Expired carbon monoxide (CO) was used for validation in another six (24%) of the trials. One study tested CO levels only amongst people followed up in person (Curry 2003). Five others used some validation but did not report rates based on biochemical validation of every self-reported quitter (Nebot 1992; Miller 1997; Froelicher 2004; Borrelli 2005; Rice 1994). Six studies (23%) did not use any biochemical validation and relied on self-reported smoking cessation at a single follow-up (Janz 1987; Allen 1996; Carlsson 1997; Bolman 2002; Hilberink 2005; Hanssen 2007) though two of these warned participants that samples might be requested for testing (i.e., "bogus pipeline"). Where both self-reported and validated quitting were reported, the level of misreporting or failure to provide a sample is typically similar across intervention and control groups. One recent study, however, reported differential validation failure rates so that the significant differences based on self-report were not found for validated abstinence (Hennrikus 2005).

Almost all the trials used convenience rather than randomly selected samples. Only one of the studies (Vetter 1990) did not let participants know initially that they were going to be part of a smoking cessation study. In most of the research, the basis for sample size was not specified *a priori,* nor was a retrospective power analysis conducted. Most studies did not report "refusal to participate" rates. Although a few studies did not report drop-out rates, most tried to account for all participants in their sample and treated "non-reporters" as continuing smokers. Drop-out rates, both before and after informed consent, varied considerably across studies. In one study 79% of usual care participants were not followed up (Feeney 2001).

RESULTS

Effects of Intervention versus Control/Usual Care

Smokers offered advice by a nursing professional had an increased likelihood of quitting compared to smokers without intervention, but there was evidence of moderate statistical heterogeneity between the results of the 31 studies contributing to this comparison ($I^2 = 54\%$). Heterogeneity was more apparent in the subgroup of 24 high intensity trials ($I^2 = 59\%$). There was one trial with a significant negative effect for treatment (Rice 1994) and two with particularly large positive effects (Canga 2000; Terazawa 2001). Pooling all 31 studies using a fixed-effect method gave a risk ratio (RR) of 1.28 with 95% confidence interval (CI) 1.18 to 1.38 at the longest follow-up *(Comparison 01)*. Because of the heterogeneity we tested the sensitivity to pooling the studies using a random effects model. This did not materially alter the estimated effect size or significance (random-effects RR 1.31, 95% CI 1.14 to 1.50). Excluding the three outlying trials marginally lowered the fixed effect estimate (RR 1.27, 95% CI 1.18 to 1.38) and almost removed the heterogeneity not attributable to chance ($I^2 = 17\%$).

We also tested the sensitivity of these results to excluding studies that did not validate all reports of abstinence, limiting the analysis to studies graded A for quality of allocation concealment, and excluding studies with less than 12 months follow-up. None of these altered the estimates to any great extent, although confidence intervals became wider due to the smaller number of studies. Excluding one study (Bolman 2002) for which we were not able to enter the numbers of quitters directly did not alter the results.

Some participants in Taylor 1990 had been encouraged to use nicotine replacement therapy (NRT). Exclusion of these people did not alter the significant effect of the intervention in this study. In Miller 1997 more people in the intervention conditions than the control used NRT (44% of intensive and 39% of minimal intervention versus 29% of control). People who were prescribed NRT had lower quit rates than those who were not, but the relative differences in quit rates between the usual care and intervention groups were similar for the subgroups that did and did not use NRT. However, because of the different rates of use of NRT, it is probable that the increased use of NRT contributed to the effects of the nursing intervention. Use of NRT was also encouraged as part of the Canga 2000 intervention, with 17% of the intervention group accepting a prescription.

Effect of Intervention Intensity

We detected no evidence from our indirect comparison between subgroups that the trials we classified as using higher intensity interventions had larger treatment effects. In this update of the review the point estimate for the pooled effect of the seven lower intensity trials is effectively the same as for the 24 of higher intensity. The difference between this update and previous versions of the review is that the confidence interval for the low intensity trials no longer excludes 1. (High intensity subgroup RR 1.28, 95% CI 1.18 to 1.39. Low intensity subgroup RR 1.27, 95% CI 0.99 to 1.62.) In the previous version we had found that the significance in the low intensity subgroup was lost when we included Hajek 2002, a study for which we were uncertain over the classification of the control group (as noted above in the *Description of studies* section). As before, including this study in the low intensity subgroup

Comparison 01. All nursing intervention vs control trials, grouped by intensity of intervention

Outcome Title	No. of Studies	No. of Participants	Statistical Method	Effect Size
01 Smoking cessation at longest follow-up	31	15205	Relative Risk (Fixed) 95% CI	1.28 [1.18, 1.38]

Comparison 02. All nursing intervention vs control trials, grouped by setting and population

Outcome Title	No. of Studies	No. of Participants	Statistical Method	Effect Size
01 Smoking cessation at longest follow-up			Relative Risk (Fixed) 95% CI	Subtotals only

Comparison 03. Effect of additional strategies: Higher versus lower intensity

Outcome Title	No. of Studies	No. of Participants	Statistical Method	Effect Size
01 Additional components at single contact. Smoking cessation at longest follow-up			Relative Risk (Fixed) 95% CI	Subtotals only
02 Additional contacts. Smoking cessation at longest follow-up			Relative Risk (Fixed) 95% CI	Subtotals only

Comparison 04. Sensitivity analysis by intensity, including Hajek 2002, with Lancaster, Bolman, Curry as low intensity

Outcome Title	No. of Studies	No. of Participants	Statistical Method	Effect Size
01 Smoking cessation at longest follow-up	32	15710	Relative Risk (Fixed) 95% CI	1.24 [1.15, 1.33]

Comparison 05. Sensitivity analysis by setting and population, including Hajek 2002

Outcome Title	No. of Studies	No. of Participants	Statistical Method	Effect Size
01 Smoking cessation at longest follow-up			Relative Risk (Fixed) 95% CI	Subtotals only

further reduced the point estimate and there was no evidence of a treatment effect (RR 1.09, 95% CI 0.92 to 1.29). Compared to the other trials in the low intensity subgroup, the Hajek trial was conducted amongst hospitalized patients with cardiovascular disease and the overall quit rates were high. The large number of events gave this trial a high weight in the meta-analysis.

The distinction between low and high intensity subgroups was based on our categorization of the intended intervention. Low levels of implementation were particularly noted in the trial reports for Lancaster 1999, Bolman 2002, and Curry 2003, so we tested the effect of moving them from the high to the low intensity subgroup. This reduced the point estimate of effect in the low intensity subgroup and increased it in the high intensity one. If these three studies and Hajek 2002 are included in the low intensity subgroup, the pooled estimate of effect is small and non-significant (RR 1.09, 95% CI 0.96 to 1.25 *[Comparison 04]*). We also assessed the sensitivity of the results to using additional participants in the control group for Aveyard 2003 (see notes in Included Study Table for details). This reduced the size of the effect in the low intensity subgroup but did not alter our conclusions.

Effects of Differing Health States and Client Settings

Trials in hospitals recruited patients with health problems, but some trials specifically recruited patients with cardiovascular disease, and amongst these, some interventions addressed multiple risks whilst most only addressed smoking. Trials in primary care generally did not select patients with a particular health problem. We combined setting and disease diagnosis in one set of subgroups *(Comparison 02)*.

Four trials that included a smoking cessation intervention from a nurse as part of cardiac rehabilitation showed a significant pooled effect on smoking (RR 1.39, 95% CI 1.17 to 1.65). Three of these (Allen 1996; Carlsson 1997; Hanssen 2007) did not use biochemical validation of quitting, and in the fourth (DeBusk 1994) we were unable to confirm the proportion of drop-outs with the study authors.

There was moderate heterogeneity ($I^2 = 50\%$) amongst seven trials in hospitalized smokers with cardiovascular disease, due to the strong intervention effect in one of the seven trials (Taylor 1990). The estimated RR was 1.29 (95% CI 1.14 to 1.45) and the effect remained significant if Taylor 1990 was excluded or if a random effects model was used. A sensitivity analysis of the effect of including Hajek 2002 in this category increased the heterogeneity ($I^2 = 60\%$), and the pooled effect was just significant whether a fixed effect or a random-effects model was used *(Comparison 05)*. Excluding Taylor 1990 again removed heterogeneity but the pooled effect was then small and not significant (RR 1.1, 95% CI 0.99 to 1.26, P = 0.23, figure not shown).

Amongst the five trials in non-cardiac hospitalized smokers the risk ratio was small and the confidence interval did not exclude no effect (RR 1.04, 95% CI 0.89 to 1.22). We included in this subgroup one trial that began the intervention in a pre-admission clinic for elective surgery patients (Ratner 2004). There was no evidence for an effect of an intervention in one trial (Rice 1994) amongst non-hospitalized adults with cardiovascular disease (RR 0.35, 95% CI 0.13 to 0.55). Subgroup analysis in that study, however, suggested that smokers who had experienced cardiovascular bypass surgery were more likely to quit, and these patients were over-represented in the control group who received advice to quit but no structured intervention.

Pooling 14 trials of cessation interventions for other non-hospitalized adults showed an increase in the success rates (RR 1.84, 95% CI 1.49 to 2.28). A sensitivity analysis testing the effect of excluding those trials (Janz 1987; Vetter 1990; Curry 2003; Hilberink 2005) where a combination of a nursing intervention and advice from a physician was used did not substantially alter this.

Higher versus Lower Intensity Interventions

Effects of Physiological Feedback

Two trials (Sanders 1989b; Risser 1990) that evaluated the effect of physiological feedback as an adjunct to a nursing intervention failed to detect an effect at maximum follow-up *(Comparison 03.01).*

Effects of Other Components at a Single Contact

One trial in hospitalized smokers with cardiovascular disease (Hajek 2002) failed to detect a significant benefit of additional support from a nurse giving additional written materials, a written quiz, an offer of a support buddy, and carbon monoxide measurement compared to controls receiving brief advice and a self-help booklet (RR 0.91, 95% CI 0.73 to 1.13) *(Comparison 03.01).*

Effects of Additional Telephone Support

There was weak evidence from pooling three trials that additional telephone support increased cessation, since the lower limit of the confidence interval was at the boundary of no effect (RR 1.25, 95% CI 1.00 to 1.56; *Comparison 03.02*).

Effects of Additional Face-to-Face Sessions

One trial of additional support from an alcohol and drug assessment unit nurse for patients admitted to a coronary care unit (Feeney 2001) showed a very significant benefit for the intervention. The cessation rate among the controls, however, was very low (1/97), and there were a large number of drop-outs, particularly from the control group. This could have underestimated the control group quit rate. In another trial (Alterman 2001), offering four nurse sessions rather than one as an adjunct to nicotine patch showed no benefit, with the control group having a significantly higher quit rate (OR 0.36, 95% CI 0.15 to 0.85). No explanation was offered for the lower than expected quit rates in the intervention group. One trial of providing additional clinic sessions and telephone support to people receiving either nicotine sublingual tablets or placebo (Tonnesen 2006) had almost identical quit rates in the high and low intensity arms (all in *Comparison 03.02*).

ANALYSIS 01.01 Comparison 01 All nursing intervention vs control trials, grouped by intensity of intervention, Outcome 01 Smoking cessation at longest follow up

Review: Nursing interventions for smoking cessation
Comparison: 01 All nursing intervention vs control trials, grouped by intensity of intervention
Outcome: 01 Smoking cessation at longest follow up

Study	Treatment n/N	Control n/N	Relative Risk (Fixed) 95% CI	Weight (%)	Relative Risk (Fixed) 95% CI
01 HIGH INTENSITY INTERVENTION					
Allen 1996	9/14	6/11		0.8	1.18 [0.61, 2.29]
Bolman 2002	103/334	110/401		11.9	1.12 [0.90, 1.41]
Canga 2000	25/147	3/133		0.4	7.54 [2.33, 24.40]
Carlsson 1997	16/32	9/35		1.0	1.94 [1.00, 3.77]
Curry 2003	4/156	3/147		0.4	1.26 [0.29, 5.52]
DeBusk 1994	92/131	64/121		7.9	1.33 [1.09, 1.62]
Hollis 1993	79/1997	15/710		2.6	1.87 [1.09, 3.23]
Lancaster 1999	8/249	10/248		1.2	0.80 [0.32, 1.99]
Lewis 1998	4/62	3/61		0.4	1.31 [0.31, 5.62]
Miller 1997	245/1000	191/942		23.3	1.21 [1.02, 1.43]
Rice 1994	24/207	16/48		3.1	0.35 [0.20, 0.60]
Rigotti 1994	22/44	22/43		2.6	0.98 [0.65, 1.48]
Taylor 1990	47/84	20/82		2.4	2.29 [1.50, 3.51]
Terazawa 2001	8/117	1/111		0.1	7.59 [0.96, 59.70]
Chouinard 2005	26/106	7/55		1.1	1.93 [0.89, 4.16]
Froelicher 2004	64/134	55/132		6.6	1.15 [0.88, 1.50]
Hennrikus 2005	66/666	68/678		8.0	0.99 [0.72, 1.36]
Quist-Paulsen 2003	57/114	44/119		5.1	1.35 [1.00, 1.82]
Ratner 2004	10/114	11/114		1.3	0.91 [0.40, 2.06]
Hilberink 2005	39/244	13/148		1.9	1.82 [1.01, 3.29]
Sanz-Pozo 2006	3/60	4/65		0.5	0.81 [0.19, 3.48]
Borrelli 2005	9/114	5/120		0.6	1.89 [0.65, 5.48]
Hanssen 2007	36/77	20/61		2.6	1.43 [0.93, 2.19]
Kim 2005	28/200	18/201		2.1	1.56 [0.89, 2.73]
Subtotal (95% CI)	6403	4786		87.9	1.28 [1.18, 1.39]
Total events: 1024 (Treatment), 718 (Control)					
Test for heterogeneity chi-square = 56.41 df = 23 p = 0.0001 I^2 = 59.2%					
Test for overall effect z = 5.88 p < 0.00001					
02 LOW INTENSITY INTERVENTION					
Aveyard 2003	9/413	3/418		0.4	3.04 [0.83, 11.14]
Davies 1992	2/153	4/154		0.5	0.50 [0.09, 2.71]
Janz 1987	26/144	12/106		1.6	1.59 [0.84, 3.01]
Nebot 1992	5/81	7/175		0.5	1.54 [0.51, 4.72]
Tonnesen 1996	8/254	3/253		0.4	2.66 [0.71, 9.90]
Vetter 1990	34.237	20/234		2.4	1.68 [1.00, 2.83]
Nagle 2005	48/698	54/696		6.4	0.89 [0.61, 1.29]
Subtotal (95% CI)	1980	2036		12.1	1.27 [0.99, 1.62]
Total events: 1.32 (Treatment), 103 (Control)					
Test for heterogeneity chi-square = 9.35 df = 6 p = 0.16 I^2 = 35.8%					
Test for overall effect z = 1.86 p = 0.06					
Total (95% CI)	8383	6822		100.0	1.28 [1.18, 1.38]
Total events: 1156 (Treatment), 821 (Control)					
Test for heterogeneity chi-square-65.74 df = 30 p = 0.0002 I^2 = 54.4%					
Test for overall effect z = 6.14 p < 0.00001					

0.1 0.2 0.5 1 2 5 10
Favours Control — Favours Treatment

ANALYSIS 02.01 Comparison 02 All nursing intervention vs control trials, grouped by setting and population, Outcome 01 Smoking cessation at longest follow up

Review: Nursing interventions for smoking cessation
Comparison: 02 All nursing intervention vs control trials, grouped by setting and population
Outcome: 01 Smoking cessation at longest follow up

Study	Treatment n/N	Control n/N	Relative Risk (Fixed) 95% CI	Weight (%)	Relative Risk (Fixed) 95% CI
01 SMOKING INTERVENTION AS PART OF MULTIFACTORIAL INTERVENTION IN PATIENTS WITH CARDIOVASCULAR DISEASE					
Allen 1996	9/14	6/11		6.5	1.18 [0.61, 2.29]
Carlsson 1997	16/32	9/35		8.3	1.94 [1.00, 3.77]
DeBusk 1994	92/131	64/121		63.9	1.33 [1.09, 1.62]
Hanssen 2007	36/77	20/61		21.4	1.43 [0.93, 2.19]
Subtotal (95% CI)	254	228		100.00	1.39 [1.17, 1.65]
Total events: 153 (Treatment), 99 (Control)					
Test for heterogeneity chi-square = 1.44 df = 3 p = 0.70 I^2 = 0.0%					
Test for overall effect z = 3.71 p = 0.0002					
02 SMOKING INTERVENTION ALONE IN HOSPITALIZED SMOKERS WITH A CARDIOVASCULAR DISEASE					
Bolman 2002	103/334	110/401		30.7	1.12 [0.90, 1.41]
Miller 1997	100/320	74/310		23.1	1.31 [1.01, 1.69]
Rigotti 1994	22/44	22/43		6.8	0.98 [0.65, 1.48]
Taylor 1990	47/84	20/82		6.2	2.29 [1.50, 3.51]
Chouinard 2005	26/106	7/55		2.8	1.93 [0.89, 4.16]
Froelicher 2004	64/134	55/132		17.0	1.15 [0.88, 1.50]
Quist-Paulsen 2003	57/114	44/119		13.2	1.35 [1.00, 1.82]
Subtotal (95% CI)	1136	1142		100.00	1.29 [1.14, 1.45]
Total events: 419 (Treatment), 332 (Control)					
Test for heterogeneity chi-square = 12.04 df = 6 p = 0.06 I^2 = 50.2%					
Test for overall effect z = 4.19 p = 0.00003					
03 SMOKING INTERVENTION ALONE IN OTHER HOSPITALIZED SMOKERS					
Lewis 1998	4/62	3/61		1.2	1.31 [0.31, 5.62]
Miller 1997	145/680	117/632		47.2	1.15 [0.93, 1.43]
Hennrikus 2005	66/666	68/678		26.2	0.99 [0.72, 1.36]
Nagle 2005	48/698	54/696		21.1	0.89 [0.61, 1.29]
Ratner 2004	10/114	11/114		4.3	0.91 [0.40, 2.06]
Subtotal (95% CI)	2220	2181		100.0	1.04 [0.89, 1.22]
Total events: 273 (Treatment), 253 (Control)					
Test for heterogeneity chi-square = 1.83 df = 4 p = 0.77 I^2 = 0.0%					
Test for overall effect z = 0.54 p = 0.6					
04 SMOKING INTERVENTION ALONE IN NON-HOSPITALIZED SMOKERS WITH A CARDIOVASCULAR DISEASE					
Rice 1994	24/207	16/48		100.0	0.35 [0.20, 0.60]
Subtotal (95% CI)	207	48		100.0	0.35 [0.20, 0.60]
Total events: 24 (Treatment), 16 (Control)					
Test for heterogeneity: not applicable					
Test for overall effect z = 3.77 p = 0.0002					

0.1 0.2 0.5 1 2 5 10
Favours Control Favours Treatment

ANALYSIS 02.01 Comparison 02 All nursing intervention vs control trials, grouped by setting and population, Outcome 01 Smoking cessation at longest follow up—cont'd

Study	Treatment n/N	Control n/N	Relative Risk (Fixed) 95% CI	Weight (%)	Relative Risk (Fixed) 95% CI
05 SMOKING INTERVENTION ALONE IN OTHER NON-HOSPITALIZED SMOKERS					
Aveyard 2003	9/413	3/418		2.4	3.04 [0.83, 11.14]
Canga 2000	25/147	3/133		2.5	7.54 [2.33, 24.40]
Curry 2003	4/156	3/147		2/4	1.26 [0.29, 5.52]
Davies 1992	2/153	4/154		3/1	0.50 [0.09, 2.71]
Hollis 1993	79/1997	15/710		17.5	1.87 [1.09, 3.23]
Janz 1987	26/144	12/106		10.9	1.59 [0.84, 3.01]
Lancaster 1999	8/249	10/248		7.9	0.80 [0.32, 1.99]
Nebot 1992	5/81	7/175		3.5	1.54 [0.51, 4.72]
Terazawa 2001	8/117	1/111		0.8	7.59 [0.96, 59.70]
Tonnesen 1996	8/254	3/253		2.4	2.66 [0.71, 9.90]
Vetter 1990	34/237	20/234		15.9	1.68 [1.00, 2.83]
Hilberink 2005	39/244	13/148		12.8	1.82 [1.01, 3.29]
Borrelli 2005	9/114	5/120		3.8	1.89 [0.65, 5.48]
Kim 2005	28/200	18/201		14.2	1.56 [0.89, 2.73]
Subtotal (95% Cl)	4506	3158		100.0	1.84 (1.49, 2.28]
Total events: 284 (Treatment), 117 (Control)					
Test for heterogeneity chi-square = 1473 df = 13 p = 0.32 I^2 = 11.8%					
Test for overall effect z = 5.63 p < 0.00001					

ANALYSIS 03.01 Comparison 03 Effect of additional strategies: Higher versus lower intensity, Outcome 01 Additional components at single contact. Smoking cessation at longest follow up

Review: Nursing interventions for smoking cessation
Comparison: 03 Effect of additional strategies: higher versus lower intensity
Outcome: 01 Additional components at single contact. Smoking cessation at longest follow up

Study	Treatment n/N	Control n/N	Relative Risk (Fixed) 95% CI	Weight (%)	Relative Risk (Fixed) 95% CI
01 IDEMONSTRATION OF CO LEVELS					
Sanders 1989b	18/376	17/375		100.0	1.06 [0.55, 2.02]
Subtotal (95% Cl)	376	375		100.0	1.06 [0.55, 2.02]
Total events: 18 (Treatment), 17 (Control)					
Test for heterogeneity: not applicable					
Test for overall effect z = 0.17 p = 0.9					
02 DEMONSTRATION OF SPIROMETRY AND CO MEASUREMENT					
Risser 1990	3/45	9/45		100.0	0.33 [0.10, 1.15]
Subtotal (95% Cl)	45	45		100.0	0.33 [0.10, 1.15]
Total events: 3 (Treatment), 9 (Control)					
Test for heterogeneity: not applicable					
Test for overall effect z = 1.74 p = 0.08					
03 ADDITIONAL SUPPORT INCLUDING CO READING MATERIALS					
Hajek 2002	94/254	102/251		100.0	0.91 [0.73, 1.13]
Subtotal (95% Cl)	254	251		100.0	0.91 [0.73, 1.13]
Total events: 94 (Treatment), 102 (Control)					
Test for heterogeneity: not applicable					
Test for overall effect z = 0.84 p = 0.4					

0.1 0.2 0.5 1 2 5 10
Favours Control Favours Treatment

ANALYSIS 03.02 Comparison 03 Effect of additional strategies: Higher versus lower intensity, Outcome 02 Additional contacts. Smoking cessation at longest follow up

Review: Nursing interventions for smoking cessation
Comparison: 03 Effect of additional strategies: Higher versus lower intensity
Outcome: 02 Additional contacts. Smoking cessation at longest follow up

Study	Treatment n/N	Control n/N	Relative Risk (Fixed) 95% CI	Weight (%)	Relative Risk (Fixed) 95% CI
01 ADDITIONAL TELEPHONE SUPPORT					
Chouinard 2005	13/53	13/53		12.0	1.00 [0.51, 1.95]
Hasuo 2004	32/60	25/54		24.3	1.15 [0.79, 1.67]
Miller 1997	100/540	64/460		63.7	1.33 [1.00, 1.78]
Subtotal (95% CI)	653	567		100.0	1.25 [1.00, 1.56]
Total events: 145 (Treatment), 102 (Control)					
Test for heterogeneity chi-square=0.79 df = 2 p = 0.67 I^2 = 0.0%					
Test for overall effect z = 1.97 p = 0.05					
02 SELF-HELP MANUAL, ADDITIONAL TELEPHONE SUPPORT					
Feeney 2001	31.92	1/97		100.0	32.68 [4.55, 234.56]
Subtotal (95% CI)	92	97		100.0	32.68 [4.55, 234.56]
Total events: 31 (Treatment), 1 Control)					
Test for heterogeneity: not applicable					
Test for overall effect z = 3.47 p = 0.0005					
03 THREE ADDITIONAL SESSIONS					
Alterman 2001	9/80	20/77		100.0	0.43 [0.21, 0.89]
Subtotal (95% CI)	80	77		100.0	0.43 [0.21, 0.89]
Total events: 9 (Treatment), 20 Control)					
Test for heterogeneity: not applicable					
Test for overall effect z = 2.27 p = 0.02					
04 ADDITIONAL FACE-TO-FACE AND TELEPHONE SUPPORT					
Tonnesen 2006	19/187	17/183		100.0	1.09 [0.59, 2.04]
Subtotal (95% CI)	187	183		100.0	1.09 [0.59, 2.04]
Total events: 19 (Treatment), 17 Control)					
Test for heterogeneity: not applicable					
Test for overall effect z = 0.28 p = 0.8					

0.1 0.2 0.5 1 2 5 10
Favours Control Favours Treatment

ANALYSIS 04.01 Comparison 04 Sensitivity analysis by intensity, including Hajek 2002, with Lancaster, Bolman, Curry as low intensity, Outcome 01 Smoking cessation at longest follow up

Review: Nursing interventions for smoking cessation
Comparison: 04 Sensitivity analysis by intensity, including Hajek 2002, with Lancaster, Bolman, Curry as low intensity
Outcome: 01 Smoking cessation at longest follow up

Study	Treatment n/N	Control n/N	Relative Risk (Fixed) 95% CI	Weight (%)	Relative Risk (Fixed) 95% CI
01 HIGH INTENSITY INTERVENTION					
Allen 1996	9/14	6/11		0.7	1.18 [0.61, 2.29]
Canga 2000	25/147	3/133		0.3	7.54 [2.33, 24.40]
Carlsson 1997	16/32	9/35		0.9	1.94 [1.00, 3.77]
DeBusk 1994	92/131	64/121		7.0	1.33 [1.09, 1.62]
Hollis 1993	79/1997	15/710		2.3	1.87 [1.09, 3.23]
Lewis 1998	4/62	3/61		0.3	1.31 [0.31, 5.62]
Miller 1997	245/1000	191/942		20.8	1.21 [1.02, 1.43]
Rice 1994	24/207	16/48		2.7	0.35 [0.20, 0.60]
Rigotti 1994	22/44	22/43		2.4	0.98 [0.65, 1.48]
Taylor 1990	47/84	20/82		2.1	2.29 [1.50, 3.51]
Terazawa 2001	8/117	1/111		0.1	7.59 [0.96, 59.70]
Chouinard 2005	26/106	7/55		1.0	1.93 [0.89, 4.16]
Froelicher 2004	64/134	55/132		5.9	1.15 [0.88, 1.50]
Hennrikus 2005	66/666	68/678		7.1	0.99 [0.72, 1.36]
Quist-Paulsen 2003	57/114	44/119		4.6	1.35 [1.00, 1.82]
Ratner 2004	10/114	11/114		1.2	0.91 [0.40, 2.06]
Hilberink 2005	39/244	13/148		1.7	1.82 [1.01, 3.29]
Borrelli 2005	9/114	5/120		0.5	1.89 [0.65, 5.48]
Hanssen 2007	36/77	20/61		2.4	1.43 [0.93, 2.19]
Kim 2005	28/200	18/201		1.9	1.56 [0.89, 2.73]
Sanz-Pozo 2006	3/60	4/65		0.4	0.81 [0.19, 3.48]
Subtotal (95% CI)	5664	3990		66.4	1.28 [1.20, 1.43]
Total events: 909 (Treatment), 595 (Control)					
Test for heterogeneity chi-square = 54.61 df = 20 p = 0.0001 I^2 = 63.4%					
Test for overall effect z = 5.88 p < 0.00001					
02 LOW INTENSITY INTERVENTION					
Aveyard 2003	9/413	3/418		0.3	3.04 [0.83, 11.14]
Bolman 2002	103/334	110/401		10.6	1.12 [0.90, 1.31]
Curry 2003	4/156	3/147		0.3	1.26 [0.29, 5.52]
Davies 1992	2/153	4/154		0.4	0.50 [0.09, 2.71]
Hajek 2002	94/254	102/251		10.8	0.91 [0.73, 1.13]
Janz 1987	26/144	12/106		1.5	1.59 [0.84, 3.01]
Lancaster 1999	8/249	10/248		1.1	0.80 [0.32, 1.99]
Nebot 1992	5/81	7/175		0.5	1.54 [0.51, 4.72]
Tonnesen 1996	8/254	3/253		0.3	2.66 [0.71, 9.90]
Vetter 1990	34.237	20/234		2.1	1.68 [1.00, 2.83]
Nagle 2005	48/698	54/696		5.7	0.89 [0.61, 1.29]
Subtotal (95% CI)	2973	3083		33.6	1.09 [0.96, 1.25]
Total events: 341 (Treatment), 328 (Control)					
Test for heterogeneity chi-square = 13.66 df = 10 p = 0.19 I^2 = 26.8%					
Test for overall effect z = 1.30 p = 0.2					
Total (95% CI)	8637	7073		100.0	1.24 [1.15, 1.33]
Total events: 1250 (Treatment), 923 (Control)					
Test for heterogeneity chi-square = 72.93 df = 31 p = 0.0001 I^2 = 57.5%					
Test for overall effect z = 5.67 p < 0.00001					

0.1 0.2 0.5 1 2 5 10
Favours Control Favours Treatment

ANALYSIS 05.01 Comparison 05 Sensitivity analysis by setting and population, including Hajek 2002, Outcome 01 Smoking cessation at longest follow up

Review: Nursing interventions for smoking cessation
Comparison: 05 Sensitivity analysis by setting and population, including Hajek 2002
Outcome: 01 Smoking cessation at longest follow up

Study	Treatment n/N	Control n/N	Relative Risk (Fixed) 95% CI	Weight (%)	Relative Risk (Fixed) 95% CI
02 SMOKING INTERVENTION ALONE IN HOSPITALIZED SMOKERS WITH A CARDIOVASCULAR DISEASE					
Bolman 2002	103/334	110/401		14.5	1.12 [0.90, 1.41]
Hajek 2002	94/254	102/251		14.7	0.91 [0.73, 1.13]
Miller 1997	100/320	74/310		13.4	1.31 [1.01, 1.69]
Rigotti 1994	22/44	22/43		8.7	0.98 [0.65, 1.48]
Taylor 1990	47/84	20/82		8.5	2.29 [1.50, 3.51]
Chouinard 2005	26/106	7/55		3.7	1.93 [0.89, 4.16]
Froelicher 2004	64/134	55/132		13.0	1.15 [0.88, 1.50]
Hennrikus 2005	66/666	68/678		11.3	0.99 [0.72, 1.36]
Quist-Paulsen 2003	57/114	44/119		12.0	1.35 [1.00, 1.82]
Subtotal (95% CI)	2056	2071		100.00	1.20 [1.02, 1.42]

Total events: 579 (Treatment), 502 (Control)
Test for heterogeneity chi-square = 19.80 df = 8 p = 0.01 I^2 = 59.6%
Test for overall effect z = 2.22 p = 0.03

0.1 0.2 0.5 1 2 5 10
Favours Control Favours Treatment

Results of Studies Not Included in the Meta-Analysis

We identified five studies (Sanders 1989a; Family Heart 1994; OXCHECK1994; Campbell 1998; Steptoe 1999) in which nurses intervened with primary care patients. All except Sanders 1989a addressed multiple cardiovascular risk factors, and all except Campbell 1998 targeted healthy patients. The latter recruited patients with coronary heart disease. Although they met the main inclusion criteria, in four of the trials the design did not allow for data extraction for meta-analysis in a comparable format to other studies. In the other (Sanders 1989a) only a random sample of the control group was followed up. We therefore discuss these trials separately.

Sanders 1989a, in which smokers visiting their family doctor were asked to make an appointment for cardiovascular health screening, reported that only 25.9% of the patients made and kept such an appointment. The percentage that had quit at one month and at one year and reported last smoking before the one-month follow-up was higher both in the attenders (4.7%) and the non-attenders (3.3%) than in the usual care controls (0.9%). This suggests that the invitation to make an appointment for health screening could have been an anti-smoking intervention in itself, and that the additional effect of the structured nursing intervention was small.

We do not have comparable data for OXCHECK 1994, which used similar health checks, because the households had been randomized to be offered the health check in different years. The authors compared the proportions of smokers in the intervention group who claimed to have stopped smoking in the previous year to patients attending for their one-year follow-up, and to controls attending for their first health check. They found no difference in the proportions that reported stopping smoking in the previous year.

The Family Heart 1994 study offered nurse-led cardiovascular screening for men aged 40 to 59 and for their partners, with smoking cessation as one of the recommended lifestyle changes. Cigarette smokers were invited to attend up to three further visits. Smoking prevalence was lower amongst those who returned for the one-year follow-up than amongst the control group screened at one year. This difference was reduced if non-returners were assumed to have continued to smoke, and if CO-validated quitting was used. In that case there was a reduction of only about one percentage point, with weak evidence of a true reduction.

Campbell 1998 invited patients with a diagnosis of coronary heart disease to nurse-run clinics promoting medical and lifestyle aspects of secondary prevention. There was no significant effect on smoking cessation. At one year the decline in smoking prevalence was greater in the control group than in the intervention group. Four-year follow-up did not alter the effect of a lack of benefit. Steptoe 1999 recruited patients at increased risk of coronary heart disease for a multi-component intervention. The quit rate amongst smokers followed up after one year was not significantly higher in the intervention group (9.4%, 95% CI −9.6 to 28.3), and there was greater loss to follow-up of smokers in the intervention group.

DISCUSSION

The results of this meta-analysis support a modest but positive effect for smoking cessation intervention by nursing, but with caution about the effects that can be expected if interventions are very brief or cannot be consistently delivered. A structured smoking cessation intervention delivered by a nurse was more effective than usual care on smoking abstinence at six months or longer post-treatment. Whilst the direction of effect was consistent in different intensities of intervention, in different settings, and in smokers with and without tobacco-related illnesses, a subgroup of low intensity studies showed small and non-significant effects. There was also some evidence of statistical heterogeneity, although this was attributable to a very small number of outlying studies. In the one study (Rice 1994) that showed a statistically significant higher quit rate in a control group, participants had been advised to quit and the control group included a significantly larger proportion of people who had had coronary artery bypass graft surgery. A multivariate analysis of one-year follow-up data in this study revealed a quitter was significantly more likely to be less than 48 years, male, have had individualized versus group or no cessation instruction and to have had a high degree of perceived threat relative to their health state.

In this update of the review, we have changed the summary effect measure from the odds ratio to the risk ratio. An advantage of this is that it is more stable across a range of control group quit rates, and it avoids the risk that an odds ratio will be interpreted as a relative risk. Estimated effects appear smaller in this version of the review largely as a result of the change in the measure. In this update the estimated effect in the primary comparison, pooling 31 studies, is 1.3 for the risk ratio, or 1.4 as an odds ratio. In the previous update pooling 20 studies the odds ratio was 1.5, whilst in the first version of the review published in 1999 with 15 studies the odds ratio was 1.4. The effect has therefore been quite stable over time, but a small number of the most recent trials have had smaller effects. The effect of the change in outcome measure is most apparent in the subgroup of trials where control group event rates are highest, such as interventions for people in hospital with cardiovascular disease. The risk ratio estimated from pooling four studies of multifactor risk reduction interventions *(Comparison 02.01)* is 1.4, but as an odds ratio it is 2.1, almost identical to the result based on three studies in the last version of the review.

Overall, these meta-analysis findings need to be interpreted carefully in light of the methodological limitations of both the review and the clinical trials. In terms of the review, it is possible that there was a publication selection bias due to using only tabulated data derived from published works (Stewart 1993). Data from the unpublished and/or missed studies could have shown more or less favourable results. Secondly, the results of a meta-analysis (based on the findings of many small trials) should be viewed with caution even when the combined effect is statistically significant (LeLorier 1997). In this analysis one study (Miller 1997) contributes 23% of the weight to the primary analysis, while the next largest contributes 12% of the weight. Finding statistical heterogeneity between the odds of cessation in different studies limits any assumption that interventions in any clinical setting and with any type of patient are equally effective.

A difference among the studies that may have contributed to the differences in outcome was baseline cigarette use. There was an inverse relationship between number of cigarettes smoked per day and success in quitting; the more addicted the individuals, the more difficult it was for them to quit. Studies that recruited a higher proportion of lighter smokers or that included recent quitters could have achieved better results. Interestingly, the studies in the meta-analysis that reported the highest cigarette use rates had the weakest effect for the intervention (Davies 1992; Rice 1994). Although some trials included recent quitters in their recruitment, there was no evidence that these trials had different results.

When this review was first prepared we found similar effect estimates for high and low intensity smoking cessation interventions by nurses, as was found in a review of physicians' advice (Lancaster 2004). Presumably, the more components added to the intervention the more intense the intervention; however, assessing the contribution of factors such as total contact time, number of contacts, and content of the intervention was difficult. Our distinction between high and low intensity based on the length of initial contact, and number of planned follow-ups may not have accurately distinguished among the key elements that could have contributed to greater efficacy. We found that the nature of the smoking cessation interventions differed from advice alone, to more intense interventions with multiple components, and that the description of what constituted "advice only" varied. In most trials, advice was given with an emphasis on "stopping smoking" because of some existing health problem. To make most interventions more intense, verbal advice was supplemented with a variety of counselling messages, including benefits and barriers to cessation (e.g., Taylor 1990) and effective coping strategies (e.g., Allen 1996). Manuals and printed self-help materials were also added to many interventions along with repeated follow-ups (Hollis 1993; Miller 1997). In some studies the proposed intervention was not delivered consistently to all participants. In recent updates the evidence for the benefit of a low intensity intervention has become weaker than that for a more intensive intervention, and the estimated effect is sensitive to the inclusion of one additional study (Hajek 2002) and to the classification of intensity of three studies. Almost all the intensive interventions were delivered by either dedicated project staff or nurses with a health promotion role. Most studies in which the intensive intervention was intended to be delivered by a nurse with other roles, reported problems in delivering the intervention consistently. None showed a statistically significant benefit for the intervention. No studies were found for the giving of brief opportunistic advice that were directly analogous to the low intensity interventions used in physician advice trials (Lancaster 2004).

In two studies in the low intensity category (Janz 1987; Vetter 1990), advice from a physician was also part of the intervention and this almost certainly contributed to the overall effect. The largest study in the high intensity subgroup (Miller 1997) produced only relatively modest results. This was due in part to the effect of the minimal treatment condition that had just one follow-up telephone call. If their intensive condition alone had been used in the comparison, the estimate of effect in the intensive intervention subgroup of trials might have been increased.

One study (Miller 1997) provided data on the effect of the same intervention in smokers with different types of illness and showed a greater effect in cardiovascular patients. In these individuals the intervention increased the 12-month quit rate from 24% to 31%, which just reached statistical significance. In other types of patients, the rates were increased from 18.5% to 21%, an effect that did not reach statistical significance. In this study patients were eligible if they had smoked any tobacco in the month prior to hospitalization, but were excluded if they had no intention of quitting (although they were also excluded if they wanted to quit on their own). These criteria may have contributed to the relatively high quit rates achieved. Also, a higher proportion of patients in the intensive treatment arm than in the minimal or usual care interventions were prescribed nicotine replacement therapy (NRT). However, the intervention was also effective in those not prescribed NRT. Those given NRT were heavier smokers (with higher levels of addiction) who achieved lower cessation rates than those who did not use NRT.

This suggests that nursing professionals may have an important "window of opportunity" to intervene with patients in the hospital setting, or at least to introduce the notion of not resuming tobacco use on hospital discharge. The size of the effect may be dependent on the reason for hospitalization. The additional telephone support, with the possibility of another counselling session for people who relapsed after discharge, seemed to contribute to more favourable outcomes in the intensive intervention used by Miller and colleagues. A separate Cochrane review of the efficacy of interventions for hospitalized patients has been recently updated (Rigotti 2007), and this supports the efficacy of interventions for this patient group, but only when the interventions included post-discharge support for at least one month. It should be noted that our subgroup analysis making indirect comparisons between trials in patients with cardiovascular disease and mixed patient populations did not distinguish by intervention intensity. The subgroup differences could be due to confounding, although both subgroups included trials of higher and lower intensity interventions. Providing additional physiological feedback in the form of spirometry and demonstrated carbon monoxide level as an adjunct to nursing intervention did not appear to have an effect. Three studies in primary care or outpatient settings used this approach (Sanders 1989b; Risser 1990; Hollis 1993). It was also used as part of the enhanced intervention in a study with hospitalized patients (Hajek 2002).

The identification of an effect for a nurse-mediated intervention in smokers who were not hospitalized is based on 14 studies. The largest study (Hollis 1993) increased the quit rate from 2% in those who received only advice from a physician to 4% when a nurse delivered one of three additional interventions, including a video, written materials, and a follow-up telephone call. Control group quit rates were less than 10% in almost all these studies, and more typically between 4% and 8%. The relative risk in this group of studies, 1.8, was a little higher than in some subgroups, but because of the low background quit rate the proportion of patients likely to become long-term quitters as a result of a nursing intervention in these settings is likely to be small. However, because of the large number of people who could be reached by nursing, the effect would be important.

The evidence is not strong for an effect of nurse counselling about smoking cessation when it is provided as part of a health check. It may be unrealistic to expect a benefit from this type of intervention. Two studies that invited smokers to make an appointment with a nurse for counselling (Lancaster 1999; Aveyard 2003) also had relatively poor results. In both cases the uptake of the intervention was reported to be poor, with participants reluctant to schedule visits.

Combined efforts of many types of healthcare professionals are likely to be required. The US Public Health Service clinical practice guideline "Treating Tobacco Use and Dependence" (AHRQ 2000) used logistic regression to estimate efficacy for interventions delivered by different types of providers. Their analysis did not distinguish among the non-physician medical healthcare providers, so that dentists, health counsellors, and pharmacists were included with nurses. The guideline concluded that these providers were effective (Table 15, OR 1.7, 95% CI 1.3 to 2.1). They also concluded that interventions by multiple clinician types were more effective (Table 16, OR 2.5, 95% CI 1.9 to 23.4). Although it was recognized that there could be confounding between the number of providers and the overall intensity of the intervention, the findings confirmed that a nursing intervention that reinforces or complements advice from physicians and/or other healthcare providers is likely to be an important component in helping smokers to quit.

AUTHORS' CONCLUSIONS

Implications for Practice

The results of this review indicate the potential benefits of interventions given by nurses to their patients. The challenge will be to incorporate smoking cessation interventions as part of standard practice so that all patients are given an opportunity to be asked about their tobacco use and to be given advice to quit along with reinforcement and follow-up. Nicotine replacement therapy has been shown to improve quit rates when used in conjunction with counselling for behavioural change and should be considered an important adjunct, but not a replacement for nursing interventions (Stead 2008). The evidence suggests that brief interventions from nurses who combine smoking cessation work with other duties are less effective than longer interventions with multiple contacts, delivered by nurses with a role in health promotion or cardiac rehabilitation.

Implications for Research

Further studies of nursing interventions are warranted, with more careful consideration of sample size, participant selection, refusals, drop-outs, long-term follow-up, and biochemical verification. Additionally, controlled studies are needed that carefully examine the effects of "brief advice by nursing" as this type of professional counselling may more accurately reflect the current standard of care. Work is now required to systematize interventions so that more rigorous comparisons can be made between studies. None of the trials reviewed was a replication study; this is a very important method to strengthen the science, and should be encouraged.

POTENTIAL CONFLICT OF INTEREST

V.H. Rice was the principal investigator in one of the studies included in this review.

ACKNOWLEDGMENTS

Nicky Cullum and Tim Coleman for their helpful peer review comments on the original version of this review. Hitomi Kobayasha, a doctoral student, for assistance with Japanese translation of a study.

SOURCES OF SUPPORT

External Sources of Support

American Heart Association USA • NHS Research & Development Programme UK

Internal Sources of Support

Wayne State University College of Nursing, Adult Health & Administration USA • Department of Primary Health Care, Oxford University UK

INDEX TERMS

Medical Subject Headings (MeSH)

*Counseling; *Nursing Care; Randomized Controlled Trials; Smoking [*prevention & control]; Smoking Cessation [*methods]

MeSH check words

Humans

REFERENCES

References to Studies Included in this Review

Allen 1996

Allen JK. Coronary risk factor modification in women after coronary artery bypass surgery. *Nursing Research* 1996;45(5):260-265. [MEDLINE: 96428548].

Alterman 2001

Alterman AI, Gariti P, Mulvaney F. Short- and long-term smoking cessation for three levels of intensity of behavioral treatment. *Psychology of Addictive Behaviors* 2001;15(3):261-264.

Aveyard 2003

Aveyard P, Griffin C, Lawrence T, Cheng KK. A controlled trial of an expert system and self-help manual intervention based on the stages of change versus standard self-help materials in smoking cessation. *Addiction* 2003;98(3):345-354. [MEDLINE: 22491185].

Bolman 2002

*Bolman C, De Vries H, van Breukelen G. A minimal-contact intervention for cardiac inpatients: long-term effects on smoking cessation. *Preventive Medicine* 2002;35(2):181-192. [MEDLINE: 22189120].

Bolman C, De Vries H, van Breukelen G. Evaluation of a nurse-managed minimal-contact smoking cessation intervention for cardiac inpatients. *Health Education Research* 2002;17(1):99-116. [MEDLINE: 21884877].

Borrelli 2005

Borrelli B, Novak S, Hecht J, Emmons K, Papandonatos G, Abrams D. Home health care nurses as a new channel for smoking cessation treatment: outcomes from project CARES (Community-nurse Assisted Research and Education on Smoking). *Preventive Medicine* 2005;41(5-6):815-821.

*Indicates the major publication for the study.

Campbell 1998

*Campbell NC, Ritchie LD, Thain J, Deans HG, Rawles JM, Squair JL. Secondary prevention in coronary heart disease: a randomised trial of nurse led clinics in primary care. *Heart* 1998;80(5): 447-452.

Campbell NC, Thain J, Deans HG, Ritchie LD, Rawles JM, Squair JL. Secondary prevention clinics for coronary heart disease: randomised trial of effect on health. *BMJ* 1998;316(7142):1434-1437.

Murchie P, Campbell NC, Ritchie LD, Simpson JA, Thain J. Secondary prevention clinics for coronary heart disease: four year follow-up of a randomised controlled trial in primary care. *BMJ* 2003;326 (7380):84.

Canga 2000

Canga N, De Irala J, Vara E, Duaso MJ, Ferrer A, Martinez-Gonzalez MA. Intervention study for smoking cessation in diabetic patients: a randomized controlled trial in both clinical and primary care settings. *Diabetes Care* 2000;23(10):1455-1460.

Carlsson 1997

Carlsson R, Lindberg G, Westin L, Israelsson B. Influence of coronary nursing management follow-up on lifestyle after acute myocardial infarction. *Heart* 1997;77(3):256-259. [MEDLINE: 1997246900].

Chouinard 2005

Chouinard MC, Robichaud-Ekstrand S. Predictive value of the transtheoretical model to smoking cessation in hospitalized patients with cardiovascular disease. *European Journal of Cardiovascular Prevention and Rehabilitation* 2007;14:51-58.

Chouinard MC, Robichaud-Ekstrand S. The effectiveness of a nursing inpatient smoking cessation program in individuals with cardiovascular disease. *Nursing Research* 2005;54(4):243-254.

Curry 2003

Curry SJ, Ludman EJ, Graham E, Stout J, Grothaus L, Lozano P. Pediatric-based smoking cessation intervention for low-income women: a randomized trial. *Archives of Pediatric and Adolescent Medicine* 2003;157(3):295-302.

Davies 1992

Davies BL, Matte-Lewis L, O'Connor AM, Dulberg CS, Drake ER. Evaluation of the "Time to Quit" self-help smoking cessation program. *Canadian Journal of Public Health* 1992;83(1):19-23. [MEDLINE: 92240528].

DeBusk 1994

DeBusk RF, Miller NH, Superko HR, Dennis CA, Thomas RJ, Lew HT, et al. A case-management system for coronary risk factor modification after acute myocardial infarction. *Annals of Internal Medicine* 1994;120(9):721-729. [MEDLINE: 94197361].

Family Heart 1994

Family Heart Study Group. Randomised controlled trial evaluating cardiovascular screening and intervention in general practice: principal results of British family heart study. *BMJ* 1994;308:313-320. [MEDLINE: 1994169709].

Feeney 2001

Feeney GF, McPherson A, Connor JP, McAlister A, Young MR, Garrahy P. Randomized controlled trial of two cigarette quit programmes in coronary care patients after acute myocardial infarction. *Internal Medicine Journal* 2001;31(8):470-475. [MEDLINE: 21577083].

Froelicher 2004

Froelicher ES, Christopherson DJ. Women's Initiative for Nonsmoking (WINS) I: design and methods. *Heart and Lung* 2000;29(6):429-437.

Froelicher ES, Christopherson DJ, Miller NH, Martin K. Women's initiative for nonsmoking (WINS) IV: description of 277 women smokers hospitalized with cardiovascular disease. *Heart and Lung* 2002;31:3-14.

Froelicher ES, Li WW, Mahrer-Imhof R, Christopherson D, Stewart AL. Women's Initiative for Non-Smoking (WINS) VI: reliability and validity of health and psychosocial measures in women smokers with cardiovascular disease. *Heart and Lung* 2004;33(3):162-175.

*Froelicher ES, Miller NH, Christopherson DJ, Martin K, Parker KM, Amonetti M, et al. High rates of sustained smoking cessation in women hospitalized with cardiovascular disease: the Women's Initiative for Nonsmoking (WINS). *Circulation* 2004;109(5):587-593.

Mahrer-Imhof R, Froelicher ES, Li WW, Parker KM, Benowitz N. Women's Initiative for Nonsmoking (WINS) V: under-use of nicotine replacement therapy. *Heart and Lung* 2002;31:368-373.

Martin K, Froelicher ES, Miller NH. Women's Initiative for Nonsmoking (WINS) II: the intervention. *Heart and Lung* 2000;29(6):438-445.

Hajek 2002

Hajek P, Taylor TZ, Mills P. Brief intervention during hospital admission to help patients to give up smoking after myocardial infarction and bypass surgery: randomised controlled trial. *BMJ* 2002;324(7329):87-89. [MEDLINE: 21645850].

Hanssen 2007

Hanssen TA, Nordrehaug JE, Eide GE, Hanestad BR. Improving outcomes after myocardial infarction: a randomized controlled trial evaluating effects of a telephone follow-up intervention. *European Journal of Cardiovascular Prevention and Rehabilitation* 2007;14(3):429-437.

Hasuo 2004

Hasuo S, Tanaka H, Oshima A. [Efficacy of a smoking relapse prevention program by postdischarge telephone contacts: a randomized trial] (Japanese). *Nippon Koshu Eisei Zasshi [Japanese Journal of Public Health]* 2004;51(6):403-412.

Hennrikus 2005

Hennrikus D, Lando HA, McCarty MC, Vessey JT. The effectiveness of a systems approach to smoking cessation in hospital inpatients. Society for Research on Nicotine and Tobacco 7th Annual Meeting, March 23-23, Seattle, Washington. 2001:47.

*Hennrikus DJ, Lando HA, McCarty MC, Klevan D, Holtan N, Huebsch JA, et al. The TEAM project: the effectiveness of smoking cessation interventions with hospital patients. *Preventive Medicine* 2005;40:249-258.

Hilberink 2005

Hilberink SR, Jacobs JE, Bottema BJ, de Vries H, Grol RP. Smoking cessation in patients with COPD in daily general practice (SMOCC): six months' results. *Preventive Medicine* 2005;41:822-827.

Hollis 1993

Hollis JF, Lichtenstein E, Mount K, Vogt TM, Stevens VJ. Nurse-assisted smoking counseling in medical settings: minimizing demands on physicians. *Preventive Medicine* 1991;20(4):497-507. [MEDLINE: 91334341].

*Hollis JF, Lichtenstein E, Vogt TM, Stevens VJ, Biglan A. Nurse-assisted counseling for smokers in primary care. *Annals of Internal Medicine* 1993;118(7):521-525. [MEDLINE: 93182891].

Janz 1987

Janz NK, Becker MH, Kirscht JP, Eraker SA, Billi JE, Woolliscroft JO. Evaluation of a minimal-contact smoking cessation intervention in an outpatient setting. *American Journal of Public Health* 1987;77(7):805-809. [MEDLINE: 87239065].

Kim 2005

Kim JR, Lee MS, Hwang JY, Lee JD. Efficacy of a smoking cessation intervention using the AHCPR guideline tailored for Koreans: a randomized controlled trial. *Health Promotion International* 2005;20:51-59.

Lancaster 1999

Lancaster T, Dobbie W, Vos K, Yudkin P, Murphy M, Fowler G. Randomised trial of nurse-assisted strategies for smoking cessation in primary care. *British Journal of General Practice* 1999;49(440):191-194. [MEDLINE: 99274889].

Lewis 1998

Lewis SF, Piasecki TM, Fiore MC, Anderson JE, Baker TB. Transdermal nicotine replacement for hospitalized patients: a randomized clinical trial. *Preventive Medicine* 1998;27(2):296-303. [MEDLINE: 98240165].

Miller 1997

*Miller NH, Smith PM, DeBusk RF, Sobel DS, Taylor CB. Smoking cessation in hospitalized patients—results of a randomized trial. *Archives of Internal Medicine* 1997;157(4):409-415. [MEDLINE: 97198917].

Miller NH, Smith PM, Taylor CB, Sobel D, DeBusk RF. Smoking cessation in hospitalized patients—results of a randomized trial. *Circulation* 1995;92(8):SS179 (abstract 855).

Taylor CB, Miller NH, Herman S, Smith PM, Sobel D, Fisher L, et al. A nurse-managed smoking cessation program for hospitalized smokers. *American Journal of Public Health* 1996;86(11):1557-1560. [MEDLINE: 97073971].

Nagle 2005

Hensley MJ, Nagle AL, Hensley MJ, Schofield MJ, Koschel A. Efficacy of a brief nurse provided nicotine management intervention for hospitalised smokers. *Respirology* 2002;7:A12.

*Nagle AL, Hensley MJ, Schofield MJ, Koschel AJ. A randomised controlled trial to evaluate the efficacy of a nurse-provided intervention for hospitalised smokers. *Australian and New Zealand Journal of Public Health* 2005;29(3):285-291.

Nebot 1992

Nebot M, Cabezas C. Does nurse counseling or offer of nicotine gum improve the effectiveness of physician smoking-cessation advice? *Family Practice Research Journal* 1992;12:263-270. [MEDLINE: 97073971].

OXCHECK 1994

Imperial Cancer Research Fund OXCHECK Study Group. Effectiveness of health checks conducted by nurses in primary care: final results of the OXCHECK study. *BMJ* 1995;310(6987):1099-1104. [MEDLINE: 95261213].

*Imperial Cancer Research Fund OXCHECK Study Group. Effectiveness of health checks conducted by nurses in primary care: results of the OXCHECK study after one year. *BMJ* 1994;308(6924):308-312. [MEDLINE: 94169708].

Quist-Paulsen 2003

Brown DW. Nurse-led intervention increases smoking cessation among people with coronary heart disease. *Evidence Based Healthcare* 2004;8:128-130.

Quist-Paulsen P, Bakke PS, Gallefoss F. Does smoking cessation improve quality of life in patients with coronary heart disease? *Scandinavian Cardiovascular Journal* 2006;40(1):11-16.

Quist-Paulsen P, Bakke PS, Gallefoss F. Predictors of smoking cessation in patients admitted for acute coronary heart disease. *European Journal of Cardiovascular Prevention and Rehabilitation* 2005;12(5):472-477.

*Quist-Paulsen P, Gallefoss F. Randomised controlled trial of smoking cessation intervention after admission for coronary heart disease. *BMJ* 2003;327(7426):1254-1257.

Quist-Paulsen P, Lydersen S, Bakke PS, Gallefoss F. Cost effectiveness of a smoking cessation program in patients admitted for coronary heart disease. *European Journal of Cardiovascular Prevention and Rehabilitation* 2006;13(2):274-280.

Ratner 2004

Ratner PA, Johnson JL, Richardson CG, Bottorff JL, Moffat B, Mackay M, et al. Efficacy of a smoking-cessation intervention for elective-surgical patients. *Research in Nursing and Health* 2004;27(3):148-161.

Rice 1994

Rice VH, Fox DH, Lepczyk M, Sieggreen M, Mullin M, Jarosz P, et al. A comparison of nursing interventions for smoking cessation in adults with cardiovascular health problems. *Heart and Lung* 1994;23(6):473-486. [MEDLINE: 95155020].

Rigotti 1994

Rigotti NA, McKool KM, Shiffman S. Predictors of smoking cessation after coronary artery bypass graft surgery. Results of a randomized trial with 5-year follow-up. *Annals of Internal Medicine* 1994;120(4):287-293. [MEDLINE: 94121392].

Risser 1990

Risser NL, Belcher DW. Adding spirometry, carbon monoxide, and pulmonary symptom results to smoking cessation counseling: a randomized trial. *Journal of General Internal Medicine* 1990;5(1):16-22. [MEDLINE: 90133025].

Sanders 1989a

Sanders D, Fowler G, Mant D, Fuller A, Jones L, Marzillier J. Randomized controlled trial of anti-smoking advice by nurses in general practice. *Journal of the Royal College of General Practitioners* 1989;39(324):273-276. [MEDLINE: 90079848].

Sanders 1989b

Sanders D, Fowler G, Mant D, Fuller A, Jones L, Marzillier J. Randomized controlled trial of anti-smoking advice by nurses in general practice. *Journal of the Royal College of General Practitioners* 1989;39(324):273-276. [MEDLINE: 90079848].

Sanz-Pozo 2006

Sanz Pozo B, Miguel Diaz J, Aragon Blanco M, Gonzalez Gonzalez AI, Cortes Catalan M, Vazquez I. [Effectiveness of non-pharmacological primary care methods for giving up tobacco dependency] (Spanish) [Efectividad de los métodos no farmacológicos para la deshabituación tabáquica en atención primaria]. *Atencion Primaria* 2003;32(6):366-370.

*Sanz-Pozo B, Miguel-Diez J, Anegon-Blanco M, Garcia-Carballo M, Gomez-Suarez E, Fernandez-Dominguez JF. [Effectiveness of a programme of intensive tobacco counselling by nursing professionals] (Spanish) [Efectividad de un programa de consejo antitabaco intensivo realizado por profesionales de enfermería]. *Atencion Primaria* 2006;37:266-272.

Steptoe 1999

Steptoe A, Doherty S, Rink E, Kerry S, Kendrick T, Hilton S. Behavioural counselling in general practice for the promotion of healthy behaviour among adults at increased risk of coronary heart disease: randomised trial. *BMJ* 1999;319:943-947.

Taylor 1990

Taylor CB, Houston-Miller N, Killen JD, DeBusk RF. Smoking cessation after acute myocardial infarction: effects of a nurse-managed intervention. *Annals of Internal Medicine* 1990;113(2):118-123. [MEDLINE: 90297441].

Terazawa 2001

Terazawa T, Mamiya T, Masui S, Nakamura M. [The effect of smoking cessation counseling at health checkup] (Japanese). *Sangyo Eiseigaku Zasshi* 2001;43(6):207-213. [MEDLINE: 21661116].

Tonnesen 1996

Tonnesen P, Mikkelsen K, Markholst C, Ibsen A, Bendixen M, Pedersen L, et al. Nurse-conducted smoking cessation with minimal intervention in a lung clinic: a randomized controlled study. *European Respiratory Journal* 1996;9(11):2351-2355. [MEDLINE: 97102844].

Tonnesen 2006

Tonnesen P, Mikkelsen K, Bremann L. Nurse-conducted smoking cessation in patients with COPD using nicotine sublingual tablets and behavioral support. *Chest* 2006;130(2):334-342.

Vetter 1990

Vetter NJ, Ford D. Smoking prevention among people aged 60 and over: a randomized controlled trial. *Age and Ageing* 1990;19(3):164-168. [MEDLINE: 90302668].

References to Studies Excluded from this Review

Andrews 2007

Andrews JO, Felton G, Wewers ME, Waller J, Tingen M. The effect of a multi-component smoking cessation intervention in African American women residing in public housing. *Research in Nursing and Health* 2007;30(1):45-60.

Browning 2000

Browning KK, Ahijevych KL, Ross P Jr, Wewers ME. Implementing the Agency for Health Care Policy and Research's Smoking Cessation Guideline in a lung cancer surgery clinic. *Oncology Nursing Forum* 2000;27(8):1248-1254.

Carlsson 1998

Carlsson R. Serum cholesterol, lifestyle, working capacity and quality of life in patients with coronary artery disease. Experiences from a hospital-based secondary prevention programme. *Scandinavian Cardiovascular Journal Supplement* 1998;50:1-20.

Chan 2005

Chan SS, Lam TH, Salili F, Leung GM, Wong DC, Botelho RJ, et al. A randomized controlled trial of an individualized motivational intervention on smoking cessation for parents of sick children: a pilot study. *Applied Nursing Research* 2005;18:178-181.

Fletcher 1987

Fletcher V. An individualized teaching programme following primary uncomplicated myocardial infarction. *Journal of Advanced Nursing* 1987;12:195-200.

Galvin 2001

Galvin K, Webb C, Hillier V. Assessing the impact of a nurse-led health education intervention for people with peripheral vascular disease who smoke: the use of physiological markers, nicotine dependence and withdrawal. *International Journal of Nursing Studies* 2001;38(1):91-105.

Griebel 1998

Griebel B, Wewers ME, Baker CA. The effectiveness of a nurse-managed minimal smoking-cessation intervention among hospitalized patients with cancer. *Oncology Nursing Forum* 1998;25(5):897-902. [MEDLINE: 1998308576].

Haddock 1997

Haddock J, Burrows C. The role of the nurse in health promotion: an evaluation of a smoking cessation programme in surgical preadmission clinics. *Journal of Advanced Nursing* 1997;26(6):1098-1110.

Hall 2007

Hall S, Reid E, Ukoumunne OC, Weinman J, Marteau TM. Brief smoking cessation advice from practice nurses during routine cervical smear tests appointments: a cluster randomised controlled trial assessing feasibility, acceptability and potential effectiveness. *British Journal of Cancer* 2007;96: 1057-1061.

Jelley 1995

Jelley MJ, Prochazka AV. A smoking cessation intervention in family planning clinics. *Journal of Women's Health* 1995;4:555-567.

Johnson 1999

Johnson JL, Budz B, Mackay M, Miller C. Evaluation of a nurse delivered smoking cessation intervention for hospitalized patients with cardiac disease. *Heart and Lung* 1999;28(1):55-64.

Johnson 2000

*Johnson JL, Ratner PA, Bottorff JL, Hall W, Dahinten S. Preventing smoking relapse in postpartum women. *Nursing Research* 2000;49(1):44-52.

Ratner PA, Johnson JL, Bottorff JL, Dahinten S, Hall W. Twelve-month follow-up of a smoking relapse prevention intervention for postpartum women. *Addictive Behaviors* 2000;25(1):81-92.

Kendrick 1995

Kendrick JS, Zahniser SC, Miller N, Salas N, Stine J, Gargiullo PM, et al. Integrating smoking cessation into routine public prenatal care: the Smoking Cessation in Pregnancy project. *American Journal of Public Health* 1995;85(2):217-222. [MEDLINE: 1995160170].

Lifrak 1997

Lifrak P, Gariti P, Alterman AI, McKay J, Volpicelli J, Sparkman T, et al. Results of two levels of adjunctive treatment used with the nicotine patch. *American Journal of Addiction* 1997;6(2):93-98. [MEDLINE: 1997279664].

McHugh 2001

McHugh F, Lindsay GM, Hanlon P, Hutton I, Brown MR, Morrison C, et al. Nurse led shared care for patients on the waiting list for coronary artery bypass surgery: a randomised controlled trial. *Heart* 2001;86(3):317-323.

O'Connor 1992

O'Connor AM, Davies BL, Dulberg CS, Buhler PL, Nadon C, McBride BH, et al. Effectiveness of a pregnancy smoking cessation program. *Journal of Obstetric, Gynecologic, and Neonatal Nursing* 1992;21(5):385-392. [MEDLINE: 1993019683].

Pozen 1977

Pozen MW, Stechmiller JA, Harris W, Smith S, Fried DD, Voigt GC. A nurse rehabilitator's impact on patients with myocardial infarction. *Medical Care* 1977;15(10):830-837. [MEDLINE: 1978009142].

Reeve 2000

Reeve K, Calabro K, Adams-McNeill J. Tobacco cessation intervention in a nurse practitioner managed clinic. *Journal of the American Academy of Nurse Practitioners* 2000;12(5):163-169.

Reid 2003

Reid R, Pipe A, Higginson L, Johnson K, D'Angelo MS, Cooke D, et al. Stepped care approach to smoking cessation in patients hospitalized for coronary artery disease. *Journal of Cardiopulmonary Rehabilitation* 2003;23:176-182.

Rigotti 1997

Rigotti NA, Arnsten JH, McKool KM, Wood-Reid KM, Pasternak RC, Singer DE. Efficacy of a smoking cessation program for hospital patients. *Archives of Internal Medicine* 1997;157(22):2653-2660. [MEDLINE: 1998189721].

Stanislaw 1994

Stanislaw AE, Wewers ME. A smoking cessation intervention with hospitalized surgical cancer patients: a pilot study. *Cancer Nursing* 1994;17(2):81-86. [MEDLINE: 1994291090].

Sun 2000

Sun C. [Roles of psychological nursing played in the course of auricle point applying to help individuals giving up smoking] (Chinese). *Shanxi Nursing Journal* 2000;14(2):69-70.

van Elderen 1994

van Elderen–van Kemenade T, Maes S, van den Broek Y. Effects of a health education programme with telephone follow-up during cardiac rehabilitation. *British Journal of Clinical Psychology* 1994;33 (3):367-378. [MEDLINE: 1995086426].

Wadland 1999

Wadland WC, Stoffelmayr B, Berger E, Crombach A, Ives K. Enhancing smoking cessation rates in primary care. *Journal of Family Practice* 1999;48(9):711-718.

Wadland 2001

Wadland WC, Stoffelmayr B, Ives K. Enhancing smoking cessation of low-income smokers in managed care. *Journal of Family Practice* 2001;50(2):138-144.

Wewers 1994

Wewers ME, Bowen JM, Stanislaw AE, Desimone VB. A nurse-delivered smoking cessation intervention among hospitalized postoperative patients—influence of a smoking-related diagnosis: a pilot study. *Heart and Lung* 1994;23(2):151-156. [MEDLINE: 1994266626].

Woollard 1995

Woollard J, Beilin LJ, Lord T, Puddey I, MacAdam D, Rouse I. A controlled trial of nurse counselling of life-style change for hypertensives treated in general practice—preliminary results. *Clinical and Experimental Pharmacology and Physiology* 1995;22(6-7):466-468. [MEDLINE: 1996172110].

References to Ongoing Studies

Chan 2005b

Chan SC, Lam TH, Lau C-P. The effectiveness of a nurse-delivered smoking cessation intervention for cardiac patients: a randomised controlled trial. *Nicotine and Tobacco Research* 2005;7:692.

Additional References

AHRQ 2000

Fiore MC, Bailey WC, Cohen SJ, et al. *Treating Tobacco Use and Dependence. A Clinical Practice Guideline*. AHRQ publication No. 00-0032. Rockville, MD: US Dept of Health and Human Services, 2000.

ANA 1995

American Nurses Association. *Position Statement: Cessation of Tobacco Use*. Indianapolis: American Nurses Association, 1995.

Cherry 2003

Cherry DK, Burt CW, Woodwell DA. National Ambulatory Medical Care Survey: 2001 summary. *Advance Data* 2003;Aug 11(337):1-44.

Cochrane Handbook

Higgins JPT, Green S, editors. *Cochrane Handbook for Systematic Reviews of Interventions 4.2.6* [updated September 2006]. http://www.cochrane.org/resources/handbook/hbook.htm (accessed 7th November 2007), 2006.

Coultas 1991

Coultas DB. The physician's role in smoking cessation. *Clinics in Chest Medicine* 1991;12(4):755-768. [MEDLINE: 92083710].

Davis 2007

Davis RM, Wakefield M, Amos A, Gupta PC. The Hitchhiker's Guide to Tobacco Control: a global assessment of harms, remedies, and controversies. *Annual Review of Public Health* 2007;28: 171-194.

Deeks 2006

Deeks JJ, Higgins, JPT, Altman DG, editors. In: Higgins JPT, Green S, editors. Analysing and presenting results. Cochrane Handbook for Systematic Reviews of Interventions 4.2.6 [updated September 2006]; Section 8. The Cochrane Library, Issue 4, 2006. Chichester, UK: John Wiley & Sons, Ltd, 2006.

DHHS 2004

Dept. of Health and Human Services. *The health consequences of smoking: a report of the Surgeon General.* Washington, DC: Centers for Disease Control and Prevention, Office on Smoking and Health, 2004.

Greenland 1985

Greenland S, Robins J. Estimation of a common effect parameter from sparse follow-up data. *Biometrics* 1985;41:55-68.

Higgins 2003

Higgins JP, Thompson SG, Deeks JJ, Altman DG. Measuring inconsistency in meta-analyses. *BMJ* 2003;327(7414):557-560.

Lancaster 2004

Lancaster T, Stead LF. Physician advice for smoking cessation. Cochrane Database of Systematic Reviews 2004, Issue 4. Art. No.: CD000165. DOI:10.1002/14651858.CD000165.pub2.

LeLorier 1997

LeLorier J, Gregoire G, Benhaddad A, Lapierre J, Derderian F. Discrepancies between meta-analyses and subsequent large randomized, controlled trials. *New England Journal of Medicine* 1997;337(8):536-542. [MEDLINE: 97390204].

Lumley 2004

Lumley J, Oliver S, Waters E. Interventions for promoting smoking cessation during pregnancy. Cochrane Database of Systematic Reviews 2004, Issue 1. Art. No.: CD001055. DOI: 10.1002/14651858.CD001055.pub2.

NIH 2006

NIH State-of-the-Science Panel. National Institutes of Health State-of-the-Science Conference Statement: Tobacco Use: Prevention, Cessation, and Control. *Archives of Internal Medicine* 2006;145:839-844.

Percival 2003

Percival J, Bialous SA, Chan S, Sarna L. International efforts in tobacco control. *Seminars in Oncology Nursing* 2003;19:301-308.

Rigotti 2007

Rigotti NA, Munafo MR, Stead LF. Interventions for smoking cessation in hospitalised patients. Cochrane Database of Systematic Reviews 2007, Issue 3. Art. No.: CD001837. DOI: 10.1002/14651858.CD001837.pub2.

Schulz 1995

Schulz KF, Chalmers I, Hayes RJ, Altman DG. Empirical evidence of bias. Dimensions of methodological quality associated with estimates of treatment effects in controlled trials. *JAMA* 1995;273(5):408-412. [MEDLINE: 95123716].

Stead 2008

Stead LF, Perera R, Bullen C, Mant D, Lancaster T. Nicotine replacement therapy for smoking cessation. Cochrane Database of Systematic Reviews 2008, Issue 1. Art. No.: CD000146. DOI: 10.1002/14651858.CD000146.pub3.

Stewart 1993

Stewart LA, Parmar MK. Meta-analysis of the literature or of individual patient data: is there a difference? *Lancet* 1993;341:418-422. [MEDLINE: 93156516].

West 2006

West R. Tobacco control: present and future. *British Medical Bulletin* 2006;77-78:123-136.

Whyte 2003

Whyte F, Kearney N. Enhancing the nurse's role in tobacco control. Tobacco Control Factsheets, UICC GLOBALink. http://factsheets.globalink.org/en/nursesrole.shtml (accessed 10th November 2007), 2003.

References to Other Published Versions of this Review

Rice 1999a

Rice VH, Stead LF. Nursing interventions for smoking cessation. Cochrane Database of Systematic Reviews 1999, Issue 3. Art. No.: CD001188. DOI:10.1002/14651858.CD001188.pub3.

Rice 1999b

Rice VH. Nursing intervention and smoking cessation: a meta-analysis. *Heart and Lung* 1999; 28:438-454.

Rice 2001

Rice VH, Stead LF. Nursing interventions for smoking cessation. Cochrane Database of Systematic Reviews 2001, Issue 3. Art. No.: CD001188. DOI:10.1002/14651858.CD001188.pub3.

Rice 2004

Rice VH, Stead LF. Nursing interventions for smoking cessation. Cochrane Database of Systematic Reviews 2004, Issue 1. Art. No.: CD001188. DOI:10.1002/14651858.CD001188.pub3.

Glossary

A

a priori From Latin: *the former;* before the study or analysis.

absolute benefit increase The absolute arithmetic difference in rates of good outcomes between experimental and control patients in a trial.

absolute risk increase The absolute arithmetic difference in rates of bad outcomes between experimental and control patients in a trial.

absolute risk reduction (ARR) The value that tells us the reduction of risk in absolute terms. The ARR is considered the "real" reduction because it is the difference between the risk observed in those who did and did not experience the event.

accessible population A population that meets the population criteria and is available.

after-only design An experimental design with two randomly assigned groups—a treatment group and a control group. This design differs from the true experiment in that both groups are measured only after the experimental treatment.

after-only nonequivalent control group design A quasi-experimental design similar to the after-only experimental design, but subjects are not randomly assigned to the treatment or control groups.

alternate form reliability Two or more alternate forms of a measure are administered to the same subjects at different times. The scores of the two tests determine the degree of relationship between the measures.

analysis of covariance (ANCOVA) A statistic that measures differences among group means and uses a statistical technique to equate the groups under study in relation to an important variable.

analysis of variance (ANOVA) A statistic that tests whether group means differ from each other, rather than testing each pair of means separately. ANOVA considers the variation among all groups.

animal rights Guidelines used to protect the rights of animals in the conduct of research.

anonymity A research participant's protection in a study so that no one, not even the researcher, can link the subject with the information given.

antecedent variable A variable that affects the dependent variable but occurs before the introduction of the independent variable.

assent An aspect of informed consent that pertains to protecting the rights of children as research subjects.

attention control Operationalized as the control group receiving the same amount of "attention" as the experimental group.

auditability The researcher's development of the research process in a qualitative study that allows a researcher or reader to follow the thinking or conclusions of the researcher.

axial coding A data-analysis strategy using the grounded theory method. It requires intense coding around a single theme.

B

beneficence An obligation to act to benefit others and to maximize possible benefits.

benefit Potential positive outcomes of participation in a research study.

bias A distortion in the data-analysis results.

Boolean operator Words used to define the relationships between words or groups of words in literature searches. Examples of Boolean operators are words such as "AND," "OR," "NOT," and "NEAR."

bracketed A process during which the researcher identifies personal biases about the phenomenon of interest to clarify how personal experience and beliefs may color what is heard and reported.

C

case control study See *ex post facto study*.

case study method The study of a selected contemporary phenomenon over time to provide an in-depth description of essential dimensions and processes of the phenomenon.

chance error Attributable to fluctuations in subject characteristics that occur at a specific point in time and are often beyond the awareness and control of the examiner. Also called *random error*.

chi-square (χ^2) A nonparametric statistic that is used to determine whether the frequency found in each category is different from the frequency that would be expected by chance.

citation management software Software that formats citations.

clinical guidelines Systematically developed practice statements designed to assist clinicians about health care decisions for specific conditions or situations.

clinical question The first step in development of an evidence-based practice project.

close-ended question Question that the respondent may answer with only one of a fixed number of choices.

cluster sampling A probability sampling strategy that involves a successive random sampling of units. The units sampled progress from large to small. Also known as *multistage sampling*.

cohort The subjects of a specific group that are being studied.

community-based participatory research Qualitative method that systematically accesses the voice of a community to plan context-appropriate action.

computer database Print database that is put on software programs that can be accessed online or on CD-ROM via the computer.

concealment Refers to whether the subjects know that they are being observed.

concept An image or symbolic representation of an abstract idea.

conceptual definition General meaning of a concept.

conceptual framework A structure of concepts and/or theories pulled together as a map for the study.

conceptual literature Published and unpublished non–data-based material, such as reports of theories, concepts, synthesis of research on concepts, or professional issues, some of which underlie reported research, as well as other nonresearch material.

conceptual model A set of interrelated concepts that symbolically represents a phenomenon.

concurrent validity The degree of correlation of two measures of the same concept that are administered at the same time.

conduct of research The analysis of data collected from a homogeneous group of subjects who meet study inclusion and exclusion criteria for the purpose of answering specific research questions or testing specified hypotheses.

confidence interval Quantifies the uncertainty of a statistic or the probably value range within which a population parameter is expected to lie.

confidentiality Assurance that a research participant's identity cannot be linked to the information that was provided to the researcher.

consent See *informed consent*.

consistency Data are collected from each subject in the study in exactly the same way or as close to the same way as possible.

constancy Methods and procedures of data collection are the same for all subjects.

constant comparative method A process of continuously comparing data as they are acquired during research with the grounded theory method.

construct An abstraction that is adapted for scientific purpose.

construct replication The use of original methods, such as sampling techniques, instruments, or research design, to study a problem that has been investigated previously.

construct validity The extent to which an instrument is said to measure a theoretical construct or trait.

consumer One who actively uses and applies research findings in nursing practice.

content analysis A technique for the objective, systematic, and quantitative description of communications and documentary evidence.

content validity The degree to which the content of the measure represents the universe of content, or the domain of a given behavior.

content validity index A calculation that gives a researcher more confidence or evidence that the instrument truly reflects the concept or construct.

context Environment where event(s) occur(s).

context dependent An observation is defined by its circumstance or context.

contrasted-group approach A method used to assess construct validity. A researcher identifies two groups of individuals who are suspected to have an extremely high or low score on a characteristic. Scores from the groups are obtained and examined for sensitivity to the differences. Also called *known-group approach.*

control Measures used to hold uniform or constant the conditions under which an investigation occurs.

control event rate (CER) Proportion of patients in control group in which an event is observed.

control group The group in an experimental investigation that does not receive an intervention or treatment; the comparison group.

controlled vocabulary The terms that indexers have assigned to the articles in a database. When possible, it is helpful to match the words that you use in your search to those specifically used in the database.

convenience sampling A nonprobability sampling strategy that uses the most readily accessible persons or objects as subjects in a study.

convergent validity A strategy for assessing construct validity in which two or more tools that theoretically measure the same construct are administered to subjects. If the measures are positively correlated, convergent validity is said to be supported.

correlation The degree of association between two variables.

correlational study A type of nonexperimental research design that examines the relationship between two or more variables.

credibility Steps in qualitative research to ensure accuracy, validity, or soundness of data.

criterion-related validity Indicates the degree of relationship between performance on the measure and actual behavior either in the present (concurrent) or in the future (predictive).

critical appraisal Appraisal by a nurse who is a knowledgeable consumer of research, and who can appraise research evidence and use existing standards to determine the merit and readiness of research for use in clinical practice.

critical reading An active interpretation and objective assessment of an article during which the reader is looking for key concepts, ideas, and justifications.

critical thinking The rational examination of ideas, inferences, principles, and conclusions.

Cronbach's alpha Test of internal consistency that simultaneously compares each item in a scale to all others.

cross-sectional study A nonexperimental research design that looks at data at one point in time, that is, in the immediate present.

culture The system of knowledge and linguistic expressions used by social groups that allows the researcher to interpret or make sense of the world.

Cumulative Index to Nursing and Allied Health Literature (CINAHL) A print or computerized database; computerized CINAHL is available on CD-ROM and online.

D

data Information systematically collected in the course of a study; the plural of *datum.*

database A compilation of information about a topic organized in a systematic way.

data-based literature Reports of completed research.

data saturation A point when data collection can cease. It occurs when the information being shared with the researcher becomes repetitive. Ideas conveyed by the participant have been shared before by other participants; inclusion of additional participants does not result in new ideas.

debriefing The opportunity for researchers to discuss the study with the participants and for participants to refuse to have their data included in the study.

deductive reasoning A logical thought process in which hypotheses are derived from theory; reasoning moves from the general to the particular.

degrees of freedom The number of quantities that are unknown minus the number of independent equations linking these unknowns; a function of the number in the sample.

delimitations Those characteristics that restrict the population to a homogeneous group of subjects.

Delphi technique The technique of gaining expert opinion on a subject. It uses rounds or multiple stages of data collection, with each round using data from the previous round.

demographic data Data that includes information that describes important characteristics about the subjects in a study (e.g., age, gender, race, ethnicity, education, marital status).

dependent variable In experimental studies, the presumed effect of the independent or experimental variable on the outcome.

descriptive statistics Statistical methods used to describe and summarize sample data.

design The plan or blueprint for conduct of a study.

developmental study A type of nonexperimental research design that is concerned not only with the existing status and interrelationship of phenomena but also with changes that take place as a function of time.

diffusion The strategy for promoting adoption of evidence-based practices.

direct observation A method for measuring psychological and physiological behaviors for the purpose of evaluating change and facilitating recovery.

directional hypothesis Hypothesis that specifies the expected direction of the relationship between the independent and dependent variables.

dissemination The communication of research findings.

divergent validity A strategy for assessing construct validity in which two or more tools that theoretically measure the opposite of the construct are administered to subjects. If the measures are negatively correlated, divergent validity is said to be supported.

domains Symbolic categories that include the smaller categories of an ethnographic study.

downlink A receiver for programs beamed from other agencies that allows a person to participate in telecommunication conferences.

E

electronic database/electronic index The electronic means by which journal sources (periodicals) of data-based and conceptual articles on a variety of topics (e.g., doctoral dissertations) are found, as well as the publications of professional organizations and various governmental agencies.

element The most basic unit about which information is collected.

eligibility criteria Those characteristics that restrict the population to a homogeneous group of subjects.

emic view The native's or insider's view of the world.

empirical The obtaining of evidence or objective data.

empirical literature A synonym for data-based literature; see *data-based literature*.

equivalence Consistency or agreement among observers using the same measurement tool or agreement among alternate forms of a tool.

error variance The extent to which the variance in test scores is attributable to error rather than a true measure of the behaviors.

ethics The theory or discipline dealing with principles of moral values and moral conduct.

ethnographic method A method that scientifically describes cultural groups. The goal of the ethnographer is to understand the native's view of their world.

ethnography A qualitative research approach designed to produce cultural theory.

etic view An outsider's view of another's world.

evaluation research The use of scientific research methods and procedures to evaluate a program, treatment, practice, or policy outcomes; analytical means are used to document the worth of an activity.

evaluative research The use of scientific research methods and procedures for the purpose of making an evaluation.

evidence hierarchy Rating system for the level of evidence a research article provides.

evidence-based guidelines A set of guidelines that allow the researcher to better understand the evidence base of certain practices.

evidence-based practice The conscious and judicious use of the current "best" evidence in the care of patients and delivery of health care services.

ex post facto study A type of nonexperimental research design that examines the relationships among the variables after the variations have occurred.

exclusion criteria Those characteristics that restrict the population to a homogeneous group of subjects.

existing data Data gathered from records (e.g., medical records, care plans, hospital records, death certificates) and databases (e.g., U.S. Census, National Cancer Data Base, Minimum Data Set for Nursing Home Resident Assessment and Care Screening).

experiment A scientific investigation in which observations are made and data are collected by means of the characteristics of control, randomization, and manipulation.

experimental design A research design that has the following properties: randomization, control, and manipulation.

experimental event rate (EER) Proportion of patients in experimental treatment groups in which an event is observed.

experimental group The group in an experimental investigation that receives an intervention or treatment.

exploratory survey A type of nonexperimental research design that collects descriptions of existing phenomena for the purpose of using the data to justify or assess current conditions or to make plans for improvement of conditions.

external validity The degree to which findings of a study can be generalized to other populations or environments.

extraneous variable Variable that interferes with the operations of the phenomena being studied. Also called *mediating variable.*

F

face validity A type of content validity that uses an expert's opinion to judge the accuracy of an instrument. (Some would say that face validity verifies that the instrument gives the subject or expert the appearance of measuring the concept.)

factor analysis A type of validity that uses a statistical procedure for determining the underlying dimensions or components of a variable.

findings Statistical results of a study.

Fisher's exact probability test A test used to compare frequencies when samples are small and expected frequencies are less than six in each cell.

fittingness Answers the questions: Are the findings applicable outside the study situation? Are the results meaningful to the individuals not involved in the research?

frequency distribution Descriptive statistical method for summarizing the occurrences of events under study.

G

generalizability (generalize) The inferences that the data are representative of similar phenomena in a population beyond the studied sample.

grand theory All-inclusive conceptual structures that tend to include views on person, health, and environment to create a perspective of nursing.

grand tour question A broad overview question.

grounded theory Theory that is constructed inductively from a base of observations of the world as it is lived by a selected group of people.

grounded theory method An inductive approach that uses a systematic set of procedures to arrive at theory about basic social processes.

H

hazard ratio A weighted relative risk based on the analysis of survival curves over the whole course of the study period.

historical research method The systematic compilation of data resulting from evaluation and interpretation of facts regarding people, events, and occurrences of the past.

history The internal validity threat that refers to events outside of the experimental setting that may affect the dependent variable.

homogeneity Similarity of conditions. Also called *internal consistency.*

hypothesis A prediction about the relationship between two or more variables.

hypothesis-testing approach Method used when an investigator uses the theory or concept underlying the measurement instruments to validate the instrument.

hypothesis-testing validity A strategy for assessing construct validity in which the theory or concept underlying a measurement instrument's design is used to develop hypotheses that are tested. Inferences are made based on the findings about whether the rationale underlying the instrument's construction is adequate to explain the findings.

I

inclusion criteria See *eligibility criteria.*

independent variable The antecedent or the variable that has the presumed effect on the dependent variable.

inductive reasoning A logical thought process in which generalizations are developed from specific observations; reasoning moves from the particular to the general.

inferential statistics Procedures that combine mathematical processes and logic to test hypotheses about a population with the help of sample data.

information literacy The skills needed to consult the literature and answer a clinical question.

informed consent An ethical principle that requires a researcher to obtain the voluntary participation of subjects after informing them of potential benefits and risks.

innovation diffusion Process by which an innovation or research findings are communicated through various channels over time among the members of a profession.

institutional review boards (IRBs) Boards established in agencies to review biomedical and behavioral research involving human subjects within the agency or in programs sponsored by the agency.

instrumental case study Research that is done when the researcher pursues insight into an issue or wants to challenge a generalization.

instrumentation Changes in the measurement of the variables that may account for changes in the obtained measurement.

integrative research review Synthesis review of the literature on a specific concept or topic.

internal and external validity threat Factor that can compromise outcomes. If these threats are not considered, they could negate the results of the research.

internal consistency The extent to which items within a scale reflect or measure the same concept.

internal validity The degree to which it can be inferred that the experimental treatment, rather than an uncontrolled condition, resulted in the observed effects.

Internet The global electronic network that links a cadre of participating networks (e.g., commercial, educational, and governmental agencies).

interpretive phenomenology Research that is "informed by interpretive phenomenology seeks to reveal and convey deep insight and understanding of the concealed meanings of everyday life experiences" (deWitt & Ploeg, 2006, pp. 216-217).

interrater reliability The consistency of observations between two or more observers; often expressed as a percentage of agreement between raters or observers or a coefficient of agreement that takes into account the element of chance. This usually is used with the direct observation method.

interrelationship/difference studies The classification of a nonexperimental research design that attempts to trace relationships among variables. The four types are correlational, ex post facto, prediction, and developmental.

interval The level of measurement that provides different levels or gradations in response. The differences or intervals between responses are assumed to be approximately equal.

interval measurement Level used to show rankings of events or objects on a scale with equal intervals between numbers but with an arbitrary zero (e.g., centigrade temperature).

intervening variable A variable that occurs during an experimental or quasi-experimental study that affects the dependent variable.

intervention Deals with whether or not the observer provokes actions from those who are being observed.

interview guide A list of questions and probes used by interviews that use open-ended questions.

interviews A method of data collection in which a data collector questions a subject verbally. Interviews may be face-to-face or performed over the telephone, and they may consist of open-ended or close-ended questions.

intrinsic case study Research that is undertaken to have a better understanding of the essential nature of the case.

item to total correlation The relationship between each of the items on a scale and the total scale.

J

justice Human subjects should be treated fairly.

K

Kappa Expresses the level of agreement observed beyond the level that would be expected by chance alone. Kappa (K) ranges from +1 (total agreement) to 0 (no agreement). K greater than .80 is generally indicates good reliability. K between .68 and .80 is considered acceptable/ substantial agreement. Levels lower than .68 may allow tentative conclusions to be drawn when lower levels are accepted.

key informants Individuals who have special knowledge, status, or communication skills and who are willing to teach the ethnographer about the phenomenon.

knowledge-focused triggers Ideas that are generated when staff read research, listen to scientific papers at research conferences, or encounter evidence-based practice guidelines published by federal agencies or specialty organizations.

Kuder-Richardson (KR-20) coefficient The estimate of homogeneity used for instruments that use a dichotomous response pattern.

L

level of significance (alpha level) The risk of making a type I error, set by the researcher before the study begins.

levels of measurement Categorization of the precision with which an event can be measured (nominal, ordinal, interval, and ratio).

life context The matrix of human–human-environment relationships emerging over the course of one's life.

likelihood ratios Provide the nurse with information about the accuracy of a diagnostic test and can also help the nurse to be a more efficient decision maker by allowing the clinician to quantify the probability of disease for any individual patient.

Likert-type scales Lists of statements for which respondents indicate whether they "strongly agree," "agree," "disagree," or "strongly disagree."

limitation Weakness of a study.

literature Print and nonprint sources such as books, chapters of books, journal articles, critique reviews, abstracts published in conference proceedings, professional and governmental reports, and unpublished doctoral dissertations.

literature review A systematic and critical appraisal of the most important literature on a topic.

lived experience In phenomenological research, a term used to refer to the focus on living through events and circumstances (prelingual) rather than thinking about these events and circumstances (conceptualized experience).

longitudinal study A nonexperimental research design in which a researcher collects data from the same group at different points in time.

M

manipulation The provision of some experimental treatment, in one or varying degrees, to some of the subjects in the study.

matching A special sampling strategy used to construct an equivalent comparison sample group by filling it with subjects who are similar to each subject in another sample group in relation to preestablished variables, such as age and gender.

maturation Developmental, biological, or psychological processes that operate within an individual as a function of time and are external to the events of the investigation.

mean A measure of central tendency; the arithmetic average of all scores.

measurement effects Administration of a pretest in a study that affects the generalizability of the findings to other populations.

measurement error The difference between what really exists and what is measured in a given study.

measures of central tendency Descriptive statistical procedure that describes the average member of a sample (mean, median, and mode).

measures of variability Descriptive statistical procedure that describes how much dispersion there is in sample data.

median A measure of central tendency; the middle score.

mediating variable A variable that is between or occurs between an independent and dependent variable and can produce an indirect effect of the independent variable on the dependent variable. Also called *extraneous variable.*

MEDLINE The print or computerized database of standard medical literature analysis and retrieval system online; it is also available on CD-ROM.

meta-analysis A research method that takes the results of multiple studies in a specific area and synthesizes the findings to make conclusions regarding the area of focus.

meta-synthesis Integrates qualitative research findings on a topic and is based on comparative analysis and interpretative synthesis.

methodological research The controlled investigation and measurement of the means of gathering and analyzing data.

microrange theory The linking of concrete concepts into a statement that can be examined in practice and research.

midrange theory A focused conceptual structure that synthesizes practice-research into ideas central to the discipline.

modal percentage A measure of variability; percent of cases in the mode.

modality The number of peaks in a frequency distribution.

mode A measure of central tendency; the most frequent score or result.

model A symbolic representation of a set of concepts that is created to depict relationships.

mortality The loss of subjects from time 1 data collection to time 2 data collection.

multiple analysis of variance (MANOVA) A test used to determine differences in group means; used when there is more than one dependent variable.

multiple regression Measure of the relationship between one interval level dependent variable and several independent variables. Canonical correlation is used when there is more than one dependent variable.

multistage sampling (cluster sampling) Involves a successive random sampling of units (clusters) that programs from large to small and meets sample eligibility criteria.

multitrait-multimethod approach A type of validity that uses more than one method to assess the accuracy of an instrument (e.g., observation and interview of anxiety).

N

naturalistic research A general label for qualitative research methods that involve the researcher going to a natural setting, that is, to where the phenomenon being studied is taking place.

naturalistic setting A setting that people live in every day.

negative likelihood ratio The LR of a negative test tells us how well a negative test result does by comparing its performance when the disease is absent to that when it is present. The better test to use to rule out disease is the one with the smaller likelihood ratio of a negative test.

negative predictive value Expresses the proportion of those with negative test results who truly do not have the disease.

network sampling (snowball effect sample) A strategy used for locating samples that are difficult to locate. It uses social networks and the fact that friends tend to have characteristics in common; subjects who meet the eligibility criteria are asked for assistance in getting in touch with others who meet the same criteria.

nominal The level of measurement that simply assigns data into categories that are mutually exclusive.

nominal measurement Level used to classify objects or events into categories without any relative ranking (e.g., gender, hair color).

nondirectional hypothesis One that indicates the existence of a relationship between the variables but does not specify the anticipated direction of the relationship.

nonequivalent control group design A quasi-experimental design that is similar to the true experiment, but subjects are not randomly assigned to the treatment or control groups.

nonexperimental research design Research design in which an investigator observes a phenomenon without manipulating the independent variable(s).

nonparametric statistics Statistics that are usually used when variables are measured at the nominal or ordinal level because they do not estimate population parameters and involve less restrictive assumptions about the underlying distribution.

nonprobability sampling A procedure in which elements are chosen by nonrandom methods.

normal curve A curve that is symmetrical about the mean and is unimodal.

null hypothesis A statement that there is no relationship between the variables and that any relationship observed is a function of chance or fluctuations in sampling.

null value In an experiment, when a value is obtained that indicates that there is no difference between the treatment and control groups.

O

objective Data that are not influenced by anyone who collects the information.

objectivity The use of facts without distortion by personal feelings or bias.

observed score The actual score obtained in a measurement.

observed test score Derived from a set of items actually consists of the true score plus error.

odds ratio (OR) An estimate of relative risk used in logistic regression as a measure of association; describes the probability of an event.

one-group (pretest-posttest) design Design used by researchers when only one group is available for study. Data are collected before and after an experimental treatment on one group of subjects. In this type of design, there is no control group and no randomization.

online database Online resource used to find journal sources (periodicals) of research and conceptual articles on a variety of topics (e.g., doctoral dissertations), as well as the publications of professional organizations and various governmental agencies.

ontology The study of being, of existence, and its relationship to nonexistence.

open-ended question Question that the respondent may answer in his or her own words.

operational definition The measurements used to observe or measure a variable; delineates the procedures or operations required to measure a concept.

ordinal The level of measurement that systematically categorizes data in an ordered or ranked manner. Ordinal measures do not permit a high level of differentiation among subjects.

ordinal measurement Level used to show rankings of events or objects; numbers are not equidistant, and zero is arbitrary (e.g., class ranking).

P

paradigm From Greek: *pattern;* it has been applied to science to describe the way people in society think about the world.

parallel form reliability See *alternate form reliability.*

parameter A characteristic of a population.

parametric statistics Inferential statistics that involve the estimation of at least one parameter, require measurement at the interval level or above, and involve assumptions about the variables being studied. These assumptions usually include the fact that the variable is normally distributed.

Pearson correlation coefficient (Pearson *r*) A statistic that is calculated to reflect the degree of relationship between two interval level variables. Also called *Pearson product moment correlation coefficient.*

phenomena Those things that are perceived by our senses (e.g., pain, losing a loved one).

phenomenological method A process of learning and constructing the meaning of human experience through intensive dialogue with persons who are living the experience.

phenomenological research Phenomenological research is based on phenomenological philosophy and is research aimed at obtaining a description of an experience as it is lived in order to understand the meaning of that experience for those who have it.

phenomenology A qualitative research approach that aims to describe experience as it is lived through, before it is conceptualized.

philosophical beliefs The system of motivating values, concepts, principles, and the nature of human knowledge of an individual, group, or culture.

philosophical research Based on the investigation of the truths and principles of existence, knowledge, and conduct.

pilot study A small, simple study conducted as a prelude to a larger-scale study that is often called the "parent study."

population A well-defined set that has certain specified properties.

population validity Generalization of results to other populations.

positive likelihood ratio The LR of a positive test tells us how well a positive test result does by comparing its performance when the disease is present to that when it is absent. The best test to use for ruling in a disease is the one with the largest likelihood ratio of a positive test.

positive predictive value Expresses the proportion of those with positive test results who truly have disease.

power analysis The mathematical procedure to determine the number for each arm (group) of a study.

prediction study A type of nonexperimental research design that attempts to make a forecast or prediction derived from particular phenomena.

predictive validity The degree of correlation between the measure of the concept and some future measure of the same concept.

primary source Scholarly literature that is written by person(s) who developed the theory or conducted the research. Primary sources include eyewitness accounts of historic events, provided by original documents, films, letters, diaries, records, artifacts, periodicals, or tapes.

print databases Indexes, card catalogues, and abstract reviews. Print indexes are used to find journal sources (periodicals) of data-based and conceptual articles on a variety of topics, as well as publications of professional organizations and various governmental agencies.

print index See *print databases.*

probability The probability of an event is the event's long-run relative frequency in repeated trials under similar conditions.

probability sampling A procedure that uses some form of random selection when the sample units are chosen.

problem statement An interrogative sentence or statement about the relationship between two or more variables.

problem-focused triggers Those that are identified by staff through quality improvement, risk surveillance, benchmarking data, financial data, or recurrent clinical problems.

process consent In qualitative research, the ongoing negotiation with subjects for their participation in a study.

product testing Testing of medical devices.

program A list of instructions in a machine-readable language written so that a computer's hardware can carry out an operation; software.

propositions The linkage of concepts that lays a foundation for the development of methods that test relationships.

prospective study Nonexperimental study that begins with an exploration of assumed causes and then moves forward in time to the presumed effect.

psychometrics The theory and development of measurement instruments.

purpose That which encompasses the aims or objectives the investigator hopes to achieve with the research, not the question to be answered.

purposive sampling A nonprobability sampling strategy in which the researcher selects subjects who are considered to be typical of the population.

Q

qualitative measurement The items or observed behaviors are assigned to mutually exclusive categories that are representative of the kinds of behavior exhibited by the subjects.

qualitative research The study of research questions about human experiences. It is often conducted in natural settings, and uses data that are words or text rather than numerical in order to describe the experiences that are being studied.

quantitative measurement The assignment of items or behaviors to categories that represent the amount of a possessed characteristic.

quantitative research The process of testing relationships, differences, and cause and effect interactions among and between variables. These processes are tested with either hypotheses and/or research questions.

quasi-experiment Research designs in which the researcher initiates an experimental treatment but some characteristic of a true experiment is lacking.

quasi-experimental design A study design in which random assignment is not used but the independent variable is manipulated and certain mechanisms of control are used.

quota sampling A nonprobability sampling strategy that identifies the strata of the population and proportionately represents the strata in the sample.

R

random access memory (RAM) A computer's memory that the user can read or change.

random error Error that occurs when scores vary in a random way. Random error occurs when data collectors do not use standard procedures to collect data consistently among all subjects in a study.

random selection A selection process in which each element of the population has an equal and independent chance of being included in the sample.

randomization A sampling selection procedure in which each person or element in a population has an equal chance of being selected to either the experimental group or the control group.

randomized controlled trial (RCT) A research study using a true experimental design.

range A measure of variability; difference between the highest and lowest scores in a set of sample data.

ratio The highest level of measurement that possesses the characteristics of categorizing, ordering, and ranking and also has an absolute or natural zero that has empirical meaning.

ratio measurement Level that ranks the order of events or objects and that has equal intervals and an absolute zero (e.g., height, weight).

reactivity The distortion created when those who are being observed change their behavior because they know that they are being observed.

recommendation Application of a study to practice, theory, and future research.

refereed journal or peer-reviewed journal A scholarly journal that has a panel of external and internal reviewers or editors; the panel reviews submitted manuscripts for possible publication. The review panels use the same set of scholarly criteria to judge if the manuscripts are worthy of publication.

relationship/difference studies Studies that trace the relationships or differences between variables that can provide a deeper insight into a phenomenon.

relative benefit increase The value that tell us about the proportional increases in rates of good outcomes between experimental and control patients in a trial divided by the control group event rates.

relative risk (RR) Risk of event after experimental treatment as a percentage of original risk.

relative risk reduction (RRR) The RRR is helpful in telling us how much of the baseline risk (the control group event rate) is removed as a result of having the intervention.

reliability The consistency or constancy of a measuring instrument.

reliability coefficient A number between 0 and 1 that expresses the relationship between the error variance, the true variance, and the observed score. A zero correlation indicates no relationship. The closer to 1 the coefficient is, the more reliable the tool.

repeated measures studies See *longitudinal study*.

representative sample A sample whose key characteristics closely approximate those of the population.

research The systematic, logical, and empirical inquiry into the possible relationships among particular phenomena to produce verifiable knowledge.

research base The accumulated knowledge gained from several studies that investigate a similar problem.

research hypothesis A statement about the expected relationship between the variables; also known as a *scientific hypothesis*.

research literature A synonym for data-based literature.

research problem Presents the question that is to be asked in a research study.

research question A key preliminary step wherein the foundation for a study is developed from the research problem and results in the research hypothesis.

research utilization A systematic method of implementing sound research-based innovations in clinical practice, evaluating the outcome, and sharing the knowledge through the process of research dissemination.

research-based practice Nursing practice that is based on research studies, that is, supported by research findings.

research-based protocols Practice standards that are formulated from findings of several studies.

respect for persons People have the right to self-determination and to treatment as autonomous agents; that is, they have the freedom to participate or not participate in research.

respondent burden Occurs when the length of the questionnaire or interview is too long or the questions too difficult for respondents to answer in a reasonable amount of time considering their age, health condition, or mental status.

retrospective data Data that have been manifested, such as scores on a standard examination.

retrospective study A nonexperimental research design that begins with the phenomenon of interest (dependent variable) in the present and examines its relationship to another variable (independent variable) in the past.

review of the literature An extensive, systematic, and critical review of the most important published scholarly literature on a particular topic. In most cases it is not considered exhaustive.

risk Potential negative outcome(s) of participation in research study.

risk-benefit ratio The extent to which the benefits of the study are maximized and the risks are minimized such that the subjects are protected from harm during the study.

S

sample A subset of sampling units from a population.

sampling A process in which representative units of a population are selected for study in a research investigation.

sampling error The tendency for statistics to fluctuate from one sample to another.

sampling frame A list of all units of the population.

sampling interval The standard distance between the elements chosen for the sample.

sampling unit The element or set of elements used for selecting the sample.

saturation See *data saturation*.

scale A self-report inventory that provides a set of response symbols for each item. A rating or score is assigned to each response.

scholarly literature Refers to published and unpublished data-based and conceptual literature materials found in print and nonprint forms.

scientific approach A logical, orderly, and objective means of generating and testing ideas.

scientific hypothesis The researcher's expectation about the outcome of a study; also known as the *research hypothesis.*

scientific literature A synonym for data-based literature; see *data-based literature.*

scientific observation Collecting data about the environment and subjects. Data collection has specific objectives to guide it, is systematically planned and recorded, is checked and controlled, and is related to scientific concepts and theories.

secondary analysis A form of research in which the researcher takes previously collected and analyzed data from one study and reanalyzes the data for a secondary purpose.

secondary source Scholarly material written by person(s) other than the individual who developed the theory or conducted the research. Most are usually published. Often a secondary source represents a response to or a summary and critique of a theorist's or researcher's work. Examples are documents, films, letters, diaries, records, artifacts, periodicals, or tapes that provide a view of the phenomenon from another's perspective.

selection The generalizability of the results to other populations.

selection bias The internal validity threat that arises when pretreatment differences between the experimental group and the control group are present.

self-report Data-collection methods that require subjects to respond directly to either interviews or structured questionnaires about their experiences, behaviors, feelings, or attitudes. These are commonly used in nursing research and are most useful for collecting data on variables that cannot be directly observed or measured by physiological instruments.

semiquartile range A measure of variability; range of the middle 50% of the scores. Also known as *semiinterquartile range.*

sensitivity The proportion of those with disease who test positive.

simple random sampling A probability sampling strategy in which the population is defined, a sampling frame is listed, and a subset from which the sample will be chosen is selected; members are randomly selected.

skew Measure of the asymmetry of a set of scores.

snowball effect sampling (network sampling) A strategy used for locating samples difficult to locate. It uses the social network and the fact that friends tend to have characteristics in common; subjects who meet the eligibility criteria are asked for assistance in getting in touch with others who meet the same criteria.

Solomon four-group design An experimental design with four randomly assigned groups—the pretest-posttest intervention group, the pretest-posttest control group, a treatment or intervention group with only posttest measurement, and a control group with only posttest measurement.

specificity The proportion of those without disease who test negative. It measures how well the test rules out disease when it is really absent; a specific test has few false positive results.

split-half reliability An index of the comparison between the scores on one half of a test with those on the other half to determine the consistency in response to items that reflect specific content.

stability An instrument's ability to produce the same results with repeated testing.

standard deviation (SD) A measure of variability; measure of average deviation of scores from the mean.

statistical hypothesis States that there is no relationship between the independent and dependent variables. The statistical hypothesis also is known as the null hypothesis.

statistical reliability An index of the interval consistency of responses to all items of a single form of measure that is administered at one time.

stratified random sampling A probability sampling strategy in which the population is divided into strata or subgroups. An appropriate number of elements from each subgroup are randomly selected based on their proportion in the population.

survey studies Descriptive, exploratory, or comparative studies that collect detailed descriptions of existing variables and use the data to justify and assess current conditions and practices, or to make more plans for improving health care practices.

survival curve A graph that shows the probability that a patient "survives" in a given state for at least a specified time (or longer).

symbolic interaction A theoretical perspective that holds that the relationship between self and society is an ongoing process of symbolic communication whereby individuals create a social reality.

systematic Data collection carried out in the same manner with all subjects.

systematic error Attributable to lasting characteristics of the subject that do not tend to fluctuate from one time to another. Also called *constant error.*

systematic sampling A probability sampling strategy that involves the selection of subjects randomly drawn from a population list at fixed intervals.

systematic review Process where investigators find all relevant studies, published and unpublished, on the topic or question, at least two members of the review team independently assess the quality of each study, include or exclude studies based on preestablished criteria, statistically combine the results of individual studies, and present a balanced and impartial evidence summary of the findings that represents a "state of the science" conclusion about the evidence supporting benefits and risks of a given health care practice.

T

***t* statistic** Commonly used in nursing research; it tests whether two group means are more different than would be expected by chance. Groups may be related or independent.

target population A population or group of individuals that meet the sampling criteria.

test A self-report inventory that provides for one response to each item that the examiner assigns a rating or score. Inferences are made from the total score about the degree to which a subject possesses whatever trait, emotion, attitude, or behavior the test is supposed to measure.

test-retest reliability Administration of the same instrument twice to the same subjects under the same conditions within a prescribed time interval, with a comparison of the paired scores to determine the stability of the measure.

testable Variables of proposed study that lend themselves to observation, measurement, and analysis.

testing The effects of taking a pretest on the scores of a posttest.

text Data in a contextual form, that is, narrative or words that are written and transcribed.

theme A label that represents a way of describing large quantities of data in a condensed format.

theoretical framework Theoretical rationale for the development of hypotheses.

theoretical literature A synonym for conceptual literature; see *conceptual literature.*

theory Set of interrelated concepts, definitions, and propositions that present a systematic view of phenomena for the purpose of explaining and making predictions about those phenomena.

time series design A quasi-experimental design used to determine trends before and after an experimental treatment. Measurements are taken several times before the introduction of the experimental treatment, the treatment is introduced, and measurements are taken again at specified times afterward.

time-sharing Several users working on one mainframe via terminals at the same time.

transferability See *fittingness.*

triangulation The expansion of research methods in a single study or multiple studies to enhance diversity, enrich understanding, and accomplish specific goals.

true experiment Also known as the *pretest-posttest control group design.* In this design, subjects are randomly assigned to an experimental or control group, pretest measurements are performed, an intervention or treatment occurs in the experimental group, and posttest measurements are performed.

trustworthiness The rigor of the research in a qualitative research study.

type I error The rejection of a null hypothesis that is actually true.

type II error The acceptance of a null hypothesis that is actually false.

U

uplink The ability to broadcast conferences so that they can be attended from a distance.

V

validation sample The sample that provides the initial data for determining the reliability and validity of a measurement tool.

validity Determination of whether a measurement instrument actually measures what it is purported to measure.

variable A defined concept.

W

Web browser Software program used to connect or "read" the World Wide Web (www).

World Wide Web (www) A conceptual group of servers on the Internet. The Web is multiple hypertext linked together in an Internet network that crisscrosses the whole Internet like a spider web.

worldview Another label for paradigm; the way people in society think about the world.

Z

Z score Used to compare measurements in standard units; examines the relative distance of the scores from the mean.

Index

Entries followed by "b" indicate boxes; "f" figures; and "t" tables.

D

E

F

J

K

L

P

Q

R